~~~~~~~~~~~~~~~~~~~~~~~~~

In this Digital Information Age – aka the Viral Age, beginning with the Age of Computers – most sources are based on fluctuating science to support their theories and experimental therapies; they begin with: **WARNING!** Do not do anything mentioned here without first consulting Your health-care provider! Using Natural Law, Common Sense and Mother Nature's Ways – the Essene tradition is based on Source, which is constant, and so prefers: **WELCOME!** Are You exploring possibilities for Self-healing? Breathe deeply. Exhale completely. Go at Your Own pace. Follow Your Inner Voice Intuition. Love, Honor and Respect the blossom unfolding within You. Lasting change in Life requires profound change**s**. Tune into Your feelings. Be aware... be mindful of what You think... and say... and... how You act. To experience change in Your Life requires serious adjustment in the Ways You do things.

> If You always do what You've always done,
> You'll always get what You've always gotten!

CHANGE begins with commitment. Treat Yourself to some TLC – Tender Loving Care – with **T**herapeutic **L**ifestyle **C**hanges. Create a new You and change how You *feel*... ultimately, how You *look* in the mirror. This is the miracle **only** You can perform! Rather than blaming others, or holding others accountable for Your health and well-being, the holistic approach recognizes the ultimate responsibility lies with the Individual... to go within... and there to discover healing for HeartMindBodySpirit as One.

> You Have the Power.
> You Are the Power.
> Be EmpOwered!

Ancient Wisdom teaches: You Are the Power. You power the One as You power the Many – at the same time of no-time, in the same space of no-space. You truly are Pure Consciousness explOring Pure Awareness... by explOring human consciousness. While honoring Your Innate Intelligence expressing Great Spirit – Divine Guidance, through Your Inner Voce Intuition – You can *feel* the Creative Forces that surge within You! What could possibly delay or destroy Your dreams? Well... for starters, Your subconscious beliefs, as well as thought-forms in the collective conscious, naysayers among Your family and associates, personal and professional. Leave the naysayers behind in their own "dys-functional comfort zone." There are **3Ds for Success** in Our 3D World!

Dedication, **D**evotion and **D**iscipline.
Dedication to Your **P**rinciples engages the *thinking* body.
Devotion to Your Heart's **P**urpose engages the *feeling* body.
Discipline with all Your **P**rotocols engages the *acting* body.
This **3D** holistic approach guarantees success in our 3D-world.

Know Thyself...
Be Aware of Yourself as Pure Consciousness explOring Pure Awareness,
as the I AM Presence *only* You can be.
Now is the time to Create the New You...
Create Your Wish Fulfilled!

Know Thyself! **How? D**iscipline is the catalyst, the enzyme that ferments and produces beneficial changes. Has discipline been a challenge for You, in the past? *Give Yourself permission to make this easy.* With the Power of Intention – eloquently discussed in Lynne McTaggart's *The Field* – affirm: I Am Now *Easily* Doing This! And, rather than beat Yourself up about perceived failure or falling short of a goal, give Yourself credit with every small success. Soon You will find Yourself saying: "I feel Great about Life! I actually enjoy being **d**isciplined in my choices... and I'm beginning to notice the **d**ifference in the mirror**!** I'm a-**maze**-d. In the Quest to Know Myself, I know *Love* for the first time – *for* Myself. I feel Love *within*!"

~~~~~~~~~~~~~~~~~~~~~~~~~~~~

Re: the logo on the cover, and in the book: "**The Unity Grid** in actuality is a 3-dimensional sphere. It is the higher order of two Platonic solids – the Icosahedron and Dodecahedron – woven together. Each triangular face contains the same angles as the Great pyramid at Giza and reflects the phi ratio, putting it in resonant relationship with all organic life and the structure of DNA itself. It creates the highest level of sacred space by aligning all the subtle bodies with the higher realms... dispelling the illusion of 3D separation. As pointed out in 'The Law of One' the center of the phi diamond is a direct portal into Intelligent Infinity. Ancient Wisdom hidden through the ages – such as the 10,800 stanzas in the Rigveda and the same number of bricks in the Indian fire altar – point toward the importance of the Unity Grid, which is one of the few forms to contain exactly 10,800 degrees." {Special thanks to Gail and Gregory Hoag. Please explore: https://iconnect2all.com/}

Table of Contents

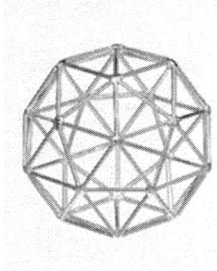

DEDICATION
Know space-time as One.
Accept and Honor the past.
Give Thanks for the Present moment.
Look forward to a Joyful future.

Life on Mother Earth, indeed the Life *of* Mother Earth, is tenuous. The question: Survival. The answer: return to Ancient Ways with heartfelt Consciousness recognizing We Are **One** with the Cosmos. Ancient ways come from the mountains north and east of Mesopotamia, most likely from Caucasus via Persia (Iran). Simple farmers living by Mother Nature's Ways migrated, discovering the Tigris-Euphrates Valley. Some of these farmers went further west, evidenced by the discovery in Qumran at the Dead Sea in 1946 – scrolls transcribed by Essenes… and their cousins to the south, the Therapeutae of Egypt, were the Coptic authors of the Nag Hammadi Library discovered in 1945. Therapeutae and Essenes lived far from the congestion and corruption found in cities, where people tend to live out of balance with Mother Nature; thereby, dis-eases flourish. Traditionally, these farmers / healers provide a retreat, a Sanctuary for those seeking balance and harmony. Learning about the Sacred Journey Within, they re-connect with the Creator of All… with Mother Earth, Father Sun… and with each other as Sisters and Brothers, nurturing Communion – Love. Healers of all traditions know the primal power of healing is: Love. Every spiritual tradition says: God is Love. After creation "God saw all that was made and, indeed, it was very good." God expresses in Creation – ultimately, expressing Love.

The Coptic Master Hamid Bey says: "Love is the Voice of God – the Master Key opening our Heart – enabling us to enter the arena of spiritual Realization. Happiness depends on the principle of Harmony and Balance. Balance makes Harmony. Harmony equals Happiness. Happiness equals Love." This site is worth exploring. <u>Our History – The Coptic Center</u>

Life's purpose is to express Joyful Love. Saints have said, "I see God in the eyes of every human being." And the Master says simply, "The Father and I are One. I Am in my Father and You in Me, and I in You!" We are all creations of Infinite Being as the Divine Presence manifests in a multitude of forms. We are All the Word made flesh! Jesus says, "Whatsoever You do to the least of these, that You do unto Me!"

Rather than pantheism – God is immanent in Nature… panentheism – God is immanent and transcendent. "Divinity is the enfolding and unfolding of everything that is. Divinity is in all things in such a way that all things are in divinity." {Nicholas of Cusa – 15th century mystic} The Divine Presence pervades all that is – OM is hOMe at every level: human, animal, plant, mineral, metal, soil, water, microbes, plasma – even fire.

Zoroaster says the purpose in life is to "be among those who renew the world… to facilitate world progress towards perfection." And in *The Dream of the Earth*, the monk Thomas Berry simply states: "The earth's evolutionary process is planetary self-education."

This book is offered as part of that process of Awarefulness and is respectfully Dedicated to:

The Divine Presence,
Creator of All Life Everywhere...
to Mother Goddess...
to Father God...
and to All Their Creations...
from Brilliant Light to Dazzling Darkness!
Infinite Mind is One.
Namaste...
Infinite Mind within Me recognizes and honors
Infinite Mind within You, within EveryOne!

PREFACE

All truth passes through 3 stages:
First, it is ridiculed.
Second, it is violently opposed.
Third, it is accepted as being self-evident.
-Arthur Schopenhauer

Read not to contradict and confute...
nor to believe and take for granted...
nor to find talk and discourse...
but to weigh and consider.
-Sir Francis Bacon

Having worked with Energy Medicine aka Vibrational Medicine since 1981, it was thrilling to see a local Detroit author, Richard Gerber, MD publish his tome: *Vibrational Energy Medicine* in 1988. While an excellent scientific resource book, I was looking for relatively simple explanations... suitable for a clever, articulate teenager. Apparently, if it's going to be it's up to me! And so... it is!

Harmonious Healing: Ancient Wisdom in Modern Times is the product of many years on planet Earth – with all that went before as my Foundation. Having seen profound changes in my own Life, my belief in reincarnation is existential. I have reincarnated again and again, in this one lifetime! For those of a Christian background who find belief in reincarnation scandalous, Matthew's Gospel (17:1-13) gives us food for thought. The scene is the Transfiguration where Peter, James and John see a vision of Moses and Elijah conversing with Jesus... and coming down the mountain the disciples questioned him. "Jesus replied: 'Elijah is to come to see that everything is once more as it should be. I tell You, however, that Elijah has come already and they did not recognize him, but treated him as they pleased; and the Son of Man will suffer similarly at their hands.' The disciples *knew* he was speaking of John the Baptist." This was hardly a

shock. Jesus *already* had told them: "It was toward John the Baptist that all prophecies of the prophets and of the Law were leading; and he, if You will believe me, is the Elijah who was to return. If anyone has ears to hear, let him listen." (Mt 11:13-15.) Clearly, Jesus refers to John the Baptist as the reincarnation of Elijah.

Please note: Quotations are from *The Jerusalem Bible*, translated by scholars at the Ecole Biblique in Jerusalem. Bible quotes, rather than being offered as proofs, are meant to be instructive. After all, Shakespeare tells us: "The devil can cite Scripture for his own purpose." {Antonio in *The Merchant of Venice*} And that is true... someone can deny the existence of God, and prove it from the Bible: Psalm 14 clearly says, "There is no God!" Actually, the Psalm begins: "The fool says in his heart, 'There is no God'!"

Harmonious Healing, rather than an argument or proof of anything, is offered in the spirit of intellectual honesty and academic integrity. Each individual can "weigh and consider" what is useful... what makes sense. Ben Franklin observed "there is nothing less common than common sense." It is time to take a common sense look at what we call Truth. How can we recognize Truth? Two questions are helpful: Is it ancient? Is it simple? Look at ancient, simple ways. Mother Nature's Ways are Truthful.

The following pages are from my first book (1998) which had the sub-title: *A Journey in Vibrational Medicine and Essene Living*. This Preface has stories and anecdotes perhaps of little interest to some, who may turn directly to the text. Others may enjoy "the rest of the story" exploring answers about what we call: Ancient... Simple... Truth. These two standards both innocently and profoundly influenced my early Life. Singing Gregorian chant and polyphony as a child, serving as an altar boy, going to seminary high school and college; another seminary for theological studies, ordained in 1967 and serving in the Archdiocese of Detroit until Ash Wednesday, 1972.

Freshman year of high school in seminary was influenced by Rosa Parks and Rev Dr Martin Luther King, Jr. **1955** was a time to consider. My culture and my community told me anyone "really different" is to be kept apart, held suspect, even feared. Yet, faith taught: "All baptized in Christ, You have all clothed Yourselves in Christ, and there are no more distinctions between Jew and Greek, slave and free, male and female, but all of You are One in Christ." (Gal 3: 27) And **in the 21ˢᵗ century**, we can add Oriental, Muslim, Arab, unaffiliated renegades, pagans, even the satanic Matrix! Being One in Christ Consciousness has little to do with Christianity, and everything to do with Divinity – expressing Infinite Mind! Unity of All Life Everywhere means: to hurt another is to hurt our Self... to love another is to love our Self. Jesus tells us at the end of this dimension of time, we will hear: "I tell You solemnly, as You did this to one of the least of these... You did it to me." (Mt 25:40)

12 years in seminary, 5 as a priest – energies oriented toward the civil rights and peace movements – really One and the same, actually: Human Rights has roots in Women's Rights, which are now blossoming as: LGBTQIA+ Rights {Lesbian, Gay, Bisexual, Trans-sexual / gender, Questioning, Intersex, Asexual+}. As patience and perseverance bring equal pay for equal work, we recognize and honor the matriarchal shift happening on Earth. Gandhi, Martin Luther King, Jr, and many others taught: *ahimsa*, non-resistance: the essence of the Christian message. Jesus said: "Love Your enemies. Love those who persecute You!" True Love is freedom *from* judgment or coercion – and freedom *for* connection and compassion. Love leads the shift in paradigms moving from the patriarchal, war-based economy of competition and joyfully moving into the *matriarchal, nurturing* economy of cooperation. https://gospelofsophia.com/2017/01/13/who-is-sophia/

In the midst of these tumultuous times... 1972 brought one of the biggest surprises of my Life. I had been nodding off at evening meetings, even afternoon appointments. Realizing many older priests took a nap after lunch, I considered the benefits; once a nap was part of the schedule, I was alert even through evening meetings. Thinking age was catching up with me: Imagine, I was only 30, at a New Year's party, I saw a friend from the seminary – from 9ᵗʰ grade through college. While I moved on to study theology, Max pursued a master's degree in education instead. He and his wife were living in Hawai'i and they both looked beautiful. Previously Max was hefty, a man of all sports. Now, sleek like an animal, he had so much energy because he explored vegan lifestyles! Vegan?

Previously dismissing Plato, Pythagoras, Goethe, Henry David Thoreau, George Bernard Shaw, and others as a bit "quirky" – I had yet to investigate. Max

mentioned two books by Austrian naturist Arnold Ehret: *The Mucusless Diet Healing System* and *Rational Fasting*. Asking about protein, Max laughed and said: "Where does a cow get her protein to produce all that muscle and milk? Grass & plants. Where does an elephant get the protein to build such a huge body? Grass & leaves. Living green plant energy is the source of Life. Rather than protein, Life is about chlorophyll."

Max and Elka further explained: while all meat-eating mammals *lap* water, all vegetarian mammals *sip* water! Carnivorous mammals have a short intestinal tract: 3-5X the length of the torso because animal protein putrefies quickly, and toxic residues must be eliminated efficiently. Vegetarian mammals have a long intestinal tract: 8-10X the length of the torso to extract the complex carbohydrates in plant matter. The human torso is <2'; the small intestine alone is over 20', large intestine 4-6' + the esophagus and stomach, the human alimentary canal adds to **30'**! Doing the math, those two simple points gave much to consider!

Their **challenge**: "Try it for 30 days and see how You feel. What's there to lose**?** Avoid meat, fish, eggs, and all white junk... especially pasteurized dairy products, refined flour and sugar products, white rice and white salt. Instead eat raw fruits and vegetables, sprouted grains and legumes, germinated nuts and seeds." Thinking some of my ancestors lived close to 80, this could make a difference in how I feel for the next 50 years! {And it did. Here I Am 80+!} Then again... I might feel little difference, and I could eat whatever.

The next morning – pardon the pun – I went cold-turkey, free from turkey sausage and eggs, among other things. Only halfway through the 30-day challenge... I went upstairs for my afternoon nap and was wide-awake! Feeling energized, the realization dawned: Life is about to change, beginning with the end of my afternoon naps. After 30 days, I clearly knew, for whatever reason, animal foods and refined foods made me sluggish. I remembered the other book Max mentioned. If eating this way can have such a profound effect, what would it be like to go without eating altogether? Explore. Ash Wednesday, '72 found me typing a letter to the bishop explaining: I had been without a decent retreat for a long time, and friends offered me a pre-civil war log cabin on 37 acres of Appalachia adjoining Shenandoah National Park. I was only bringing a copy of *Rational Fasting* and *The Jerusalem Bible*. "I'll see You at Easter!"

The cold mountains during February delayed the fast. I carried water gushing from the mountainside, and kerosene from the corner gas station / post office / general store. I was on delightfully friendly terms with Randolph Jenkins who ran the complex, and in contrast to my long hair and beard he had short hair, shaved every day, wore flannel shirts, bib overalls, a cap, and kept a corncob pipe between his teeth, reminiscent of Uncle Harold – we had instant rapport. One day after picking through a dozen seed packets and going to pay... Randolph smiled, "You wait another week or so, and I'll have bulk seeds out. That way You buy what You'll really use." Thinking, this man is in business to sell and make a profit, now he's telling me to wait a week and save some money. Impressed and pleased, I spent more time at the store. Randolph asked about my experience in the garden. I come from a line of farmers who left the Rhineland and settled in southeast Michigan in 1849. Grandfather taught me to plant things that grow above ground from the New Moon to the Full (waxing) and things that grow below ground from the Full Moon to the New (waning).

Randolph said that was good for a start. "In these parts, farmers do everything by the moon, even get married! If You put on shingles when the moon is waxing, a strong wind can get under the corners and You'll be repairing the roof before You know it. Put on shingles when the moon is waning and they stay put even through violent storms!" He asked if I wondered why the split rail chestnut fences have lasted >100 years. Why? "Fenceposts went in at the waning moon; then they waited two weeks until the moon was waxing, and placed the first split rail along the bottom; they waited another two weeks until the moon was waning again to stack the rest. The fenceposts and the bulk of the fence were set when the moon had a downward influence holding the fence secure. The first split rail, placed with the moon's upward influence, energetically held it away from the moisture of the ground, keeping it – along with the rest of the fence – from rotting... to this day!" Amazing. Ancient Wisdom in modern times.

Randolph referred to a book that was my next purchase: Llewellyn's annual *Moon Sign Book*... I have one to this day. The moon phase changes every 2.5 days and the book has times and dates for cutting hair to increase or inhibit growth, to increase thickness; times to have teeth filled or pulled; times to do garden chores, either to stimulate or slow growth; when to sign contracts, advertise, etc.

Llewellyn warns: "**Not All Almanacs Are the Same!** For *astronomical* calculations the Moon's place in most almanacs is given as the constellation. For *astrological* purposes the Moon's place is figured in the zodiacal sign... which is its true place in the zodiac, and nearly one sign (30°) different from the *astronomical* calculation. To illustrate: if the common almanac gives the Moon's place in Taurus (constellation) on a certain date, its true place in the zodiac is in Gemini (zodiacal sign). Thus, it is readily seen that those who use the common almanac may be planting seeds, or engaging in other endeavors, when they think the Moon is in a fruitful sign, while in reality it would be in one of the most barren signs in the zodiac! Common almanacs are worthless to follow for planting purposes. Some almanacs even add salt to the wound, inserting at the head of their columns 'Moon's Sign' when they mean 'Moon's Constellation' which brings much unmerited discredit to the value of planting by the Moon. *Constellations* form a belt outside the zodiac, yet do not conform to the signs in position or time. To obtain desired results, planting must be done according to the Moon's place in the signs of the *zodiac*. Therefore, using Llewellyn's *Moon Sign Book* for all of Your planting and planning is really best!"

Knowing all things happen in Perfect Divine Order, it was clear: more than cold weather kept me from the fast. Reading portions of the *Moon Sign Book*, it made sense to begin the fast at the next New Moon, a time for new beginnings... and to conclude at the Full Moon, a time for completion. Living by myself in the mountains, in sync with cosmic rhythm was thrilling. Those two weeks opened many windows, bringing a breath of fresh air to my feeling body, my thinking body and my acting body. With pure water gushing from the mountainside to wash externally and internally: drinking 3 quarts/day and taking an enema every other day to assist in releasing toxins... my first enema since having a high fever as a youngster. Welcoming my 2nd childhood, I stripped down, stretching out on a sheet in the warm meadow – morning and afternoon, warmed by the sun, feeling: I Am so blessed!

With intention, it is easier to go without food than one might think. The first 3 days I felt somewhat edgy and sluggish. *Rational Fasting* was clear. "When fasting You are on Mother Nature's operating table. Rest as much as possible." On day five, surprised at the amount of energy I dropped my inhibitions and began cleaning between the cabin and the apple orchard.

It was wonderful to get some exercise while fasting. Waking up on the tenth day, feeling emotional peace, mental clarity and physical energy, standing at the doorway – overlooking the meadow now filled with spring flowers, melodious birds harmonizing with the softly rushing river – the thought seriously came: "I feel so great, why should I eat again!?!" It definitely was a Natural High, and I knew food would only bring me down. Yet, with the Full Moon I was ready to complete my fast. Taking another enema, it was amazing how much was being eliminated while only drinking water for the previous two weeks. I washed, peeled and pitted 2 lbs of red grapes without even a nibble, and sat for a meditative feast. Fasting continues to be the most Liberating Experience of my Life. What else is possible? I'm ready!

Every fast presents an opportunity to connect with core realities. With that first fast, actually a few years before Alex Haley's book, there was a definite yearning to get in touch with my *Roots*. Returning to Detroit, I informed the bishop and my family about my Spiritual Pilgrimage: first to experience the village of Rech-am-Rhein, and the cathedral at Köln built by my ancestors, experiencing the centers of Europe considered the cradle of Western Civilization, visiting Rome, the Holy Land and Egypt, where Jesus studied with the Essenes during the hidden years. I applied for my first passport. It would take four weeks to arrive at my rural PO # address. The journey of a thousand miles begins with a single step! It was done... exhilarating!

I began going into town to check my mail every day after 3 weeks. I was ready to travel. Four weeks came and went without the passport. I called and they apologized for the mix up; someone should have notified me. I had submitted my birth registration rather than my birth certificate. I jumped in the car and drove to Detroit. With the paper work straight, they promised priority, so I returned to the mountains and waited. Experiencing all things happen in Perfect Divine Order... leaving the country was delayed so I could see a long-time friend from the peace movement who talked about his meditation experiences and invited me to a meeting at a Washington, DC ashram – the Sanskrit word literally means: Shelter of Rama, the House of the Lord. We walked up the steps and walked around a pile of shoes, which I thought strange – entering there was a table covered with a white cloth, laden with flowers, incense and pictures... with people bowing and prostrating. Whispering about my recent

Freedom from such obsequious formalities... How long will this be? "Listen for a few minutes." I'm glad I did; it made perfect sense. Each spoke of a gift received from their Guru Maharaj ji. In Hindi, *gu* means darkness and *ru* means dispeller; *maha* means great and *raj* means king. 15-years-old, Prem Pal (Savior of Love) Rawat was proclaimed the Great King who would dispel darkness by leading us into the Light.

Actually, it sounded attractive. Trained in scholastic philosophy and theology based on Aristotelian logic, I always felt Truth was obscured by the deluge of dogmas and intricate moral codes, such as the Principle of Double Effect: leading to rationalizations for just about anything. Maharaj ji says he could *show* You God... free from dogmas, free from moral codes, and free of charge.

What I heard was familiar. At my first assignment one of the parishioners shared a book written by Ramakrishna, comparing the life and teachings of Jesus with Buddha, and similar comparisons of Jesus with Krishna. The book pointed out when it comes to the fundamental beliefs of most scriptures, they all agree: God is Love. God is Light. God is in the Kingdom of Heaven, which is *within* You. The Light within may be experienced through meditation. Reading Christian mystics and mystics of other religions, who shared the same *inner* experience.

From birth our senses pull us outward, where society tells us we can find happiness: "I love my gorgeous home... and check out my car; it's the ultimate in engineering and comfort! Come indoors and listen to the sound system – stealth speakers with so much volume and yet, perfect overtones. Please make Yourself comfortable; this lovely couch is a blend of fine organic cotton and linen; perhaps we could do yoga on this ancient Persian rug... and if You have some time, we'll have delicious organic juice and snacks." While the finer things of life are wonderful and can lead to magical moments, all of these things tend to wear out or rust out, and loved ones sometimes move on or die. The bottom line is: all that society encourages us to accumulate is only temporary, transient happiness.

Ancient teachings are simple. According to the Vedas, if You are looking for permanent happiness, practice Raja Yoga. Whenever You choose to focus *inside*... You can *see* the Light within... You can *hear* the

Celestial Harmonies... You can *taste* the Sweetness that flows from the Well Within... You can *feel* the Vibration sustaining All Life Everywhere. Inner Happiness and Peace are available anytime – anywhere – whenever You choose. Through meditation – focusing on the central core of Your Energy – You experience permanent happiness because You are in the Here & Now... and *nOw is fOrever*. Through meditation You nurture Your Conscious Awareness of the Source of All radiating Light, Harmony, Sweetness and Vibration. When scientists split the atom – there was a flash of light... a sonic boom... radiation rained down accompanied by tremendous vibration. Fractal geometry and other scientific disciplines show how the Macrocosm relates to the Microcosm – getting larger to infinity... and getting smaller to infinity. We can experience these energies whenever we choose to focus within. Pure Energy is Ever Ready.

"Very intriguing &... I'm really ready to travel; when my passport comes, I'm off. If I'm meant to experience what this is all about, I'm sure I will." He asked where... Ireland, England and Europe. There was a group in London. While traveling through the gorgeous Emerald Isle, thoughts were about... London, and details of the four techniques turning the senses within. Self-Knowledge is referred to in the Vedas, and scriptures such as the Koran and the Bible. Jesus says, the Kingdom of Heaven is within You. If Your eye is single, Your whole body shall be filled with light. Drinking from the well within, You shall never thirst again. When You make a spectacle of prayer or fast so others may see You, You already have Your reward – so go behind closed doors. Closing the doors of Your outer *senses*, opening Your *inner* senses, You experience the sweet reward of the Kingdom of Heaven within You.

My former experiences with meditation were actually contemplation. For example, a typical "meditation" would be something like this: Patience is a virtue characterized by [point A...B...C]. I now resolve to increase the virtue of patience in my life by [resolution 1...2...3]. Rather than being meditation, this is intellectual consideration, proper contemplation. Meditation bypasses the intellect with its details, focusing Monkey-mind on the inner experience. The Book of Enoch says: "Be still and know I Am God." Meditation facilitates experiencing Great Spirit within the Self, knowing Spirit is also within *each* One of us.

The Sanskrit word *Namaste* literally means: The Divine within me recognizes and honors the Divine within You! Visiting ashrams in Europe, enthralled while discovering ancient disciplines beginning with a plant-based diet, fasting and meditation, "new" in the 70s, another profound discovery in Amsterdam: *the first book of Dō-IN – guide pratique* – a 30 page bi-lingual booklet by Jacques de Langre [1971] on the Oriental approach to energy meridians and foot reflexology; then later: *Second Book of Dō-IN 2: Art of Rejuvenation through Self-massage*, [1974] – massage with awareness of the breath. Dō-IN is a transliteration of Dao (Tao) Yinn, literally: The Way of the Voice of Nature – explOring Ancient Wisdom in modern times.

In the ashrams: meditation, service and *satsang*, which means: keeping company with those on the Path of Love... my service joyfully became foot reflexology. All these explorations with the vegan diet, fasting, meditation, bodywork, expanded my consciousness. Receptive to ancient, simple ways... happy to find what works... while experiencing inner Harmony and Peace. The first to receive foot reflexology was the middle-aged House-mother of the Amsterdam ashram, where I found the booklet; with a tender spot on one foot, and the chart indicating the right kidney, she asked if that would explain the dull ache in her right lower back, pointing to her kidney area; the relationship seemed clear to both of us. "What else can be done besides reflexology," she asked. Having a vague understanding of the power of herbs, I found Jethro Kloss' *Back to Eden* in the ashram library listing well over fifty herbs for the kidneys. Reading about several, my intuition settled on nettles; when she asked how much, again, following my intuition: make a quart and a half in the morning, and drink half a cup throughout the day. My left-brain existence began to experience right-brain energetics. After a few days, her pain was lessening; after 10 days, pain in her low back *and* foot were gone. She was pleased. I was in awe!

While basic books on natural health were enriching, hands-on experiences are always the most rewarding. The healing power of human touch goes to core issues, facilitating Holistic Healing of our Feeling body, our Thinking body, and our Acting body. The General Rule: Touch is dysfunctional when forceful and functional when inviting. Thrilling! My next discovery in the library was the science of iridology. Like the feet and hands, the iris also serves as a veritable template for the organs of the body. Dr Bernard Jensen's

Science and Practice of Iridology was quite revealing. Current iridology is truly holistic, going far beyond the acting body, delving into our feeling body and thinking body, which actually affects our Spirit. His daughter-in-law Ellen Tart-Jensen, PhD, D-Sc continues his work. https://bernardjensen.com

Journeying to Rome was truly exciting... being so close to the Holy Land. Originally intending a pilgrimage to Jerusalem and Egypt then returning home, arriving in that part of the world, war had escalated. Instead of going from Greece to the Holy Land, Spirit led me from Crete to Türkiye, by bus from Izmir to Istanbul / Constantinople, I was literally in another world. Traveling Europe gives a sense of history, Rome being the pinnacle. Traveling overland through Türkiye, Iran, Afghanistan and on to India, experiencing other ancient cultures, my "sense of history" became quite tangible. On this journey I had 1 change of clothing and a few personal effects tucked in a small shoulder bag, not even a backpack. {Boarding Aer Lingus in DC, the agent declared it was the least luggage ever on an international flight, and out of curiosity she asked to weigh my bag – 13 lbs!} Arriving at the Türkiye / Iran border, I went straight to a tailor trading my western clothing for two Afghani suits: long-sleeve shirts worn outside the trousers coming to mid-thigh, and bloomer-like trousers – wide tops, 3X my waist – tapering to tight fitting ankles. These and my turban were lightweight white cotton; local custom dictates a medium-weight blanket as protection from the heat of the day, as well as the night chill. In this regalia and in simple flip-flops, some would approach and begin a conversation in their native language, or what they guessed might be mine – taken for Punjabi, because of reddish highlights in my dark beard, I was able to blend in easily. Happy to be traveling alone, often invited to their homes to meet and sometimes stay with their families, brought cherished memories... as well as delightful, delicious meals. Most cultures eat a plant-based diet and, discovering I am vegan, they showed admiration for a Westerner who honored and respected animals. Love was their secret ingredient.

Most cultures experience *tourists* who think they see the world from chain hotels, and *travelers*, backpackers who move about in small groups – staying in hostels or small, clean hotels owned by oriental entrepreneurs. Chain hotels, as their ads say, offer: No Surprises! and they can be boring. You can always blend-in using their dining and other facilities.

My journey continued... exploring other cultures and how they relate to Mother Earth and each other... sleeping in primitive beds – such as a simple mat on the floor – or on the rooftop listening to the symphony of dogs, roosters and critters... thrilled with the wonderful Adventure of Life.

In Iran and Afghanistan - Ramadan '72 - the muezzin sang from the minaret calling everyone. Entering exquisite mosques... meditating as they chanted in Arabic... prostrating toward Mecca... I realized the *Koran* extols the Light within: where we all experience Divine Presence, the Creator of All. In my Heart of Hearts, I began to realize the Facts of Life: I AM! SitaRam! Jai Sat Chit Anand! Baruch Hashem! Praise the Lord! Praised be Jesus Christ! Allahu Akbar! In La'kech! All, indeed, celebrate and honor the same Basic Reality: Singularity... Oneness... best captured in the Sanskrit: *Namaste* – the Divine within Me recognizes and honors the Divine within You!

Traveling by bus and the occasional oxcart, it was exciting to arrive in New Delhi on the way to Haridwar for Hans Jayanti Festival. Seven jumbo jets from Australia, Europe and North America brought most devotees; a few came overland. Within a few days, amoebic dysentery was wide-spread and having moved more slowly overland, I had immunity... or so I thought. Yet after 3 weeks, in the middle of the night... that knowing feeling. At the clinic, a centenarian with a scant white beard said, if garlic fails... he would give homeopathic *Kurchi*; so, first chew two cloves and wash it down with tea; it worked. Garlic eases both diarrhea... as well as constipation! By festival's end, everyone was excited about going home for Christmas. On the road for 6 months, that nostalgia resonated with me. The travel agent said, even though it was a one-way journey, the most economic flight {$500} would be an excursion ticket; the return ticket had a narrow window of time: it could be used only after 90 days, and expired after 120 days. My intention to stay in the States was firm... until hearing in Detroit of Baisakhi Festival for Indian devotees celebrating Spring harvest of winter wheat. This would be a rare opportunity to experience another aspect of Indian culture! The ticket in my passport revealed two days before the window of time closed forever, and the Air India agent pronounced me "Lucky" having secured the last seat... a long flight from New York to New Delhi... so they provide delicious vegetarian food every four hours... London... Frankfurt... Beirut.

Excitement growing... we were grounded due to the hydraulic system; first class accommodations were provided, and the next day a Pan Am plane came to complete our journey. Since they had a minimal crew, I offered my services as steward. After serving drinks and dinner, I chatted with a general contractor in his early 60s. He realized it's wise to travel when You can, hence his pre-retirement Odyssey. Traveling a few years now, he would go back to work when he felt good and ready – when his travel funds were depleted. He asked, where after India? Realizing this is half-way around the globe... I may as well continue to Hawai'i and thank Max and Elka for challenging me to experiment with the vegan lifestyle. The veteran traveler coyly whispered: "If You get to Indonesia, be sure to visit Bali; go to Kuta Beach, find *The Garden* restaurant, and order 50 mushrooms with vegetable soup. Have lunch and enjoy an amazing day!" He referred to psilocybin, which the dictionary defines as a strong hallucinogen, yet other cultures use to cleanse mucus and to sharpen, rather than distort, one's focus! Having been to India, I knew what to expect. And, simply being away for only a couple of months, it was still culture shock: Taxi! Change money! the usual deals. No thanks. Off to the Ashram. Baisakhi Festival is about Life. Winter wheat, harvested in Spring, leaves plenty of room to pitch tents; thousands take buses, taxis, ox-carts, bike or walk to see their Guru; they stand in long lines to see him for a moment... thanking him for the Gift he freely shares: Showing the Way Within. There were forty westerners and we were treated as honored guests; we were allowed to sleep in the ashram, using the indoor facilities. Amazed at the determination of the devotees – standing in long lines, slowly moving in the hot sun – we found stainless steel pails and ladles in the kitchen and brought them water. Many touched our feet and brought their fingertips to their foreheads honoring the Divine within Namaste. Their eyes spoke volumes, clearly a lesson in Singularity – bringing water to mySelf.

After the festival... a slow journey from the Himalayas to Chennai and then by ship to Penang, Malaysia – 5 days to cross the Indian Ocean – precious time for meditation and contemplation. Malaysia is rich with abundant water and greenery, a veritable paradise. After heading north through Thailand, thoughts began of Malaysia again, Singapore... and Bali. Traveling through these cultures is a vegan delight. While Americans recognize a few varieties of papaya, there are multiple shapes, sizes and tastes, ranging in color from yellow to orange to deep red; some cultures skin a green papaya, cube it and curry it; this is *one* fruit, the same applies to mangos. Delectable offerings such as jackfruit and mangosteen when ripened on the tree, have a completely different taste from the fruits picked green for transport. Carambola known as starfruit because of its shape... Canastel known as eggfruit with the looks, taste and texture of hard-boiled egg yolk... exquisite flavors abound!

Singapore is a cosmopolitan island / city / country blending cultures and nationalities, old ways along with new... a perfect introduction to Indonesia – a string of islands under the Malay Peninsula. Bali is Hindu and the rest of the islands are Moslem; it is a spiritual center, a haven for artists. Spirit brought me to a delightful lodge... the family lovingly cared for me, seeing each guest as Krishna in disguise. Their teeth were stained red from chewing betel nut, which they offered (it was bitter) saying one would have to chew regularly to get the effect. Asking for directions to *The Garden*, she smiled: "after dinner, be sure You go to the *barong*."

I arrived on the Full Moon and each New and Full Moon there is a tribal dance to protect the village. After my 50 mushroom / vegetable soup, it was an intense experience, a delightful moonlit tribal dance. The men gather dressed in loincloth with a necklace of shells... displaying daggers in each hand, showing how ferocious they are as the sentinels of the village, warding off the Spirit of Evil with their bellowing and antics. Then sudden stillness. The Spirit of Evil undaunted, *dared* to make his presence known. Even though this was a ritual dance performed 1000s of times, the trepidation throughout the crowd... mostly locals... was quite real.

The Spirit of Evil was ugly, loud and fearsome. The men at first cowered; building their courage, they showed how tough they were by forcefully ramming pointed daggers under their collarbones! What kept them from piercing the flesh? Perhaps they were in a trance. The men and the Spirit of Evil intimidated each other back and forth... and just when it seemed the Spirit of Evil had gained control – the Spirit of Good arrived exuding such a feeling of peace and strength, the Spirit of Evil ran away... leaving the village. The Spirit of Good and the men danced and sang triumphant, exuberant. What an introduction to the island of Bali! I spent the next month meditating in the mornings, lunching at *The Garden*, wandering in the woods and mud-bathing, followed by body surfing in the late afternoon... sometimes having vegetable soup for dinner as well. After sunset... when the streetlights went on... back to the lodge for reading and conversation enjoying the beauty of radiant beings who knew the simple Life – present in the Here & Now.

How to get to Hawai'i? Slowly by ship through the south Pacific islands? or fly up the Orient? I had an address for a Japanese priest who studied in Detroit and helped out on weekends living at Holy Name parish in Birmingham. His family sent many Care Packages and he brought seaweed and other goodies to our dinner table. We had great rapport; I looked forward to seeing him again. Knowing that I would be on Bali for thirty days, the length of the visa... I wrote Paul Tago at his last known address. A couple of weeks later, going to General Delivery in Denpasar... there was a letter from Osaka. After the Bali experience, returning to Singapore, I found a dream ticket for $550: Singapore... Hong Kong... Taipei... Osaka... Tokyo... Honolulu... LAX... and... I had a year to complete the journey on China Air in 1973.

Hong Kong seemed much like Singapore – wonderful folks, warm and friendly – it was a thrill to ride junkets in Kowloon Bay... and walk in Mainland China. Even though heavily influenced by the West, it's quite an experience. Someone has an idea for every dollar in Your pocket! The morning ritual in Taipei is Tai Chi in the park. Business people dressed in suits, briefcases in the baskets on their bikes, converge on city parks. Removing their ties and dress shirts, they do the dance of martial arts then dress again, and cycle to their offices – inspiring: people of all ages doing "moving meditation." Touring the island of Taiwan proved simply spectacular.

Making reservations for Osaka & sending Paul a note – he was at the airport in all his glory, radiating his famous smile... with a parishioner, a fireman, who brought us hOMe to family and friends, enjoying a vegan feast. Paul was interpreter; they knew I was enjoying vegan living, and questioned my dietary habits... wondering. Why prefer brown rice – suitable for pigs – while refined rice is suitable for humans**?** Were your travels based on the pendulum**?** I was astonished, quizzically thinking of a grandfather clock... they excitedly shared this source of information – the pendulum – as a simple way to connect with High

Self. They asked if I had a five-yen piece in my pocket. Pulling out my change, sure enough. Think of a nickel with a hole in the center. They found a piece of string and made an instant pendulum. They asked if I had a picture in my wallet of someone dead and someone alive. I had a picture of someone who was quite alive – my meditation teacher – but dead? Realizing I had a new dollar – George Washington definitely fit the category.

Showing me how to hold the pendulum, sliding the bill underneath... it stood perfectly still. I wondered: is this a reflection on the vitality of George, or the 1973 dollar? Replacing the bill with the teacher who was alive and energetic... the pendulum began moving briskly in a clockwise direction! Skeptical... suggesting somehow nerve impulses were being transferred from my brain, knowing who was dead and who was alive... they laughed & reached into their wallets bringing out pictures. As the pendulum swung or stood still, they verified who was actually dead and who was alive. Totally amazing! I began practicing with the pendulum making statements I already knew: I have more than one brother, I have more than two brothers... watching the response... making other statements... intuitively feeling in my Heart, and Knowing... this **is** a way to connect with High Self, to **know** the Truth.

Japanese cities and country-sides are distinguished by graciousness and hospitality. Their produce sections are astonishing: twice as big as ours – half dedicated solely to delectable ocean vegetables, aka seaweed. They have a voracious appetite for all kinds of algae... fresh, dried and fermented. Algae are rich in vitamins, minerals, trace elements and micronutrients – providing a source of complete protein. Their taste for macroalgae and microalgae, with brown, green and blue-green varieties, may well be the reason Japan ranks among the top 5 countries with the highest average IQ in the world {105} and the lowest amount of white hair! In the top 5 are other SE Asian countries where seaweed is common, such as Hong Kong and, #1 – Singapore {108}. The US has an average of 98, with lots of white hair & bald heads. Seaweeds and ocean-vegetable salads offer a treat for brain health!

Approaching Hawai'i from the Orient is spectacular... tropical mountains and valleys, volcanoes, whales, and a magical mixture of humankind combine to make it as close to Paradise as it gets on planet Earth. The next few years were spent exploring islands, meeting *kahunas* and teachers, learning Johrei {Purification of the Spirit} as well as Reiki {Universal Life Force Energy} opening to Inner Voice Intuition, offering unconditional Love – being completely Detached from Results, being present in the moment for whatever growth is taking place.

Mr Ting, a Japanese / American / Hawaiian kahuna from Wailuku, taught how to recharge Your energy batteries day or night. Simply go outdoors, away from motors such as a/c, refrigerators, TVs and other electronic devices, *and* away from overhead wires. With hands stretched above Your head, similar to antennae... turn slowly until You feel tingling in Your palms. It took a few minutes to feel, and only a few seconds for the skeptical mind to surface: "Wait a minute... of course, You feel tingling in Your hands... they've been over Your head for a few minutes and the blood's drained down Your arms, silly!" So, keeping my arms stretched to the heavens... turning away from that direction, the tingling immediately disappeared; returning, so did the tingling... turning the other direction, it disappeared; returning, so did the tingling. I smiled and asked for clarification.

Mr Ting laughed. "Skepticism is quite normal... that's the direction of Your birthplace!" Fortunately, a clear night... checking the North Star – I was facing east-northeast... a fairly accurate direction from Maui to Detroit. "And when in Detroit, You will find the tingling in the direction of the hospital or home where You were born. Except for all the electrical interference in a hospital, You could find the room where You first saw the light of day... if it's a home, You can find the actual room!" To easily Reboot Your HeartMindBodySpirit... simply find Your direction. Surround Yourself with Love. Breathe slowly and deeply, caressing the roof of Your mouth with Your tongue for a few minutes as Your energies re-calibrate. All–ways Give Thanks... Feel Love... Be Empowered!

Nu'uanu Valley, Oahu: Stanley Burroughs introduced me to color healing and Vitaflex Foot Reflexology. His Master Cleanse was intriguing, as well as his commitment. He shipped in Maple syrup from Canada, in gallon tins, by the pallet! He encouraged me, and I began a 7-week fast. {I half consumed the second gallon.} Every 90 minutes I had 2 oz of juice from a lemon or lime in a glass of rain water – which You could do in those days – stirred with a Tsp of maple syrup, topped with a generous sprinkle of cayenne. {Today,

substitute a drop of Stevia to keep the blood sugar stable.} This concoction sustained me for 39 days. With the digestive system shut down... my feeling body, my thinking body and my acting body could rejuvenate. Eventually, my bowels eliminated copious dark material... actually resembling the inside-out lining of the large intestine – shiny, black, complete with sacculation – indicating aluminum and heavy metals being discharged.

I had weighed 196 lbs when I first experimented with vegan living, and lost fifty pounds in two years. The climate and circumstances were favorable for a thorough cleansing. Thinking I was taking in vitamins and minerals with the citrus and maple syrup, I committed to fast until my tongue "turned pink like a dog's" as suggested by Mr Burroughs. By that time, I had gone down to 119 lbs and felt like skin and bones. When the sun went down, I bundled in layers to keep warm; the next day greeting the warmth and energy of the sun, both morning and late afternoon. Browsing the produce section at the health food store in Kainaliu, wondering how to conclude the fast... I saw a friend from another island. Explaining I'd been fasting for 39 days and now that my tongue is pink, I'm ready to eat... he responded, "I know what I'd do if I fasted for 39 days. I'd drink some blood cleansing teas for ten days." Immediately thinking, that would bring it to 49 days – 7 weeks of 7 days – hmmm... a nice ring to that. Brilliant! I left with a pound each of burdock root, red clover flowers and wood sanicle bark. After that, papaya and avocado from the orchard for a few days, and then salads from the Garden of Eatin' out back.

After Hawai'i, I spent a year in a meditation community known as The City of Love and Light in San Antonio. Our days were spent in service, mine being at a sawmill making end-cut parquet flooring from mesquite; the wood is oily. Spare time was spent working with and learning from other natural healers. One day someone donated ½ ton of organic grapefruit, so I began a fast. Bringing some to work, sitting on the woodpile at lunch, grapefruit juice dripped down my arm – cleansing mesquite stains that had marked me as part of the sawmill crew. What a delightful discovery; we put away the chemical cleansers, and began using citrus as soap. Surprising even myself by fasting for a week while doing heavy work – I actually did a modified fast, eating 6 grapefruits each day along with copious water – grateful to be in a supportive and meditative, albeit noisy, environment.

Realizing I had gathered unusual yet practical knowledge, hanging a shingle as a "reflexologist / herbologist / iridologist" would be speaking a foreign language... at least in the 70s. So, to acquire society's official sanction, I went back to school and became a doctor. Most doctors deal with drugs and invasive measures; my option was to become a Primary Care Physician as a Doctor of Chiropractic: Sacral-Occipital-Technique – S.O.T. – the oldest, most respected of the gentle approaches to chiropractic. S.O.T. encourages more time spent with the person exploring reflex points, especially on the cranium. S.O.T. is a holistic approach to health that goes beyond the physical, and sees connections with the emotional, mental and spiritual aspects of life. It was fascinating to learn from the basic S.O.T. texts of Dr DeJarnette, DO, DC, and the cranial text of Dr Sutherland, DO. These two gentlemen were long-time friends; they would meet at the pub on a Saturday night, and discuss their unusual cases, many times finding results with what the other one had suggested; they published their books on craniopathy a year apart. Equally fascinating, Dr M.L. Rees discovered specific correlations between cranial misalignment, organ stress and emotional involvement. Doctors came from around the world to spend time with Dr Rees – from the US, CA, UK, EU, JP & AU – to Sedan, KS... town of 2000 people! Dr. M.L. Rees Archives | SOTO USA (soto-usa.com)

Receiving my diploma as Doctor of Chiropractic, my chief mentor was Jaroslava Odvarko, the first female craniopath, who encouraged me to attend Dr Rees' next seminar, whenever that might be. Waiting for FL state board results, I heard Dr Rees was coming to Atlanta, where he introduced his system of Harmonics: balancing the bones of the cranium as well as the energy of the organs... and bringing emotional healing using crystals, colors, sounds and affirmations. Grateful to have studied with Dr Rees for a few years, Vibrational Energy Medicine has been the heart of my practice since 1981 – Harmonious Healing for HeartMindBodySpirit – working from my hOMe-office, a small cottage in Coconut Grove.

As a respite from intensifying nuclear threats US<>USSR, a year-sabbatical felt appropriate. Heading Down Under the equator, '84-85 was spent in the bush with Native Fijians, rather than Indian Fijians who lived in the cities. Living near Sele-sele Falls was sheer joy... a mile up the mountain from the nearest village, which itself was a two-hour hike from the main road and the bus. For a mere $300 they built a palm-thatched hut (20x30) with a platform bed (8x8) having a traditional mattress made of shredded coconut husks, and enclosed by mosquito netting. The floor of the hut was woven pandanus mats covering a thick layer of dried, wild grass... like walking on a mattress. It was an Honor to be inducted as members of the Dranu tribe – drinking kava-kava to make it Official. They would bring papayas, bananas, young coconuts and other treats... thrilling to live as the Fijians, experiencing their culture back in the bush: going to bed soon after dark, and up at dawn... outside the village of Draunaleka, Toki, Nakorotubu, Ra, Fiji.

Returning to the States, Viktoras Kulvinskas invited me to share Harmonious Healing with the guests at Hippocrates Health Institute. In Boston for >30 years under the direction of Dr Ann Wigmore and Viktoras, HHI moved to West Palm Beach in '86. With a 30-year history of amazing recoveries from catastrophic situations... people could build self-esteem and re-gain control over their lives. Some were in terminal situations, and a few chose to make their transitions there in a peaceful, supportive environment.

Practicing Harmonious Healing in various holistic centers offering yoga, meditation, self-empowerment classes, and mind / body detox, one thing became perfectly clear: the true panacea is within – so set aside time-in... meditation, and set aside time-out... with Mother Nature. Enoch says: Be still... and know... I Am God! After Viktoras Kulvinskas was consecrated an Essene bishop, with Gabriel Cousens, MD and Patricia Bragg, he offered to ordain me a minister of the Essene Tradition. At first my reaction was: No thanks; been there, done that. He persisted saying by teaching the Essene lifestyle and honoring the relationships of All Life Everywhere, this would simply give recognition to the fact. So, on Valentine's Day '92, I gratefully accepted his invitation. Currently, Viktoras Kulvinskas, DD, PhD offers Sanctuary in the only Blue Zone in the tropics: the Nicoya peninsula – in Montezuma, Costa Rica. Viktoras Kulvinskas

After Hurricane Andrew, my intuition led me to a sabbatical in London – providing time for research and writing, teaching and treatments, and offering an opportunity to reassess Life's Goals. Returning to FL, my chiropractic license had expired; calling to renew, I discovered State laws had changed. Malpractice insurance was now required, rather than optional.

Then I was told all chiropractors must now offer the "same standard of care" which means, for litigation purposes, x-rays for everyone. A good chiropractor can make an assessment through palpation, orthopedic and neurological tests. X-rays are redundant – for the most part, they are a moneymaker. They do harm more than they do good. Finally, the State said I could have in my office *only* those things that were taught in chiropractic school! Since that excluded 75% of my practice, it was: "Strike 3, yer out!" It was such a Blessing to be relieved of the insurance games, and all the complicating, counterproductive regulations.

As an Essene physician and minister, I trust the process of Life. Rather than seeing people – or the system – as the source of my livelihood, the Universe orchestrates and choreographs the Dance, providing support for my ministry. **The Universe conspires for my success!** Indeed, Life itself supports me. I trust the Power that sustains the Universe. As we choose our Path on this Sacred Journey, we actually experience our very own creation. We do it all through the workings of our feeling-thinking body. Pure Consciousness expresses our *Attention* as our *Intention*… and creates our *chosen* Reality. Be Cautious about the thoughts and feelings You entertain! Each of us… individual Aspects of the Divine Presence, the Source of All… is exploring various experiences of human consciousness. Plutarch says: What we achieve inwardly changes our outer reality**!** How? Powered by our feeling-thinking-body. Indeed, we do it all. In fact, astronaut John Mitchell explains succinctly:

"Our attitude toward Life determines Life's attitude toward us."

Essene tradition provides places for people to rejuvenate – getting their hands in the soil… connecting with Source… with Father Sun and Mother Earth… and with Each Other as Sisters and Brothers. From ancient times, Essenes were the primal holistic healers, observing and teaching the inter-relationships between our feeling body, our thinking body and our acting body – which we heal as One: HeartMindBodySpirit. The Dead Sea Scrolls and the Nag Hammadi Library represent a small portion of the Essene Impulse that currently pervades the planet.

Rather than being a religion, cult or even a philosophy, Essenes share Unity Consciousness. Most people live in the world of duality; they are deep into judgments of right and wrong, good and bad. They proudly say there are two sides to every coin. Essenes, on the other hand, know there are many sides to every coin: the head, the tail, the side, the inside, the outside – head, tail and side as one – and, the holographic unit. Essenes see all things in terms of Unity – Aware of Relationships with All Life Everywhere, and Within.

Unity is the experience of Conscious Communion – the experience of Infinite, Divine Presence in every*one* and every*thing*. Being full of Love and Compassion means freedom from judgment or coercion of any sort. Unity is the essence of Enlightenment… Singularity.

In our world of polarity, the illusion of separation is the Origin of Suffering, the Original Sin. The serpent implied *separation* by saying: "Eat this and You will be *like* God!" A treacherous lie… You *are* God! Each One *is* a Divine Expression of Infinite Imagination. Each One equally *is* the Source of All… the Word made flesh… exploring human consciousness – the One.

Realizing One is the Source of All, the Source of the Universe, the Source of the Cosmos, One with All That Is – even Monkey-mind! – what suffering is possible? Essenes are dedicated to the experience of Unity… now and all–ways… freshly sprouting all around us.

Great Spirit… Father Sun… Mother Earth...
every Sacred Breath is my re-birth...
every day a chance to be…
Love and Compassion with all I see, including Me.
I see with loving eyes. I love what I see. I see clearly.
I see the truth.
I hear with loving ears. I love what I hear. I hear
clearly. I hear the truth.
Perfect Divine Order takes place in my Life all–ways.
Only growth comes from each experience.
It is safe to grow and mature, growth means Life.
I welcome what is useful in my Life.
I now comfortably and easily release the rest.
I heal my feminine energies and my feeling body.
I heal my masculine energies and my thinking body.
I Am now One. I Am whole and complete.
My feeling body, my thinking body and my acting
body are now in total balance, my system *is* in order.
My glands and my organs are happy,
doing an excellent job keeping me healthy.
I Am a Pure Being of Radiant Energy – the Divine
Presence sustains All.
I Am Pure Awareness exploring human
consciousness.

I Am the delightful expression of the I Am Presence
that I Am.
My Life Continues to Be One Blessing after anOther!
I Am so Blessed!
So Be It. And So, It Is. And It Is Done.
And I Am One with All, and All Is One!

As primal holistic healers in terms of Unity, some are unaware of being Essenes – even though helping birth New World Awakening – truly, Ancient Consciousness many are now discovering. In *Sacred Contracts*, Caroline Myss mentions Sir George Trevelyan, Father of the modern Essene movement in England. Good fortune allowed me to spend time with him at his hOMe – The Barn in Hawkesbury, Badminton, Avon. Sir George has been fondly referred to as "GrandFather of the New Age Movement" – rather than cult, fad and woolly notions, it is a non-sectarian, holistic, scientific, practical, mystical, compassionate, Essene perspective... pertinent today. Before the manuscript of this book was complete, he said:

"Yours is a brilliant book. It will nourish the
imaginations of those who are birthing the new
consciousness. From the seeds of the past... come
the plants of today that are blossoming... for the
survival of Our Beloved Mother Earth."
https://www.sirgeorgetrevelyan.org/

Consciousness expands. Constraints imposed by social and religious mores are simply control mechanisms. Realizing major Matrix media carefully craft continued control – contriving to maintain the status quo as though it's all in our best interests – it is uplifting to see so many freeing themselves. As awareness grows, we free ourselves from the control mechanisms of guilt and fear that sustain the old paradigm of separation and competition. Love, the liberating factor, returns us to the paradigm of Unity Consciousness and co-operation. Learning respect and compassion for others, listening, encouraging them to listen to their own Inner Voice Intuition... we recognize and honor Infinite Beauty within All.

Our precious space-time has Infinite Possibilities. Choices we make have more consequences than ever before, and will assure either the demise... or the survival of our Beloved Mother Earth. Blending Ancient Wisdom with the tools of Modern Times nurtures survival for Our Sacred Journey. Everything **is** in **P**erfect **D**ivine **O**rder... PDO... Breath by Sacred Breath! ~.~*

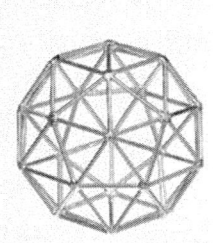

THE ART AND PRACTICE OF VIBRATIONAL ENERGY MEDICINE

1 – YOUR VERBAL DIET IS THE FOUNDATION

How can You attempt to cure the eyes
without treating the head
or the head without treating the body as a whole?
So, how can You treat the body
without treating the soul?
And the treatment of the soul, my good friend,
is by means of certain charms...
and these charms are words of the best sort.
By the use of such words
is temperance engendered in the soul,
and as soon as it is engendered and present...
one may easily secure health to the head
and to the rest of the body also.
Charmides, Plato

Like apples of gold in a silver setting
is a word that is aptly spoken.
Proverbs 25:11

"In the beginning..."
Diet and exercise are recognized as vital components for healing and for maintaining optimal health. Of equal importance are the words You use and hear. Your **Verbal Diet** determines Your Reality. As Your feelings reflect Your emotions Your words reflect Your thoughts and these comprise the building blocks – the vibrational foundation – upon which You create! Your Verbal Die-t becomes Your **Verbal Live-it!** Living Food, to feed and empower Your Life.

Vibrations have two basic components, wavelength and frequency: each scientifically measured. Recent studies in water coherence and intelligence prove everything is vibration – from medicines to thought-forms. Medicine means: to mediate balance and harmony – homeostasis – and is usually understood as something that influences or alters the blood chemistry. Medicine may be preventive or a remedy.

Going far beyond drugs – be they prescription, OTC, recreational: whether shots, pills or ointments – medicine also includes herbs, from which a number of pharmaceuticals are derived... as well as foods and juices, colors and sounds, crystals and metals, fresh air and water, and ultimately – Your thoughts, which reflect Your feelings.

To understand how this can be, and how it can make a difference, let's begin at the beginning of the book by John the Evangelist. "In the beginning was the Word, and the Word was with God, and the Word was God." What is the profound Word that John mentions? Christians would say the Word is Jesus. Jews, however, would say the Word is so sacred it is left unpronounced! When the Tetragrammaton YHWH appears in their readings, the lector pauses for a second and everyone knows in that pause, the Word Yahweh is understood. Muslims say the Word is Allah. Hindus say Sat Nam. The Vedas say: "In the beginning was Brahman – I Am – with whom was the Word." So, what **is** the Word**?**

"In the beginning" gives pause to reflect. Alphabets... languages... even the lips to pronounce any of these Names, simply were a twinkle in the Eye of Infinite Mind. In the beginning was only Infinite Mind. John tells us: "and the Word was God." In English, the word GOD may be seen as an acronym describing the Essence of Infinite Being: **G**enerator – **O**perator – **D**estroyer. When one cycle is complete, another cycle begins. Divine Presence simply is... and continues... throughout every dimension.

We are still left wondering what is the Word that was in the beginning... before alphabets, languages and lips came into being? Scriptures shed some light. The book of *Genesis* says we are literally "made in the image and likeness of God!" This means we can learn something about God by looking at ourselves and something about ourselves by looking at God.

If we truly *are* "made in the image and likeness of God" – and we observe both women and men – then Infinite Being *must* reflect those Qualities and Energies. Essenes go back to Sumer millennia before the time of Jesus and the Jewish People. Essenes consider the Divine as Infinite Being – the I Am Presence – Creator of All Life Everywhere or simply, Great Spirit. Imagining a world of polarity, the first offspring Infinite Being created was: Mother-Goddess and Father-God.

I Am represents Infinite Being, Source of All. Mother-Goddess represents the aspect of Vision and Imagination. Father-God represents the aspect of Being and Action. Within this trinity, Essenes recognize the Energy we call God is a point of Unity... Singularity. {While Christian theology acknowledges the feminine principle as the Holy Spirit – the Dove of Peace, another theology in our world of polarity goes a step further: if there is God the Father... God the Son... and God the Holy Spirit – there must be God the Mother... God the Daughter... and God the Holy Sophia!}

Likewise, if we truly are "made in the image and likeness of God" then we can learn something about ourselves by looking at God, the Creator of All Life Everywhere. We *also* must be creators. How do *we* create? We create the same way as God – through Vibration. How long the creation process took – several seconds... several days... or several eons – is a curious question, yet of little *practical* consequence.

Noteworthy in the book of *Genesis*, When the time came for creation – rather than **thinking**: hmmm... Maybe light would be a nice way to start – "God **said**: 'Let there be light!' and there was light." Now, whether the Creator of All had vocal cords with which to speak, is another curious question for the religious speculators. Yet the Scripture clearly teaches: God creates... creation happens... with the spoken word – through *Vibration*. Spoken words show up as creative energy... again and again... and so with us... we create through Vibration!

When God gave the command to Moses to bring the tribes of Israel out of Egypt, Moses was terrified. Thinking the people would only laugh at him for such a preposterous idea, he asked, "Who shall I tell them is sending me?" And God said as succinctly as possible: "I Am That I Am. You must say: 'I Am has sent me to You'!" The word **I** connects with Source, God's Pure Energy. **Am** connects Source with Be-ing, God in Action. Every utterance of **I Am** is an expression of Infinite Being – being infinite in this finite world – where the spoken word is Powerful and Creative.

What exactly is the spoken word? Essentially, each word has vibrations; when You speak Your vocal cords vibrate... projected from Your mouth... the vibrations are then funneled into receptive ears and vibrate 3 tiny bones of the inner ear... the brain deciphers those vibrations and – Communication Happens.

20

Since we are made in the image and likeness of God... and understand *our* words as vibrations... we can understand what John is saying. "In the beginning was the Vibration, and the Vibration was with God, and the Vibration was God." The Word is the Vibrational Frequency of Infinite Mind that Sustains All – Great Spirit – Infinite Being – expressing God in Action.

Created in the image and likeness of God, You *also* express vibrational frequencies and exert creative energy. That is why Your thought-forms... which result from and govern Your feelings, as well as expressions going through Your head and Your heart are of utmost importance – especially those that pass through Your lips habitually. Some thought-forms are so powerful, simply being in Your head or feeling them in Your heart... Communication happens.

Walking through a tough part of town thinking and feeling: Oh, this is terrible; this is a good place to get mugged! – translates into one's gait and countenance. The cowering person is a walking ad: Come and get me! Yet walking the same street thinking and feeling: OK, this is a time to be especially alert and careful, surrounding myself with Love and trusting in the Divine! – translates into the gait and countenance as well. Confident, shoulders back, head held high, alerts would-be muggers: Be cautious. Back off!

Your thought vibrations and feeling vibrations are so powerful they often stand on their own. Communication happens... and when You add the power of the spoken word, Your thoughts and feelings take on a powerful dimension. For this reason, pay close attention to what You think and say, especially what You think and say *habitually.*

The way You think is the way You feel.
The way You feel is the way You vibrate.
The way You vibrate is the way You attract.
Language shapes Your Reality, focusing and directing Your energies. Since the subconscious mind accepts Your thoughts and Your language *literally*... use *only* those words You choose to Create in Your Life.

With these power-filled forces – *the **vibrations** of Your thoughts and feelings* – Your words actually do create Your Reality. Rather than being gibberish or a magical incantation like: Open, Sesame! or Open! Says!! Me!!! **Abracadabra** is from ancient Aramaic – abra'q ad habra – **Abra'qadhabra** literally: **I create as I speak!** We Do! Every One of us. Ancient Wisdom tell us:

"What You achieve inwardly
changes Your outer reality!"
Plutarch

"You are what You think.
With Your thoughts You make Your world."
Buddha

PC or PE – That is the *Real* Question!
When speaking of the words we use especially in conversation, many are conscious of being politically correct, so no group takes offense. While this can be the source of many jokes, it is a serious matter; the issue goes far beyond being politically correct. It is a question of personal *empowerment* leading one to personal *responsibility*. I... both letter and word... connects us with Source, with Pure Energy, which affects our Conscious Awareness.

Denial of self is a denial of Your Divinity. For those who feel such a statement is bold at best, and blasphemy at worst, Jesus quoted Psalm 82:6, "I once said: You, too, are gods – all of You!" A little later Jesus said: "I Am in the Father and the Father is in me. I tell You most solemnly – Whoever believes in me will perform even greater works than I." And perhaps Jesus' most profound statement: "Understand, I Am in my Father and You in Me and I in You." Another translation reads: "I and the Father are One, and You are One with Me as I Am One with You." Singularity Consciousness. When You deny the self You deny an aspect of Your Divinity Your creativity suffers at the subconscious level. When You align with Great Spirit feeling in Your Heart – I Am That I Am – Your Creativity soars; Dreams unfold. Empower Yourself with Words of Power:
I Am... I Can... I Change...
I Choose... I Create...
I Empower... I Encourage...
I Enjoy... I Experience...
I Feel... I Have...
I Know... I Love...
I Recognize... I Recreate...
I Understand... I Will...
Words of Power promote nurturing feelings, and in Your Heart call forth to the subconscious to shape wonder-full Blessings leading to Your New Reality!

Conversely, whenever You say I and follow with a negation, You deny the self and You deny Your Divine creative power! A typical question: Would You like to go to a movie? can elicit a totally disempowering

21

response: Oh, I don't know; I don't think so; I don't feel like it! This is a triple denial of Your Divine Power. Saying I don't know, aligns Yourself with ignorance. I don't think, denies Your cognitive capabilities. I don't feel, denies Your emotions. Be empowered: I'd rather do something else; what else can we do?

What if You really *don't* know something, like the time? You can always phrase Yourself positively. I don't know, easily can be transmuted into personal empowerment: That's a good question, or… I wonder, or I will find out. Why say I don't know about anything?

Rather than saying what You don't think, say what You *do* think. I don't think I'm in the mood for a movie! becomes… I'm in the mood for a walk. I don't think that makes any sense! becomes… I think that's illogical! What sense does that make? I don't think I need say more! becomes… I think it is clear! And, rather than saying what You don't feel, say what You *do* feel. I don't feel like sitting here any longer! becomes… I feel like being in the garden! I don't understand! becomes… Help me understand this; I choose clarity! And, I really can't tell You how happy I am to be here! becomes… I Am *so* happy to be here! I won't know until later this afternoon, becomes… I'll know this afternoon! I don't want, becomes… I'd rather have. I don't recommend, becomes… I recommend You avoid. I haven't ever seen, becomes… I have yet to see. I didn't notice until later, becomes… I only noticed later! I don't have much time, becomes… Since time is of the essence… Stop. Think of something You habitually say. Re-write the script making it empowering for all concerned.

While saying **I** followed by a negation is dis-empowering it is always acceptable to say No or No, thank You, at appropriate times. Are You going to the movies? Rather than No, I'm not! simply say No! or No, I'm doing something else! Do You care for more salad? Rather than No I don't, thank You! Say: No, thank You!

The words we use definitely make a difference. As a young chiropractor with a home office in Coconut Grove, FL, early one morning someone called saying he had a tough day ahead and would like me to "fix" his neck. Arriving, he said he "slept wrong". Had he been traveling and slept in an uncomfortable bed? Did he sleep on two pillows instead of one? "No, everything was normal. I just slept wrong!" So… how's life been?

Within a few minutes he said his boss was a real pain in the neck, and he had to go in early to re-design a whole project that was a real pain in the neck in the first place! When he also referred to his girlfriend as a pain in the neck, a look of knowing came to his eyes. We talked about the power of the spoken word, encouraging him to speak only those words he chooses to manifest in his life. As for the tough day ahead, if that's what he claims, if that's what he owns, then that's what it shall be. His neck was adjusted, and his mind as well. Dr B.J. Palmer referred to the latter as the adjustment of the subluxation above atlas.

Expressions such as a pain in the neck, or another part of the anatomy, are examples of things said out of habit. It takes a conscious person to speak Conscious Language. Fortunately, there are a couple of phrases to redeem a disempowering situation. When something comes out of Your mouth that is less than Your highest choice, You can say: **Cancel / Clear** – in Your head, or in comfortable surroundings You can say it aloud. Both have the same effect. This empowering phrase takes its origin from the early days of computers. After typing for a while, the operator may be frustrated, look at the screen and say: Let's start over! and then hit the button at the bottom corner of the keyboard which used to say: Cancel / Clear. The screen is wiped clean… and the operator begins with a fresh start. Today we hit Ctrl/Z. Also effective: Cancel / Cancel, Erase / Erase, Delete / Delete, or Escape / Escape. In this manner You honor the brain as the Master Computer – wiping it clean from disempowering thoughts and expressions, then expressing Yourself consciously… and masterfully.

Another phrase that can redeem a disempowering situation is, **in the past**. When someone says, what a disorganized slob! they claim that as current reality, which only serves to re-enforce and prolong the situation. If something disempowering slips out, You can alter the meaning and intent. What a disorganized slob… he has been in the past, and I empower him to establish order in his life! Or, I really hate the way my life is going… in the past, and I empower myself with Conscious Language to create my New Reality!

After going through these games for a while, the brain – being an efficient organ – soon begins to express itself masterfully simply out of habit. With a soft Cancel / Clear, those committed to Conscious Language can coach each other in a friendly and playful way when something less than our highest choice is spoken. Growing attentive to Your Verbal Diet, You speak slowly, thoughtfully; thinking, feeling, being, and acting – delightfully different. Your conscious Verbal Diet expresses and creates Your Life's true Purpose, as You endeavor to express Your true human nature of Love and Compassion.

An Examination of Consciousness

"If I have lost confidence in myself,
I have the Universe against me!"
Ralph Waldo Emerson

"Whether You think You can
or think You can't
You are right!"
Henry Ford

"Stand up for Your limitations…
and surely You shall own them."
Robert Tennyson Stevens

We have many words and expressions to consider for disposal. Some are obvious; others are subtle. Feel the difference. Say the common expressions *out loud*, then the suggestions. Compare how You *feel* with each.

Two words that clearly express lack are: **need** and **want**. To need is to lack. To say: For my home office I need a new computer and printer, claims a lack of said items and *owns* that condition. I get to have or I can use, is acceptable or quite simply, Basic requirements for my home office are… While to need is to lack, it's empowering to get things. We all have requirements for food, clothing and shelter. When we want a new house, we are affirming we lack it. It is my highest choice to have a new house by the end of the year, stating it clearly. Proper usage of want is: I saw the new exhibit at the museum, and for *want* of a better word – it's a type of post-modern expressionism.

Advertisers sabotage themselves in their 60-second time slot by telling us how **incredible** their product is. Actually, the script-writers would be better off to simply say: it's supercalifragilisticexpialidocious! At the very least, say it's wonderful, marvelous or amazing! Incredible means un-believable, and the subconscious suggestion is: too good to be true… why even bother?

To **try** to do something is self-sabotage. Do You think trying is going to get something done? Try to touch

Your nose. You are either doing it, or You are not. If You are doing it, You are not trying; if You are trying, You are not doing it. To try to do something that is negative is a *real* challenge. Some people have said: This time, I'm really going to try to **quit** smoking! Mark Twain tells us: Quitting smoking is the easiest thing I have ever done. I've done it hundreds of times! Why? He kept trying. Rather than trying to quit, positively affirm Your outcome: I choose to be free from tobacco! I choose fresh air for my lungs!

Many have said: I'm really going to try to lose weight! Here is a triple sabotage: **try**ing… to **lose**, which is a negative concept… **weight**, which is a part of us! This goes against our subconscious mind, and all the training we've had since we were kids: You go back down the street and get Your wagon. You've got to keep track of Your things or You'll lose them! Thus, we have been programmed to hold onto our "stuff" and here we resolve to lose weight – to lose a part of us! The subconscious says, **No way!** To facilitate Your desire: I choose to tone my body! See Yourself in the mirror and *feel* Yourself in Your outcome. Be **there** now: I Am fit and trim. My body is toned. I Am beautiful.

I'm really **helpless** When it comes to this sort of thing! is easily transformed to: I can use help with this! I can't help myself when it comes to food! can change to: I get to create discipline in my life, especially when it comes to food! While this begins the journey, it still involves process rather than outcome. My **choice** is to **have** discipline in my life! **I Am** in charge of my life. My choices are clear! These statements firmly establish outcome-oriented thinking and speaking. Or simply: I have an easy time with discipline and food! Some people are discouraged after years of trying; there is an antidote: I choose to make this easy, and fun! If brought up in authoritarian surroundings: I give myself *permission*, and I choose to make this easy – and fun!

Many PBS pledge-drives make comments like: Every year it is such a **struggle** to meet our operating expenses! This merely serves to foster that as on-going reality. They would be wise to say: We are so grateful to You. We appreciate Your continued support helping us meet our expenses on time. Thank You!

When paying bills, why **grudgingly** say: There goes another $100 to the power company; they sure gouge us! Give thanks for all the uses You've had with their services… & You can pay the bills in a timely manner!

Some words are quite subtle in their consequences. Have a **terrific** day! invites the experience of terror. As First Lady, Mrs. Clinton was asked if she would like a second child and she answered: It would be terrific! Since lawyers know the significance of words – arguing what the meaning of *is* is – one can only conclude, the idea struck terror in her heart.

Other common words and expressions are obvious. Gimme a **break**! invites osteoporosis, which is a precursor for a fracture and a fall, or invites an accident resulting in a fracture. Let's take a break! offers a similar invitation. It's time for a kidney break! is really devastating. It is both empowering and polite to say: It's time for intermission! We'll pause now, and resume in ten minutes! Are these examples too extreme or inconsequential? Some say a little humor is good for You. While laughter may be the best medicine, remember the subconscious takes things literally. Habitual expressions have a way of showing up.

Using **but** or **however** weakens or totally negates what You say. Imagine how You feel when someone says: I love You! Now imagine how You feel when someone says: I love You, but You make such a mess in the kitchen! Change *but* to *and*... now You are poised to express two positive statements: I love You, and I encourage You to clean the kitchen after making food!

To answer the phone and say: I'm **afraid** she's not here, or to say: I'm afraid I can't do that... affirms fear as Reality in Your Life. You can easily say: She's out right now, can I take a message? and: I have a busy day tomorrow. Can we make other arrangements?

We have used **sorry** – in the past – to the point where the true meaning: a painful situation causing intense sorrow, is both obscured and weakened. At a funeral, the words come out, yet they have lost the luster of their meaning. Only say I'm sorry! when truly sorrowful. Say what is meant. Oops! suffices in most situations. Excuse me! or: Pardon me! are to the point, respectful and empowering. Rather than feigning sorrow and making complicated excuses, simply say: I apologize for being late! And... to honor time-integrity in the collective subconscious: I apologize for being late, and I re-commit to being on time!

Do You **mind** if I open the window? also opens the way for a disempowering response. No, I don't mind! in effect negating the mind. Rather: That's a great idea!

Or: I'm comfortable the way it is, actually! Both, empowering responses. Isn't this mind-blowing? No, thank You I love my mind: this is mind-expanding!

To say: If I don't slow down, I'll have a nervous breakdown! Or: I'm overwhelmed! *owns* and promotes *that* as reality. Rather: I have so much going on, I'm going to take a deep breath, surround myself with Love and clarify my focus! I didn't realize how powerful this could be! becomes: I'm only now beginning to realize how powerful this can be!

After a tall tale, someone may say: I can't swallow that! Or say: Please, change the channel. I can't stomach that! These are open invitations to esophageal or digestive challenges. At a pre-prandial conversation, a guest used these expressions. Wondering how these negative thought-forms were programmed into his subconscious, as we sat at the table passing food, he bypassed a certain item saying: I can't digest that! reinforcing his thought-forms – I can't swallow that. I can't stomach that! – further disempowering the person. Say: Thank You! and pass the dish.

Seemingly innocent negative expressions can be transformed into conscious thoughts by changing a declaration to a question. You can't unscramble an egg! becomes: How can You unscramble an egg? Don't cry over spilled milk! becomes: Why cry over spilled milk? Why we talk the way we do is a question for scholars. As custodians of proper Verbal Diet, it is wise to "Live-it" and speak up when hearing truly offensive words – usually those attacks are based on gender, skin color, ethnicity or religion, meant to degrade, harm and divide in the most personal way possible. Speak up. Be Compassionate. The fact that people use negativity daily, reflects lazy habits as well as an undernourished vocabulary. Vulgarity simply means: talk of the commoners. We all succumb. As we actually begin to Live-it, we become aware of shades of meaning of various words, we expand our vocabulary, and express ourselves masterfully.

One thing that is mystifying... why the hell in hello? Professor Laurence McNamee, author of *A Few Words: a cornucopia of questions and answers concerning language, literature, and life,* says hello is attributed to Thomas A. Edison, who used it to answer the telephone. The Professor says hello is a corruption of hallow, a word of greeting common in the time of Chaucer, just as good-bye is a corruption of God be with You. He relished in telling me a form of "hello" was used to call or get someone's attention, quoting Shakespeare's *The Twelfth Night*, Viola to Olivia: "I will make me a willow cabin at Your gate, and halloo Your name to the reverberant hills!"

So, why the hell be in hell consciousness? How about, Heaven-o... or simply Hi! This latter word is a contraction of How are You, and etymologists find this greeting as early as the 12th century, perhaps as a corruption of Ahoy or Hoy! It is said that Alexander Graham Bell used this greeting all his life, rejecting Hello – being credited to his rival, Mr Edison. With respect to both, when answering the phone, a polite: Good morning / Good afternoon / Good evening!

Sometimes things are projected upon us, so be observant and swiftly clear any negativity. A sadistic professor walked into the first day of class in advanced calculus, threw his books on the desk and announced: Ladies and gentlemen, this is going to be the **toughest** class You've ever had. So, get ready for some hard work! Everyone immediately tenses and every time the students open their text, these negative thoughts are embedded in their subconscious. The clever student takes a deep breath and affirms: Cancel / clear. It may be tough for some... and... I choose to make this easy!

A considerate professor walks into the same class and announces: Ladies and gentlemen, this class presents a real **challenge**. Apply Yourselves with diligence, ask about anything less than clear, and You will do well! Who prefers a tough or difficult situation? On the other hand, the subconscious loves to deal with a challenge.

At another school, an educator told the student body: At this school we **stress** quality! which makes quality a stressor. Say: At this school we **encourage** quality!

Another projection: You **can't imagine** the traffic today! Everyone has seen gridlock and crazies on the road, and we sympathize. When driving affirm: I Am a safe driver and I surround myself with safe drivers; traffic flows smoothly and the police are busy with something else! And: I thank the Divine for the perfect parking space! It works wonders or it's an opportunity to **meditate**, stretch Your legs: perfect *space*, indeed!

Another similar projection: This picture really *captures Your imagination*! No thanks. Who can capture Figment? My imagination runs free! A common

projection foisted on others: *Don't forget!* The simple remedy is: **Remember!** Saying don't forget implies the person forgets a lot. Saying remember implies the person does remember things. Remember Your appointment this afternoon! Why say: I **almost forgot** to return that book! Congratulate Yourself: I **just remembered** to return that book! This embeds itself in the subconscious and You do tend to remember, sometimes even obscure things. Always *congratulate Yourself* whenever You remember anything... it's an honest boost to self-esteem and with repetition, becomes self-fulfilling prophecy. Affirm with a smile how wonderful it is – I **have a great memory!** – Your synapses become engaged... endorphins flow... and Your subconscious and conscious mind are alert... ready for the next *thrill* of remembering!

I *hate to think* about it, but it's really *driving me crazy*! In the first place, why hate? Is that Your highest choice? or is loving Your highest choice? Often people say: I hate it when... or, I really hate being here! The metaphysical principle is: **What You resist persists! What You allow changes!** Why hate anything? Hating hatred only buys into it... feeds and fuels it. Scores of great masters teach the simple power of Love. Saying: I hate it when... owns hatred as a part of Life. I hate to think... degrades Your cognitive powers, and the person subconsciously begins to own that as well. And to say: **but** it's really driving me crazy! So, even though I hate to think about it... *but* says, I'll do it anyway, even if it *does* drive me crazy! This is self-sabotage. Empower Yourself: I fill my memories with Love! I will think about something else! *Feel* the difference.

One final projection – pardon the pun – You'll die laughing! How many times have we heard: Laugh? I thought I'd die! Actually, laughing – simply smiling – is strengthening for Your immune response system. The "dessert to die for" – "Paradise Pie is to live for!"

Someone asks: Are You finished? In the past, I might have said: No, I'm not finished yet! Knowing the power of words – especially words denying power: No, I have yet to finish! What a difference it makes to use the word *yet* in its proper place. Rather than say: I haven't read it yet! I haven't met her yet! Say: I have yet to read it! I have yet to meet her! I haven't read it yet says: I'm so busy; it's another project on hold! I have yet to read it! puts the subconscious on high alert. I *really* get to create the time! And, things start getting done. In fact, You *do* meet her; she shows up at the perfect time!

Verbal Diet and Children

We are born little geniuses...
and educated to mediocrity.
Buckminster Fuller
{In the past, Bucky... in the past!}

Everyone knows children are little monkeys in so many ways, imitating what they see and what they hear. Science recognizes infants are sensitive to the vibrations of words, even tones of voice, during the 1st trimester! Raising children is a huge responsibility and, therefore, of paramount importance. Let them see and hear only things that facilitate them to experience their own power, and to affirm the wholesome aspects of Life – such as being out in Nature. If You are constantly checking Your devices, their curiosity and their desire will be naturally stimulated in that direction.

In the first years of life, it is best to avoid TV, monitors, and any sort of screen-time, especially under the guise of "toys"! Fleeting images program the supple mind for a short attention span. The same is true for rides in the car. Little ones are sometimes taken on errands so the other parent can have some space. Whenever it is necessary, turn the baby seat to face the rear of the car. Rather than seeing Life whizzing by, let the focus be on a colorful book or creative (**non-digital**) toys.

Infants do many challenging things: scratching, pulling our hair or slapping. Scratching is merely a reminder: time to trim, best when sleeping. Pulling hair may be an automatic response to keep balance, as when You are holding the child and bend to pick up something, or like slapping it may be a way of getting Your attention. Rather than scowling or growling: Don't do that; it hurts! which teaches the child that You, their Love Connection, are angry with them... with a big smile, even if feigned, say with *enthusiasm*: Oh, You'd like to play the hair-pulling game (slapping-game)? Keeping Your smile, give a decent tug of their hair or slap them briskly where they slapped You. Keeping the smile: Sure, we can play that game if You choose... or would You rather play a different game? Most often the child chooses to do something else. If the choice is the game, and the child pulls or slaps again... keep Your smile and be even firmer in Your response. Are You sure You enjoy this game? I'd rather do something else! Keep responding in a cheerful, gamely way until the choice is something else. The child learns: Actions have Consequences... and rather than angry or upset, You are experienced as happy and playful.

When the child crawls and stands, child-proof the house. Crayons, felt markers, pens and pencils are brought out only when it is time for drawing. Anything and everything You truly care about is always to be put out of reach. What understanding do children have about value? At this age, they take delight throwing things on the floor, perhaps to see how many pieces they can create. When the child has something inappropriate, it is because someone left it in an inappropriate place. The child is acting out of healthy curiosity – noticing certain items are always put up high... when left within reach it is intriguing to see how they feel, what they taste like, and... whether they bounce. The temptation? It's time for a playpen! This is strongly contraindicated for three reasons:

1) The child feels isolated. When You have chores, put the child in a highchair nearby with a toy or a treat: a spear of cucumber or, surprisingly, a stick of Spring onion – perhaps the spiciness is a distraction from the pain of teething. The two of You can then communicate during chores. Children love to have conversations, even before they can talk; this is how they learn. In this regard, while it may be endearing when a baby says: ba-ba-goo-goo, make sure **You** always speak properly – using baby talk only serves to confuse the child.

2) The child stands too soon. The playpen is a small space to explore and quickly is a bore – the only place to go is up... also the only way out; the baby stands for extended periods on legs barely capable of the weight.

3) The child misses the opportunity to completely develop neural pathways. Now is the time to crawl; to deny it has consequences. Many adults experience emotional as well as physical challenges, and the therapist many times recommends cross-crawl exercises. Getting down and scooting around the floor with the kids or the dog is a **remedial** form of neural development – the optimal way: the opposite arm and leg move forward, as in walking. The length of the stride is proportional to the benefit. Given opportunity, children love to crawl and explore.

Allow the child freedom in a safe environment – child-proof the area and close the door or gate. Provide plenty of creative, colorful options: visuals on walls, mobiles from the ceiling, with creative toys on the floor... or on the lawn. Avoid plastic toys and musical instruments – they look and sound cheap. A wooden recorder is an optimal choice for a young child. Quality instruments have quality sounds – providing an investment lasting for years. Electronic instruments are best avoided since they emasculate the overtones and diminish therapeutic value, which is why many professional musicians are returning to **vinyl** in the 21st century. Nurturing acoustic instruments and sounds include: drums, flutes, gongs, ocarina and strings.

Interact as much as possible reading, singing, playing music, playing games. They love make-believe games, expanding their imaginations as well as Yours. Playing games outdoors with children presents adults with an opportunity to show superiority or, an opportunity to develop ambidextrous skills. This lesson came through my 4-year-old nephew; while he was finding his pitching legs, I began pitching back to him using my left arm. I was surprised how soon I could throw a fairly decent pitch. It was win-win for both of us. The same applies to lawn darts and other games. They can tell when You are pretending to do Your best and flubbing; keep Your integrity. Let them know You are developing Your skills by using Your other hand. You will have planted a seed... and You both will have fun.

Why Say No?
No! cuts creativity, stifles imagination, inspires rebellion, and can create a power conflict that lasts a lifetime! When the child grabs something dangerous, *give* something else... along with a comment or question distracting from the object taken from the other hand. Yes, an ideal scenario... Life often happens otherwise – the child may object. Rather than being negative: No. You could hurt Yourself! Say: That's Your mom's (dad's) and we'll put it up here until she gets home because she knows where it belongs!

If the child gets a knife, simply pick up the child; now, by extension, You are in control of the knife; bring the child to the sink: Please put it in the sink. I can wash it! If the child refuses, rather than grab the knife Yourself which teaches "might makes right" lovingly say: Either You put it in the sink, or else I will take it and put it in the sink *for* You! Either way the knife is in the sink, and You gave a choice. She can do it herself or she can allow You to do it for her. If she complains: I gave You the choice; You could have put it in the sink if You really chose to do that! If she still complains: A sharp knife is for another age group. There are other things You can do to help. Would You like to do this... or would You rather do that? Always give children choices.

Children understand certain things are allowed for certain age groups. They understand age makes a difference. When children race and ask: Who won? Perhaps reply: You won in the ten-year-old category and You won in the six-year-old category! or whatever the case may be... the big ones and the little ones... all–ways can win together. Tempering the fierceness of competition teaches Life can be Win-Win... helps them relate differently... and plants seeds for healthy, wholesome relationships in their lives. Relating this way is a boon for creativity, influencing other aspects and relationships in Your life, as well as theirs.

No! can easily create anxiety and/or poverty consciousness. The child asks for another apple. You look and see none. There are no more apples! merely accentuates the desire and emphasizes the emptiness. We'll get more apples when we go to the store! says there are plenty of apples, and more are on the way. When asked for another apple close to mealtime, there are choices. No, You'll spoil Your appetite! It's too close to supper, You can't have another apple! Rather: Save Your appetite; it's almost time to eat! Let Your tummy digest what's in there; dinner will be ready soon! Or: You can have more apples another time. Now it's almost time for dinner – this is a great time to have a glass of water. Here, I'll join You! We teach by example.

This same principle applies to other occasions. The child asks to go to the park / beach / playground and time factors say otherwise. Rather than: We don't have enough time! which breeds a severe form of poverty consciousness, say: We can do that another day, right now I have this to do. Would You like to help, and spend some time with me? Or would You like to play in Your room? In this way, another choice is given... and the room is experienced as being useful for something other than sleep and time-out. It's a safe, private space to play or read. Subliminally, being told: You can take care of Yourself, builds healthy self-esteem. It's OK to be alone; often, that's when creativity happens.

Avoid electronic devices as long as possible... perhaps teenage! Those devices scramble young brain-waves: 20 minutes of use, takes 2 hours to normalize the brain!

The human skull fully *thickens*
and is fully *wired* neurologically
at age *26*!

Children asking for something expensive, is a perfect opportunity to counter poverty consciousness, and instill prosperity. Rather than: We can't afford that! a wise response is: After I get to the bank and pay the bills, we'll see what's left to play with! A woman raised her family without them realizing how close they were to living in abject poverty by making such comments. Her bank account was with the Bank of Universal Love and Trust. Both her children grew to be quite successful. With a little imagination You can use positive phrases and thinking – Conscious Language – to create Your highest choices... among which is healthy, happy, balanced children.

Finally, why say **no** when the human brain – especially the brain of a child – ignores the word**?** Don't touch that; it's wet paint! The child hears: Touch that and You'll see, it's wet paint! Don't go there! The child hears: Go there! Rather say: Please leave that alone; it's wet paint! Please stay away from there! And always remember to say: **Thank You!**

Awareness Performs Wonders
Children crave our attention – as well as from our proxy: grandparents, aunts, uncles, nanny or baby-sitter – the **optimal designated guardian will avoid "screen-time"** and be thoroughly versed in Verbal Diet and Conscious Relationships. This teaches children that others also treat them with respect – relating as a human being – sharing their own unique gifts and perspectives.

For a young child, the most dangerous rooms are the bathroom and kitchen. While the bathroom door may be closed or hooked, the kitchen is usually more accessible. The kitchen may be gated or simply designated off limits at certain times. During those times, always give a choice: Would You like to draw, or practice learning the recorder? Or we could play outside; let's go barefoot in Our Garden of Eatin'!

Time-out or off limits can be either punishment or choice. If the child does something inappropriate and You impose a time-out, it is perceived as punishment. When the child does something, teach the child it is dangerous or inappropriate while informing: If You do that again, You will have time-out and that means You'll have to say good-bye to Your friend (or stop what You're doing)! If the child repeats the behavior always follow through with the designated consequence. Otherwise, what value do Your words have? The child

learns You are a pushover, setting the stage for a lifetime of struggle. Always follow through with designated consequences.

When the young child repeats the behavior the next day, perhaps the next, *and* the next, this is only a test. The child is exploring boundaries, and wonders if it may be allowed under some circumstances, or on another day. Consistency and patience teach that Your love is always there, and that You are always fair. So, when behavior is repeated, treat it as a fresh day: Remember, that is inappropriate behavior! If You do that again, You will have time-out (or whatever the natural consequence is.) If the behavior continues day after day, it's fair to give a warning when circumstances present themselves. When a friend comes over to play. Make the consequence relate to the action.

Unless blood is drawn or bones are broken, it is usually prudent to let children settle their own differences. Otherwise, they will constantly vie for Your attention. Once the baby goes beyond the stage of the hitting game, the child learns about inappropriate behavior... hitting that leaves a mark is understood as an automatic time-out. If a child comes crying: He pushed me, or: She's being mean to me, respond with a question: Why would You choose to be around someone like that? I'd find something else to do! Allow children to fend for themselves. It relieves You of unnecessary interruptions and builds character for all.

Many power struggles are initiated because the parent or guardian feels the child must eat *now*... or *finish* everything on the plate. This is simply erroneous. If the child turns away from nutritious food, it's OK. If You are alarmed that food may be wasted, eat it Yourself or put it away for later. If the situation goes on for an extended period... then emotional issues could be investigated. Normally, children eat when hungry. Why get involved in a power struggle over how much, when or what kinds of foods to eat? When a nutritious variety is presented, the child does well. More or less eaten one day or another is normal. When the child leaves the table, make it clear: Nibbling is for parties; the next meal will be served at 1 o'clock, when we'll have lunch (or, 6 o'clock when we'll have dinner.) Or: It's OK if You'd rather eat another time. Or: If You feel hungry now, have a big glass of water... dinner will be soon, at 6 o'clock. Here, let me join You. Teach by example.

When parents say: My kids only eat junk foods; it's hard to get them to eat nutritious foods! The answer is simple; children eat what's available. When junk foods are in the house, they eat them. Leave the junk foods in the store. When they complain: I prefer to spend my money on wholesome foods. You get enough junk foods at school and over at Your friends. What I bring into this house is my choice. We do have our occasional parties and feasts... so it all works out! This way, You avoid the tangled web of judging them or their friends for what they eat and enjoy. Instead, You are making a statement... declaring Your choice, Your preference. At the same time, You teach an important lesson: if what You eat every day is nutritious and wholesome, that's what really matters; what You eat on special occasions has little consequence, other than a possible upset tummy, relieved with enzymes.

Special occasions happen once a month, maybe twice, except for the extended Holy-Days at year's end – beginning with Hallowe'en and Thanksgiving until the New Year. Next is Valentine's Day – a full 6 weeks away – then Passover and Easter, Memorial Day, July 4th, Labor Day... with a sprinkling of birthdays and anniversaries in between. Eating differently at special times is a healthy jolt for Your immune response system – as long as Your immune response system is strong – especially when taking extra enzymes. Love Yourself. If Your immune response system is challenged, give special occasions careful thought before celebrating, even with extra enzymes and probiotics. If on these special occasions we think or say: I'm really being naughty, but it tastes SOOO good! we connect naughtiness and fun, resulting in Guilt. Rather than feel naughty, recognize reality. Today, I Am Celebrating Life and having Fun! Life is truly wonderful with wonder-filled choices! As You Voice Your Choice: Abracadabra!

With children of all ages, choice is key. With peer pressure the child may ask to see something on TV – if so, a house meeting can determine the time factor. At such a meeting everyone's viewpoint is honored and respected, and the best interest for all concerned can be determined. This scenario presumes that television – **T**ell-lies-with-**V**ision – is part of Your daily routine. Television programs are exactly that... *programming*... from basic values to food choices... most of which are far less than Your highest choice, and for Mother Earth. Commercials and promos add insult to injury.

Thoughtful books present varied viewpoints: TV makes us spectators of life, rather than participants in Life. The house-meeting – all those who live in the house discussing together and coming to consensus – may determine, for instance, one hour of TV on school nights after homework is done; two hours on weekends, exceptions being made for any unusual program. After the allotted time, the child usually tests the limits to see if they can be stretched. But this is one of my favorite shows! Rather than negative terms: You can't watch any more tonight, but You don't have to go to bed! Be positive: You can watch more TV tomorrow. Or, is this so important You'd like to take ½ hour from tomorrow's time and use it today? Oh, there's something important on tomorrow, too? Well, the choice is Yours. What else can we do?

If the child pouts or cries: It's OK to feel sad or even cry. Please do so in the privacy of Your own room! Saying big girls and boys don't cry is more than nonsense, it is frankly **abuse** – suppressing their feelings and creating guilt, which can get repressed as hidden anger. An acceptable way to vent steam is in the privacy of one's room: to cry, or punch the pillow.

Let *Them* Own *Their* Experiences
With a smile, the child proudly presents a drawing or painting. Thinking to build the child's self-esteem, many say: Oh, I really like that... it's beautiful! Well... with the next drawing, the groundwork has been set for the child to wonder: if this will be as pleasing to You as the last one - anxiety actually can set in early. Now the child is doing something to please the parents, setting the stage for co-dependency. An *empowering response*? That's beautiful. I see You really enjoy drawing. You really have a talent for the use of colors. You're so creative! The same applies to something like piano playing. I really like Your piano playing! nurtures co-dependence. Instead? Your piano playing is wonderful! The love You put into the piano really comes through and fills our house! If the child counters: I make so many mistakes! That's OK... mistakes are part of life. We learn from our mistakes.

Another situation presents itself with grades at school, or awards. How many parents co-opt the child's experience: I'm so proud of You! An appropriate and empowering response? You must be so proud of Yourself! I know I'm proud to be Your mother / father / friend. Life is exciting... how shall we celebrate?!? With awards or grades in school, always praise the *effort* the child makes rather than intelligence. Praising effort encourages more effort, increasing their success in all aspects of Life: Congratulations! You really know how to *apply* Yourself! You get things done on time, and stay ahead of the game... kudos for You!

When children are drawn to things that cause You to gasp! or take a deep breath! use reason – discussing with them, *as You always have in the past*, explaining things. Ballet can end with crippled feet... boxing or soccer, a crippled mind. Why would anyone choose continued abuse only to end later in catastrophe? Refer to history and learn with them. Hopefully the stage for this conversation has been set... letting them know as they grow, certain things are *dangerous* or for another age group... beginning with **EMF**s: using digital gadgets in place of a wooden teething toy, or as mere amusement, is child endangerment and abuse! Hold back as long as You can, especially in the early years; do research and always use some protection. https://www.giawellness.com/23215/products/energy/

The principles of Verbal Diet for Children apply to *all* relationships. Relating to Your children, other children, or other adults in Your Life as responsible persons – creates exactly that. Talking down to people is disempowering. Talking on an equal basis... readily listening to their thoughts, feelings and opinions, and sharing Your own... You avoid judgment and build self-esteem. Imagine how I felt when my four-year old son looked up at me and said: You know what Dad? I'm really a big man. I'm just growing up!

Words used with children and with each other have profound impact. When You choose Your words with care... You tend to breathe deeply, and speak slowly. You say what You mean, and mean what You say. Your words, tone, pitch and volume clearly convey the Vibrations You intend to create. Expressing Your thoughts and feelings through conscious Verbal Diet sets the stage to Live-It... creating Your Wish Fulfilled. You begin to experience Life as One Blessing after anOther. Thus, You teach others they can achieve Satisfaction as well by simply observing Rule #1:
If it's Going to Be... it's Up to Me!

Verbal Diet Sprouts Fresh Consciousness
Conscious Language supports Your feeling body, Your thinking body and Your acting body. As personal and planetary Consciousness expand, "Fear" is transmuted into "the World Vision" where Love and Compassion abound. Consciousness offsets the current fear-based MainstreamMatrixMedia: news and yellow journalism concentrate on the negative and the outrageous. We are "entertained" with violent digital "games" and action movies, serial murder, violence and bigotry. These are depressing enough, yet comedians numb our sensitivities further saying: Life is an endless swirling of despair, with a few bright shining moments of false hope, as we move toward a black hole! Embracing Awareness... many laugh and rejoice, knowing white light is on the other side of the black hole... realizing there all–ways are conscious choices based on Love.

As Scriptures foretold: people are beginning to separate the wheat from the chaff – recognizing there are many wolves in sheep's clothing offering books and seminars at a hefty profit, leading one down the Primrose Path to the collectivist agenda... summarized in UN Agenda 2030... which – in the fine print – seeks an end to private property, and the Bill of Rights! A significant number take the other fork in the road: claiming God-given Independence and Freedom as their birth-right... the cherished foundation stones of the American Republic offer Hope for the world.

The Tenth Insight teaches we are all souls in growth. We all have an original Intention that is positive and we can all remember. Your responsibility is to hold that ideal for everyone You meet. Called the true Interpersonal Ethic, how You uplift... that's the contagion of the New World Awakening encircling the planet. The choice is clear: either *fear* that human culture is falling apart... or *hold* the Vision that the world is awakening. Either way, Your expectation goes out as a *force* that tends to bring about the end *You* envision – in Your *own* Life. We consciously and constantly choose between these two visions and possible futures – either by shallow breathing, or consciously: Breath by Sacred Breath.

Living Your Verbal Diet with conscious *feelings*, create Your own "Force Field" and color Your *own* experience of Reality. You can choose to paint Your Life with shadow and dark color like Rembrandt... brightly colored like Van Gogh... get wild like Picasso... go beyond-beyond like Dali... or paint Your Life with flowery delights like Georgia O'Keeffe. Go For It! One thing *absolutely* certain: Create You *will*, that is part and parcel of the human experience. Pause, reflect, and *consider*: How will I create and color my Life?
Affirming Your Reality

Often – in the past – much of what is spoken affirms and prolongs a negative reality. Rather than speak out of habit, speak consciously. I'm so tired, can be replaced with: I can use some rest. I'm sick and tired of hearing about that, with: Let's talk about something else. Saying: I have a bad kidney, *owns* a malfunctioning kidney… continuing as our thought-form, claiming that as our reality… from that thought-form our subconscious creates! Our kidney is being a *good* kidney – following our direction – by being a *bad* kidney. I have a challenge with my kidney… sends a different message to the subconscious. My kidney is presenting me with an opportunity for healing, tells the conscious mind to look beyond the physical, and search for metaphysical causes. Kidney issues may relate to fear or forgiveness – left kidney of a female figure or feminine issues, right kidney of a male figure or masculine issues.

Saying or even thinking: My husband is so inattentive to my needs! Or: My boss is so nerve-wracking! are forms of communication reinforcing that reality. Rather: My husband gets to learn sensitivity, and really pay attention! I get to breathe deeply around my boss, and thereby keep my focus. I do have control over my life! Positive thoughts bring marvelous results… changing Your experience and Your *feelings* about outer reality.

Saying: Johnny has ADD – especially in the presence of the child – firmly locks that thought-form in everyone's subconscious. Even saying that outside of his presence has an effect because that communication reaches the Grid that surrounds Gaia. The same applies to saying: Mary has such a hard time with math! An entirely different thought-form is projected to the Grid, as well as to the subconscious, with: Johnny has challenges that require extra attention. Mary can use extra help with math! Extra help can come in surprising ways. ADD often means **A**lgae **D**eficient **D**iet. Trace elements and minerals abundant in *uncooked* algae significantly nourish the brain! This includes all varieties of dried and reconstituted *macroalgae* or seaweed aka ocean vegetables… as well as *microalgae* such as aphanizomenon-flos-aquae from Klamath Lake and spirulina, as well as green algae such as chlorella. These dry powders taken orally stimulate saliva production and creates a gummy substance that, spread across the teeth and gums, feeds the mucosal membranes. Every edible form of algae provides abundant sources of complete protein, vitamins, minerals and trace elements with a nutritional profile similar to Mother's milk – supporting synapses, and is rejuvenating for children of all ages!

The Hundredth Monkey and the Information Grid
Science confirms the existence of the Information Grid with the 100th monkey. Studying macaque monkeys on some of Japan's uninhabited islands, sitting offshore monitoring their behavior… the monkeys were eating sweet potatoes and since they were covered with dirt, they would break them in half, eat the insides, and throw away a good portion. One day they noticed a young female brought her sweet potato to a stream to wash off the sand. That was a first! The next day they noticed a few others followed her, doing the same. Did she go to her family that night explaining they dealt with 3 potatoes for her one? Did she explain how efficient it was – as well as tasty – to wash the sand away? Monkey see - monkey do, they said. The next day more monkeys began washing off the sand. When about 100 monkeys were performing this new ritual, they noticed *all* the monkeys – as well as monkeys on a neighboring island – began doing so. Macaques only bathe in water and avoid swimming, so they discounted the notion one of them swam a mile to share the secret.

Scientists heard of this remarkable event and quickly devised studies with rats using a series of different mazes. They timed the rats and found that once several rats learned the route, others of the *same species* found their way much more quickly. Using another series of mazes, scientists worked with others around the globe. Much to their surprise, once several rats learned a maze in one part of the world, rats *worldwide* somehow tapped into this knowledge – finding their way ever so quickly. It was a-maze-ing!

Then a British team devised another scheme: If this works for rats and monkeys, what about homo sapiens? They commissioned a 2'x3' painting that at first glance had roughly a dozen faces; all together there were more than a hundred. One face found on the knot of a man's tie, another on a woman's earring, another in the contours of a woman's hair, some in the background drapes. Scientists took this painting to the streets of England and Australia stopping people.

Excuse me, what do You see here? Faces. How many do You see? In both countries, the response was in the neighborhood of 8-12; the survey went on for several days with the same results. Then on British only CCTV

– as opposed to being beamed around the globe – they spoke of the intricacies of art and used a pointer to show the faces without reference to the monkeys, the rats or their study. The next day they were back on the streets of England and Australia. Now people were seeing multiple faces. How many? Answers varied from 60-80 and up.

Scientists could only agree: there is some kind of Grid around planet Earth. Once information is embedded in the Grid, it can be accessed around the globe.

Knowing this... people are coming together in meditation groups, and empowerment seminars to offset "the Fear" that is so prevalent, and to establish in the Grid "the World Vision" of Compassion and Love. How many people does it take? Eye-opening studies in Transcendental Meditation were done in multiple cities. Crime rates were seriously reduced when the square root of 1% of the population were engaged in meditation.   We can collectively participate in birthing a truly conscious humanity... a New World Awakening is here & now... with Sacred Breath – in this mOMent.

The reality of this Grid was known long before these studies. Ancient Wisdom recognized the Akasha as Knowledge recorded in the ethers. Rudolph Steiner talks a great deal about our etheric body – the body of formative forces – in *Knowledge of the Higher Worlds and its Attainment*. Edgar Cayce and others could access those records. Energy Grids are well-recognized. Power plants are situated where they are so they have less resistance to the flow of electricity. Dowsers have been able to locate underground streams and underground energy lines. Cathedrals of Europe, and other ancient structures, were built on top of an auspicious energy vortex – intersections of several ley lines crossing underneath and overhead. Fascinating studies about nature, science and consciousness, and the Essene perspective of Singularity are readily found: Bruce Lipton, Caroline Myss, Gregg Braden, Lynn McTaggart, and Rupert Sheldrake to name a few.

Standing In Your Wish Fulfilled

Without visions of the future, You re-create the past. Neville Goddard of Barbados, renowned New York lecturer in the 1940s and 50s, spoke of the Energy Grid that surrounds the Planet and wrote brilliant books: *The Power of Awareness*, *Awakened Imagination*, *Your Faith is Your Fortune*, *Seedtime and Harvest* and

The Law and the Promise being among his major works. He often referred to the words of Florence Scovel Shinn: *The Game of Life, and How to Play It*, like Neville, she shows how You create Your *own* Reality... by the way You *think*, the way You *speak*, and the way You *feel*... or vibrate.

In a lecture one day, a woman raised her hand and said: Neville, I know what You teach is true. It has worked in many aspects of my life. For some reason my boss seems impervious to this teaching. Can You help me understand what is going on? Neville questioned her. She used his techniques to create a good paying job within walking distance from her newly created residence and had a comfortable life. So, Neville asked, what is the issue? She worked at an opera house on Broadway designing sets and costumes. Every time she brought drawings to her boss' desk he would start nitpicking. She wrote out her Wish Fulfilled and used it before going to bed for 3 months. Yet his behavior remained steady. Please, what's wrong? Neville probed: Do You stand in Your Wish Fulfilled as soon as You get up? Yes, I do. And then what? I do meditation and have breakfast. And then? I walk to work. And at that, her eyes lit up... suddenly realizing her moment of self-sabotage.

During her fifteen-minute walk to work, she canceled her creative powers by negative thoughts and feelings about her boss. Rather than continue in her Wish Fulfilled, she got caught up in her feeling-thinking body – how her boss may not like this or that aspect of the work she would present that day... or what a nasty personality he has... or frustration at how such an immature person could be in such a responsible position! With that revelation, she continued her Wish Fulfilled morning, evening and on her way *to* and *from* work. She returned a couple of months later and told Neville she was delighted to report that her boss now treats her with respect, and compliments her work. Standing in Your Wish Fulfilled really works!

Real Life... Doing It

It is totally delightful to stand in Your Wish Fulfilled and watch it unfold. Shortly after passing my State Board exam, there was an ad for a chiropractor to join a holistic health center in Liberty City, Miami. My years as deacon and priest in the inner city of Detroit and Wayne County Jail primed me. I could be quite comfortable in the Heart of Miami. Meeting a podiatrist, a dentist and the ophthalmologist-coordinator who was looking for a chiropractor and medical doctor, I felt aligned with a holistic center and so I joined. Several months later, my practice building nicely, he announced: The clinic will be open only on Saturdays from 10-2. Shocked! I have so many clients, many twice a week; what You are asking is absurd. What's going on? He said his wife was suing for divorce, and if the clinic seems like a small-time operation, the judge would give a lesser settlement. So much for dealing with a conscious person whose heart was in service to the indigent!

Making a few calls, I spoke with a macrobiotic woman I had known from my first days in Coconut Grove. She had her irons in many fires... aware of what was happening locally in the field of holistic health care. Saying a certain doctor was leaving his partnership practice to write some books, and since we did similar energy work with Vibrational Energy Medicine {known as Harmonics} she suggested: Call the office; meet the remaining partner. He may be thrilled to have someone walk in – and take over where the other left off! She mentioned another office to contact, and then said: You know what You *really* must do. Sit down and compose Yourself. Then write down where You see Yourself five years from now. Write a paragraph and be specific. Then write down where You see Yourself 3 years from now... one year from now... one month from now... and what You see Yourself doing to create all that, a week from now... and tomorrow! And so, I did. When I came to a week from now: This week I will come in contact with the person who will help me find my niche in the holistic field. For tomorrow: I will call the doctors Kay recommended, trusting my life is Divinely guided and everything *is* in **P**erfect **D**ivine **O**rder. Yes... **PDO**... I Am Ready!

I called the one doctor offering to step in and he sounded intrigued... "it certainly would fill a void", he said... and leaving town for a weeklong seminar, he asked me to "call next week when we could get together and work out the details." Exciting! Can things happen that fast? He sounded warm and receptive, and I was confident, so I spent the week relaxing, reading and meditating at the ocean. When I called him the next Monday, it was an entirely different energy. He was trying to place my name... and remember our conversation. How humbling! Feeling confident he could handle the practice by himself: Thanks for calling! I hung up... how can this be?

Intuition told me to meet him, and shake his hand... looking in his eyes, I could tell if we were meant to work together. I offered to meet at the end of his workday to show him my protocol. He said OK, and we agreed on the time. Arriving, the secretary said he had an emergency patient and would be delayed ten minutes. I took a deep breath. He poked his head out long enough to say: Hi! and shaking hands, I knew I belonged someplace else. I accepted his invitation to go to the adjoining office where he held yoga classes. There was a grand piano, artwork, and a table with books and magazines.

I played the one piece of Gregorian chant I still remember: *Ave Verum Corpus Natum.* Then browsing the table, I picked up the current local holistic magazine. Flipping through the pages, my attention was drawn to an ad that took up a third of a page consisting of a wide white border with a short paragraph set in the middle: We, the family at the Center for Effective Living, are looking for a holistically oriented chiropractor to join our staff. The candidate must be licensed and aware of nutrition. If You are that person, or if You know of such a person, please contact us! Heart leaping with joy... I ran to the front desk and asked to make a quick call. The receptionist answered and said it was the end of a long day, in fact a long weekend... could I call another time? Replying I was in the area, could I have fifteen minutes? She checked, and asked if I could be there in a half-hour. Sure! My heart and mind were elsewhere, so I did an abbreviated session and shook his hand thanking him... he probably wondered for what... and ran out the door. And that's how it happened. During that week, I *did* come in contact with the person who would help me find my niche in the holistic field – at another office!

Everyone at the Center radiated with gleaming eyes and open spirit. One other doctor called preferring part time. Quickly outlining my training and experience, they said to call in a couple of days. I had stopped on a magical day. They concluded a seminar in Body Electronics with Robert Tennyson Stevens of Mastery Systems... working on a young man they had worked with for months, paralyzed from the waist down due to a car accident. His legs moved enough to signal nerves were making connections once again. Everyone was thrilled. That evening there was a double rainbow which they took as a sign from above. My Wish Fulfilled – my New Reality – materialized!

When Your Wish Fulfilled is written, let it ripen a couple of days... then do any necessary editing. When perfect... write it out using Your finest stationery, perhaps parchment, Your finest blue ink pen, and Your finest cursive – whatever that may be – all of which enhances creative energy and flow. This step is *essential* for success. Doing so, there is a holistic connection between Your eyes – extensions of Your brain – the muscles of Your fingers and hands writing the words, and Your subconscious mind. A deep impression is made; every cell vibrates yearning for completion of Your New Reality. Once written, keep it on Your nightstand. Every night before going to bed, begin this creative experience with **Mirror Therapy**. Get close. Look deeply into Your eyes... with Your tongue gently *caressing* the roof of Your mouth, loving Yourself... breathe deeply... exhale completely. Looking deeply, *caressing*, see Your Divine Self within, at play. Visualize Your creative power and Your Happiness manifesting with 3 Sacred Breaths.

Then meditate 10 minutes in whatever posture suits You. Perhaps *savasana* – the receptive pose of yoga – on Your back with arms and legs slightly apart, with a small pillow under Your knees taking pressure off the low back – or sit with spine erect, either on a mat or the edge of a chair. Give full attention to the sounds of Your Breath. Then, read Your Wish Fulfilled aloud – with excitement –as many times as it takes to *feel* Yourself *being* there, so much so You are smiling! Go to bed totally embracing that excitement – see it and *feel* it as a Done Deal! Let a smile once more bless Your Beatific Being as You drift off into sleep regenerating Your HeartMindBodySpirit.

Upon awakening, focus on Your Sacred Breath. Give Thanks for another day of conscious creation. As soon as possible, repeat Your routine as above beginning with Mirror Therapy. Before and after sleep are powerful times to contact and influence the subconscious. Going about Your day... as much as possible... keep Your focus on Your Sacred Breath... *caressing* the roof of Your mouth... loving Yourself. Know You are Pure Awareness, a pure being of radiant energy. This diverts any harshness You may encounter as You move about Your day – perhaps purposely directed toward You to "push Your buttons" seeing if You buy into another pugilistic waste of time and effort – all brought to You by the one and only... magnificent Monkey-mind.

Learn to laugh loudly and ignore those flagrant attempts. Simply smile and move to a safe, quiet space... or, keeping Your focus on Your Sacred Breath, say: That's pure bs and You know it! and then immediately focus on Your Sacred Breath – and Your Wish Fulfilled. If someone persists, simply smile and say: I'm amazed You have such an emotional charge about this! As many times as possible throughout the day, look out the window at trees or the sky; better yet, step out in the garden for a few minutes in bare feet. Remember to be *there* now... *in* Your Wish Fulfilled... *feel* it in Your Heart of Hearts.

Drifting off to sleep... waking for the day... and throughout the day... think and *feel* in Your Heart of Hearts: I choose to be and I choose to express Love and Compassion in every situation, *especially* with myself, and the various characters in my life – yes, including my Monkey-mind, which I have learned to nip in the bud! Simply be aware of Your Sacred Breath and experience the fullness of Your Reality, especially during lovemaking. With focus on Your Sacred Breath, *feel* the Force within You. Be *aware* of Divine Presence within, *powering* Your experience of Reality. We are here with Free Will as it relates to expressions and experiences of the Heart. Enjoy Your Sacred Journey.

OM is Home... so be in the comfort of Your true hOMe. The inner experience is All–Ways there, ready and available for easy access. Know: if it's going to be... it's up to Me! Maintain the *feeling* of being *there* now, *in* Your Wish Fulfilled. Be patient. Some things take longer... sometimes the outcome is much more than anticipated. Whatever it is... it is... in Perfect Divine Order. You are on a Sacred Journey. Smile. The subconscious follows instructions precisely. How it gets done is none of Your business. Concern and worry are forms of self-sabotage that *slow* the work down, maybe even *cancelling* the work order altogether! With Your Wish Fulfilled being *precise* and *complete* – and deeply *experienced* in Your Heart of Hearts – Your subconscious, Your faithful servant, does what it can to Create according to Your wishes.

Sometimes repeated expressions may be *vague*, yet the subconscious still does its best to create accordingly. Those who repeatedly say: It's always something, always something to deal with! will find themselves dealing with issues again and again. Constant repetitive worry certainly creates as well! Remember... **Abracadabra! = I create as I speak!**

How many people in nursing homes say: I always knew it would end like this someday! Why did it? They spent years of worry that their life would happen precisely this way! Constant attention and focused energy about *any* experience... results in its Creation! Only speak words You choose to create, like Rose Mae.

Rose Mae's Story... Creating Her Wish Fulfilled
"Lord, Give Me Strength!"

I Am blessed with parents in a loving, happy relationship caring for me as I transitioned from the Spirit World to this physical reality... and I have been ultimately blessed to have cared for them during their transition back to the Spirit World.

One day Mother asked to visit a friend of her sister in a nursing home; it was shocking for both of us to see Mona bedridden, surrounded by people in wheelchairs in the halls, drooling and nodding. I promised both parents, their experience would be different. Father was tired of all the medical poking and prodding... the perennial tests. In the end, he was ambulatory and he'd even have an occasional Manhattan... often enjoying a menthol cigarette outdoors. His end-of-life mantra was: Dear God, please take me. Dear God, please let me die! He went peacefully in a hospice bed in his living room, in a week.

Comparatively, Rose Mae had only a few encounters with the medical establishment... she did suffer a few times from dehydration... even *C. diff*! Several times while my siblings prepared for her passing, I told her antibiotics would get the "bad guys" – Father was a detective, and she related to that terminology – and I would give her enzymes and probiotics – "friendly bacteria" – to restore her health. She recovered again and again... with zest for Life... looking forward to seeing her 21 great-grandchildren. Rose Mae was lucid and happy... and she went on her own terms.

In addition to raising 6 children, Rose Mae was a seamstress... making her own dress for family occasions. She was also a perfectionist; if the machine somehow missed a stitch, she'd rip out the whole seam and do it over. Although no one would ever notice, she would know of the imperfection and her Mother taught her precision... she was clearly detail oriented. And with that rigor, she firmly held to her Vision for her final days – repeatedly saying she would like to pass in her own bed, or her pink chair.

Rose Mae only ate when truly hungry, usually after 10 am... only had small portions... and chewed her food well – always the last one to leave the table. She celebrated Thanksgiving as she usually did, having two helpings, and came home with leftovers for Friday and Saturday, which she immensely enjoyed. Sunday, she had a normal breakfast – 1 egg fried in bacon drippings, 1 sausage, 1 toast, and decaf with her meds; she had a normal day and went to bed early.

Monday morning, Rose Mae woke with severe pain in her chest and refused to even consider ER, asking for a nurse. Dr Shishu recognized reality and understood, having talked with Mother, and so she ordered a hospice nurse... we thought perhaps for a week, as with Dad.   By the time the nurse arrived, Mother's pain was intense. It took 3X the normal dose of morphine to make a dent in the pain. After the nurse had given instructions – every two hours this, every four hours that – and was about to leave, Mother rang her bell. The nurse went up and called down that the bottom sheet was a bit soiled, asking me to replace it while she tended to Mother. I thought I'd wash her favorite beige marble sheets and pillowcases, and get them back on the bed the next morning for her final days.

Rose Mae, however, had written the script differently! On top of the pile was an old set of pink sheets with lace on the pillowcases and top sheet. She was cold, so I brought her a choice of flannel nightgowns... saying they were too heavy, she asked for a simple long-sleeve nightgown. I grabbed the first I saw – her favorite pink nightgown and she said: Perfect! Later, I gave the meds as instructed and went to bed. I heard her steady breathing as she rested through the night.

Waking at 7 am and hearing sounds of her breathing, I went downstairs to wait for her bell to ring and read the morning *Detroit Free Press*, with the headline: "Today Is Thanksgiving Tuesday!" After Black Friday and Cyber Monday, the Salvation Army thanking the upscale donors for their generosity – offer 50% discount + 10% going to the charity of Your choice! Finishing the paper, I started up the stairs to check... and immediately heard deafening silence. I knew.

Walking in her room, I saw her mouth slightly open and her chest motionless. I felt her forehead – still warm. I went to the foot of her bed, realizing she was up in the corner of the room looking down – as many NDEs claim – and I invoked an Essene Celebration of Life:

Great Spirit... Divine Presence... Creator of All Life Everywhere, Thank You for the Love that flows through Our Hearts... for it is with this Love that We are able to see You in the eyes of every Being before Us and as the Essence of All that Is. Thank You for sending all those Angels Who stand firm in Love, Truth and Beauty, Trust, Harmony and Peace, throughout the Cosmos – those Who work with Us, and are here with Us now. Thank You for opening Our Minds and Our Hearts as We manifest Love upon the Earth. And, Thank You for blessing, cleansing and purifying our feeling bodies, our thinking bodies and our acting bodies... that the Radiant Energy of Eternal Life flow freely through them and through Us. We are grateful to be One with You... Great Spirit... here and now. Now is forever. So Be It. And So It Is!

And that is how Rose Mae created her Wish Fulfilled – through repetition. She passed in her own home... in her own bed... on her pink sheets... in her pink nightgown... on a day celebrating her life of Gratitude – Thanksgiving Tuesday – November 29th also happened to be her own Mother's birthday! Rose Mae was buried on Saturday December 3rd, her husband's birthday. She was lucid and happy to the end. Blessed at 101! To celebrate, as her casket was about to leave the church, we played her favorite song... played at the end of every Lawrence Welk Show:
    "Goodnight, goodnight, until we meet again...
    Adios, Au Revoir, Auf Wiedersehn 'til then...
    And though it's always sweet sorrow to part...
    You know You'll always remain in my heart...
Goodnight, sleep tight, and pleasant dreams to You...
        Here's a wish and a prayer
        that every dream comes true...
        And now, 'til we meet again...
    Adios, Au Revoir, Auf Wiedersehn...
        GOOD NIGHT!"

Rose Mae created her Reality through steady repetition of her Wish Fulfilled. You, too, can create Your Wish Fulfilled – to the last detail!

Use Your Senses – Be Specific!
Once upon a time... someone's Wish Fulfilled was a new car by the end of the year – in fact, a brand-new Mercedes-Benz, 4-door sedan. Sounds reasonably straightforward. Wait and see.

Toward the end of the year, he was getting frustrated. Where is the car? Then, it was time for B-I-N-G-O! And the prize? You guessed it: a brand-new Mercedes-Benz, shiny and bright! It will look lovely on the mantel, or a shelf in the library. Alas, it was a model! Yet, it *was* a brand-new Merc 4-door sedan, *and*... before the end of the year! There is a moral to the story.

Involve all the senses... and *all* their aspects. Why be limited to seeing, hearing, tasting, smelling, touching? Using the example of the Mercedes: *see* Yourself *in* the car... *listening* to Your favorite music... *smelling* that new car fragrance... *feeling* comfortable in the seat... put Yourself in *motion* down Your favorite country road... *feel* the *heat* of the day and the *cool* from the a/c... *feel* the car's *weight* giving You *balance* on the road... *see* and *feel* whatever You can: the *color* and *texture* of the upholstery... the *direction* of Your travel down the road... the *pressure* between Your body and the seat of the car... different aspects of *light* and *dark*, such as shaded windows and a clear moon roof... *feel* what is happening both in Your *internal* and Your *external* environments... Be *in* Your Wish Fulfilled! In this way, You invoke the metaphysical law:
Specificity + Feelings = Creation!

Enhancing Your Right Brain Energies
According to https://www.heartmath.com, signals from the heart to the brain influence our perceptions... emotional processing... and high cognitive functions. The heart is 100,000X stronger electrically, and up to 5000X stronger magnetically than the brain! And so, while Your Egoic brain likes to *Think* it makes things happen... Your Heart and *Feelings* direct Your subconscious in the creation of Your Reality!

Your **Left**-brain energies love to labor over alliterative lists linking Your logical, linear, analytical, mathematical, masculine levels of Life. Your **Right**-brain energies look at this lugubrious litany – laughing... knowing You can playfully alleviate the lullaby of Your left brain by releasing Your radiant, creative forces through romantic images of poetry and color, through baroque recordings – such as the **Red Priest**, and Verdi's operas... coruscating composers, such as Gabrieli, Scarlatti, Monteverdi, and George Frederic Handel... also reptilian and bird recordings... rumblings of a rambling creek, rhythmic, crashing waters at the shore, and the restful rhythm of a waterfall. In addition to radiant colors and sounds, right brain stimulators include roundness and curves... in furniture and surroundings. A modern example is Rudolph Steiner's architecture, gracefully clear in the Swiss city of Dornach, which provides continuing inspiration to creative architects... Waldorf teachers and students... and other students world-wide.

For a different perspective on Life...
rouse Your right brain...
and Create Your New Reality!

Creating Your Reality

Having written Your Wish Fulfilled... You can fine-tune and re-enforce that Reality through Mind-mapping and Treasure-mapping... enhanced by right brain forces such as baroque music and/or nature sounds... stimulating Creative Forces – clarifying and bringing things into tangible focus.

The tools of Mind-mapping consist of poster board or a plain piece of paper, colored pencils, pens or crayons. At the center draw a symbol of the main theme... if things seem nebulous and You are exploring, draw a cloud. To use a basic example, create Your ideal home. Draw a house in the center of the page. From the house draw several lines, each a specific room with its own color: yellow for the kitchen, green for the library, red for the living room, lavender for the bedroom, brown for the yard. Write Your vision for each in flowing lines, stimulating right brain energies. Your subconscious grasps the Vision easily when using **3** words per line... longer thoughts may be written on flowing lines sprouting underneath the previous 3-word line. Subconscious stimulation is also aroused by symbols and abbreviations: hearts and flowers, B4 2C $ # ~.~*! Such elements allow You to easily apprehend the Vision. Stimulating the mind's creative forces, originality flows... awakening Your Heart of Hearts, and... Creation Happens.

The tools of Treasure-mapping consist of poster board, glue, tape, scissors, pictures, graphics and headlines. At the center of Your collage, have a picture or use crayons, colored pencils or paints to convey the theme. Around this focal point, display various aspects of Your New Reality. Find a conspicuous place where You will see it several times a day, and spend a few moments throughout the day *feeling* Your feelings *standing in* Your Wish Fulfilled! That is the Key. And when You are away from this collage, spend as much time as possible looking out a window – perhaps over water or looking in the distance at trees or sky. Stand *in* Your

Wish Fulfilled! *Feel* how gloriously wonderful it is, how joyful to be *there*. Wrap Yourself in those feelings throughout the day. According to Neville, more time spent in Your Wish Fulfilled, means less time spent in Your current, frustrating reality.

The Power of Your Subconscious Mind is a classic by Joseph Murphy, 1963; and a recent classic is found in: *The Aladdin Factor,* by Jack Canfield and Mark Victor Hansen, with these two amazing, true stories. In 1983, the Australian sailing team won the America's Cup for the first time. When the coach of the team was interviewed about the victory, he explained that he had read the book *Jonathan Livingston Seagull* which inspired him to make a cassette of the Australian team beating the American team. He had recorded a narration of the winning race over the sound effects of a sailboat cutting through the water. He then gave a copy of this tape to all the members of the team and asked them to listen to it twice a day, for 3 years – that's 2,190 times! Yes, before they ever set sail in San Diego harbor, they had beaten the American team 2,190 times. The flame of belief had been deeply instilled in each member of the team. They were *feeling* those feelings... *feeling* the excitement... the emotions of winning! And so... their Wish *Was* Fulfilled!

For the four years leading to the Olympics, Peter Vidmar, U.S. Olympic gold medalist in gymnastics, and his training partner would stay in the gym for an additional 15 minutes of practice after everyone else had left. They *imagined* the Olympic gymnastics meet was down to the wire – the last event, they were about to perform, decides the gold medal. They would *visualize* themselves performing a perfect 10... *winning* the medal *standing* on the victory platform *receiving* their gold medals... every day for four years. The flame of belief got stronger every day. Is it any wonder they won the gold?

Go for the Gold! Be Daring! What else is possible? Compose Your Thoughts and Feelings. Write it down. Stand *in* Your Wish Fulfilled. *Feel* the joy!

When You have done everything imaginable to create Your Wish Fulfilled, and it is still elusive... the Universe is saying: for the growth of *all concerned*, another plan is in order – reminding us of C.S. Lewis:

Imagine Yourself as a living house.
God comes to rebuild that house.

At first, You can understand what He is doing.
He is getting the drains right,
and stopping the leaks on the roof and so on.
You knew that these jobs needed doing,
and so, You are not surprised.
But presently He starts knocking the house about
in such a way that it hurts abominably
and does not seem to make sense.
What on earth is He up to?
The explanation is: He is building
quite a different house
from the one You thought of:
throwing out a new wing here,
putting on an extra floor there,
running up towers, making courtyards.
You thought You were going to be
made into a decent little cottage:
but He is building a palace.
He intends to come and live in it Himself!

Such is the magnificence of Great Spirit within...
Imagine and *Feel* it in Your Heart of Hearts... *Be* **there** n**O**w! George Bernard Shaw says:
Life isn't about *finding* Yourself.
Life is about *creating* Yourself!

Imagine it... Write it out... then **Voice** Your **Choice**!
As You speak... and as You **feel**...

ABRACADABRA – Your Wish *IS* Fulfilled!

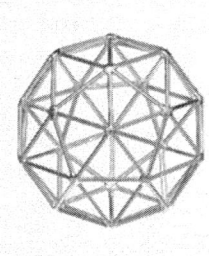

2 – FOUNDATIONAL ELEMENTS OF VIBRATIONAL ENERGY MEDICINE

Vibrations were vaguely understood until the mid-1800s. In 1869 arranging his periodic table of elements, Dmitri Ivanovich Mendeléev, a Russian chemist, predicted the discovery of a missing element... with the atomic number 32 and atomic weight 70... to fill the gap between the elements of *silicon* and *tin* in his periodic table. He named the missing element eka-silicon. Then in 1886, German chemist Clemens A Winkler discovered the missing element in a sample from a silver mine, known as argyrodite, contained 6-7% – a significant amount – of an *unknown* element. This new element belonged to the eka-silicon category which he called germanium from the Latin *Germania* – some say means *siblings*, from the same parents – also named after the country where Winkler was born, and discovered the missing element – only 1.6 ppm germanium available in the Earth's crust.

As for the uses of this element... as with most discoveries, they happen on different parts of the planet, relatively close together in time. Marconi, Stubbleman, and Tesla... all discovered a piezo-electric crystal of germanium possessed the unique ability to receive the vibrations of radio frequencies – electromagnetic waves – the "wireless" suddenly became popular everywhere.

Crystal radios operate without electricity, batteries, or solar... free energy! The power source is the crystal of germanium and a spool of copper wire. Without volume control, the earplug is sufficient. Moving up / down the spool of copper wire, distant radio stations are heard.

Crystals are pervasive; every electric motor has a crystal chip. The computer communication revolution creating Silicon Valley is based on silicon dioxide – quartz crystal – as is laser surgery and fiber optics. Crystals can be programmed with specific vibrational frequencies, and can transmit this information. Colors and sounds also transmit vibrational frequencies – like crystals, bringing balance and harmony – influencing our immune response and endocrine energy systems.

Vibrational Energy Medicine works through the principle of sympathetic vibration. Strike the A key on the middle octave of a piano and, in a small enough room, the A string on a violin will begin to resonate. Recognizing its vibration, it leaps for joy... much like when we hear a special song, we may hum along, tap our foot, or jump up and dance!

Vibrational Energy Medicine also works through amplitude resonance – the vibration of a body, secondary to a force of a particular magnitude. Simply explained: observe the lines of force within a magnetic field. By placing a bar magnet beneath a sheet of paper and then sprinkling fine metal filings on top of the paper, the filings assume elliptical and symmetrical lines on both sides of the magnet between north and south poles. Strike the paper with a specific force, the filings become asymmetrical; they would cease to be in the neat elliptical lines because of the intrusion of an extraneous force – in a word, *stress*. Strike the paper again harder, even more stress, there would be further disruption to the neat pattern originally observed. To return the filings once again to their exact original state of homeostasis – *gently* tap the paper. This light tapping is a visible example of what is meant by amplitude resonance. Subtle energetics!

Vibrational Energy Medicine – like the gentle tapping – normalizes the Great Motherboard of the brain, the hypothalamus, directing the endocrine glands to produce optimal hormone levels restoring Order and Harmony. Balance is achieved physically, emotionally, mentally and spiritually blending HeartMindBodySpirit as One. Discovering Infinite Being within... we find Harmony at the center of our being. Peace with the Creator of All. Peace with All Life Everywhere.

All things exist in Perfect Divine Order. While things may appear imperfect, they are actually... perfectly imperfect. For example, while most of us are born healthy on the physical, emotional, mental and spiritual levels... most of us have "all our fingers and toes" and a small % are born with physical and/or mental challenges. These situations are part of Life's Opportunities for that individual, as well as for family and friends – a special opportunity to express compassion, patience and, ultimately... Love.

We learn our own lessons in life; some lessons we are learning together. As we grow and assume responsibility for our lives, we are exposed to traumas, toxins, negative thoughts and tension, or stress. Depending on strengths / weaknesses of our genetic inheritance, the epi-genetics of our thoughts and feelings nourish our spirit and our acting body... *we* create our environment, and various states of health.

Disease or injury indicates imbalance at the physical level... metaphysically reflecting imbalance at the emotional, mental and spiritual levels – the latter affected by *feelings* of *separation* from the One. As holographic beings... each One is here to experience hOw we fit together as a whOle... and hOw we heal as a whOle: feeling body, thinking body, acting body, social body... as One. Disease is a Soul Lesson. Your expression of Spirit promotes the process as progress for Your maturity... feeling One once again, learning the Main Lesson of Life: I AM that I AM. The Power

sustaining the Universe is the Power that sustains You. Powerful words shook Moses and Earth to the core: I AM that I AM – **You Are that I AM** – in the flesh!

It took thousands of years of evolutionary process for humankind to begin to understand the true meaning of "I AM that I AM." Thomas Berry, monk and cultural historian, claims: the matriarchal period of Old Europe extended from 6500 BCE to the Aryan invasions around 3500 BCE. We have been in a patriarchal period for 5000 years. Now post-patriarchy is being birthed with ecological and ecofeminist influences. Eventually: balancing matriarchy and patriarchy!

"One of the main characteristics of the emerging ecological, ecofeminist period is the move from a human-centered norm of reality and value, to a nature-centered norm. We cannot expect life, the earth, or the universe to fit into our rational human designs of how life, the earth, or the universe should function. We must fit our thinking and actions within the larger process, moving from democracy to biocracy. We require a constitution for the whole continent... not simply a constitution for the humans occupying this continent... a United Species, rather than a United Nations.

"We came into being within the life community through the billions of years that it took to shape a world into which humans could be born. It has been a creative maternal process throughout... with all the violence of the primordial fireball, the supernova explosions, and the volcanic eruptions from within the earth herself. Terrifying as these transitional moments may have been, they have consistently been birth moments. What we are now experiencing is another birth moment, the labor being that the patriarchal period is too poignant in its past memories as well as its present realities for us to fully understand what is happening, or what will emerge in the years to come. Much of what we are doing appears irreversible. What we can say is: Mother Earth seems to be rising in defense of herself and her children after this long period of patriarchal dominion." (*The Dream of the Earth*, Thomas Berry)

Planetary Consciousness ebbs & flows in Grand Cycles. With Patriarchal consciousness, there is a sense of history, linear time, and dogma based on rationality; the focus is on waking reality and science. With Matriarchal consciousness, there is a sense of eternity, cycles of time, and ritual based on magic; the focus is on altered states of consciousness and the arts. While the Planet may be in one phase of consciousness, we can align... or disengage. We have Free Will. To be fully cognizant of the birthing process Earth is involved in... we look at all aspects of Life in their simplest terms, to discern what our choices are, what is our highest choice, and the highest choice for all concerned. We begin to understand Who we Are and... Our relationship with All Life Everywhere.

Whether You believe You are a physical being who strives for, and sometimes has *psyche-delic* {*soul-revealing*} spiritual experiences... or whether You believe You are a spiritual being having a spiritual experience in a physical body... or whatever *else* You may believe... we all must come to terms with our physical body – which is the densest of our levels: HeartMindBodySpirit. Then we begin to understand the relationships with our emotional, mental, etheric, astral, causal and spiritual bodies. Through these relationships, we begin to appreciate the Sacredness of Life... and learn what Life is all about.

Whatever one's philosophy or spirituality... we recognize and honor the physical body. We take excellent care of our cars and other things, now it is time to indulge in some **TLC** for ourselves – **T**herapeutic **L**ifestyle **C**hanges.

Body Dynamics

In the past**...** we have thought of the human body in static terms. Truth is quite another matter. When asked the temperature of the human body, most will say 98.6°F or 37°C. Actually, that is the *average* temperature under the tongue in the morning; in the evening, the average is one degree higher. Under the armpit, the average is 97.6°; rectally, 99.6°; the stomach likes to be 101° to secrete digestive juices; the intestines 105° for assimilation.

Showing the Creator has a sense of humor... the testicles prefer 95° to produce sperm. {The Creator could have tucked them inside, like the ovaries, and have them produce sperm at a warmer temperature!} So, on a cold day, the scrotal muscles contract drawing the testicles to the warmth of the body; on a hot day, the scrotal muscles relax allowing the testicles to be away from the heat of the body. The reason: maintain 95° to produce sperm for the continuation of the species. This is a graphic example of the fantastic dynamics of the human body.

The Seven Major Endocrine Energy Centers

As we have different *temperatures* for different purposes, so... different energy *vibrations* for different purposes. Ancient Wisdom speaks of seven major energy centers in the body. Some were clairvoyant and spoke Sanskrit, naming them *chakras* meaning *spinning wheels*, which they perceived at each center – each, one of the seven colors of the rainbow – corresponding to seven endocrine glands: gonads, adrenals, pancreas, thymus and heart, thyroid, pineal, pituitary. Each gland is surrounded by a nerve bundle and a vascular network, together creating a vortex of energy directed by the hypothalamus with a feed-back loop from the Heart as chief choreographer. These glands, nerves and vessels keep us in balance until times of trauma, toxins, negative thoughts or stress. Traditionally, these seven hormonal energy centers were harmonized or recalibrated using the seven colors of the rainbow: red, orange, yellow, green, blue, indigo & violet. The Ancients saw a further correspondence to the seven tones of the musical scale: C D E F G A and B.

Energies of color, sound, fragrances, vibrational energies of words we use, as well as our visualizations, blend to recalibrate the spin of each vortex – restoring harmony to our endocrine glands and the nerve bundles and vessels that support them – promoting hormones of happiness and health... bestowing balance, strength and vitality.

Besides the seven endocrine glands, the human body contains other focal points of concentrated energy, such as the palms of our hands and the soles of our feet. In addition, every joint – fingers, toes, wrists, elbows, shoulders, ankles, knees, and hips – as well as the areas between the vertebrae, between the sternum and ribs are minor energy centers – with a metaphysical message.

From a holistic point of view – where all things are perceived in relationship – each center is recognized as a focal point of Life Force relating to physical, emotional, mental and spiritual energies. These centers of force located within our etheric body receive, transmit, and process Life Energy known as chi, ki, prana, animation of soul or spirit, and they create a network where Heart and mind and body and spirit are experienced as One... HeartMindBodySpirit. The Heart is the coordinator, and each one corresponds to aspects of consciousness and unconsciousness.

Working with and understanding our energy centers creates integration of the various aspects of our being, and facilitates our experience of Life as a whole being. In this way we transmute the various aspects of unconsciousness into consciousness... integrating all levels of our being – physical, emotional, sexual, mental, social, etheric, astral, and spiritual. Facilitating the process of our unfoldment, these centers are doorways for our consciousness through which emotional, mental, and spiritual forces flow into physical expression. They are openings through which our attitudes and belief systems enter, and create our mind-body structure. Energy created from our mental attitudes, feelings and emotions run through these centers, reaching our cells, tissues and organs. Knowing this brings insight into how we ourselves – thoughts, and especially feelings – deeply affect our bodies... our minds... and our circumstances. Understanding the relationship of the energy centers to our consciousness, we clearly understand Who We Are... enabling us to choose with Awareness.

Metaphysics

When Aristotle catalogued the works of his beloved mentor, Plato – who himself was a student of Socrates – he undertook a monumental task. In addition to the sheer volume of material, Plato was operating from a right-brain perspective: he thought in terms of ideas that exist apart from reality and <u>form</u> – reality as we perceive it – being a *shadow* of the world of <u>ideas</u>. Plato used inductive reasoning and a priori principles, based on intuition and insight... putting us in touch with the world of soul and spirit. Plato heavily influenced the early church thinkers and scholars, especially Augustine – and the roots of mystical Christianity.

Aristotle, on the other hand, was operating from a logical, left-brain perspective; he thought in terms of substance and form, cataloging and ordering everything according to their logical pieces. Aristotle operated with deductive reasoning, based on the syllogism: a major, a minor, and a conclusion. Aristotle influenced scholastic philosophers and theologians, especially Thomas Aquinas – and the roots of the legal and regulatory aspects of Christianity.

Looking at the works of Plato... Aristotle began with the physical world. Physics is the science of matter and energy, and the interactions between the two – grouped in fields of optics, acoustics, mechanics, thermodynamics and electromagnetism; in modern times we include atomic, nuclear, and quantum physics, cryogenics, solid-state physics, particle physics and plasma physics. Who knows what else is to come? After all, we are Infinite Being, Infinite Mind exploring infinity.

After cataloguing Plato's Physics, Aristotle began to look at other aspects of Plato's work – things to do with the nature of **first principles** and the problems of **ultimate reality**. These systematic investigations had to do with the study of the nature of being (ontology), the study of the nature of truth (epistemology), the study of the structure of the universe (cosmology), as well as the study of the nature of the soul (philosophical psychology).

When Aristotle set these works on his bookshelf, so to speak, he wondered how to categorize them. Rather than call them non-physics, as though they were somewhat less than real – he thought it appropriate to simply say these works are "other than" physics or "after" physics, perhaps "next to" physics on his bookshelf. The Greek word *meta* succinctly says all of that, so he simply called these works Metaphysics.

Commonly used today, metaphysics is based on speculative or abstract reasoning, involving imagery and symbolism touching on the supernatural. With this in mind, remembering the classic search for *the nature of first principles*, and *the problems of ultimate reality* – we explore the physical *and* metaphysical aspects of the major energy centers.

Understanding and Energizing the Seven Major Energy Centers

The Root or Basic Endocrine Energy Center is located at the perineum – between the genitals and the anus – where the Central and Governing Vessels of the acupuncture chi system both originate. According to Vedic tradition, Kundalini {coiled energy} rises from the perineum and goes through the sacrum... up the spine... to the brain... bringing enlightenment. The root energy center vitalizes the physical body reflecting our level of life force... nurturing instincts of survival and self-preservation. The primary body part is the pelvis as well as the legs and feet – extensions of the pelvis, which is the true foundation of the body reflecting both our grounding and our security.

Metaphysically, symbolically, pelvic imbalance indicates imbalance at other foundational areas of Life

– usually relating to our parents, or others in our house, our spouse or lover (present or former), our job; whatever gives us a feeling of security in our lives... or feelings that threaten our security. The operative word here is *feelings*... true security comes from within. Our parents, our house, our spouse, our job, only give temporary, transient security. Imbalance is noted with those who habitually stand on one leg, shift their weight from one foot to the other, or experience low back pain or pain running down the leg. This can indicate a strain of the sacroiliac ligament, which can be brought back to a point of balance through physical support and metaphysical awareness.

Imbalance on the right side (controlled by the left brain) indicates challenges with masculine energies – father, grandfather, influential uncle or teacher, brother, husband / lover, boss, or all of the above. Perhaps none of the above... it may indicate getting in tune with masculine issues: standing on Your own two feet, taking charge of Your life, providing for self and others.

Imbalance on the left side (controlled by the right brain) indicates challenges with feminine energies – mother, grandmother, influential aunt or teacher, sister, wife / lover, boss, or all of the above. Perhaps none of the above... it may indicate getting in tune with feminine issues: enhancing Your creativity, compassion, intuition, sensitivity... developing nurturing qualities.

Lessons of the Root Energy Center relate to success in the material world. This entails mastery of the physical body with particular emphasis on grounding and stability leading to feelings of safety and security. At this level we express stillness... recognizing we are One with All... One with the Source of All. There is only Infinite Being. Learning this lesson, we are patient with ourselves and we stand up for ourselves, taking courage to accomplish our goals, as we take care of the necessities of daily life. Experiencing contentment and peace within ourselves, we are compassionate with others, encouraging them to attain their highest choices. With an Attitude toward Life free from judgment and coercion... we experience Health and Wholeness, Balance and Harmony.

Challenges of the Root Energy Center are tendencies toward insecurity, self-centeredness and greed, or toward anger and violence. This begins with **FEAR** which truly is **F**alse **E**vidence **A**ppearing **R**eal, leading many to **F**orget **E**verything **A**nd **R**un... while also leading others to **F**ilch **E**verything **A**s **R**eserves, rather than **F**ace **E**verything **A**nd **R**ise! Fear may express itself as concern with physical survival and well-being... rigidity in the spine, tension in the back muscles and constipation – the latter being a fear of letting go... fear of there being enough to replenish supplies. This can show up as low back pain, sciatica, varicose veins, colorectal tumors, immune challenges. The element of the root energy center is the earth, so working in the garden or working with the soil enhances our ability to sink our own roots into Mother Earth, feeling contentment and security. Foods that enhance these root energies include: red fruits... cherries, goji, strawberries, other red-skinned fruits... apples and lychees, as well as red vegetables... beets and purple cabbage... rich in minerals and trace elements, macroalgae in seaweed, also called ocean vegetables; microalgae from Klamath Lake are superior being wild grown... also, spirulina and chlorella are nutrient-rich foods with Mother Nature's own formula... all of which have a nutritional profile much like Mother's milk and, therefore, support our grounding.

Traditionally, the primary color is red, secondary is black; the tone is C; stones to enhance these energies include ruby, red jasper, bloodstone; onyx, obsidian, black tourmaline. The endocrine, hormone-producing glands are the gonads: ovaries or testes; associated influences: spine, colon, legs, bones (blood production), feet, and the immune response system.

The Emotional Endocrine Energy Center is located between the navel and pubic bone, where we assimilate and eliminate on the physical level and – metaphysically – on the emotional level. It is common to see someone walking around holding this area at the scene of a tragedy, serving the dual purpose of exerting a calming influence to prevent nausea and vomiting, and holding the person together emotionally. The focus of this energy center is balance between stress and calm – reflected in the quality of the fluids of procreation. As we assimilate our food, we increase our physical force, our vitality... and express our sexuality to continue the species and for the continued expression of Divine Love. Imbalance at this level indicates challenges in the emotional arena.

Lessons of the Emotional Energy Center relate to giving and receiving... especially working creatively and harmoniously, both personally and professionally. Emotional love is experienced at this level with the

42

elements of desire, pleasure and sexuality. Lessons here require openness to change, assimilation of new ideas, tolerance and surrender enhance the lessons.

Challenges of the Emotional Energy Center are tendencies toward over-indulgence in food, drink and sex, which can lead to a sense of confusion about the purpose of Life, showing up as a more intense desire to possess others... with the associated negative emotions of envy and jealousy. As this only serves to intensify the confusion, challenges often appear regarding the sexual organs: frigidity, impotence or urinary tract infection. Issues revolve around blame and guilt, money and sex; either, relates to power and control – power over? or power with? This shows up as low back pain, sciatica, and pelvic challenges.

The element of the emotional energy center is water, so working with water enhances our ability to feel our feelings, restoring emotional balance. Sounds of a fish tank, a waterfall or the ocean serve to calm our emotions and bring peace. Foods that enhance these energies include: fresh fruit and/or vegetable juices, reconstituted dried fruit along with the soak juice, and persimmons. Macroalgae found in ocean vegetables or seaweed, and microalgae from Klamath Lake are superior being wild grown; spirulina and chlorella, also rich in nucleic acids similar to Mother's milk, nurture neuropeptides, emotional balance and well-being.

Traditionally, the color is orange; the tone is D; stones to enhance these energies include carnelian, peach aventurine, coral and amber. The endocrine, hormone-producing glands are the adrenals; resting on top of the kidneys, our water filtering stations, the adrenals register stress or calm as our emotions fluctuate. Excess salt, especially salt with aluminum and/or sugar, upsets the adrenals; associated influences: lumbo-pelvic area; testicles, tubes and prostate; ovaries, tubes and uterus; kidneys and bladder; the blood and circulatory system.

The Solar Plexus Endocrine Energy Center is located between the navel and the rib cage where the organs digest and assimilate food – liver, gall bladder, pancreas, stomach and spleen work together to facilitate vital support for the physical body. Imbalance in this area indicates challenges with the harmonious use of power.

Lessons of the Solar Plexus Energy Center relate to power and energy, expressing through mastery of desire and self-control. Here we find awakening of immortality transforming itself in humor and laughter, resulting in a feeling of radiance and bliss... expressing peace on the physical level. Self-esteem, self-confidence and self-respect are seen in the care we show ourselves and others – especially with issues of intimacy and trust.

Challenges of the Solar Plexus Energy Center are tendencies to place excess emphasis on power and recognition. Often this is more than one can reasonably assimilate so there can be a mixture of anger, fear and hate that leads to digestive challenges... caused by challenges digesting seemingly incompatible segments of reality; specific messages relate to their functions.

The element of the solar plexus energy center is fire, so working around these energies is conducive to balance... with the exception of the pyromaniac-fireman type. Working in a foundry, as a mechanic or jeweler provides a connection. Foods that enhance these energies include: starches, especially millet, as well as protein in quinoa and amaranth; yellow fruits – such as grapefruit, lemon, yellow melons, yellow apples, bananas, passionfruit, and guava. Ancient Wisdom says greens are beneficial to the liver / gall bladder complex, because of their high chlorophyll content; macroalgae found in ocean vegetables or seaweed... and microalgae from Klamath Lake are superior for wild grown chlorophyll, as well as commercially-grown spirulina and chlorella.

Traditionally, the color is yellow; the tone is E; stones to enhance these energies include citrine, gold topaz, and tiger eye; the metal is gold. The endocrine, hormone-producing gland is the pancreas. When we experience sweetness in our lives, our pancreas is balanced and calm, our body is free from cravings. Things that stress the pancreas are caffeine, refined foods, sweets and sodas; associated influences: the entire digestive, nervous and muscular systems.

The Heart Endocrine Energy Center is located within the rib cage, where we experience personal, perhaps sexual, love as well as universal, pure love for All Beings, beginning with Self. There are two endocrine glands: the thymus gland produces T-cells, indicating our immune strength based on love of Self. The second endocrine gland is the heart itself. Electron microscopy discovered the hormone Atrial Naturetic Factor, made by the atria of the heart, facilitating heart communication with the brain, the hypothalamus and the pineal... mediating our emotional state, regulating our sleep cycle, aging process and our energy level. Imbalance in the Heart Center indicates a challenge with proper love of Self. {Ancient Wisdom traditionally knew of two heart centers in the Heart Energy Center. This is the only center with two separate endocrine glands – and we only discovered that recently – this is reminiscent of the Dogons who knew there was Sirius A as well as Sirius B, thousands of years before we did – another mystery of Ancient Wisdom.}

Lessons of the Heart Center relate to Pure Divine Love given freely and spontaneously... experiencing Oneness with Life. Recognizing our human condition, we are moved toward compassion and understanding. This openness and acceptance for self and others create feelings of contentment, harmony and balance.

Challenges of the Heart Center are tendencies toward fearful repression of love, due to issues of low self-esteem, bitterness, resentment, inordinate grief or loneliness... indicating self-centeredness. Emotional instability may result in heart, circulatory, breathing, upper back and shoulder challenges, or breast cancer.

The element of the heart center is air; working outside – surrounding ourselves with the green energy of the trees – opens our hearts to the Love that is all around us. Foods that enhance these energies include: green fruits and vegetables: the darker the leafy green, the more minerals – raw or dehydrated kale reigns supreme having all essential amino acids plus 9 others. Wild-grown macroalgae, ocean seaweed, and microalgae from Klamath Lake as well as spirulina and chlorella offer enzymes and chelated minerals, vitamins, all essential fatty acids, all essential amino acids – the complete spectrum of nutrition – in a ratio found in Mother's milk; edible algae are excellent wild-grown foods for the heart.

Traditionally, the primary color is green, secondary is pink; the tone is F; stones to enhance these energies include emerald, malachite, green aventurine, green jade, green and pink tourmaline, rose (pink) quartz. The endocrine, hormone-producing glands are the thymus and heart {Source: Endocrine cardiomyocytes, *Journal of Submicroscopic Cytology*, 19(4), 683-694, 1987}; associated influences: circulatory, lungs, ribs, diaphragm, shoulders, arms and hands.

The Throat Endocrine Energy Center located in the neck, shows flexibility and our ability to see both sides of an issue; this is Communication Central. An imbalance in this area indicates a challenge with openness and acceptance for others and their ideas.

Lessons of the Throat Energy Center relate to clear and concise communication. Understanding the true power of the spoken word, we are led to creative expressions in our speech, our writing, even in the arts. We use our personal power to create our dreams... with Love, Truth and Beauty, Trust, Harmony and Peace... Knowledge leading to Wisdom, Honesty leading to Loyalty, Kindness leading to Gentleness – all of these foster Strength, Tranquility, Responsibility and resonate with a clear voice.

Challenges of the Throat Energy Center are tendencies toward secretiveness, and knowledge used unwisely... ignorance and lack of discernment often being excuses; less than truthful communication in speech and writing may result. This can lead to depression and/or thyroid hormone irregularities. Challenges affect mouth, throat and neck.

The element of the throat energy center is ether... in Vedic tradition called the akasha, the unwritten record of all. Working in a spiritual capacity fosters honest and open communication. Foods that enhance these energies include: blue fruits such as all blue berries, especially concord grapes, plums, and blue corn; macroalgae found in ocean vegetables or seaweed... and microalgae from Klamath Lake are superior being wild grown; also, spirulina and chlorella.

Traditionally, the color is blue; the tone is G; stones to enhance these energies: Queen Anne's blue lace agate, turquoise, sodalite, lapis lazuli. The endocrine, hormone-producing glands are parathyroid & thyroid; associated influences: hypothalamus, throat, mouth, teeth, gums, salivary glands, neck and esophagus.

The Third Eye Endocrine Energy Center is at the center of the forehead, above the eyebrows. Focus there in meditation, and the pineal gland is activated. We can experience the Light of Love. Scientists scratch their heads wondering why, in the *center* of our head, the pineal gland is composed of light-sensitive, corneal tissue… complete with rods and cones! Interestingly enough, scriptures from different cultures *all* say in common: God is Light… God is in the Kingdom of Heaven… the Kingdom of Heaven is *within* You!… therefore, that Light *is* within You! The Book of Matthew says, "The lamp of the body is the eye. It follows that if Your eye is single, Your whole body will be filled with light!" with the standard commentary: keep Your vision focused; go about Your business.

Catherine of Siena, John of the Cross, Teresa of Avila, and other mystics throughout the ages of **all** religions, actually *experienced* the "single eye" – the Light within – through meditation! With their Third Eye opened, they all witnessed and experienced the Divine Presence within… All That Is. That experience is open to everyone. Free from expectations… humbly sit in quiet meditation; focus on Your inner vision while caressing the roof of the mouth with the tongue. Witness the Kingdom of Heaven… which *is* within You! {Ch 10: **Tongue Awareness**}

Lessons of the Third Eye Energy Center relate to our intuitive nature. Honoring innate instincts and insights stimulates our imagination and facilitates creation of our highest choices. Meditation enhances our Third Eye energies; we develop concentration, clairvoyance, peace of mind… and Wisdom, of which Hermann Hesse speaks in *Siddhartha*: "Wisdom is a capacity of thinking, feeling and breathing thoughts of Unity at every moment of Life." The lessons at this level bring us beyond dichotomy and duality, which can only lead to comparison, judgment and condemnation. We begin to appreciate Singularity and the relationship of all things to one another – the One and the Many, actually are the same manifestation.

Challenges of the Third Eye Energy Center are tendencies toward fear, leading to unconsciousness and cynicism that blurs concentration. This can be seen as habitual practical jokes and apathetic remarks that tend to scatter energies; also tension headaches, vision, hearing and neurological challenges.

The element of this energy center is light, so working outdoors is nurturing; indoors use full spectrum, incandescent lighting. Fluorescent lights turn on and off hundreds of times a second and tend to scatter our energies as well as our focus; many get headaches from exposure to them. Foods that enhance this energy center include: purple fruits and vegetables, the macroalgae from the ocean and the microalgae from Klamath Lake, as well as spirulina and chlorella, and all foods rich in chlorophyll. Leafy greens and sprouts capture the sun's Light energy.

Eating these foods in their raw, enzyme-rich state… we feed our Light Body, raising emotional integrity. These living energies facilitate the experience of and expression of… Divine Love.

Traditionally, the color is indigo; the tone is A; stones to enhance these energies include indigo, blue sapphire, sodalite, lapis lazuli. The endocrine, hormone-producing gland is the pineal; associated influences: the neurological system, especially the cerebellum, eyes, ears and nose.

The Crown Endocrine Energy Center is located at the top of the head. The Vedas – ancient scriptures forming the basis of Hinduism – describe it as a thousand-petaled lotus flower dripping with Nectar. Raja Yoga teaches techniques of meditation that turn our senses inward: *see* Celestial Light, *hear* Harmony, *taste* Nectar, *feel* the Sacred Vibration that supports All Life Everywhere. With the tip of the tongue at the roof of the mouth, we complete the microcosmic circuit between the central and governing vessels; caressing, Nectar flows from the thousand-petaled lotus flower at the crown energy center and the facial sinuses.

Lessons of the Crown Energy Center relate to process, trusting in Life… feeling safe… knowing and experiencing Awareness… seeing Self as One with All. Accomplishing this we unite High Self, Middle Self and Low Self. Our perceptions go beyond space-time. Continuity of consciousness goes from microcosm to macrocosm… repeating itself again and again, from one level to the next. Lessons in altruism lead to loving Service based on Spirituality, Wisdom, Understanding, Love… and Compassion.

Challenges of the Crown Energy Center are tendencies toward confining one's energies to the Low and Middle Self, focusing on the material world… and the emotional drama that surrounds it. Issues of fear and self-esteem can result in feelings of alienation and confusion regarding the purpose of Life, depression based on resentment, and perhaps feelings of complete helplessness / hopelessness.

The element of the crown energy center is the power of thought based on free will; choices bring consequences. A cerebral occupation enhances this energy center. The more we know, the more we know there is to know. Thomas Merton says: "There is in all visible things...a hidden wholeness." Einstein and other scientists intensely realize the Divine Presence in All. Foods that enhance spiritual energies include: flowers and leaves of plants, especially violets: delicious and energizing; also, macroalgae in ocean vegetables or seaweed, the wild grown microalgae from Klamath Lake and spirulina and chlorella all support neurological and spiritual energies.

Traditionally, the color is violet; the tone is B; stones to enhance these energies include amethyst of a light violet to lavender shade, quartz and luvulite; purple fluorite opens receptivity to energies of other stones. The endocrine, hormone-producing gland is the pituitary; associated influences: cerebrum, central nervous system, muscles and skin.

The Auric Endocrine Energy Center is primarily located a hand's length from the top of the head, all around the body and below the feet. Other auric fields go beyond: a secondary auric field is 4-12' from the body, depending on one's consciousness; a tertiary auric field, verified by NASA, is 55' from the Heart Center of every individual. The primary Auric Energy Center is referred to as the eighth energy center. {Egyptian sacred geometry has thirteen energy centers: the distance between them being the distance from the tip of the nose to the tip of the chin – actually, the same distance between the pupils! That adds up between the crown and root centers.} Actually, the auric energy center engages the whole body. In meditation visualize toroidal energy coming through the perineum *and* the crown of the head – flowing out the heart center. This Spherical Breathing enhances Christ Consciousness, which is Unity Consciousness leading to the Awareness and Pure Universal Love for everyOne and for All Life Everywhere.

Lessons of the Auric Energy Center relate to Unity Consciousness and our relationship with All Life Everywhere. Denying this Consciousness, the aura is tight and dark; accepting and living by it to the best of our ability, the aura is expansive and bright... as our ego begins to feel and express Love and Compassion.

Challenges of the Auric Energy Center are tendencies toward acute, sometimes chronic, I-itis – inflammation of the Ego, looking out for **#1**. Some prefer to think of this life as an accidental collision of gases – even so, where did the *gases* come from**?** They think we are caught on planet earth, in an ever-expanding universe on its way to destruction. It's easy to grasp the corollary: Get what You can from the earth and each other. Destroy what You must; step on all the toes You must. Eat, drink and be merry; get it while You can; it won't last forever. These egoic challenges revolve around issues of Love and Trust.

The element of the auric energy center is *creation* and *expression* of Universal Love from Your Heart of Hearts. Foods that enhance these energies include: sprouts, fresh juices, fresh nut and seed milks, fermented nut and seed cheeses. Macroalgae in ocean vegetables or seaweed and microalgae from Klamath Lake are superior, wild grown; spirulina and chlorella are also excellent sources. Fasting is recommended.

Traditionally, the primary color is white, secondary is yellow gold; the tone is C#; stones to enhance these energies include rutilated quartz, diamond, Herkimer diamond, selenite. The hypothalamus, in a feedback loop from the heart controls all endocrine, hormone-producing glands and is associated with the Auric energy field; associated influences: DNA, RNA.

Color Influences Our Vibrations
Interestingly, my virginal experience with color therapy happened while I was a priest working in the early 70's with the National Lawyers Guild in Detroit, taking to court the officials of Wayne County and Wayne County Jail regarding inhuman conditions at the jail... conditions in violation of the Michigan Housing and Penal Codes. Following the admonition of Jesus: "I was in prison and You came to see me," spending time behind bars counseling and doing whatever to relieve the anxiety of the prisoners calling their families, I began exploring the operations of other prisons, such as a prison in Colorado with an innovative psychologist and a warden who was receptive to new ways of doing things. In the past, whenever a prisoner would go berserk – as happens from time to time given the intense nature of prisons – he would be put in a straitjacket by several guards and thrown into a padded cell where he would bounce around until exhausted. After a few hours he would be released. The prison psychologist had read about color therapy

and talked the warden into painting one cell entirely pink, including pink sheets on a pink bed. Whenever any prisoner became unruly, he was put in this cell without a straitjacket. They saw him cool off within minutes – because pink has a calming effect. However, leaving the prisoner too long, would re-produce the previous bizarre behavior. Why? Too much – excess!

That experiment reminded me of two other instances regarding color. As a young boy helping paint the kitchen, "Mother, why do we always paint the kitchen yellow, why not another color for a change, maybe peach?" "Well," she said, "my mother always had a yellow kitchen, and I like yellow, so I'm going to keep that color." Smiling, painting... what's the difference? Several years later, I went ice fishing and caught a mess of perch. Bringing some to Grandma and Grandpa, in the kitchen with Grandma cleaning the fish, I stamped my feet a few times to get the circulation moving. Grandpa called in from the living room, "What's going on, Bobby?" "Well, my feet still feel like the ice I've been standing on all day; I'm just warming them up." Without a moment's hesitation, Grandpa called back: "Didn't You have on red socks?" While I knew he wore red long-johns from Labor Day until Memorial Day that was the first inkling of some rhyme or reason beyond the insulating benefits. Resolving to get red socks... the next weekend standing on the same ice... same boots... my feet were quite comfortable. If red is too bright for You, brown is a mixture of red and green.

How can color make such a significant difference? Red, as a warming and stimulating color, increases circulation. At the opposite end of the spectrum, blue is cooling, soothing and relaxing. Some blind people among others, can *feel* the difference through their palms between the energies radiating from red and blue colored paper; some being so sensitive they can perceive all major colors!

Businesses are quite aware of the power of color. In the car when we are cold, we move the dial to the red; when we are hot, we move the dial to the blue. Accident? Is it an accident that McDonald's arches are yellow? Or that basic colors of fast-food restaurants are red and yellow? Red is a color that is at once warming and inviting, as well as stimulating... it gets You moving; red is a perfect color for fast-food places; get them in, get them out. Yellow is the color traditionally associated with the solar plexus...

including the pancreas, liver / gall bladder, spleen and stomach... governing digestion.

The use of color in the kitchen and dining area goes back long before the red and white checker tablecloths or oilcloths of yesteryear. We find healing with color... stimulating organs and glands with corresponding colors... in the origins of every culture. Grandmother may have read Goethe, who wrote about the power of color and stones. Had mother then absorbed this knowledge?

Advertisers know we gravitate toward red packages... being a warming, stimulating, inviting color. Red is the color of the first energy center and relates to feelings of grounding, foundational security and survival. Restaurants with color themes at the other end of the spectrum... blue, purple and violet, even though well appointed... soon realize people feel more comfortable eating elsewhere – unless there is a spectacular view.

Caution: at the bottom of the spectrum, red can trigger imbalance at the other end of the body. A baseball player went from doctors to psychiatrists asking why he got headaches at every away game... separation anxiety? His answer came when he met a color therapist who questioned him; he wore a white cap at home games and a red cap away. At the other end of the spectrum, red was emanating the opposite vibration. Why weren't all the players experiencing the same thing? Different points of tolerance.

For this same reason people find it challenging to think diet has much to do with health. Everyone sitting around the table on Thanksgiving has different symptoms; since they all eat basically the same, how can diet be a contributing factor? Each one has inborn strengths and challenges; stressed beyond their tolerance level, symptoms show up. Stress may further confuse the issue. The fact is, the young man began wearing his white hat at away games and has been free of headaches ever since. Is it all in his head? Who knows? He may have been living in the fast lane. A congested liver or over-burdened digestive system can be a contributing factor to headaches; a congested pancreas can bring on skin sensitivity – even to color.

What is Color?
We point to an apple and call it red. We tend to think of redness as being in or on the object. This is true to a certain extent... the cause of the redness is in the

surface that we see; the effect, our sensory response to that color is in the brain. Color sensation is aroused in the brain by the way the eyes and brain respond to wavelengths of light reflected to the eyes after striking the surface of an object. To understand the effect of color on human response it helps to consider color's dependence on light – because color begins with light.

Visible light is merely one form of radiant energy that makes up the electromagnetic spectrum. At one end are long, invisible waves: electric power transmission waves, radio, TV, radar waves and the infrared waves of heat. While at the opposite end of the electromagnetic spectrum are the short, UV waves, also invisible: x-ray, gamma and cosmic ray waves. Between these bands of invisible energy is a small span of visible wavelengths we call light... these light waves stimulate the human visual mechanism producing sensory effects we call color. If the entire spectrum of light energy were a yardstick... visible light would be 1/16th of an inch!

The exact mechanism of color vision remains a mystery. We only see color where there is light because surfaces reflect varying proportions of different wavelengths of light. When making color choices of paint, wallpaper and fabric, always check under the lighting in which they are to be used. Different types of lighting make for strikingly different effects of color.

The Psychological Power of Color

Color is a powerful emotional stimulus. Psychologists know these waves of electromagnetic energy transmitted to the eyes and brain affect human behavior in diverse ways. Color may be used to create an atmosphere of comfort and well-being... making us feel warmer in a cold environment and cooler when temperatures rise. Color can depress or irritate, as well as stimulate and inspire. Used in other ways, color can change the distance, appearance and size of things... help see things clearly, or make them less distinct... even make things seem to weigh more – or less.

Red is a hot, vibrant color that stimulates, activates and energizes, when used in the proper amounts and places. Orange has many of these attributes. Although a creative color, an excess of orange can over-activate – leading to tension, and producing fatigue. An accent wall in soft orange, properly located, can be quite effective. Yellow is bright and fresh, producing feelings

of gaiety. Perceived as the color of sunlight, yellow produces the same positive, psychological effects. Yellow as a color produces activity. Green is considered neutral, with a tendency to make us feel cool, it has more of a quieting energy – reminding us of the peace found with Mother Nature. Blues, like greens, are subdued colors that bring to mind sunlit skies and tranquil lakes. Light blues are cool colors that contribute to a feeling of relaxation, yet vibrant blues can be somewhat disturbing. Purple and dark violet have characteristics of the reds and blues. Excess can create depression: a purple and/or dark blue room.

Looking at objects of the same size in different colors, we notice light colors appear larger and dark colors appear smaller – hence people have a propensity to wear black. In the linear dimension, the use of unbroken areas of color can give a special effect adding to the apparent length or depth; broken areas of color can be used to give the appearance of shorter distance or depth. Contrast also plays a part in the overall effect of color.

Colors through the Cultures

Every ancient culture used color. Specific color therapy was applied for the benefit of internal organs... emotional, mental and spiritual balance as well as symptomatic relief. These systems have their subtleties and are detailed in readable form in *The Healer's Manual*, by Ted Andrews. According to the ancients, the healing attributes of color can be divided into two types: Red, orange and yellow stimulate, bring warmth, alkalinize and dilate. These are *advancing* colors and make a room seem smaller. Traditional Wisdom calls them yang. Blue, indigo and violet refresh, contract, acidify and act as astringents. These are *receding* colors and make a room seem larger. Thus, they are yin.

Green, a combination of yellow and blue, is neutral... nurturing peace and harmony for the physical and emotional heart. Green is so important Leonardo suggested it as one of the basic colors in the 15th century. In 1914, Wilhelm Osterwald eliminated green as a primary color; obviously, it is a mix. Vibrations of the 3 primary colors compose the first chord of music: Red = C, Yellow = E, Blue = G.

25 centuries ago, Pythagoras, well-versed in ancient knowledge of his time, used colors to facilitate healing. And 3 centuries ago, Sir Isaac Newton proposed the

first theory concerning color. He used a prism to show that sunlight was comprised of seven different colors: red, orange, yellow, green, blue, purple or indigo, and violet. When these seven colors were in turn passed through a second prism, they again became light.

Ancient Egypt and Greece

With quantum physics and explorations into space-time, our consciousness is expanding and we are beginning to experience the wisdom of our ancient ancestors who had an intricate knowledge of colors, the planets... the signs of the zodiac, parts of the body – and their relationships:

Sun Orange / gold: Vitality, heart and circulatory system.

Moon Silver and green: Body rhythms, ovaries, breasts, and stomach.

Mercury Metallic blue: Nervous system, respiratory system, hands.

Venus Pastel blue, pastel green: Reproduction, hair, skin, nails.

Mars Scarlet and magenta: Blood, muscles, testicles.

Jupiter Deep blue or purple (indigo): Liver, cellular nutrition, hips, thighs.

Saturn Black, dark brown, dark green: Bones, teeth, joints, skin, hearing.

Uranus Electric blue, electric silver: Eyes (cones / rods).

Neptune Sea green, smoky gray: Endocrine glands (especially pineal).

Pluto Magenta: Regenerative forces and reproductive system.

~~~~~~

Aries Red: Head, brain, face.

Taurus Light blue, pastels: Neck, throat, thyroid.

Gemini Slate blue, lemon: Lungs, shoulders, arms, hands.

Cancer Silver and green: Breasts, stomach.

Leo Orange and gold: Heart, back.

Virgo Deep blue: Intestines.

Libra Soft pink, soft blue: Kidneys, ovaries.

Scorpio Bright red, deep yellow: Reproductive organs, bladder, nose.

Sagittarius Deep blue: Hips, thighs, muscles.

Capricorn Black, brown, dark green: Knees, joints, skin.

Aquarius Electric blue, pale yellow, pale green: Calves, ankles, eyes.

Pisces Sea green, silver: Feet, toes, lymphatic system.

NOTE: When pendulum, muscle test or intuition says a particular endocrine energy center is <u>under</u>-active... apply the appropriate color; when <u>over</u>-active... apply the complementary color. The after-image of a color is known as the complement of that color; prolonged staring at any bright hue reduces sensitivity of the receptors to that particular color... and correspondingly, heightens receptor sensitivity to the complementary color. Stare at a red disc, and then look at a blank white page or wall; You see a green disc exactly the same size; stare at a blue disc and the after-image will be orange. Practice develops the ability to perceive auras.

Color... Complement

Red... Green
Orange... Blue
Yellow... Violet
Red-orange... Blue-green
Red-violet... Yellow-green
Yellow-orange... Blue-violet

Creating Colors... Filters or Gels

Scarlet... 2 reds
Red-orange... 2 red, 1 yellow
Orange... 1 red, 1 yellow
Yellow-orange... 2 yellow, 1 red
Yellow-green... 2 yellow, 1 blue
Green... 1 yellow, 1 blue
Blue-green... 3 blue, 1 yellow
Turquoise... 2 blue, 1 yellow
Indigo... 2 blue, 1 red
Violet... 1 red, 1 blue
Blue-violet... 2 blue, 1 red
Red-violet... 2 red, 1 blue
Magenta... 3 red, 1 blue
Purple... 1 red, 1 blue, 1 yellow

Color Correspondences

Ted Andrews' *The Healer's Manual* offers ancient, time-honored correspondences between certain conditions and beneficial colors by presenting color schematics for the four worlds – spiritual, mental, astral, physical – as applied to the ten levels of the Kabbala. "By sending energy along the ancient 'Path of the Flaming Sword' You activate a powerfully creative force. You draw it down through the body, affecting all systems and all levels of energy." His system is called Awakening the Tree of Life.

Dr Dinsha P Ghadiali, who contributed much to the modern renaissance of color therapy, taught the correlation between colors and glands. Red: liver. Scarlet (vivid red to reddish orange): gonads. Orange: thyroid and mammary glands. Yellow: pancreas and thymus. Green hypothalamus. Blue: pituitary. Indigo: parathyroid. Violet: spleen.

Rudolf Steiner taught how to understand color through feelings. Colors that have *luster* have <u>activity</u>: red, blue and yellow. Colors that have *form* have <u>image</u>: white, black, green and peach blossom. Green is the image of life; peach blossom, the image of soul; white, the image of spirit; black: the image of death – the doorway to the next dimension of consciousness. Through the images of life, soul, spirit & death sense perception is experienced. Steiner felt dis-ease indicates a rift between earthly consciousness and the high self.

To understand Steiner, who organized and catalogued the works of Goethe: *The Wholeness of Nature: Goethe's Way Toward a Science of Conscious Participation in Nature*, by Henri Bortoft. Synthesizing 6000 lectures and writings of Steiner: *The Imagination of Pentecost: Rudolf Steiner & Contemporary Christianity*, by Richard Leviton.

Color Potentiation
M.L. Rees, DC, recognized and honored in Sacral-Occipital-Technique for cranial discoveries as well as Vibrational Energy Medicine with Harmonics, offers the following relationships between the vertebral levels and organ involvement, along with other common challenges and their balancing colors:
D1: Heart Muscle... Medium Lemon
D2: Heart Valves... Crystal
D3: Respiratory... Rose
D4: Gall Bladder... Dark Burgundy
D5: Stomach... Violet
D6: Pancreas... Deep Blue
D7: Spleen and Immune Function... Pale Lavender
D8: Liver... Light Rose Purple
D9: Adrenals... Dark Burgundy
D10: Small Intestine... Mist Blue
D11: Duodenum... Pale Yellow Green
D12: Kidneys... Fire – red, orange, yellow, green, blue
L1: Ileocecal Valve... Ultraviolet
L2: Cecal... Surprise Lavender
L3: Ovaries / Testes... Middle Rose
L4: Colon... Lavender
L5: Uterus / Prostate... Frost

S1: Bright Yellow Green
S2: Light to medium Blue
S3: Bright Yellow
S4: Jade Green
S5: Pastel Pink
Coccyx: Pink
Sacroiliac: Light to medium Blue
Sciatica: Light Straw;
Cranial: Pink; Allergies: Medium Pink; Bursa: Medium Pink, and Dark Burgundy; Cell Salts: Violet; Infections: Medium Pink; Negative Energies: Pale Lavender; Vascular Enhancement for Pulmonary and Mitral: Blue; Aortic and Tricuspid: Pink.
<u>Dr. M.L. Rees Archives | SOTO USA (soto-usa.com)</u>

Colors and Their Influences
Robert Tennyson Stevens, author: *My Word Made Flesh* and *Conscious Language*, teaches about auras and what aura photography can reveal:
Clear bright red: Vibrant, stimulated, excited about Life
Muddy bright red: Withheld intense anger with judgment
Bright orange-red: Willful self-pride
Bright rose: Love and human affection
Pure brilliant pink: Divine Love
Pale faint pink: Tentative, shy, divinely inspired love
Clear, bright orange: Wisdom and reasoning power
Orange with muddy red: Self-serving, intellectual pride
Light orange: Emerging intellectual strength
Golden sparkles: Ascension energies, enthusiasm
Clear bright yellow: Highest intellect, knowing & radiating
Light, clear green yellow: Sympathy & empathy
Light, clear green: Compassion with understanding
Medium, clear green: Adaptable, rebirth – Spring
Green with reds, browns and blacks: Jealousy
Green with gray: Deceit
Muddy green: Sickness
Olive green: Selfishness, envy
Clear blue: Passionate spirituality, pure spiritual purpose
Dark blue: Power
Blue with dark reddish brown: Selfish religious tendency
Blue with gray: Sadness and despair, tendency toward religious fear
Blue with black: Tendency toward resistance, fear of evil
Turquoise: Pure spiritual belief
Blue with lavender: High idealism
Indigo: Spiritual integrity, sincerity, wisdom

Gray: Love of formality, convention, lacking imagination
Silver: Volatile; tends toward unreliability, inconsistency
Brown: Orderliness, convention, ambition, power
Brown with green tinges: Selfishness
Black: Negation of color – isolation, hatred, discord
Black with crimson: Viciousness
White: Godliness

Dr Jacob Liberman, *Light: Medicine of the Future* and *Luminous Life*, uses a pulse-meter or measures the breathing response to determine the color that irritates, and applies that color via strobe light, medium setting, through the open eyes. After a few sessions, balance and harmony are restored; symptoms recede and disappear. However, another point of view Dr B. Bhattacharyya, *Science of Cosmic Ray Therapy*, treats with the complimentary color. Muscle test to know.

Reuben Amber in *Color Therapy* offers a wealth of information, and some cautions. When in doubt, always underexpose. Individuals experiencing exhaustion or fever after using a red bulb to energize the system for the purpose of toning the body and achieving a reduction of weight, and individuals with tachycardia or hypertension are advised to switch to an orange bulb which stimulates and raises the pulse rate w/o raising the blood pressure.

Dr Bernard Jensen, respected chiropractor who revived the Art of Iridology, talks about "the amazing eye" saying the human eye is able to perceive around 9 million colors! The thought astounded me; my logical mind rebelled at 9 million colors; maybe I could handle 900, stretching the imagination, and I thought: "No wonder medical science scoffs at chiropractors and others who make such outlandish claims!" Shortly thereafter, there was an ad for the latest computer printer that, depending on software, can create 16.7 million colors! Calling technical support, they assured me this was no typo... it is possible through the magic of dot matrix and other technology. We are beginning to re-claim our appreciation and respect for the diversity of colors as well as chiropractic approaches to holistic healing. The influence of colors is phenomenal, certainly worthy of exploration and experimentation.

Sound: Primordial Vibration

"Natives who use incantations and drumming
to drive out evil spirits
are objects of scorn to smart Americans
who yell epithets and honk horns
to break up traffic jams." -Anon

All things exist in vibration. The vibrations of color and sound are easily measured; differences can be subtle. Other vibrations are substantially different: wood, water, rock, metal, cloth, glass, and plastic. Whatever the differences they share a commonality: all are supported by the One Vibration, the Source of All that sustains everything, every person, and every universe. Movement and sound are essential to vibration, essential to Creation. Both sound and light are consequences of *movement*.

"In the beginning, God created the heavens and earth. Now the earth was a formless void, there was darkness over the deep, and God's spirit *hovered* over the water. God *said* 'Let there be light' and there was light." (Gen. 1:1-3) Spirit *hovering* implies at least minimal movement and sound. Among the first movements creating sounds by humankind were: stone against stone, wood against wood, wood against stone - the beginnings of percussion. Then our ancestors noticed sounds of hollow bamboo, then the first flute carved with stone or cut with blade, then someone carved varying lengths & diameters of bamboo to create various tones! Imagine the excitement as music began filling the air. Communion with Infinite Being was an Inspiration for all the sisters and brothers. Blessings of pre-history continue through the present.

As **color** exists in precise visible mathematical frequencies measured in angstroms (Å), **sound** exists in precise audible mathematical frequencies measured in hertz (Hz). Tuning forks and musical instruments can create healing sound vibrations. While electronic instruments make the sounds, the healing *overtones* are missing. In the 21st century, acoustic instruments are preferred; many musicians do analog recordings.

The human auditory system is capable of hearing close to 10 octaves. We hear between 20 Hz and 20000 Hz. The musically usable octaves of frequencies are between 40 Hz - 5000 Hz. Below 40 Hz, things become muddy in a mix. Above 5000 Hz, the fundamental tones become piercing in the high registers.

There is a correlation between color / light and sounds. Below 40 Hz is the infra-red spectrum, big, slow waves. The octave of 40-80 Hz is seen in the spectrum as red. 80-160 Hz orange. 160-320 Hz yellow. 320-640 Hz green. 640-1280 Hz blue. 1280-2560 Hz indigo. 2560-5120 Hz violet. 5120-20000 Hz are akin to the ultra-violet spectrum, small, extremely fast waves.

Solfeggio – a tad short of being truly ancient – is an Italian word meaning musical scale developed by Benedictine monk, Guido D'Arezzo (991 – 1050 CE) believing singers could learn chants more easily. We know the Solfeggio as 7 ascending notes assigned to the syllables Do-Re-Mi-Fa-So-La-Ti – which is forever emblazoned in both the Akasha and in Universal Mind as *Doe a Deer*. The original scale was six ascending notes assigned as Ut-Re-Mi-Fa-Sol-La.

Physicist, inventor and engineer, Nikola Tesla said:
"If you only knew the magnificence of **3**s, **6**s and **9**s, then you would hold a Key to the Universe."

Those 3 numbers form the vibration of the six Solfeggio Frequencies when reduced to a single number!

UT – **396** Hz – transforms grief into joy, and guilt into forgiveness.
RE – **417** Hz – clears negativity & removes subconscious blockages.
MI – **528** Hz – stimulates love, restores equilibrium, and repairs DNA.
FA – **639** Hz – strengthens relationships, family and commUnity.
SOL – **741** Hz – cleanses the physical body from all types of toxins.
LA – **852** Hz – awakens Intuition, and balances HeartMindBodySpirit as One.

Syllables for the scale are from Vespers for the Nativity of John the Baptist: **Ut** queant laxis **Re**sonare fibris **Mi**ra gestorum **Fa**muli tuorum **So**lve polluti **La**bii reatum, Sancte Iohannes! (*Liber Usualis*)

Throughout history things became nebulous as **A** has been tuned between 430>460 Hz depending on various musical or philosophical viewpoints. Proponents of A=444 Hz claim the resulting C=528 Hz is the frequency of the sound of the sun... as well as the yellow-green color of chlorophyll. {Quintessentially exemplified with *wheatgrass*, having a bright yellow lecithin-rich base supporting a bright green stem!} In

this theory, the 528 Hz frequency is part of The Complete Circle of Sound, which ranges from: 174, 285, 396, 417, 528, 639, 741, 852, 963 Hz. While this is attractive to mathematicians like Marko Rodin, critics argue 111 Hz intervals are less than optimal for brainwave entrainment without the use of an Epsilon carrier wave – hence the imbalances in those who use them. Epsilon waves – <0.5 Hz – are associated with high states of consciousness. Epsilon brainwave patterns have HyperGamma {40-100 Hz} or Lambda {100-200 Hz} patterns modulating within them. The former reflects high levels of brain organization... 40 Hz common among Tibetan monks during meditation – reflecting ecstatic states of consciousness. HG and L patterns ride on the super-slow Epsilon modulation, cultivated by rhythmic breathing – especially caressing the bump at the roof of the mouth, connecting the microcosmic circuit – worthwhile to cultivate as a daily habit for energy flow, and bringing focus to One's Life. Proponents of A=432 Hz claim it is the frequency of Mother Earth – 7.83 / 8 Hz – being the fundamental "beat" of the planet. The heartbeat of Earth is better known as the Schumann Resonance after Winfried Otto Schumann physicist, who mathematically proved in 1952 a global electromagnetic resonance, from electrical discharges of lightning within the cavity existing between the Earth's surface and the ionosphere. This cavity resonates with electromagnetic waves in extremely low frequencies of 7.86–8 Hz. Taking 8 Hz as our starting point and working upwards by five octaves, the seven notes in the scale five times, we reach a frequency of 256 Hz in which A is 432Hz – matching the Sitar tuned to C#, considered to be the sound of OM in Vedic cultures.
https://www.sonicgeometry.com

According to harmonic principle, any sound automatically calls to action multiples of that frequency. When we play C at 256 Hz... the C of all other octaves vibrate in sympathy; 8Hz also vibrates... which is why, along with other mathematical reasons, the musical pitch A tuned to 432 oscillations per second is the "scientific tuning" called the Vivaldi or Verdi tuning. Proposed by physicists Joseph Sauveur and Felix Savart, and the Italian scientist Bartolomeo Grassi Landi, approval was given at the Congress of Italian Musicians in 1881, seemingly settling the matter.

In sharp contrast, when A=440 Hz, the note C is at 261.656 Hz completely out of sync with Mother Nature; since every other number is 6, some say this frequency was chosen for nefarious purposes in London in 1953 to be the worldwide "reference frequency" and defined as "disharmonic" – without scientific relationship to physical laws that govern our universe – promoting frustration, anger and fear in our modern world.

From ancient times, music based on mathematical proportions brought healing sounds and vibrations. Wherever A may be tuned, it's glorious as part of Creation. As a musician, experiment with tunings... and feel what resonates in Your Heart with Your message. For the mathematical basis of sound: Michael Schneider's *A Beginner's Guide to Constructing the Universe: The Mathematical Archetypes of Nature, Art and Science* – Ch 7; *Cymatics: a study of the structure and dynamics of waves and vibrations* by Dr Hans Jenny dedicated to the memory and research of Dr Rudolf Steiner. See also: Ch 10: **Humming for Holistic Health**.

Classical, Jazz and Beyond: Holistic Harmonics

The language of music is universal. Through music we experience healing for the heart... mind... body... spirit. Whatever happened to wholesome entertainment such as Mitch Miller and Gang with their TV sing a-longs? With the words at the bottom of the screen we could follow the bouncing ball and play the most beautiful instrument of all – the human voice. Camaraderie, conviviality, great exercise for the heart and lungs, and with a little movement the lymphatic system has a workout as well... bringing healing benefits to all the hormone-producing glands and all the organs. A smile on Your face tells Your subconscious all is well, so the brain produces hormones of happiness and contentment, and... we *are* well! "Those were the days, my friend..." In lieu of Mitch, gather 'round the piano, guitar or ukulele... sing to Your heart's content.

The following system known as **Harmonics** was gifted to M.L. Rees, DC in 1980. Dr Rees was from Sedan KS, a tiny town of 2000 at the time, and doctors would come from AU, EU, JP, NZ, and all of North America to work with him; patients drove for an hour or more!

He and Major Bertrand DeJarnette, DO, DC were geniuses promoting Sacral Occipital Technique. At a seminar in Atlanta in 1981, Dr Rees – conservative, on the religious right – told us he had his eyes opened by his granddaughter regarding the channeling of Spirits. Guided by her Guardian Angels for a couple of months with remarkable results, she was filled with Gratitude.

One day they admitted working with her to "get through" to her grandfather, whose work they deeply respected.

"They said to tell You about a tough case You have. You've done everything You know, with zero results – so here are two things they said would work." Applying the techniques... they actually worked! Then the angels asked to speak with him, revealing what we now call Harmonics – using variously programmed crystal chips arranged in specific patterns. They were all set in 3" discs, >200 of them! Various affirmations, colors, metals being used along with an Omnichord – together, offered an experience in Vibrational Energy Medicine. It was an amazing discovery for this respected gentleman who had previously discovered many cranial healing techniques relating to tender spots on the sagittal suture connecting to various emotions! Dr. M.L. Rees Archives | SOTO USA (soto-usa.com)

Condition: Key... Melody...Tempo...Color
Adrenals: E maj... Latin... Fast... Burgundy
Allergies: F min... Waltz... Slow... Burgundy
Blood: F flat 7th... Slow rock... Fast... Red
Bones: A maj... Latin... Medium... Yellow/Green
Bursitis: C 7th... Latin... Fast... Med. Pink
Cecum: C min... Swing... Fast... Lavender
Cell Salts: A maj... Waltz... Medium... Violet
CNS: B flat min... Swing... Medium... White
Cervicals: D min... Slow rock... Fast... Blue
Chakras, lower: C maj... Waltz... Medium... Red
Chakras, middle: D maj... Waltz... Medium... Yellow
Chakras, upper: A min... Waltz... Medium... Blue
Colon: F min... Fox Trot... Slow... Lavender
Cranium: C min... Rock... Medium... Pink
Duodenum: G min... Slow Rock... Medium... Yellow/Green
Energy: B flat maj... Latin... Mod. Fast... Burgundy
Gall Bladder: E flat maj... Latin... Medium... Burgundy
Heart Muscle: A maj... Waltz... Medium... Lemon
Heart Valves: F maj... Swing... Medium... Crystal
Aorta: B flat min... Rock... Mod. Fast... Crystal
Mitral: G maj... Rock... Mod. Fast... Crystal
Pulmonary: G maj... Rock... Mod. Fast... Crystal
Tricuspid: B flat min... Rock... Mod. Fast... Crystal
Hormonal Balance (Pituitary): F maj... Latin... Medium... Purple
(Thyroid): F maj... Slow Rock... Medium... Blue
Ileocecal Valve: D 7th... Rock... Mod. Fast... Ultraviolet

Infections: F min... Waltz... Slow... Pink

Kidney Dissolve Stones: E maj... Fox Trot... Medium... Fire

Kidney Drainage: E flat min... Latin... Medium... Fire

Kidney Energizer: F maj... Slow Rock... Fast... Fire

Liver Drainage: C min... Waltz... Medium... Burgundy

Liver Energizer: G maj... Swing... Slow... Rose/Purple

Lung Drainage: F min... Waltz... Medium... Rose

Lung Energizer: G maj... Waltz... Medium... Rose

Migraine: G 7th... Fox Trot... Medium... White

Negative Energies/Entities: F maj... Latin... Medium... White

Nutrition: A maj... Waltz... Medium... Yellow

Ovaries: E maj... Swing... Medium... Rose

Pain Control (deep): B flat maj... Slow Rock... Medium... White; followed by: B maj... Fox Trot... Medium... White

Pain Control (superficial): B flat maj... Slow Rock... Medium... White; followed by: D maj... Swing... Medium... White

Pancreas: B maj... Slow Rock... Mod. Fast... Blue

Parkinson's: C min... Waltz... Medium... Burgundy; followed by: G maj... Fox Trot... Medium... Burgundy

Prostate: B flat min... Slow Rock... Slow... Frost

Skin Challenges: F min... Fox Trot... Medium... Blue

Small Intestine: F 7th... Fox Trot... Slow... Mist Blue

Spleen: F 7th... Waltz... Slow... Lavender

Stomach: G maj... Waltz... Medium... Violet

Systemic Lupus: F min... Fox Trot... Fast... Gold

Testes: E maj... Swing... Medium... Rose

Uterus: B flat min... Slow Rock... Slow... Frost

Aromatherapy: Balance for the Emotions, thus – HeartMindBodySpirit

The term aromatherapy was coined in the 1920's... when Rene-Maurice Gattefosse, French chemist / perfumer, burned himself quite seriously in his laboratory. He turned quickly and stuck his arm in the closest vat of cool liquid. Much to his amazement, the pain lessened remarkably. When he took his arm out, he realized the lavender oil helped heal a serious burn he thought would surely scar; he was amazed at the lack of blisters, inflammation, and redness... even heat. After that he spent his life experimenting with essential oils, studying and reviving the ancient, almost forgotten, art of using oils to enhance Quality of Life.

Ancient cultures used fragrances... sprinkling herbs on hot embers creating incense, soaking petals creating rose water, adding flowers to fragrant oils. To this day, Egyptians anoint their bodies with botanicals. In India sandalwood is traditionally used in religious and spiritual practices. The Chinese use jasmine to venerate their ancestors. Hebrew law prescribes a one-year purification process with myrrh and other fragrant oils before the maiden is presented to the royal court. African brides and grooms coat their bodies with special oils to beautify, and to deter evil on their wedding day. Aromatherapy is particularly beneficial with challenges in a synthetic world; with subtle benefits from inhaling the fragrances, to stimulate deep healing: emotionally, mentally and spiritually.

Analogies are made between sound and smell. We speak of sounds as high, low, harmonious, and discordant. Perfumers and aromatherapists borrow the musical vocabulary to describe aromas and speak of essential oils as having a high or low note. This was elaborated in the mid-1850s into a theory of Top, Middle and Bass Notes by scientist / perfumer G.W. Piesse who arranged frequencies of fragrances on a staff, like a musical scale. Chemist, perfumer and prolific writer, he wrote among his scientific books, *The Art of Perfumery* – the first modern book about perfumery in 1857. Another early modern researcher, Roland Hunt, in 1937 published *Fragrant and Radiant Healing Symphony: An enquiry into the wondrous correlation of the healing virtues of Colour, Sound and Perfume – a consideration of their influence and purpose*. His research found these elements blend together creating balance and harmony.

Robert Tisserand, *The Art of Aromatherapy*, takes us to the Next Order of Magnitude doing remarkable studies in the '70s using an EEG – noticing influences of aromas on brainwave patterns. Interestingly, the EEG was **unphased** with synthetic fragrances!

Helpful Hints

Use Caution with straight essences. Certain oils can irritate sensitive skin. Usually, essences are diluted in a carrier oil – traditionally: almond, apricot, grapeseed or jojoba; today fractionated coconut oil seems superior. These can be applied to the skin safely. With any hesitation, follow Your Inner Voice Intuition... apply a little to the underside of Your forearm. Keep oils away from Your eyes. Use cold-water wash for any irritation. Certain oils are to be used only when *well* diluted. Even if diluted, avoid exposure to sunlight when skin is treated with oils of angelica, bergamot, citrus including mandarin, ginger and peppermint.

You deserve pure organic or therapeutic essential oils. Inexpensive means synthetic. Ask the person in the shop to tell You about the sources. There are choices: Commercial essential oils can be natural, yet perhaps grown with Roundup, or from a polluted country; a blend of natural with synthetic, or pure synthetic. Organic essential oils are grown according to the Moon, free from chemicals, while nurturing the soil with compost. BioDynamic essential oils follow organic principles, adding detailed instructions set forth in Rudolf Steiner's *Agriculture* – initially developed in 1924, as the first book of the organic agriculture movements {see: Chapter 10}. Therapeutic essential oils are from plants that were planted by the Moon's phase, and harvested according to the Moon's phase, some in the early morning before the dew dries – others at the end of the day.

Use only glass containers. Except when being used, keep the bottles snugly capped and out of sunlight. When mixing a recipe, follow drop for drop. Better one drop less than one drop in excess.

Inhale essential oils for short periods, as frequently as Spirit moves; a few drops in a tissue lasts awhile.

Contraindications
Epileptic challenges: avoid clary sage, fennel, hyssop, mugwort, rosemary, sage and thyme.

High blood pressure: avoid hyssop, mugwort, rosemary, sage and thyme.

Pregnant: avoid basil, cedarwood, hyssop, jasmine, juniper, marjoram, mugwort, myrrh, peppermint, rosemary, sage and thyme.

Taking homeopathic remedies: avoid basil, camphor, and eucalyptus altogether. Avoid peppermint a half-hour before and after remedies.

Essential Oils and Their Qualities
Angelica supports connection with Guardian Angels, Spirit Guides and the High Self... supporting harmonious integration of various aspects of Your being – physical, emotional, mental and spiritual. It facilitates insight and self-understanding, promoting a sense of stability in relation to all of life. Angelica aids detoxification of the blood and lymphatic system, relaxes nerves and relieves tension headaches. Stimulating the glandular, hormonal system, it restores strength and vitality, which supports convalescence. Two-parts frankincense and one-part angelica energizes the auric energy field.

Basil builds confidence and courage... energizing brain functions, especially concentration and memory... enabling a leader to express authority with dignity and to make clear decisions. It relieves head challenges, such as migraines or colds; as a nerve tonic, it relieves depression; in the bath it relieves sore muscles. Basil refreshes sluggish, congested skin... and repels insects.

Benzoin energizes the root energy center bringing stability and balance. Excellent for the physical and emotional heart; releasing anger and emotional tension, it brings balance and comfort. Benzoin clears negativity from the aura and environment and has circulatory benefits rejuvenating the skin; it resembles vanilla in color, consistency and fragrance.

Bergamot promotes confidence and discernment, opening the heart to love, light and life. Strengthening digestive, immune and nervous systems, bergamot is excellent for challenges relating to menses and menopause. As an antiseptic balm for the skin, one undiluted drop on a boil, cold sore or pimple does wonders. Bergamot eases depression and anxiety... with the terminally ill, resolving old issues, opening the heart for what is to come. It is useful both before and after transition. A sweet, citrusy, warm, floral top note... it blends well.

Black Pepper serves as an eye-opener for day-dreamers and a Third Eye-opener for drowsiness during meditation. Profound mental stimulation makes it a great aid for studying and taking tests. As a physical stimulant to get You moving when You feel stuck, it alleviates the fear of speaking... encourages self-expression... and improves communication. A common aroma molecule or terpene, beta-caryophyllene (BCP), is abundant and functions as a cannabinoid. Similar to other plant-based cannabinoids, BCP binds with the CB2 receptors, reducing inflammation. Research suggests BCP assists the treatment of arthritis and osteoporosis, and likely increases effectiveness of anti-cancer drugs.

Carrotseed restores confidence where there is doubt or confusion. It serves as a tonic for the liver and gall bladder detoxifying the body by purifying the blood, having beneficial effects with the skin: rashes, eczema, even psoriasis. Carrotseed rejuvenates dry, aging skin, and relieves menses and menopause challenges.

Cedarwood erases aggression, anxiety and tension… supporting our connection with the Divine, inspiring faith, optimism and wisdom. Cedarwood cuts through congestion that clogs our noses and our minds… helping see things clearly while retaining composure. Toning the kidneys, it affects glandular, nervous and respiratory systems. Useful as a chest rub for breathing challenges, and a tonic for the skin, it strengthens the hair shaft stimulating growth; it is also an insect repellent, especially for moths.

Chamomile calms and soothes physically and mentally, decreases anxiety with an experience of TLC for children… and adults doing inner child work. An immune response system stimulant, it soothes the kidneys, liver and spleen, aids digestion, lowers blood pressure and induces restful sleep. Purifying the complexion, chamomile rejuvenates the skin – delaying the wrinkling process; it eases painful muscles and joints, and is excellent for sprains – a few drops do wonders. Mild to moderate asthma or exercise-induced asthma can be relieved with a blend of blue chamomile, lavender (anti-inflammatory and anti-spasmodic), cypress (dilates bronchial tubes), and bergamot (relieves anxiety and depression). Chamomile dispels anger relaxing the heart, opens the door for honesty, integrity in communication. Blue chamomile has a special charm alleviating the fear of speaking, and encourages self-expression.

Cinnamon enhances digestive energies physically, emotionally, mentally. It is a stimulant, and a warming antiseptic, normalizing oily skin and reducing acne.

Clary Sage is a confidence booster, easing impotence and frigidity, a relaxing aphrodisiac. Encouraging vivid dreams, enhancing dream recall… avoid alcohol a few hours before and after, or there may be nightmares. Exceptionally exotic and erotic dreams may suggest some aspect of sexuality requires clarification. Relaxing muscles, with lavender and peppermint, it eases tension headaches; it stimulates the scalp to support hair growth. A whiff dispels anxiety with breathing challenges. While pregnancy is a contraindication, after birth it is restorative for convalescence and post-partum blues – especially combined with massage; equally relaxing with massage during menses and PMS.

Clove antiseptic for teeth and the gums. Place a clove between gum and cheek for relief, rather than the oil.

Coriander blended with rosemary and ginger is thought to be an aphrodisiac.

Cypress offers comfort, self-assurance and strength… especially during times of transition: job, relationships, house and life. It relieves challenges associated with menses and menopause, and aids concentration. Dilating bronchioles, relieving breathing challenges, it helps control crying fits. Restoring circulation and lymphatic drainage, cypress relieves cellulite and fluid retention; normalizing oily skin and acne, a natural deodorant, a soothing footbath… and insect repellent.

Eucalyptus disperses negative energies. Burned or vaporized in the sickroom, the antiseptic, antibiotic and antiviral qualities speed recovery, helping prevent the spread of infection around the house. Eucalyptus heals the heart and opens the lungs so we can take in the essence of life. A major heart-healer on the emotional level, it relieves grief and sorrow… defuses anger… and clears the air after arguments or physical fighting. Eucalyptus stimulates circulation and relieves breathing challenges. Used in massage, it relieves arthritic / muscular pain; it is an excellent insect repellent.

Fennel relieves digestive challenges… and used with cypress facilitates the relief of cellulite. Fennel increases sexual desire; yet, regular use can permanently numb erotic sensations… and impair the sex drive. By rubbing a few drops at the solar plexus, fennel can dispel negative entities or psychic attack. Place a drop on each hand, rub them together and smooth them over Your body and Your aura – front, back and sides – let each stroke of the hands touch the ground completing the circuit… optimal with bare feet on the ground, receiving the negative ions and free electrons from Mother Earth.

Frankincense promotes peaceful sleep and pleasant dreams, relieves breathing challenges, rejuvenates skin and assists in healing wounds. Frankincense enhances connection to Spirit, expanding intuition, opens our hearts to inner guidance and has the ability to deepen and slow the breath, facilitating the meditative state. It breaks ties with the past, especially those that interfere with personal and spiritual growth; use a few drops in the bath with conscious intention.

Geranium as a normalizer can be stimulating or sedating promoting hormonal balance, balance in communication, encouraging self-expression alleviating fear of speaking. Antiseptic and antifungal properties help with burns and wounds, as well as rejuvenating for the skin. It can regulate and relieve menses, and eases menopause. Anxiety and stress respond well to a blend of geranium and tangerine. Geranium, a strong yet soft, green, rose-like floral, blends well.

Ginger warms and energizes the digestive system, and facilitates digesting things on the emotional level as well. As an aphrodisiac, it ignites desire and potency. Relieving menstrual, muscular, arthritic and rheumatic pains, ginger is excellent for sprains; always dilute as it can irritate the skin.

Grapefruit eases depression / moodiness with cheerful, confident energy; strengthens liver, gall bladder, kidneys and pancreas, soothes nerves and the mind. Grapefruit promotes circulation and lymphatic drainage, relieving fluid retention, cellulite. For anxiety and stress, blend grapefruit / orange.

Helichrysum provides quick relief from spasms and coughs, strengthens and protects the immune and nervous systems, eases depression and stress, and relieves thickening of the blood – clearing blood clots resulting from hemorrhage. The therapeutic variety is *Helichrysum angustifolium italicum*, with a honey-like, sweet fragrance having green undertones... usually pale yellow in color, with some red tints. It has been studied by Italian natural product chemist Giovanni Appendino, who presented at the International Cannabinoid Research Society: cannabinoid-like compounds are made by plants, starting from an aromatic acid... which is different from the normal cannabinoid biosynthetic route. This South African daisy has strong cannabigerol (CBG), also found in the cannabis plant. Helichrysum is used in ritual ceremonies making fumes with potential psychotropic, soul-nurturing effects similar to other cannabinoids.

Hyssop has been used to purify spaces for meditation, blessing or healing. Most consider hyssop dangerous, and since there are safer oils like cedar, juniper,

lavender and sage, it is wise to leave hyssop alone. Contraindications are epilepsy, high blood pressure, and pregnancy. Avoid hyssop if You have these situations or if such a person is likely to be in that area. Be safe; use something else.

Jasmine with exquisite sensual qualities opens the heart for romance as a gentle aphrodisiac, eases emotional challenges, and melts frigidity or impotence. Dispelling anger, decreasing anxiety, promoting calm energies, jasmine unites sensuality, sexuality and spirituality. It stimulates creativity, dreams, fantasy and imagination, eases depression, especially post-partum, and imparts confidence... sensitivity... and emotional balance. While soothing for dry skin, jasmine promotes uterine contractions – avoid during pregnancy; it may be used once labor begins.

Juniper promotes a sense of well-being and inner strength encouraging us to step beyond our comfort zone to expand our mental and emotional boundaries, perhaps to embrace new ideas or perspectives. Juniper enhances the memory and clears the mind of clutter; it strengthens the glands and nerves, beneficially affecting the immune function; it balances the kidneys and the urinary tract; it is also used as an antiseptic spray. Juniper has been used from time immemorial by diverse cultures for clearing negative energies from one's aura, and from the environment.

Lavender is the most versatile of oils: anti-bacterial, anti-depressant, anti-inflammatory, anti-septic, and anti-spasmodic – bringing pain relief even at childbirth. As the pre-eminent remedy for physical, emotional and psychic first aid, lavender prevents scarring from burns and wounds at these levels. Lavender has a cheerful nature and a cooling energy that at once sanitizes and relaxes; it is a sedative that balances and calms: cleansing all levels. It facilitates deep meditation, integrating spirituality and daily life. With lavender we realize unity between the ordinary and the sacred. It cleanses negative energies and keeps bacteria in check. Soak crystals and gems in water with a few drops of lavender. It can be used undiluted on the skin by most people. Antiseptic, beneficial for acne and oily skin, it normalizes secretions of the sebaceous glands. Blended with peppermint: useful for headaches. It provides a clean, fresh floral with a top note.

Lemon infuses HeartMindBodySpirit with solar energy, enhancing optimism and humor. Clearing the sinuses as well as the mind, lemon eases worry and depression. As a tonic for the liver, gall bladder, nervous and circulatory systems, lemon enhances the immune function. Lemon acts as an astringent for the skin, and provides antiseptic healing for boils and insect bites. Like all citrus oils, lemon can irritate the skin; always dilute, avoid direct sunlight. It has a green, fruity fragrance.

Lemon Eucalyptus obtained from the lemon-scented gum eucalyptus tree is a great insect repellent. Used widely for catarrh, colds, cold sores and coughing, fever, flu, poor circulation, and inflammatory conditions such as arthritis, bronchitis and sinusitis. Lemon eucalyptus has a pale, yellow color and thin consistency; fresh, lemony, sweet with a woody hint.

Lemongrass is a general stimulant that has anti-septic qualities. Organic beekeepers use just a hint on their hives, because it mimics the honeybee's pheromones. **Lime** serves as a general stimulant and tones the body. More fresh and green than lemon, it blends well.

Mandarin brings joy to children and the child within. A tonic for the liver and stomach, it aids digestion and promotes peaceful sleep, especially with children. Mandarin is safe and soothing during pregnancy. Avoid sunlight after use.

Marjoram as an emotional diffuser can be used with lavender and peppermint for emotional headaches. Marjoram alone is associated with celibacy – whether desired by choice... or forced by circumstances such as a temporary or permanent separation, perhaps death. A few drops in the nightly bath can diminish the desire for sexual contact. On the emotional level, marjoram can have a comforting, warming effect to ease loneliness and grief, of particular value with the transition of a loved one. Caution: prolonged use of this oil can eventually inhibit normal response. Consider marjoram only if committed to life-long celibacy, and fully realize it may deaden the emotions.

Melissa dispels fear and regret, and encourages acceptance and understanding by creating a feeling of spiritual unity. It has a special value at the time of death, especially when it is sudden – adding shock to grief, offering great support to those individuals and their families confronted by an impending transition. Melissa helps some to remember past lives and others to have a vague recollection. It is good for devitalized,

dull, flabby skin. Lemongrass and lemon verbena are often substituted for true melissa which is >$1/drop.

Mugwort as an herb – with cedar, juniper and sage in a smudge stick – is used to purify people and places. The herb is used to make dream pillows. While these are safe, the oil is a hazard; avoid during pregnancy.

Myrrh gives confidence, courage, stability and strength; like frankincense, it strengthens and enhances spirituality. Facilitating benediction and meditation, it has special value for those who choose to move forward emotionally as well as spiritually. The anti-septic, anti-fungal qualities of myrrh assist in healing cuts and wounds. Especially good for throat, mouth and gums... two drops in 8 oz of water: gargle; beneficial for respiratory challenges.

Neroli aka **Orange Blossom** connects with High Self, facilitating an open heart, blossoming with love and joy. Enhancing the aura, it spiritualizes sexual union. Use a single drop in 1 oz coconut oil to anoint the body. A single drop inhaled from a tissue or 3 drops in the bath while holding the visualization of this sacred union is an ideal preparation. Neroli brings relief from anxiety and emotional stress... eases fear, grief, shock or hysteria. Rejuvenating for the skin, it promotes restful sleep.

Orange essence is derived from the rind by simple pressure. Orange essence nourishes feelings of joy and creates a cheerful atmosphere. It promotes mental and emotional balance, dispels gloom, restores positive feelings, and facilitates easy assimilation of new ideas. Orange promotes digestion... fluid and lymphatic drainage... and restful sleep. Revitalizing and energizing, orange essence is a good skin toner.

Palmarosa enhances the energies of the healing area with a single drop on a quartz crystal or generator crystal cluster – emanating anti-septic and anti-viral properties. With dry skin, it rejuvenates skin cells. It provides a fresh, rose-like floral that blends well.

Patchouli facilitates fluid flow – physically, emotionally and sexually. It grounds and integrates our energies; keeps us in touch with physical self. So powerful it is used in a blend. Small amounts of patchouli stimulate the nervous system; larger amounts act as a sedative. Anti-bacterial, anti-fungal and anti-septic qualities make it useful for skin conditions; an insect repellent.

Peppermint dispels pride, which is often a mask for feelings of inferiority... awakens the inner child inspiring excitement and enthusiasm, clears negative energies, and stimulates all aspects of the mind: concentration, decisiveness, discernment, and memory. A general stimulant, peppermint has a sedative effect in times of shock or hysteria. Excellent for nausea and headaches, blended with lavender for digestion and elimination. Anti-septic for the skin; astringent tonic for oily skin. Dilute for sensitive skin. One drop in water for mouthwash.

Petitgrain aka **Orange Leaf** brings clarity to the mind by easing fatigue, and enhancing memory. It strengthens our recuperative abilities, promoting easy digestion and sleep. It provides a fresh, invigorating floral of a bitter note that blends well.

Pine particularly invigorates male endocrine energies, cleansing and promoting feelings of energy and balance. A strong anti-septic, it enhances breathing, digestion and urinary function. Pine is beneficial for skin prone to acne, although it can be a skin irritant; always dilute; a fresh, woodsy, balsamic fragrance.

Rose expresses the quintessence of Love... healing the heart – both Personal Love and Universal Love. A gentle aphrodisiac spiritualizing the sexual experience. Rose helps wrinkling skin. Anxiety and stress respond to rose and jasmine; if severe, add a drop of marjoram.

Rosemary enhances concentration, mental clarity, memory and creativity. The invigorating aroma alleviates physical, emotional and mental lethargy. It strengthens the liver and gall bladder, the heart and lungs, and the immune response system. Beneficial for the scalp and oily hair, and for the skin increasing circulation; as a tonic it can prevent pimples and blackheads, and is an antiseptic for wounds and burns. Used in the morning, rosemary serves as a psychic protector and a stimulant. Used later in the day, it can lead to sleeplessness.

Rosewood enhances meditation. A drop at the temples and forehead alleviates headache. A gentle aphrodisiac, it eases the symptoms of menopause. Rosewood rejuvenates the skin and serves as a deodorant. It provides a sweet, slightly woodsy, rose-like fragrance that blends well.

Sage connects with wisdom, and is used in conjunction with meditation and visualization. It helps dry skin recover elasticity. A bit harsh, it is strongly aromatic.

Sandalwood enhances connection to the spiritual world by quieting the mind and the emotions; it supports an experience of deep meditation and healing work. Enhancing the sexual experience, especially for men, sandalwood strengthens our immune response system, and tones the skin. It is at once persistently woodsy, with a sweet and spicy oriental fixative.

Spikenard intensifies spiritual feelings and embodies the feeling of generosity and altruism. Comforting for those who work with charities and those experiencing pain over sufferings of those involved in disasters.

Tangerine relieves tension and stress, aids sleep, helps adjust to life's changes. Avoid sun after use.

Tea Tree is the most effective, non-toxic, anti-bacterial and anti-fungal oil; good for acne, burns, dandruff, gums, rashes, bites and stings. It can alleviate athlete's foot, candida, ringworm and warts. Tea tree, blended with lavender, eucalyptus and bergamot... (all anti-virals) brings relief to oral and genital herpes, especially when applied at the first signs of an itch or sore. This blend is also helpful for shingles, which is associated with the herpes zoster virus. Other skin challenges – abscess, fungus, infection, psoriasis and rash – can be drawn out and/or relieved with a blend of tea tree, lavender and eucalyptus. Some are sensitive to tea tree oil; apply a little to the underside of the forearm as a test.

Thyme strengthens the physical, emotional and mental bodies, yet it can have the side effect of closing down the intuitive, psychic mind. It can help those who tend to be dreamy or involved in their spiritual life, to the detriment of their functioning in the everyday world. When returning to work after a long retreat or an intense time with a spiritual master, a few drops in the tub or a single drop inhaled from a tissue can facilitate re-entry into mundane reality. Thyme normalizes secretions of the sebaceous glands, yet can be aggressive; use sparingly. Thyme, lemon and coriander together can enhance the memory and increase concentration; use together or individually, while studying and before a test. Inner soles impregnated with thyme oil to kill bacteria are available; or, wipe a few drops inside Your shoes.

Vetiver is the quintessential grounding oil promoting security and stability at the root energy center, easing fear, insomnia, tension and worry. Extracted from the *roots* of a tropical grass – hence grounding qualities – it has a deep, earthy aroma. Used at the solar plexus as protection for sensitivity to "psychic junk" from others: use a single drop at the solar plexus counter-clockwise.

Ylang-Ylang flower-of-flowers fragrance releases anger, fear, frustration and shock. Anxiety and stress respond well to a blend of ylang-ylang, orange and patchouli. As such it calms the mind and promotes a meditative state; for some, it can have a soporific effect. Ylang-Ylang enhances one's sensuality and sexuality with its exotic and sweet aroma, especially appealing for men in this regard... and for women too, with the added benefit of easing PMS. Excellent for the hair and skin; it provides a voluptuous, sweet floral of the top note.

Using Essential Oils

During the Middle Ages spice merchants stole money and jewelry from the bodies of those who died from the plague, remaining healthy by rubbing their bodies with essential oils of cinnamon, clove, frankincense and lemon strengthening the immune response system. Essential oils are powerful and to be respected. Always use Caution... yet, be brave. Be Aware.

If You are unsure about the application of any oil, put it on the palms of Your hands and the soles of Your feet. The largest pores on Your body, the oils absorb quickly, positively and non-intrusively impacting health. In a few seconds, the energies are in Your bloodstream; after a half hour, they circulate through Your entire body; similarly, a clove of garlic in the shoe will be apparent on Your breath in a short time.

Air Purifiers: Bergamot, Cinnamon, Lemon, Orange, Pine.

Anti-bacterial: Lavender, Patchouli, Tea Tree.

Anti-fungal: Myrrh, Patchouli, Tea Tree.

Anti-inflammatory: blend Blue Chamomile = Lavender.

Anti-septic: Lavender, Lemongrass, Myrrh, Palmarosa, Patchouli, Peppermint, Pine.

Anti-spasmodic: blend Blue Chamomile = Lavender.

Anti-viral: blend = Bergamot, Eucalyptus, Lavender, & Tea Tree; add a drop or two of Palmarosa, if available.

Aphrodisiac Qualities: Clary Sage, Jasmine, Neroli, Patchouli, Rose, Rosewood, Sandalwood, Ylang-Ylang.

Astringent: Lemon, Peppermint.

Blood pressure: Lavender, Ylang-Ylang.

Bruises: Fennel, Marjoram.

Burns: Lavender.

Cardiovascular system: Benzoin, Bergamot, Eucalyptus, Grapefruit, Lemon, Rosemary.

Children / Inner Child Issues: Chamomile, Mandarin, Orange, Peppermint.

Cellulite: Cypress, Fennel, Grapefruit, Juniper, Lavender, Lemon, Rosemary.

Circulation: Cypress, Ginger, Juniper, Lavender, Lemon, Orange.

Constipation: Fennel, Marjoram, Rose, Rosemary.

Depression: Basil, Bergamot, Chamomile, Clary Sage, Geranium, Grapefruit, Jasmine, Lavender, Lemon, Neroli, Orange, Patchouli, Rose, Sandalwood, Ylang-Ylang.

Digestive system – Spleen / Stomach / Pancreas: {Ancients see these as one.} Chamomile, Ginger, Grapefruit, Mandarin, Orange, Peppermint, Pine.

Dreams: Clary Sage, Frankincense, Jasmine.

Endocrine energy systems (all): Angelica, Cedarwood, Geranium.

Female Issues: {Underline = Menopause; *Italics* = PMS} Carrotseed, *Cedarwood*, Chamomile, Clary Sage, *Cypress*, Eucalyptus, Fennel, *Frankincense*, *Geranium*, Jasmine, *Juniper*, Lavender, Neroli, Patchouli, Rose/wood, *Sandalwood*, Ylang-Ylang.

Gingivitis: Cypress, Myrrh, Tea Tree.

Hair: {Underline = dandruff; *Italics* = head lice} Cedarwood, Chamomile, Clary Sage, *Eucalyptus*, Juniper, *Lavender*, *Rosemary*, *Tea Tree*, Ylang-Ylang.

Headache: Angelica, Chamomile, Clary Sage, Lavender, Marjoram, Peppermint, Rose, Rosewood.

Immune response system: Bergamot, Chamomile, Juniper, Lemon, Rosemary, Sandalwood.

Insect bites: Lavender, Tea Tree.

Insect repellent: Basil, Cedar, Cedarwood, Citronella, Cypress, Eucalyptus, Geranium, Lemon, Lemongrass, Lemon Eucalyptus, Patchouli, Peppermint, Vetiver.

Joint and Muscle Aches: Chamomile, Cypress, Eucalyptus, Ginger, Juniper, Lavender, Lemon, Marjoram, Pine, Rosemary.

Kidneys: Cedarwood, Chamomile, Ginger, Grapefruit, Juniper, Pine.

Liver: Carrotseed, Chamomile, Ginger, Grapefruit, Lemon, Mandarin, Rosemary. To energize the liver and kidneys, add two drops of Carrotseed, Chamomile, Geranium, Grapefruit, Juniper, Lemon and Mandarin to 2 oz olive oil for a massage; add to a tub of soak water.

Lymphatic System: Angelica, Cypress, Grapefruit, Orange.

Masculine Issues: Clary Sage, Eucalyptus, Fennel, Frankincense, Jasmine, Pine, Sandalwood.

Meditation: Angelica, Black Pepper, Cedarwood, Frankincense, Juniper, Lavender, Myrrh, Peppermint, Pine, Rose, Rosewood, Sandalwood, Ylang-Ylang.

Mind Enhancement: Basil, Black Pepper, Cardamom, Cypress, Juniper, Lemon, Peppermint, Petitgrain, Pine, Rosemary, Sage, Thyme.

Mood Elevators: Bay, Bergamot, Clary Sage, Grapefruit, Neroli, Orange, Rosemary, Sandalwood, Vetiver, Ylang-Ylang.

Mouth Ulcers: Cypress, Myrrh, Tea Tree.

Negative Energy: Frankincense, Juniper, Pine.

Nervous system: Bergamot, Cedarwood, Lemon, Patchouli.

Pain: Chamomile, Eucalyptus, Ginger, Lavender.

Protection: Chamomile, Rosemary, Vetiver.

Purification: Cedar, Juniper, Lavender, Pine, Sage.

Respiratory system: Basil, Cajeput, Cedar, Cedarwood, Chamomile, Cinnamon (room fumigant only), Cloves, Cypress, Eucalyptus, Frankincense, Garlic, Juniper, Lavender, Lemon, Marjoram, Myrrh, Peppermint, Pine, Rosemary, Sandalwood, Thyme.

Sacred Sexuality: Frankincense, Jasmine, Lavender, Neroli, Patchouli, Rose, Sandalwood, Ylang-Ylang.

Sedative: Bergamot, Chamomile, Lavender, Mandarin, Marjoram, Neroli.

Skin: {Underline = rejuvenating benefits; *Italics* = acne or oily skin.} Basil, Benzoin, Bergamot, Carrotseed, *Cedarwood*, Chamomile, *Cinnamon*, *Cypress*, *Eucalyptus*, Frankincense, Geranium, Jasmine, *Juniper*, Lavender, Lemon, Melissa, Myrrh, Neroli, Orange, Palmarosa, Patchouli, *Peppermint*, Pine, Rose, *Rosemary*, Rosewood, Sage, *Sandalwood*, Tea Tree, Ylang-Ylang. Use special care with all citrus, Ginger, Pine and Peppermint; dilute and keep out of direct sun after use. For dry skin: Carrotseed, Jasmine, Palmarosa, Sage. For infection, fungus or rash: equal parts Eucalyptus, Lavender & Tea Tree. For eczema: Chamomile, Lavender; weeping eczema: Juniper.

Sleep: Chamomile, Frankincense, Lavender, Mandarin, Neroli, Orange, Petitgrain, Rose, Sandalwood, Tangerine, Ylang-Ylang.

Strains & sprains: Chamomile, Eucalyptus, Ginger (always dilute), Lavender.

Stress: blend: Geranium & Tangerine, or Grapefruit & Orange, or Jasmine & Rose; severe: a touch of Marjoram or Orange, Patchouli & Ylang-Ylang; individually, use Bergamot, Chamomile, Clary Sage, Cypress, Geranium, Frankincense, Juniper, Marjoram, Neroli, Patchouli, Tangerine, Ylang-Ylang.

Transitions: <u>Bergamot</u>: for the terminally ill & the family before and after death; <u>Cypress</u>: for everyday changes – house, job, relationship; <u>Marjoram</u>: for death of a loved one; <u>Melissa</u>: for sudden death, shock, grief, families facing the impending death of a loved one; <u>Tangerine</u>: for everyday changes. Sudden transitions: homeopathic *Ignatia amara* (30C); gradual: *Gelsemium* (30C).

Crystals and Stones in Vibrational Energy Medicine

Now dawns the Age of Aquarius awakening to Love, Light and Hope – the Age of the Crystal – friend, teacher, tool for change and growth. For millennia we valued and cherished crystals: their inherent beauty, their physical, their astrological and esoteric properties. Respected by shamans – Wise Women & Men – from primeval times, ancient history, through modern civilizations, frequencies of crystals facilitate commUnication with High Self, focus mental energy for telepathy, increase inner vibrations, amplifying / stimulating mental abilities to heal Yourself, others and Earth, our hOMe. The word ecology derives from *eikos logos*, study of the home. Think Globally – Act Locally is the mantra of the ecological movement. Ecology reflects our relationship and our responsibility – collectively and individually – with Mother Earth, the Universe and Cosmos. Crystals and stones resonate with and emanate Consciousness.

Clear quartz can amplify and transmit subtle vibrations. Quartz is the symbol of Elemental Wholeness, containing Four Elements of Creation. <u>Fire</u>: piezoelectric qualities; <u>Earth</u>: from which it was born; <u>Water</u>: contained within its structure; <u>Air</u>: the clarity of quartz allows passage of light. Rutilated quartz magnifies those powers.

Quartz crystal has diverse uses and properties. We make use of its piezoelectric properties in energy transmission, control and storage, and its abilities to vibrate at precise frequencies, as in oscillators. It assists purification of air by absorbing positive ions and emitting negative ions. Quartz crystals are all-purpose power tools: balancing spiritual energies at all levels of human consciousness.

Even without conscious awareness, association with quartz brings the gift of positive energies embellishing the light of Love... facilitating the growth of awareness in the freshly awakening mind. Quartz assists as we focus, direct, amplify, store and transmit physical, mental and spiritual energies. Quartz can expand Your aura, giving protection against negative energies and the debilitating effects of fluorescent lights, TV, microwaves, cellphones, laptops, any source of EMFs. Crystals improve the quality of Life as do Your dearest friends. Your existence is enhanced in their company. There are various reactions to the current use of crystals and stones: New Age? Ephemeral? A fad that will pass? Actually, this is Ancient Wisdom rediscovered. Yet some consider it the work of the devil – astonishing; something so beautiful, so spiritual; bizarre allegations!

Responding to these reactions, consider Ex 28:15-22. Yahweh instructs Moses regarding vestments for his brother Aaron, the High Priest: in their tradition, healer and mediator between God and Humankind. "You are to make the pectoral of judgment (known as the breastplate of Israel) finely brocaded, of the same workmanship as the ephod. You are to make it of gold, purple stuffs, violet shade and red, crimson stuffs, fine twined linen. It is to be square and doubled over: a span in length and a span in width. In this You are to set four rows of stones. Sard (chalcedony), topaz, carbuncle, for the first row; emerald, sapphire, diamond the second row; the third row, hyacinth (zircon), ruby, amethyst; the fourth row, beryl, onyx, jasper. Mount these in gold settings. They are to bear the names of the sons of Israel, each engraved like seals with the names of the 12 tribes of Israel."

Obviously, stones and crystals are neither new age nor the work of the devil! Crystals have been and are used in every culture. Surprisingly, every electric motor has a crystal as a basic component. Microcomputer chips utilize crystal energy; laser surgery and fiber optics are based on pure quartz crystal. Crystals hold amazing amounts of information. Crystal energy does wondrous work at the speed of light... and beyond.

Having a crystal radio in the late 40s, I'd crawl under the covers at night, while the family radio played in the living room. Mother and Dad thought I was asleep, yet, I had my own contact with the world of thought and music. Imagine a radio seemingly without a power source of electricity or batteries. Solar power had yet to be developed. Formerly known as a crystal set, it can still be purchased from hobby shops as a crystal radio kit. The only power source is a piece of germanium crystal that slides up and down a coil of copper wire, tuning into various radio frequencies. As for volume control, the earplug serves quite adequately. Especially at night, You can pick up stations from around the country. Crystal energy is fascinating. Today we are adding to our basic understanding of energy, exponentially.

All things exist in vibration. As solid as things may seem, matter is comprised of countless atoms choreographing with their quirky quarks and other minutiae, engaged in molecular structures... vibrating at specific frequencies. As for the Big Bang: dust & gases must have come from some Source: known by the Ancients as Great Spirit – the Divine Presence. Big Bang implies an explosion and mayhem, contrary to what we see. More accurately, creation is a Big Breath – exhaling Perfect Divine Order. Whatever the source, timing, or any other question, in the aftermath, we recognize the major elements of creation: helium, hydrogen, carbon, oxygen, silicon, etc. Every element differentiated by wavelength and frequency – in a word: vibration – such as color, matter, and sound.

Color is an expression of light; all light, all Life, comes from our star. Light is a vibration of the ether and travels with an *average* velocity of 186,000 mi/s – implying some rays are faster and others slower. Most rays, ultraviolet & infrared, are invisible. If light rays were a yard-stick... we can see <1/16th of an inch. We call the rays within the visible spectrum: color. Color is differentiated by vibratory frequencies. Red: 0.0000256" – Violet: 0.0000174" with other colors in between. Below red: infrared, invisible heat rays. Above violet: ultraviolet, invisible chemical rays. Proper instruments measure these frequencies.

The various organs of our body are also differentiated by their wavelengths and frequencies... together known as vibrations. We all take our origins from the primordial vibrations of ovum and sperm. Joining, they exchange chromosomes forming the zygote and multiply. Microscopically, embryologists notice changes taking place. A primary streak forms the notochord, developing into the central nervous system. Then a cluster of cells begins to pulsate, forming the first organ – the Heart; as the circulatory system develops, so does the digestive, skeletal, muscular system, and all the rest, resonating at their own vibrations harmoniously weaving together.

After birth, there are various experiences of Life; we are exposed to traumas... toxins... tensions... and stress. Our lives may be compared to a piano. Someone playing gentle lullabies may have their piano tuned once a year. Playing ragtime, boogie-woogie requires more frequent tunings. Question: How do You play Your Piano of Life? As we experience Life with various amounts of stress, our vibrational harmonics may require re-calibrating from time to time. Vibrations of various crystals, along with the vibrations of affirmations, colors, fragrances, and tuning forks, refresh our cellular memory with frequencies of balance and harmony... restoring homeostasis. Crystals have been used from time immemorial to Reboot integrity of HeartMindBodySpirit.

The most well-known crystal is quartz: a crystalline glass-like mineral composed of silicon dioxide. It has a variety of colors from which it derives many names. Amethyst varies: lavender to purple, depending on the amount of minerals. Aventurine is popularly seen in green or peach. Citrine is yellow gold. The Herkimer Diamond is a type of clear quartz. Other types of quartz are chalcedony, flint, opal and rock crystal.

Chalcedony is milky quartz arranged in slender fibers of parallel bands including agate, which has color banding or irregular clouding with almost two-dozen varieties. Other chalcedony: bloodstone, carnelian, chrysoprase, onyx, and tiger eye. There are 3 separate categories of quartz: rock crystal is transparent, although it sometimes has inclusions; flint is hard, fine-grained quartz giving sparks when struck; opal is a translucent mineral of hydrated silicon dioxide.

Cleansing of Crystals and Stones
Whether purchased or received as gifts, it is wise to cleanse all stones. Depending on the negativity they are exposed to, clean them from time to time. One way: bury them for several hours or overnight in a bowl filled with Epsom salts. This draws out negativity, much like a salt bath draws acids and toxins from Your body. Then fill the bowl with water; let it run over the sides until the salt and negativity dissolve, and everything runs down the drain. Caution: salt may tend to pit metals and soft stones such as azurite, lepidolite, malachite, moldavite and selenite. Affecting appearance, the healing powers remain intact.
There are options: stones may be placed overnight on the earth in Your houseplants, necklaces draped over the branches; on the ground, or in water receiving

energies of indirect sun, the moon and the stars; on a large crystal cluster for a few hours to cleanse and energize them, or inside a pyramid, perhaps on a pyramid tray – containing small pyramids side by side.

Stones may be cleansed conceptually. With Intention, in meditation. Be the stones. Be in commUnion. Visualize. Give Thanks for their pristine radiance... their integrity... their coherence with Singularity... being Divine Presence in this Precious Form, at Your Service. Stones also may be cleansed through the power of Benediction. Hold Your intention / focus:

Great Spirit, Creator of All Life Everywhere... Thank You for blessing us with the gift of these stones dedicated to healing. Thank You for these reflections of Your Love, and Thank You for filling them with Your Mercy and Compassion, that they may be used as tools to heal Your children, and to honor our Beloved Mother Earth. We are grateful to be One with Divine Presence... expressing the Sacred Spirit of Love... Peace... and Harmony. So Be It. And So, It Is!

The following benediction from the Essene tradition may be adapted for other purposes – commitment ceremony, blessing a journey or new house – substituting words for those between {brackets}:

Great Spirit, Creator of All Life Everywhere... Thank You for the Love that flows through Our Hearts... for it is with this Love that We are able to see You in the eyes of every Being before Us, and as the Essence of All that Is. Thank You for sending all those Angels who stand firm in Love, Truth and Beauty, Trust, Harmony and Peace, throughout the Cosmos, those who work with Us, and are here with Us now. Thank You for opening Our Minds and Our Hearts as We manifest Love upon the Earth. And, thank You for blessing, cleansing and purifying {these stones... tools of healing.} May the Radiant Light of Eternal Life shine brightly through them, and through Us... Grateful to be One with You... here and now...   nOw is forever. So Be It. And So, It Is!

Crystals, Stones and Their Qualities

Some stones come in one color... others a variety. Whenever You have the choice of color, remember as a general rule: red, orange and yellow have a stimulating and warming action; green is neutral; blue, purple and violet have a sedating and cooling action. General effects: **Red:** physical grounding; **Orange:** emotional balance; **Yellow:** digestive balance; **Green:** opening the Heart; **Blue:** communication skills; **Purple** or **indigo:** spiritual vision; **Violet:** spiritual grounding. Rough stones have more facets, more reflection of their energy, than polished – pretty as they may be.

Agate embodies the spirit of: "God, grant me the Serenity to accept the things I must... the Courage to change the things I can... and the Wisdom to know the difference." Types of agate include green moss agate – said to bring in the energy of mountain air, devic forces of the plant kingdom... fairies, gnomes and elves, especially around the garden. Grounding energy of agate strengthens the physical body, giving courage to the mental body.

Alexandrite restores self-esteem helping appreciate the inter-relationship of all aspects of Creation, being One with Source, enhancing the pancreas / spleen / stomach complex and nervous system. It facilitates regeneration of the internal, external and spiritual bodies.

Amber is liquefied golden light electrically charged: fossilized resin from pine trees, it may be enhanced with inclusions of insects. Energizing the endocrine energy system, amber draws toxins from the body... awakening inclinations to altruism and Universal Love.

Amethyst leads us from darkness of illusion to the light of Divine Love... enhancing powers of healing, intuition, meditation and psychic abilities. Amethyst is quartz with a small amount of iron; it clarifies our feeling body and strengthens our thinking body as we experience spiritual awareness. Amethyst has beneficial effects for the throat, lungs, blood, endocrine and immune response systems. Especially healing for someone making the transition, and for those left behind to handle their grief.

Aquamarine helps meditation, promotes tranquil courage and brings clarity for creative self-expression, strengthens and optimizes liver and kidneys. Antidote for fear and phobias, aquamarine balances all levels.

Aventurine brings confidence and builds feelings of self-assurance...   fostering   faithfulness   to commitments. It transmutes anger, anguish, grief and jealousy... promoting tranquility, and alignment with Life's Purpose. Green aventurine benefits the physical heart, and balances personal love when faced with adversity. Orange aka peach aventurine brings awareness and stability to our feeling body, balancing our sentiments with the light of reason - energizing our muscles & organs by cleansing the blood, thus strengthening the heart.

Azurite helps creativity, clarity at the mental level, psychic abilities, promoting meditation, confidence, and heart-felt communication. The copper component gives strength, restoring sexual balance and facilitates electrical flow throughout the nervous system.

Beryl includes aquamarine, emerald and golden beryl. The latter promotes confidence, and inspires purity of intent. It can ease cranial trauma and spinal injuries.

Bloodstone raises our energies from the root to the heart center, with courage to take a deep, caressing breath in the present moment. Bloodstone is a type of chalcedony, enhancing physical and mental energies, vitalizing our bones, our heart and our bloodstream, normalizing iron excess or deficiency!

Boji Stones grow on stems at the bottom of a natural earth pyramid, uncovered as the earth erodes from them. Smooth bojis are female; protruding platelets are male. Together they support rejuvenation, balance female and male energies, and clean the aura.

Calcite promotes awareness of and appreciation for the creative forces of Mother Nature, helpful when studying the arts and sciences; helps the feeling body appreciate balance with female and male polarities, helps the thinking body remember astral experiences, and helps the acting body with cellular memory of its true state of perfection during challenges.

Carnelian facilitates tissue regeneration, energizes the blood, with a beneficial influence on the thinking and acting bodies. It resolves confusion and forgetfulness, bringing clarity to the present. Carnelian dissolves envy, fear, rage and sorrow, opening our heart to accept... respect... and honor our inner child with warmth and joy.

Celestite tunes into high states of awareness, cleansing the aura. It facilitates seeing and hearing clearly, both physically and mentally. Energizing the throat center, it prepares for clear communication.

Chrysocolla aka **Gem Silica** promotes strength and balance in matters of the heart and communication, giving courage to be silent when appropriate. It activates our feminine energies: compassion, creativity, humility, intuition, sensitivity and tolerance. As such it is beneficial for all female challenges: menses, childbirth, miscarriage and menopause. Chrysocolla assists men who suppressed their feeling body, enhancing sensitivity and intuition, nurturing what it means to be vulnerable in a wholesome way.

Chrysoprase supports compassion and clemency, and instills a meditative state. Imparting a feeling of joy and a light heart, chrysoprase restores sexual balance... helps see issues clearly... and readily helps recognize our talents, putting them to use.

Citrine facilitating alignment with High Self, brings cheer, hope, and feelings of warmth – raising self-esteem and attracting abundance. Promoting function of digestive organs, heart and kidneys; self-cleansing, dissipating, and transmuting negative energy. Most citrine is heat-treated quartz –> look for uniform color.

Diamond facilitates alignment with High Self, promoting abundance, energy, faithfulness and purity – all the while maintaining pure innocence. A Master Healer, it purifies and balances all aspects of our feeling body, our thinking body and our acting body.

Dioptase promotes full-spectrum holistic healing for HeartMindBodySpirit, especially benefiting the central nervous system and cardiovascular system. Instilling feelings of abundance on all levels, it promotes balance for the feeling body and peace for the thinking body. It facilitates being in the present: excellent with affirmations, healing sessions and meditations.

Emerald promotes rhythmic breathing bringing tranquility to the heart – with feelings of abundance and love as we recognize our Inner Divinity. Emerald brings life, nourishment, healing, especially for the physical body: strengthening and harmonizing mind and spirit.

Fluorite brings order out of chaos. Strengthening teeth, bones, and blood vessels, it assists in the absorption of nutrients. When used regularly this "genius stone" develops concentration and even raises IQ. Commonly used as protection for those who work either with violent people or with virulent infections, the ones so afflicted also derive benefit. Depending on the color, it works with various energy centers. Purple fluorite increases receptivity to other stones.

Fuchsite brings out the inner child, sparking enthusiasm, joyful Youth, bringing tranquility to heart and mind. Fuchsite, a green mineral often found with ruby inclusions, energizes the endocrine glands, stimulates immune function, promotes cellular regeneration and rejuvenation – affecting all tissues.

Garnet promotes compassion and love... and is used to prevent and repair RNA / DNA damage. Powerful for regeneration especially for spinal and CSF challenges, it intimately influences the bloodstream. Garnet comes in a variety of colors, the most common being red.

Granite reveals the big picture. In partnerships it is an antidote for negativity, promotes abundance, offers protection. Rich in silica, it nourishes hair and scalp.

Hematite energizes blood and circulation, feeding the brain, facilitating the thinking body – promoting courage and enhancing personal magnetism. It assists in spinal alignment, and healing breaks and fractures.

Herkimer Diamond protects from radioactive material balances RNA/DNA, and metabolism. The "attunement stone" and "dream crystal" amplifies other stones.

Jade balances the emotional body by instilling wisdom, confidence and universal love. It strengthens the eyes, heart, immune response system and the kidneys. Jade is known as a "dream stone" and a "stone of fidelity."

Jasper influences all aspects of the physical body; a valuable protector keeping one grounded on the physical plane while exploring the etheric. Jasper has a variety of colors, each with its own energy. Leopardskin jasper has an energy that attracts... inviting whatever for emotional and physical balance.

Kunzite helps addictive challenges dissolving negativity and promoting joy based on feelings of peace and love. It brings peace and balance to HeartMindBodySpirit. Kunzite can be given to children exposed to negativity and stressful situations. It helps rebuild the RNA / DNA and provides protection from radiation and microwaves.

Lapis Lazuli enhances vitality and virility facilitating connection with High Self and Spirit Guides expanding intellect, intuition and awareness. Beneficial for throat, thymus, thyroid, and the immune response system; lapis lazuli enhances communication on all levels, especially between our feeling body and our thinking body; a penetrating stone... it is an amplifier.

Lepidolite is the "calming stone" the "stone of transition." Many teachers have a grid of these stones in the classroom – a large piece in each corner. Such a grid can be useful in a board room, meeting room, treatment room, bedroom or shop. It helps re-structure RNA / DNA, and provides balance and stability... both emotionally and physically.

Malachite promotes harmonious communication and fidelity in love, relationships and partnerships; it brings to the surface what is impeding spiritual growth. Malachite helps balance the RNA / DNA, as well as the heart and circulatory system. This "stone of transformation" balances the endocrine energy system, especially the heart, pancreas, pineal and pituitary glands, spleen and thymus.

Moldavite helps connect with High Self and Spirit Guides, possibly opening other dimensions. Moldavite means molten, found in Czechoslovakia. Extra-terrestrial in origin and of gem quality, it enhances energies of other stones.

Moonstone is the guardian at the gateway to the subconscious, and balances our feminine energies. It enhances the stomach / spleen / pancreas complex, influencing the immune response system... balancing the emotional body. Moonstone alleviates female challenges associated with menses and hormonal / emotional balance, regulates the water element, skin and hair as well. Moonstone helps men tune into their feminine side.

Obsidian facilitates grounding, and offers protection internally and externally... physically and emotionally. It disperses negativity by grounding spirituality in the physical realm. Obsidian, a lustrous volcanic glass rich in silica, facilitates clarity of vision in determining the issues... and how to resolve them.

Onyx relieves stress by saturating the energy centers with frequencies of Love helping connect with High Self. Balancing the feminine and masculine polarities, it harmonizes the feeling body. Onyx imparts integrity to bone marrow and soft tissue structures.

Opal influences the pineal and the pituitary, connecting us with High Self. It enhances the function of the pancreas, kidneys and liver, benefiting the skin and eyes. It is the "stone of happy dreams and changes" and is especially comforting during childbirth.

Peridot aka **Olivine** is an excellent healing stone, accelerating personal growth by enhancing intuition. Balancing the endocrine energy system, especially the adrenals, it influences the entire body facilitating tissue regeneration, and regulating biorhythms. Peridot reduces stress and gives confidence to open the doors of opportunity: excellent for the birth process.

Petoskey Stone hexagonerie or colony coral fossilized marine life from 350m years ago, during the Devonian period, Michigan was covered with a shallow 600' sea; with a warm tropical climate, sea animals thrived. This coral was so named because it grew in colony heads that were 6-sided having an eye in the center. They broke off occasionally, falling into mud and sediment at the bottom and are found in Michigan especially around Petoskey in the Ottawa language it means "rays of dawn" or "sunbeams of promise". Used for Third Eye awakening, psychic awareness, and emotional balance... it brings consciousness of the Ocean – the origin of all life forms.

Pyrite facilitates the understanding that all things are Perfect Divine Order. Offering protection for all levels of being, it helps us to work harmoniously with others and maintain a positive outlook. Aiding intellectual pursuits enhancing memory. It helps repair RNA/DNA.

Quartz the Mother of All Crystals in its clear form influences all aspects of our HeartMindBodySpirit. It is the quintessential amplifier, enhancing the work of other stones and metals; quartz can be programmed with thoughts and frequencies dispelling negativity. Its full spectrum energy influences all levels of consciousness. Facilitating communication with High Self / Spirit Guides, quartz is excellent for meditation.

Rhodochrosite balances Divine Love, love of self and love of life. It enhances the workings of the heart, circulatory system, liver, eyes, kidneys and the intellect. This "stone of love and balance" dissolves denial /delay.

Rhodonite balances feminine and masculine energies, and enhances self-esteem and confidence; it builds the immune response system. Rhodonite grounds our heart energy putting love into action as we express our highest choices. This "love stone" brings light into dark places.

Rose quartz instills compassion, mercy and love; dissolving anger, fear, guilt, jealousy and resentment, bringing peace to relationships. The "stone of gentle love" enhances self-confidence creative expression.

Ruby assists the heart in making our highest choices. It enhances the circulatory and immune response systems, healing the physical heart – especially for controlling high blood pressure. Also good for the emotional and spiritual heart; ruby replaces any sense of limitation with courage, devotion, integrity, joy, power and service.

Rutilated quartz is silicon dioxide with inclusions of titanium dioxide or rutile, making it more electrical – intensifying everything clear quartz does. By facilitating communication with High Self and Spirit Guides rutilated quartz dispels density and negativity. Excellent for emotional, mental, physical and spiritual regeneration.

Sapphire inspires confidence replacing confusion with clarity, enhancing communion with High Self and Spirit Guides, and promotes loyal love. Sapphire influences the circulatory and endocrine energy system, benefiting all aspects of HeartMindBodySpirit.

Sardonyx provides courage by dispelling hesitation. Encouraging self-control, the "stone of virtue" attracts healthy relationships, true friends, and rich blessings.

Selenite is gypsum crystal that occurs on every continent, the most common of the sulfate minerals. Selenite calms and clears confused states of mind; beneficial for meditation, clear thinking and composing. It expands awareness, grounding spirit in Love and Light. Selenite removes energy blocks from physical and etheric bodies and other crystals and stones excellent for enhancing their properties, clearing, and charging them; excellent for protection grids, it ameliorates EMFs.

Selenite is water soluble and will dissolve if left in liquid... likewise it melts exaggerated emotions with the light force of our true essence. Selenite crystals are storehouses of information; alchemists of old are said to have recorded information to be retrieved at a later time. Selenite develops intuitive telepathic powers, strengthens the bones and teeth, soothes nerves, and enhances concentration and clarity.

Shungite has extra-terrestrial origin, and is gem quality. Between 600 million and 4 billion years ago, a meteorite crashed in Karelia, Russia – either in, or later forming beautiful Lake Onega. It is now mined for its many qualities, including its content of (Buckminster)fullerenes, soccer-ball shaped molecules found no-where else on Earth (but plentiful in space). The fullerenes in this high-carbon mineral literally draw negative energy from a person... as well as pollutants from water and foods, harmful waves from cellphones, TVs and computers, even relieves aches and pains. Shungite is an extraordinary positive stone; the only natural material known to contain fullerenes: powerful anti-oxidants brought to our attention by a Nobel Prize have a shape reminiscent of Buckminster Fuller's geodesic dome. Fullerenes in shungite cleanse water, and then infuse it with a potent healing vibration. With its active physical and metaphysical healing powers, the energy embodied within this stone is said to absorb and eliminate anything that is a health hazard to human life.

Smoky Quartz regulates the water elements in the body dissipating congestion, bringing relief especially to the hands and feet. As a protector, it facilitates recognition of who we are & our purpose in life. Smoky quartz enhances dreams and connections with our psychic powers. <u>Caution</u>: if uniformly gray, it is irradiated clear quartz.

Sodalite unites spiritual and physical, feminine and masculine; clears thought-forms from the subconscious to make way for rational, conscious thinking. Sodalite cuts through dense layers of fear and illusion... brings clarity to mind and heart and integrity to communication. It normalizes the metabolism of the pancreas / spleen / stomach complex.

Sugilite aka **Royal Azel** and **Luvulite** promotes healing by clearing negativity from all endocrine energy centers. With a special resonance for the heart, it enhances universal love and service on the earth plane, serving as a protector for those doing healing work. For children... and those doing inner child work, it helps keep or reclaim the innocence, wisdom, and magic of childhood.

Tiger Eye unites the elements of the Sun and Earth. Strengthening for the teeth and bones... it brings the energy of light to our digestive organs, helping digest and assimilate things on the physical level. By promoting tranquility and responsibility, Tiger Eye influences the emotional and mental levels. It enhances creativity... aiding spiritual awakening. Tiger Eye balances the brain, benefiting those with mental or personality challenges.

Tiger Iron a mix of tiger-eye, jasper and hematite, it puts the "tiger in Your tank." An antidote for procrastination, it increases productivity... helpful whenever expressing artistically... composing music... writing... or choosing to let creativity flow.

Topaz enhances the action of the endocrine energy system, supporting tissue regeneration on all levels. Topaz promotes confidence, creativity, joy and love – known as the "stone that brings success to all endeavors" and "stone of true love".

Touchstone helps recognize truth and deception, providing balance between steady stability and progress. It is chalcedony as a velvet-black siliceous stone; this "stone of purification" releases negativity, hostility and anger, and is readily activated by rubbing to create friction... then rubbing the stone on the area of pain. Be patient... the pain will disappear.

Tourmaline balances the endocrine energy system, bringing balance to our male and female energies emotionally and mentally. It aligns us with the forces of light, and radiates those energies to us... to those around us... and to the planet. Its high electromagnetic charge makes it a powerful healer, especially using the colors individually enhancing the purity and the splendor of their different energies: <u>Green</u> rejuvenates the masculine self, relieving fatigue, attracting abundance and prosperity. <u>Pink</u> aka <u>Rubellite</u> rejuvenates the feminine self – dissolving past emotional pain... and encouraging trust in the power of love. <u>Pink</u> Tourmaline together with Rose Quartz and Kunzite develop healthy self-love enhanced with joy... expressing enthusiasm to the world. <u>Brown</u> Tourmaline gives extra stamina during stress, and a deep acceptance of self... especially the dark side of self; it is both soothing and grounding. <u>Black</u> Tourmaline deflects negativity, resolving neuroses... gently assisting one through the "dark night of the soul".

Turquoise especially relates to the powerful expressions of the heart. It enhances the workings of the respiratory, cardiovascular and nervous systems. Should this "stone of loyalty" turn color, it is said to indicate infidelity – some say, even the *thought* of infidelity; it can also indicate imminent danger.

Wulfenite promotes the acceptance of various "other" energies at work in the world, so we can transmute them by the power of love. Enhancing our connection with High Self and Spirit Guides, it facilitates the knowledge and practice of white magic. Wulfenite facilitates transitions from the physical to the psychic, astral and etheric planes – promoting connection with ancient civilizations, as well as future civilizations; it serves as a bond among those who have agreed to meet again on Earth at this time.

Zircon promotes union at every level, and facilitates understanding that each One is a reflection of All That Is. Symbolizing innocence, purity and constancy, it is known as the "stone of virtue". In addition to healing bones and muscles, zircon is also used in the treatment of vertigo, and heals the peripheral nervous system, especially the sciatic nerve.

Uses of Stones

Abundance: Citrine, Diamond, Dioptase, Emerald, Granite, Sardonyx, Tourmaline.

Amplifiers: Herkimer Diamond, Lapis Lazuli, Moldavite, Rutilated or Clear Quartz.

Balance: Aquamarine, Aventurine, Azurite, Boji Stones, Calcite, Chrysocolla, Chrysoprase, Diamond, Dioptase, Jade, Kunzite, Lepidolite, Malachite, Moonstone, Onyx, Peridot, Rhodochrosite, Rhodonite, Tourmaline.

Birthing: Chrysocolla, Moonstone, Opal, Peridot.

Cardiovascular system: Amethyst, Aventurine, Bloodstone, Carnelian, Citrine, Dioptase, Emerald, Garnet, Hematite, Jade, Malachite, Rhodochrosite, Sugilite, Turquoise.

Children and Inner Child Issues: Carnelian, Chrysocolla, Fuchsite, Kunzite, Lapis Lazuli, Lepidolite, Malachite, Sugilite, Tourmaline.

Communication: Azurite, Celestite, Chrysocolla, Lapis Lazuli, Rutilated or Clear Quartz, Sapphire, Sodalite.

Creativity: Azurite, Chrysocolla, Topaz.

Digestive system (Spleen / Stomach / Pancreas): Alexandrite, Citrine, Moonstone, Opal, Tiger Eye.

Dreams: Opal, Smoky Quartz.

Endocrine energy system: Amber, Amethyst, Malachite, Peridot, Sapphire, Topaz.

Feminine Issues: Aventurine, Boji, Chrysocolla, Chrysoprase, Lapis Lazuli, Moonstone, Onyx, Opal, Peridot, Rhodonite, Rose Quartz, Sapphire, Sodalite, Sugilite, Pink Tourmaline, Turquoise.

Fidelity: Aventurine, Diamond, Jade, Malachite, Turquoise.

Hair: Granite, Moonstone.

Immune response system: Amethyst, Jade, Lapis Lazuli, Moonstone, Rhodonite.

Kidneys: Aquamarine, Citrine, Jade, Opal, Rhodochrosite.

Liver: Amber, Aquamarine, Opal, Tiger Eye.

Love: Amber, Amethyst, Aventurine, Emerald, Garnet, Jade, Kunzite, Malachite, Rhodochrosite, Rhodonite, Rose Quartz, Sapphire, Sugilite, Topaz, Tourmaline, Wulfenite.

Masculine Issues: Aventurine, Boji, Chrysocolla, Chrysoprase, Lapis Lazuli, Moonstone, Onyx, Rhodonite, Rose Quartz, Sapphire, Sodalite, Sugilite, Green Tourmaline, Turquoise.

Meditation: Amber, Amethyst, Aquamarine, Aventurine, Azurite, Bloodstone, Carnelian, Chrysoprase, Diamond, Dioptase, Emerald, Fluorite, Lapis Lazuli, Moldavite, Clear, Rose or Rutilated Quartz, Sapphire, Selenite, Sodalite, Tourmaline.

Memory: Calcite, Fluorite, Pyrite, Selenite.

Mind Enhancement: Agate, Aquamarine, Calcite, Celestite, Fluorite, Hematite, Jade, Pyrite,

Rhodochrosite, Rutilated Quartz, Selenite, Sodalite, Sugilite, Tiger Eye, Tiger Iron, Tourmaline.

Nervous system: Azurite, Beryl, Dioptase, Garnet, Turquoise, Zircon.

Pain: Touchstone, Tourmaline.

Protection: Fluorite, Granite, Herkimer Diamond, Jasper, Kunzite, Pyrite, Smoky Quartz, Sugilite, Zircon.

Regeneration: Alexandrite, Fuchsite, Garnet, Peridot, Rutilated Quartz, Tourmaline.

Rejuvenation: Boji Stones, Citrine, Garnet, Rutilated Quartz, Topaz (Blue or Gold), Turquoise.

Relaxation: Agate, Aventurine, Bloodstone, Dioptase, Lepidolite, Pyrite, Rose Quartz, Selenite.

RNA/DNA: Garnet, Herkimer Diamond, Kunzite, Lepidolite, Malachite, Pyrite.

Sexual (Sacred Awareness): Amethyst, Azurite, Chrysocolla, Chrysoprase, Diamond, Dioptase, Emerald, Jasper, Moonstone, Obsidian, Onyx.

Skin: Moonstone, Opal.

Stress: Kunzite, Onyx, Peridot.

Teeth and Bones: Fluorite, Lapis Lazuli, Onyx, Rutilated Quartz, Selenite, Tiger Eye, Zircon.

Transitions: Amethyst, Tourmaline, Wulfenite.
Associated with grief: Amethyst, Aventurine.
Associated with fear: Aquamarine, Carnelian.

Marcel Vogel on the Healing Power of Crystals

Marcel Vogel, senior scientist with IBM for 27 years until 1984 and the most prolific inventor in the history of IBM's San Jose General Products Division Laboratory, studied energy conversion in crystal solids, liquid crystals, magnetic coating systems, phosphor technology, optical microscopy and luminescence. A leading authority on the healing properties of crystals, his work demonstrates crystals can accelerate bone and wound healing, relieve pain, and bring remission to catastrophic illnesses. Psychics have pointed out and scientists have shown, when a person is under

emotional duress... weakness forms in the subtle energy body... and dis-ease may soon follow. Mr Vogel's life work proved crystals and other forms of subtle energy can and do release stored negative energy patterns, allowing the physical body to return to a state of wholeness.

When asked if there could be any conflict with his work and the teachings of spiritual masters such as Jesus, Mr Vogel recalled a remarkable interview in 1960 with Pope John XXIII changing his life forever. The Pope reminded Mr Vogel: The Church, the Kingdom of Heaven, is within. Mr Vogel understood when we learn to lovingly direct super-sensory forces into matter... we act in accord with Jesus' teachings: "as I have loved You, also love one another." Mr Vogel's experiences consistently led him to believe the same Divine Consciousness... the same Divine Presence... imprinted in the human Heart – is imprinted in the heart of the crystal.

Like the ancients, Mr Vogel recognized: entering into the perfection of the crystallographic form – becoming one with the inherent, coherent sacred geometry – we experience the mystical perfection of the Divine. Crystal is the most perfectly organized state of matter due to its precision, regularity and freedom from imperfections and impurities. Mr Vogel says the Heart of Healing is Love – opening to Spirit, opening our hearts in Service.

Crystal Meditation

With an attitude of Compassion, Dedication, Devotion and Gratitude... inviting Infinite Possibilities... place the terminated end of the crystal as indicated.

{Center of the Forehead} I have an image of myself, as a reliable, trustworthy person full of confidence in my future. With all my being, I believe everything is Perfect Divine Order. Total faith, free from suspicion, is bestowed upon my Pineal Gland.

{Center of Sacrum} In my mind's eye, I clearly see myself as a courageous person, strong and determined... doing those things that are mine to accomplish in Life. I have the strength and the voice power to achieve all those things that are mine to accomplish.

{Navel} I picture myself filled with... and expressing Universal Love. Any fault I notice in another that carries an emotional charge... reflects something in myself... something to work through. I relax and let go. I relate to others free from judgment and coercion. I have loving thoughts for all. I Am an expression of Divine Wisdom. I Am a reasonable, thoughtful, understanding person... full of inspirational Wisdom.

{Center of Sternum} My Innate Intelligence now freely expresses total love for all. I now picture Love for All. Divine Love. I love You. I bless and praise You.

{Front base of Neck} I imagine myself as a person who uses my voice to speak only of good things. My Word is my power. I speak only those things I choose to create. I know the power of my Word is to create what I decree. I will to use this power constructively.

{Between the Eyebrows} I know whatever I picture in my mind with feelings... I cause to come to pass. I will to use this image power to vision only wonderful things. I know once I have imagined my outcome... I have already willed the means to create that choice. I know image and feelings are the most creative of powers. I picture myself as using this image power for Love and Compassion.

{Center of Forehead} I now visualize the Light of Understanding. Divine Understanding is mine. Enlightenment is understanding in action. I always interpret Life's Divine Plan in the Light of Love. Intuitively knowing Infinite Being expresses through me... I know I Am the Light of the World. I Am always ready to follow my Inner Voice Intuition with a spiritual knowing. Knowing instinctively what to do... I willingly do it. I will to be well... and to emanate wellness.

{Below Sternum} My Life is established in Divine Order and Harmony. I Am peaceful and poised. I picture myself as being systematic in my Life Plan. I will to express my Life in a systematic, organized manner. Divine Order and Harmony are mine. I Am happy with and grateful for Divine Order and Harmony in my Life.

{Center back of Head} I picture myself as enthusiastic, eager and dynamic in doing those things that are mine to accomplish in life. I do those things with enthusiasm as an expression of awarefulness. Praise every sign of enthusiasm; encourage enthusiasm. Praise all things.

{Center of Sacrum} I picture myself as releasing all thoughts, emotions, feelings and experiences that are less than wholesome. Gratefully, I purge myself from those things that interfere with my power to heal to be whole. I willingly release every thought, condition or relationship that in any way compromises my healing. I now fill my entire being with harmonious frequencies.

{Pubic Bone} I Am full of endurance and animation... filled and thrilled with vitalizing forces of Divine Energy. I Am the ever renewing, ever blooming expression of Infinite Mind... conscious with every Sacred Breath... I Am alive... I Am alert... I Am awake... I Am joyous... I Am enthusiastic about Life and what it is all about!

Metals

Copper is highly electric. As copper wires conduct the flow of electricity, copper influences the flow of blood, bringing energy to the body, mind and emotions. Whether one feels lethargic or restless, copper brings balance... detoxifying body as well as mind... raising self-esteem. Copper facilitates the release of restrictions on the path to Self-discovery.

Gold is highly stimulating. Whether yellow or white, gold reflects the heat and energy of the sun, enhancing our masculine energies. Gold facilitates regeneration of the endocrine energy system, influencing all levels of being; it balances the hemispheres of the brain, the mind and the heart... amplifying our thought-forms.

Platinum facilitates cellular memory and RNA / DNA function. It stimulates the pineal, enhancing intuition and psychic abilities. Platinum facilitates our digestive powers, brings nutrients to all tissues, especially brain and eyes, and nurtures Consciousness of Who We Are... and... Our relationship to All Life everywhere.

Silver is calming and soothing. An excellent energy conductor, it reflects the cool energy of the moon... supporting feminine energies. From the physical to the astral, silver enhances thought, speech, communication on every level. Silver influences the liver and nurtures the eyes and skin.

Stainless steel is neither stimulating nor sedating. Traditional acupuncture uses 3 sets of needles: gold to stimulate... silver to sedate... and stainless to provide neutral energy. Neutralizing "foreign" energy such as EMFs, stainless steel necklaces also may be worn around the waist, as well as having bare feet on the ground.

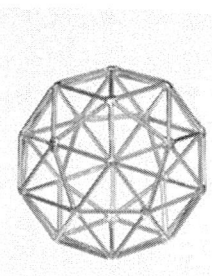

3 – PRACTICING VIBRATIONAL ENERGY MEDICINE

Vibrational Energy Medicine facilitates transformation of frequencies, bringing together energies to create Harmony and Balance, providing Harmonious Healing for the feeling body, the thinking body and the acting body. Energy Medicine recognizes and honors the choreography of frequencies on the several levels of our Be-ing. On the physical level, each cell has positive, negative and neutral energies – at the cellular level we are electrical beings. Water and metal conduct electricity. Practicing Vibrational Medicine, be well-hydrated with foods rich in minerals to facilitate.

From time immemorial doctors have said 8-10 glasses of water daily. Even with a diet rich in raw fruits, vegetable salads, vegetable juices, sprouts... these liquids are busy carrying nutrients. Several glasses of re-mineralized, re-energized distilled or r/o water between meals facilitate digestion, giving the body an opportunity to rinse. To adequately rinse toxins – to allow free flow of electrical nerve and cellular energy – it is wise to experiment: see how You feel when You drink 1 oz water per Kg of body weight. Easy to figure: divide Your weight in lbs in half, and drink that many ounces of re-mineralized and re-energized distilled or r/o water... throughout the day.

Many Hawaiian kahunas begin their day mixing 1Tbs of sea salt in a quart of water as their morning constitutional. **Experiment**. Drink an 8 oz glass of re-mineralized and re-energized distilled or r/o water **1** hour before breakfast, another **20** minutes later and a third **20** minutes before breakfast. **Repeat that before *each* meal**. What do You notice after several days? Thirty days? Improved clarity, feeling and thinking... as well as improved digestion? Freedom from headaches? Freedom from constipation? These are the common side-effects of proper hydration.

Minerals and trace elements are electrical conductors. The most abundant source: macroalgae or seaweed with many textures and tastes, growing at pH 8+. Microalgae are found in chlorella (green algae) and spirulina (blue-green algae) as well as Aphanizomenon flos-aquae – blue-green algae growing wild in Klamath Lake which has a natural pH 9-10. {Ch 10: **AFA**}

Setting the Stage for the Bodyworker

The first half of this chapter engages the left-brain for those wishing to expand their knowledge of bodywork. The second half, **The Experience of Vibrational Medicine**, engages the right-brain with holistic treatment: re-calibrating the spin of the endocrine energy centers according to Ancient Wisdom – using frequencies of colors, crystals, fragrances and sounds, including vocal cords: with affirmations. The treatment may be utilized as a Benediction of Thanksgiving and Empowerment, apart from the left-brain analysis.

Vibrational Energy Medicine is holistic: harmony and balance both physically, emotionally, mentally and spiritually. While the subconscious knows the issues we are here to resolve, and knows the relationships between various aspects of our existence, the conscious mind is mystified by the whole affair. The subconscious makes everything clear through our thought-forms and our expressions, verbally and physically. Putting together the pieces of the puzzle... we see the Big Picture. The challenges we experience with our HeartMindBodySpirit, decipher the message the subconscious is expressing.

In its basic physical expression, the body speaks about Balance in Life. Many people habitually stand with the majority of their weight on one leg... or they continually shift, one side to the other... indicating pelvic instability, many times it is pelvic rotation caused by strain at the sacroiliac ligaments. Understanding the cause... we can address the basic issues... restoring balance physically and metaphysically.

Our legs and feet are appendages; the pelvis is the true foundation, with the sacrum integral to pelvic balance. The ancients saw this triangular bone at the base of the spine as being special, that's why they named it as they did – "os sacrum" – *the* "sacred bone." In anatomy class, the professor thought sacrum meant a shovel or a spade due to its shape. He was surprised at the meaning, and suggested the ancients saw a symbol of the Trinity with its 3 sides. Plausible if they were all Christians, and were united in expressing religious devotion... highly doubtful. There is much to be learned with the Sacred Secrets of the Sacred Bone.

Eastern mysticism refers to the sacrum as the source or seat of *kundalini* – meaning coiled energy – a spiral of life force similar to the double helix of DNA – rising from the sacrum, the root energy center to the top of the head, the crown energy center. When the kundalini, coiled energy, flows we are Enlightened, as we Experience Universal Consciousness – recognizing our relationship with All Life, All Things, Everywhere as Many-festations of the One. We recognize ourselves to be an expression of All That Is. We are indeed, recognizing it or not, Infinite Being exploring... Divine Presence in action.

The significance of the sacred bone is subtle – actually, subtle action. While the cranio-sacral rhythm is separate from the respiratory rhythm, there is a subtle relationship. Inhale, and the spine extends – we become slightly taller. Exhale, and the spine flexes – we become slightly shorter. As we breathe in and out, the sacred bone gently moves, facilitating flow of cerebrospinal fluid (CSF). Electron microscopy shows CSF insulates and protects *all* nerves of the body... "to Your fingers and Your toes"! When the pelvis is torqued, rotation interferes with the free movement of the sacrum and thus, the free flow of CSF. Torquing of the pelvis frequently happens when one of the sacroiliac ligaments is strained or sprained. Ligaments, similar to bones, have limited blood supply, so allow at least 2 moon cycles to heal.

When the pelvis, as the foundation of the body, rotates... the structure resting on the pelvis – torso, neck and head – all go off center, resembling the leaning Tower of Pisa. Rather than relate to the world like this, the brain directs neck muscles *on the one side* to tighten, making the eyes level; back muscles tighten making the shoulders level. Comfortable now with how we present ourselves to the world... we go about our business. Unfortunately, the muscles on the one side of the body are tightened cables, holding the individual upright. Due to pelvic rotation, the muscles have lost their normal physiology, and are now engaged in *defense physiology*.

With chronic situations other challenges appear; long-term challenges can exhibit one eye socket larger than the other, due to a shift in the cranial bones! This can happen when muscle fibers from the cervical area interact with the tentorium – muscles covering the skull – shifting bones to one side. All this... initiated by pelvic rotation! Some people are symptom free... merely feeling out of sorts, or fatigued.

Principles for Metaphysical Applications

Reading the body, we can decipher subtle messages. Through *physiognomy* we can visually observe **signs** of organs and structures under stress. With *reflexology* the individual feels **symptoms** of pain relating to organs and structures under stress.

Some people exhibit balance in their lives on all levels. Their lessons are sometimes subtle, leading us to consider astral and etheric levels. The holistic viewpoint sees HeartMindBodySpirit as One – when the body exhibits imbalance on the physical level, we know the subconscious is telling us something. The subconscious knows everything and communicates to some extent with the conscious mind. When we tell the conscious mind what we perceive the subconscious is expressing through physical form, the conscious and subconscious can then communicate on a deeper level. Perhaps in a quiet moment we gain insight into what our challenges are – and how we can resolve them... a dream, during meditation, sitting by the fire, during a quiet walk in the woods, or precious moments before falling asleep or fully awakening.

To check for stability and balance in the person's life, it is necessary to consider the pelvis. Is there pain in the low back or running down the legs? This may be deceptive because sometimes it is absent, or the pain comes and goes. With the pressures and stresses of life, our bodies go out of alignment with some regularity; for the most part we are self-correcting. We all experience a popping or clicking sound once in a while when we bend or reach for something. The body usually repositions itself. When the body is on stress overload, when muscles are tight, when there is severe or chronic trauma or repeated micro-trauma – assistance from a bodyworker, chiropractor or osteopath may be beneficial.

Some people pay attention only to symptoms. Having pain that lasts for a few days and then goes away, they believe they *got better* as one might recover from a cold. Then... subjected to a blast of emotional stress, physical exertion or mental tension... the pain flares up again for a few days; as the exertion or tension subsides, so does the pain. We chalk it off as a sort of cold that we got over. Sometimes we have pain that stays several days, or can last weeks or months. This is generally the body's way of telling us to love ourselves: get off our feet, get bed rest. Some ignore the message and push themselves enduring severe pain… which ultimately, damages self-esteem.

Pain tells us: Do something. Some look for a pain reliever taking OTC or prescription drugs which only mask the symptoms and the cause gets buried; with continued use there are side effects. Consider the pain. Does it come and go? For how long? How long does it last? What makes it better or worse?

Listening to Body Messages
For the metaphysical causes of physical challenges, basic principles guide us. Due to crossover of nerve fibers, the right side of the brain controls the left side of the body. Challenges in these areas can relate to feminine issues: creativity, intuition, receptivity and sensitivity. Challenges can relate to feminine relationships: mother, grandmother, influential aunt or another relative such as sister, daughter, spouse, lover (former spouse, former lover) and/or our own feminine side. Perhaps self-esteem… inability to receive based on feelings of unworthiness, or imbalance in expression: reticence or verbosity, or inhibitions relating to originality and creativity following one's Inner Voice Intuition.

The left side of the brain controls the right side of the body. Challenges in these areas can relate to masculine issues: being assertive, being in charge, providing the basics in life for self and others, and bringing ideas into action. Challenges can relate to masculine relationships: father, grandfather, influential uncle or another relative such as brother, son, spouse, lover (former spouse, former lover) and/or our own masculine side. Perhaps self-esteem… inability to give based on fear or poverty consciousness, or imbalance in expression: timidity or pomposity, going to extremes as workaholic / playaholic.

The Upper Half of the Body relates to creativity and communication on the mental and spiritual levels. Challenges here relate to repression of our creative, spiritual expression.

The Lower Half of the Body relates to creativity and communication on the physical and emotional levels.

Challenges here relate to instability with our physical body and emotional life.

The Head represents the way we think… about ourselves, about others… as well as our outlook on the world, and Life. The head is in charge of the rest of the body, taking information bits from our senses, collating them and prioritizing our actions. Hippocrates taught that a blow to the head could cause bruises on the mind. He studied the effects of brain injuries and thought the mind is centered between the eyes. Romantics thought the mind is centered in the heart. Millennia later, electron microscopes and brain scans show the mind / brain connection is sophisticated. We know the brain of the cell, rather than being the nucleus, is the **mem-brane**; we also know of an intimate connection between the heart and the brain; the heart has a magnetic field 5000X that of any other organ, including the brain! HeartMath offers amazing research focused on psychophysiology, neurocardiology and biophysics… as well as clinical, workplace, and organizational studies.

While injuries to the brain can affect the mind, repeated data say changing the mind – changing thought-forms –can alter the physical brain. The mind and the brain are really two sides of the same coin. When we change our thought-forms, we change the brain's input… and output! Psychosomatic illnesses, while caused by negative, disempowering confirmations, really is a *con* job. Psychosomatic wellness is the natural corollary, brought about by positive and empowering *affirm*ations. We can overcome negative programming, and we can become empowered when affirming our highest choices with ***feeling***. Quite simply, either way – we Voice our Choice through our thoughts and through our words!

Using affirmations can affect all the senses, stimulating our feeling body and our creative forces. The vibrations of the therapist's voice rattle the tiny bones of the ears, sending vibrations along neural pathways to the brain. Knowing the affirmations, words are remembered. Speaking aloud… the person's vocal cords and ears vibrate and absorb what they are saying. Whispering, smiling, engages the feeling body. Vibrations are expressed and perceived on various levels; electrochemical oscillations redirect neurotransmitters much the same as drugs. Signals of the hypothalamus, the Great Motherboard of the Brain, communicates with the endocrine glands influencing hormonal production: pituitary, pineal, thyroid, thymus / heart, pancreas, adrenals and gonads. Known as the interbrain, the hypothalamus is part of the diencephalon, controlling visceral activities regulating metabolic processes, deeply influencing emotions, all orchestrated through a feedback loop from Your Heart of Hearts.

Head challenges indicate challenges of alignment with Divine Wisdom and Universal Love... perhaps being overly attached to our own will... or being judgmental, of self or others. Balance is possible using affirmations for confidence and trust in Divine Order... placing ourselves as instruments of Divine Will... going beyond faults... focusing on the love and compassion that invariably is to be found in every situation.

The Face reflects who we are and who we appear to be... sometimes two different entities which can express conflict. The Greek word *persona*, from which we derive the word *persona*lity, refers to *masks* that actresses and actors would wear. In early Greek vaudeville, the same individual played various parts, with a change of mask and a change of voice. Transliterated into Latin *persona* or *mask* becomes per-sonare... to sound through. This part of the body reflects our ability to face ourselves, and to face our responsibilities in Life. Masking our true selves... or our true feelings... our face is conflicted.

The ancient science of physiognomy explores messages of facial features. Facial lines indicate challenges: across the forehead = digestion and circulation; single vertical line between the eyebrows = spleen; double line = liver; horizontal line at the bridge of the nose = liver; lines from nostrils to the corners of the mouth = congested liver; lines from corners of the mouth to the jawbone = liver degeneration.

Puffiness under the eyes = swollen kidneys; swollen upper lip = irritation of the spleen / pancreas; swollen lower lip = congestion in the lower intestine. The cheeks relate to the lungs; the nose relates to the heart. Veins indicate hypertension in the associated organ.

The Eyes reflect our ability to see life – and life's issues. Clear, bright eyes indicate love and light being expressed; dull, shifty eyes indicate deception, perhaps confusion about Life's Purpose. Challenges with the eyes may indicate challenges with perceptions

of reality... caused by abandonment, emotional trauma, fear, guilt, low self-esteem and/or lack of motivation. Nearsighted tend to be introverted, focusing concern on self and what goes on from day to day; their challenge is seeing the big picture, especially relating to spiritual aspects of life. Farsighted tend to be extroverted, focusing concern on the future, and tend to procrastinate; their challenge is seeing personal relationships clearly and being close to others, taking responsibility for their choices and actions.

Lover and Beloved say: Eyes are the windows to the soul. Eyes are also the windows to the body. In the study of iridology and sclerology, the eyes serve as a map for various organs and parts of the body. *Iris* is the Greek Goddess of the Rainbow. Each iris {L. plural: *irides*: double rainbow} reflects what is going on physically, emotionally and mentally. The iris is the colored portion of the eye minus the pupil, which appears to be a part of the eye. The pupil, rather than being a structure, allows light to enter so we can see. Shining light through the pupil and observing the structures at the back, inside of the eye, we can see the condition of our circulatory and nervous system. The optic nerve is the only nerve we can see without cutting into the body. Cloudiness or clarity reflects varying states of nerve integrity.

The eyes relate to the liver. Jaundice is first apparent in the eyes with yellowing of the sclera. When the sclera has a blue shade = intestinal parasites or kidney challenge. Puffiness under the eyes, or when blue or red = swelling and congestion in the kidneys. Purple under the eyes = adrenal stress. Sties = excess protein. Discolored spotting between the eyebrow and eyelid indicates possibility of gallstones. Discolored spotting under the eyelid indicates possibility of kidney stones. Tenderness on the bony orbit around the eyes can be massaged to relieve headache and/or indigestion, the latter causing of the former.

The Ears reflect our ability to hear and to listen – to take in and assimilate communications. Ears represent ability to be open to opinions of others. Ear challenges may indicate unwillingness to hear, consider other opinions. This may indicate apathy, guilt, repression or spitefulness. Ear reflexology reflects the holographic image of the body. Acupuncturists who focus their energy on the ears are said to practice auriculotherapy. Excess wax = excess fats. Red ears = excess salt or kidney infection. Red only at the periphery = spleen. Gently massage the whole ear to relax and relieve body tension and stress. The earlobe is magnificent. Many times, pain can be relieved by firmly pinching the earlobe. A crease in the earlobe suggests challenges with the heart. Long earlobes indicate inner wisdom, and strong constitution – liver and kidneys. Our ears continue to grow as we age.

The Nose and Cheeks reflect constitutional vitality. Long, slender nose = delicate constitution. Wide nose, especially as wide as the mouth = strong constitution. Oily or shiny nose = excess animal protein. Nose and cheeks refer to heart and lungs. Bulbous nose = congested heart. Veins showing on the nose = high blood pressure. Cleft at the nose = heart murmur. Cleft at the chin = over-all vitality. Sallow cheeks = challenges with respiratory system. Full rosy cheeks = strength and vitality. Veins on cheeks = lung stress.

The Mouth and Tongue reflect ability to communicate through words… and to nourish through liquid and foods we consume. Challenges may result from inappropriate speech… feelings of resentment… or anger from withheld communication. Thin lips = frail constitution. Thick lips = strong. Peeling lips = sloughing of the intestinal wall. Cracks or blisters at corners of the mouth = possible ulcer or colitis. Jaws indicate beliefs regarding: acceptance… will… action… and reaction: lower jaw at the subconscious level… upper jaw, the conscious level.

The Neck reflects connection between spiritual and physical dimensions of being, our ability to be flexible, to see both sides of an issue. Vocal cords are the power center through which we express creatively. Challenges indicate imbalance in these areas.

The Shoulders reflect ability to carry, and to shoulder our responsibilities. Shoulders whether rounded or squared away indicate levels of self-esteem. Shoulder challenges indicate imbalance: feeling of bearing too much responsibility or carrying burdens of others. Left shoulder = imbalance with feminine responsibilities: compassion, nurturing, creativity, following one's intuition. Right shoulder = imbalance with masculine responsibilities: caring for self and others.

The Arms and Hands extend from the shoulders and the heart center, reflecting ability to handle everyday affairs of life, fulfilling responsibilities; they also indicate our ability to give and receive. Arms and hands reach for our goals, embrace life, and hold on to what we cherish. Challenges indicate an imbalance in one or more of these areas. Left arm and hand = challenges on the feminine, receptive side. Right arm and hand = challenges on the masculine, giving side. Left thumb relates to our creative will. Right thumb relates to our rational, active will. Index fingers = management and direction. Middle fingers = God-given talents and self-qualifiers. Ring fingers = helping others. Little fingers = desires, often related to sex and money.

Physiognomy tells many tales. Thumbs = lungs. Index = liver. Middle = circulation / sex. Ring = kidneys. Pinky = heart. Large moons = excess protein. Small to no moons = energetic. Short or square nails = strong constitution. Red spots = pinworms. White spots = sweets, or zinc deficiency. Vertical lines = parasites. Horizontal line = changes in environment: near the nail bed = recently; near the end = two months ago. Concave nail = parasites. Rounded nail = strong corresponding organ. Flat nail = weak corresponding organ. Biting nails = parasites.

The Lungs reflect our ability to take in the essence of Life, and to release what is toxic or stale. Shallow breathing indicates a superficial experience of life, or a desire to be someplace else. Deep breathing indicates calm, contentment and confidence. Challenges with lungs can relate to issues of repression, resentment, resistance, self-esteem or stress. Other challenges may be profound grief, or lack of inspiration.

The Breasts reflect the ability to give nourishment, and express nurturing. Breasts strongly relate to self-image and mothering energies. Challenges may indicate over-mothering… or unwillingness to provide physical or emotional nourishment. Challenges with the right breast giving nourishment, the left breast receiving.

The Heart reflects our ability to express and receive love. Being at the midpoint of the body, the heart center is the etheric connection between Middle Self and Low Self. The heart is the neutral point between the Low energy centers with their warming colors of red, orange and yellow… and the High energy centers with their cooling colors of blue, indigo and violet. The neutral color of the heart center is green, combining yellow and blue. There are two heart centers: the lower end of the sternum relates to personal love; the upper end of the sternum relates to universal love. The heart is the center of compassion and sensitivity relating to self and others. Challenges relate to anger, anxiety, fear, grief, hostility or resentment. Understanding and compassion are healing for the heart.

The Solar Plexus reflects our ability to digest food and to digest life. Liver, gall bladder, pancreas, stomach and spleen work together for harmonious digestion.

Liver >700 known functions. Only the brain and the eyes – extensions of the brain – consume more energy and have more importance. The liver is involved in desires and emotions, such as anger, and associated resentment. Compassion transmutes these feelings.

Gall Bladder stores bile created by the liver, and releases it to emulsify fats, providing warmth and energy. Challenges with the gall bladder may relate to a buildup of anger or resentment.

Pancreas, at the center of the solar plexus, reflects our balance in giving and receiving love, and assimilating sweetness in our lives. Challenges indicate loneliness, sadness, self-pity, abandonment, or possessiveness. Gratitude and joy transmute these feelings.

Stomach reflects ability to take in and process nourishment – at both physical and emotional levels. When emotionally upset due to anger, fear, grief or worry – rest or go easy on, the stomach…otherwise it can lead to indigestion and/or ulcers.

Spleen reflects our ability to handle things less than our Highest Choice. The spleen is intimately involved with digestion and immune function, creating cells that devour and eliminate toxins and wayward cells. Challenges may relate to issues of self-esteem, and may affect our desire to go on living.

The Lower Abdomen reflects ability to digest and assimilate, even on the emotional level; connected to the water element… the organs allow life to flow freely.

Small Intestine is responsible for *assimilating* nutrition through the villi, the hair-like projections, extending through the 20' of its length; stretched out, the villi would cover a basketball court.

Large Intestine is responsible for *reclaiming* necessary water (1st third) and *eliminating* waste.

Kidneys are *filtering* stations, retaining what is useful, *releasing* excess.

Bladder is a *holding* station, associated with repressed feelings, holding back one's feelings.

Genitals reflect *relationships…* to self and others, especially regarding sexual aspects of our being. Issues are desire and pleasure, power and surrender, based on commitment and responsibility. Challenges relate to the full spectrum of emotions.

The Back and Spine reflect self-esteem relating to responsibility and support regarding both self and others; on the mental level: bringing ideas into action.

The Legs and Feet reflect ability to move ahead, to be self-supporting, sustaining our existence. Challenges are based on self-esteem or fear, perhaps reflecting challenges on other levels such as confidence, courage, freedom, strength and support.

The Bones and Blood reflect foundation and support systems. Hard tissue in bones and teeth, represent condensed and crystallized forms of energy, the most energetic expression of life. Bones support flesh and fluids, while spiritual energy supports thoughts and feelings – which show up clearly in mental images, emotions and communications. A break indicates tension in the spiritual body – a challenge to continue the present state. Change is in order… refer to the associated body part. Blood forms in the bone marrow; challenges reflect stability and fluidity in life.

The Muscles and Skin reflect our inner and outer support systems. Muscles are the underlying structure providing the basis of movement for our physical form, which are covered by the skin, relating to self-image. The skin is our largest organ; its principal function: protection from outside elements and when intestines are over-burdened – elimination of excess toxins from within. Rash = irritation. Boils or pimples indicate anger or unexpressed emotions boiling from the inside.

Healing Our Challenges

Some challenges in life bring about mental or emotional pain that can show up as physical dis-ease. Causes may be wide-ranging: challenges understanding the meaning and purpose of life; issues of honesty, integrity relating to self-esteem; expressing understanding or love for self or others, or challenges with repressed emotions.

Healing means removing the causes of the challenges. Causes find roots in thoughts, expressions and feelings. Conscious thoughts, belief systems, unconscious thoughts, all combine to create our feelings – which *more than anything else* affect us at the cellular level. When we affect the cells, and we affect the tissues and organs of our physical bodies. Feelings also influence and affect our experience of the world around us.

Choosing to heal the body or circumstances of life begins by healing our feelings. Often it can be as simple as choosing to feel differently. Changing how we *feel*, changes the way we *think* on the conscious level, influencing unconscious thoughts and belief systems... and changes our Reality. Changing our attitude toward others, they change their attitude toward us. Changing our attitude toward life, life treats us differently. "What we achieve inwardly, changes our outer reality." –Plutarch

1st Step: identify the causes of our challenges. Focus to transmute them. This requires an attitude of gratitude, nourishing feelings of love, understanding and compassion. Practice with Yourself first, and then move outward to include others. The following formula can be handwritten, and spoken aloud with feeling.

"My challenge is, I feel (anger, anxiety, apathy, fear, grief, pain or unconscious – choose one of these negative emotions or insert Your own) because / about (here write the circumstances that prompted the experience of the negative emotion) and my choice is to transmute the (name the negative emotion again) into (awareness, enthusiasm, courage, joy, peacefulness, power, or understanding – each of these is an aspect of Love that transmutes everything) and I empower (myself / others) with (name the qualities / feelings You choose to instill)."

With feelings of negative emotions, especially when they creep in and distract You from being fully and completely present, use this formula. Repeat as required: fully aware of Your Sacred Breath, aware of the energetic charge. This tool helps regain focus. Awarefulness brings rejuvenation and enthusiasm.

"My challenge is, I feel grief because my wife of many years has departed, and my choice is to transmute the grief into joy. I empower myself with the knowledge that we were together for the perfect length of time for both our souls' growth... and I further empower myself knowing my life is divinely guided...always going in the optimal direction at the optimal time."

Deep breathing is a powerful tool to be in the moment. Here and nOw. Practicing 5-10 minutes at a time creates a habit for daily living. Warm-up. Stretch Your lungs with 3 deep breaths, exhaling completely. Caress the bump at the roof of Your mouth with Your tongue. Practice allows You to be fully and completely present at other times through the day: driving, chopping vegetables, etc. During times of stress simply say: "Here is another opportunity to take a deep, caressing breath!"

Holistic Health: Curing or Healing
People looking for a cure search for Dr Fixit. Jonathon Swift says "develop a close relationship with Dr Diet, Dr Exercise and Dr Merriman to experience healing for what ails us." There is a difference between curing and healing.

Curing seeks to reduce physical symptoms, remove disease or correct injury. It may involve drugs, surgery or lifestyle changes recommended by a doctor, who is seen as the primary person responsible for our health.

Healing 1st affects the person spiritually... then mentally, trickling down to the emotional level... which "directs" the denseness of the physical body. Our innate intelligence – inborn knowledge – guides us to balance, harmony or homeostasis. With spiritual energy compromised by congesting lifestyle choices, there is susceptibility to health challenges. With spiritual energy supported by TLC – Therapeutic Lifestyle Choices – there is optimal energy, and we easily return to health.

Healing is being whOle once again. Putting our spiritual house in order, we regenerate healing powers for our feeling body... and our thinking body. We feel One with All and we assume our rightful role as an equal partner with Mother Nature. This is in keeping with current studies, and advice from the National Institutes of Health: "Why medicate? Meditate!" NIH recognizes Lifestyle Medicine which, interestingly enough, grew from a paradigm shift in Consciousness in the 60s... *psyche-delic* – literally, in Greek, *soul-revealing*! New World Awakening came to humankind and forced Western culture to look at the Perennial Questions from an ancient, holistic perspective.

From time immemorial, there have been retreats where the afflicted could return to Mother Nature's Ways. Essene communities understand, respect and honor the primal, holistic relationship between our thinking bodies... our feeling bodies... and our acting bodies. Explained today through fractal geometry, Essenes perceive our Body on the planet a microcosm for the macrocosm: Earth a microcosm for our Galaxy, which is a microcosm for All Life Everywhere!

Plasma physics show macrocosm – microcosm are holographic in the physical and singular in the spirit. When germinated mustard seeds can pick up a signal from Ursa major, or any other "singular point" out there, we must recognize plants and planets communicate. Everything simply is an Expression of I AM that I AM! Nicholas of Cusa, 15th century mystic, says "Divinity is the enfolding and unfolding of everything that is. Divinity is in all things in such a way that all things are in divinity." Such is the nature of Divine Presence... such is the Essene Tradition.

An Essene Farm, Retreat, or Center can range from grandiose to simple, perhaps an individual, or welcoming family answering the call for Compassionate Service and an expression of Singularity. The movement, the shift happening today with the expansion of Lifestyle Medicine as a comprehensive approach to Health Care, has grown exponentially from a tiny seed... a wheat seed... actually multitudes of them... grown for healing wheatgrass juice by Dr Ann Wigmore, who had a triple PhD – Divinity, Psychology and Metaphysics. Rather than surgery, she reversed her colon cancer taking this juice both orally and rectally. Viktoras Kulvinskas, DD, PhD, was advised by Norman Walker, ND, to seek out Dr Ann's healing juice... which opened his scientific eyes and as Director of Research, Viktoras developed the concept of sunflower & buckwheat greens... significantly adding to the consciousness of chlorophyll and enzymes, as well as fermented foods being sources of friendly bacteria, aka probiotics.

Together they created an Essene Retreat dedicated to healing... making whole... the feeling body, the thinking body and the acting body. After 30 years offering those who came to Hippocrates Health Institute in Boston the possibility of healing HeartMindBodySpirit, HHI moved to West Palm Beach, and Ann Wigmore Natural Health Institute moved to Puerto Rico. These two have inspired other Essene retreats such as Dr Gabriel Cousens' Tree of Life Center in Patagonia, AZ and Optimum Health Institute in San Diego and Austin TX.

Holistic healing opens Your innate healing powers, demonstrated where the outcome predicted by medical science is different from what happens. Many do recover from terminal illnesses, and recover physical abilities that were supposedly lost forever. Could it be a mis-diagnosis? a miracle? or self-healing: being emotionally, mentally and spiritually open to miracles. Even when people are challenged with a terminal situation on the physical level, healing can take place emotionally, mentally and spiritually... enhancing Quality of Life, and their perspective for the future – reducing medications... affecting clarity and attitude.

Ability to self-heal depends on how You feel and think about Yourself... and Your place in the Universe. Being angry or upset with Yourself for experiencing the traumas of Life delays Your self-healing. Sometimes You can easily transmute Your anger or Your pain, learning Lessons of Life, enhancing Your healing powers. Holistic health is accepting responsibility for Your Own Healing Journey by nurturing and experiencing balance in Your feeling body, Your thinking body and Your acting body. This process is Holistic or Harmonious Healing.

When choosing Harmonious Healing Be Confident... Breathe... You are Infinite Being creating, Here and Now, in this space and time on Earth. Feel Love for Yourself. Feel Love for All Life Everywhere. **Mirror Therapy** is a wonderful place to begin healing. Most give only a casual glance at the mirror... adjust make-up or tie... hair or mustache. How frequently do You take the time to smile at Yourself? This registers in Your subconscious *and* conscious mind. You are worthy of a greeting, building self-esteem You open the Doorway of Possibilities.

Go deeper... look into Your eyes. Get close to the mirror, close to Yourself. Look in Your eyes looking back at Yourself... and say out loud: "I love You. I Am so blessed." Pause. Reflect. "You Are so Blessed!" Listen. "Be still... and know... I Am God!"

"I Am a wonderful person" speaks to Your thinking body; "You are a wonderful person" speaks to Your feeling body. Take the time to speak to both. This applies to all affirmations. The side-effects: healthy self-esteem, leading to collateral expressions of kindness.

When You experience true love of Self... when You experience Yourself as being whole and complete... within Yourself... You are then capable of entering a mature relationship. Looking for the other person to complete some emptiness within Yourself will always be frustrating. Completeness is from within. **Know Thyself!** Then when You love, You Gift Your whole complete Self – Light side and Shadow side – to the Beloved.

When Lover and Beloved experience themselves as whole and complete, freely sharing the Gift of Self with the Other, the stage is set to experience ecstatic, spiritual dimensions of human Life that can only be found in **Special Relationship**. Many are happy and blessed "until death do they part". Others become acutely aware that the person they are with, is different from the person they married; they were together for the perfect amount of time for *both* of them to learn some of Life's Lessons, and now it may be time to move on... expanding Consciousness. Others choose "living together" for various amounts of time. Still others are "players." Choice... be free from judgment; everyOne is learning Lessons required for growth along their Sacred Journey.

Consider frequencies and vibrations: Hearts inter-mingle and entwine, and carry each other's vibrations – subtle energy fields – for 30 days. The corollary is profound.   If Your Special Someone was intimate with others, her/his subtle energy field is also carrying the vibrations of everyone else who *they* were romantic with in the previous 30 days! Be Wise. Be Aware.

Avoiding the helter-skelter... cleanse the subtle energy fields. Many simply choose to be Born-Again Virgins. A hug and a kiss are in keeping with the cleanse; anything romantic that gets juices flowing is best avoided. Allow 30 days for Your subtle systems to return to normal with complete integrity.

Be patient... do Your M.E.D.S. and hold the Vision of Your Wish Fulfilled! Some have been Born-Again Virgins 10-20 years before finding the Special Someone they'd be comfortable living with to enjoy their Sacred Journey. Know Thyself first, as a Way of inviting that Special Someone to appear; it happens in Perfect Divine Order!

Caution: if Your 1st experience together is alcohol / drug-related, it will tinge the purity, and set the *tone* for what is to come in Your Relationship. Likewise passionate, wild sex... which is certainly fun, on occasion. Let the choice for Your **1st** Encounter be Sacred Sexuality. Courting... Your Sacred Relationship may be enhanced with a seminar in Tantra Yoga, before entangling and entwining forever!

Physical Balance: Checking the Foundation
Bodyworkers and massage therapists play detective. Before putting the puzzle together, gather the pieces. Look at their gait and standing posture from the front, back, and sides. Trust Your Inner Voice Intuition. Since You are in Loving service, Your High Self guides You. Relax and let Your senses do their work. Take Your time... Observe... Breathe... Feel Love.

Beds are best avoided; they are soft, and more important: the energy of the bedroom is sleeping and making love. While laudable and great sources of healing, they differ from healing energy work we pursue at this time. Ask the person to lie on the treatment table face-down in the neck cradle, breathing comfortably. Stand on the right side – Intention: Focus – take a deep, caressing breath. Prepare the person for muscle testing by checking for a strong muscle group. Have them extend their right arm straight out to the side. Place Your right hand on their forearm below the wrist and tell them "I am going to gently pull Your arm toward Your feet, and I'd like You to resist... hold it right there." Then pull for 1 second with 4-5 lbs pressure. Muscles will either lock in place or be spongy; if the latter, find a muscle group that is strong... or use energy work to create one. With leverage You can overpower anyone. Rather than being about strength, it's muscle response with light pressure, for a short period.

With a strong muscle group, ask the person their name. When they respond, say: Hold, and pull for 1 second with 5 lbs of pressure. It will lock in place. Then: "Say: I am Albert Einstein or Helen Keller." When they respond, say: Hold, and pull. It will be spongy, perhaps totally weak. This shows we can communicate on another level – the level of Truth! The person, in the subtle recesses of the mind, may think the muscles were slightly fatigued, so have them repeat their real name and say: Hold, and show them the difference between... what is True... and what is False. Then briefly explain You will be asking non-verbal questions. {To explain the **physiology of muscle testing**, see: *Your Body Doesn't Lie*, by John Diamond, MD, 1989. From a holistic perspective, *Power V/s Force*, as well as the complete works of David R Hawkins, MD, PhD.}

Given the importance of the sacrum, check there first. With the person lying face down, gently rest Your left hand on the upper sacrum and say Hold. Strength indicates a balance of energy between the sacrum and the lumbar vertebrae. A spongy response indicates interruption of the flow of energy. The question is: has the sacral base moved forward or backward, in relationship to the fifth lumbar vertebra?

Most instances doing this test, when You place Your left thumb on the sacral base and gently push headward, You will find a weak muscle response, because that accentuates the shift of the sacral base moving *anterior* in relationship to L5. Next with Your thumb, gently pull the sacral base toward the feet. You will find a strong muscle response indicating the sacral base has shifted forward in relationship to L5, and pulling in that direction brings integrity to the L5 / sacral junction.

Gently coax the pelvis to the point of balance; roll up two small towels to act as 2-3"wedges. Place them under the iliac crest of both hipbones at the front, pointing down and toward the center – along the inguinal ligament. These wedges provide a fulcrum; the body weight gently shifts the pelvic structure, moving the pelvis toward the direction of balance and well-being.

To verify the body is happy with this arrangement, begin again: rest Your left hand on the sacrum, testing the person's right arm with Your right hand. When You get a strong muscle response, the body is pleased. Otherwise, remove the wedges... it is always preferred to do nothing or too little, rather than something inappropriate.

If when You place Your left thumb on the sacral base and gently push headward You get a strong muscle response, the sacral base has moved posterior in relation to L5. Gently coax the pelvis to the point of

balance; place the two small towels under each femur head, pointing up and toward the center.

To verify the body is happy with this arrangement, begin again: rest Your left hand on the sacrum, testing the person's right arm with Your right hand. If You get a strong muscle response, the body is pleased. Otherwise, remove the wedges.

Accentuate the work of the wedges: move to the left side of the table; have them grab the head of the table or the face cradle and gently pull headward breathing in, and relax breathing out. Place Your left hand on their occiput, and Your right hand on their sacrum, pointing toward their feet. Breathing in, gently stretch Your hands apart, manual traction on the spine. As they breathe out, relax Your hands and repeat 5 times. Remove the wedges.

Have the person turn from prone to supine to accurately ascertain pelvic balance or pelvic rotation. Go to the foot of the table and extend the feet to the sides. Say, "Hold Your legs apart, as I pull them together." Let them tense the leg muscles for 1-2 seconds, then say, "OK, bring them together." Then quickly bring the feet together with Your thumbs underneath the medial anklebones. Are the thumbs even... or is there a difference between them? If the thumbs are even, there is no gross rotation of the pelvis; there may be something on a subtle level, so continue Your search. With a difference... ¼ – ¾" is common... there clearly is rotation of the pelvis; the foundation of the body has shifted. This indicates a strain on the sacroiliac ligament on the side of the short leg. There may be a short leg from birth or from some trauma, so do the following checks. Compare tension, tenderness or ticklishness on the inside of both legs where the muscles of the thigh insert, immediately above the knees; then check the outside of both legs, immediately above the knees. If there is true rotation of the pelvis, the classical indicators are a difference of feeling on the *inside* of the short leg, and the *outside* of the other.

Check whether rotation is localized at the pelvis from the head of the table. Have them place both hands on their tummy, keep the legs straight and raise both legs at the same time. Observe any sway, usually to the side of the short leg; observe how challenging it appears. Then tucking the chin slightly to the chest and pushing gently on the top of the head, ask to do that again. If it is more challenging, it is a simple pelvic rotation; if easier, there is pelvic rotation & complications of cervical involvement. Normally with this orthopedic / neurological test: they are equally easy to perform.

Verify Your assessment, checking integrity of the inguinal ligaments running diagonally from the pubic bone to the iliac crest on both sides. There is an upper and lower part, each about four fingertips wide. Keeping their eyes open, breathing evenly... stand on one side facing the person's opposite shoulder; have them hold their arm straight to the ceiling. Say, Hold and gently pull toward their feet, to verify a strong muscle group. Then place Your four fingertips snugly together at the upper inguinal area below and diagonal to the anterior superior iliac spine. Push down gently and say Hold, at the same time. Repeat at the lower inguinal area above the pubic bone. Do the same test on the opposite side.

The inguinal ligament is strong and can generally withstand slight pressure; with a balanced pelvis, the muscle response will be strong. When the pelvis is rotated, the inguinal ligament is already under strain, and the additional pressure of Your fingertips is enough to cause a weak muscle response. It can be weak at one, or all four inguinal areas.

Balancing the Foundation
Following logic based on Your assessment... and using principles of physics... which were both applied by Pythagoras and Hippocrates to bring about pelvic balance, place a wedge under the iliac crest to support the sacroiliac on the short leg side... and another wedge on the opposite side where the head of the femur joins the acetabulum – pointing to the sacrum.

This sends a signal to the brain that realignment of the pelvis is in process. Verify the accuracy of Your assessment and placement of wedges, repeat the four inguinal tests making sure they are strong in all four areas. Acting as a fulcrum, the wedges send a message to the muscles of the low back, reminding them of their proper role in pelvic balance. At this point, place a bolster under their knees.

Further enhance the power of the wedges and the flow of energy; go to the head of the table and gently stretch muscles of the upper back and neck. Simply take the head in both hands bringing the neck through the

normal range of motion. The Cervical Stair-step has four levels influencing first the motor unit of C7-T1, then C5-6, C3-4 and finally C1-2. Cradling the head in both hands and keeping as close to the table as possible to influencing C7-T1, keep the head straight with the ears maintaining a parallel plane to the shoulders and move it from side to side. Then bring one ear toward the shoulder, gently stretching; then do the same on the other side. Then turn the person's head to one side, as though looking over their shoulder; then do the same on the other side. Return the head to the original position on the table and watch the person as they take in a deep breath.

Then as the person exhales and relaxes... lift the head 1" off the table to influence C5-6; repeat the same procedure. Then lift the head 2" off the table to influence C3-4; repeat. Then lift the head 3" off the table, this time slightly tucking in the chin, to influence C1-2; repeat. Then gently stretch the neck muscles obliquely to both sides. Finally, hold the head in both hands and ask the person to take 3 deep breaths. Gently pull the head with inhalation... and push toward their feet with exhalation. When complete, Ask the person to inhale deeply; as they exhale... slowly remove the wedges if any were used, keeping the bolster under the knees.

Now, physically balanced, relaxed and receptive, we can let the subtle energies flow.

The Experience of Vibrational Energy Medicine
The following attunement is offered for Your consideration. Bodyworkers may share this experience as part of their session. Consciously reading the script alone, is a Blessing for Your Journey!

Suggested music: *The Ultimate Brain: Opening the Heart*, Tom Kenyon, MA in the key of F – Heart – connects right and left hemispheres of the brain. Nature's Symphony: Chakra Balancing Aromatherapy Kit – with gemstones: www.NSaroma.com. Quality tuning forks are found at https://tama-do.com. The gold-plated, Woven Spiral Star with Light Ring and the Golden Rectangle: https://https://iconnect2all.com/

Placement of Stones – Explaining the Process
Use stones You may have with corresponding colors, or quartz, rutilated quartz or even selenium, and whatever tools You are comfortable with, such as a

pendulum. As a rule, rough stones are more energetic than polished.

Other stones may be helpful. With purple fluorite at the foot of the table on the left side, our receptive side... we become receptive to the energies and workings of other stones in general. Snowflake obsidian at the foot of the table on the right side, our out-going side, grounds us. Near the feet, lepidolite – the calming stone; at the head of the table, a cluster of amethyst, strengthening the mind – influencing the hormone-producing endocrine glands, and immune functions; celestite and dioptase near the head, influence the auric field.

When introducing someone to the experience of Energy Medicine, share the information found in Ch 10: **Thymus Thump** and **Tongue Awareness**. Explain the energy tool – although the Woven Spiral Star is 2-dimensional, it gives energy of a 3-dimensional double star tetrahedron within a sphere. Some see the 6-pointed star and recall the Star of David, thinking it is a Jewish star. Actually, this symbol was used in Sumerian Temples, 2000 years before the time of Abraham. One triangle points up, the other down, symbolizing as above, so below. In the middle we have the Golden Mean Rectangle, which is the basis of Sacred Geometry, based on the phi ratio: 0.618. This ratio was used building Greek Temples and upscale homes, as well as placement of the Sphinx and Pyramids, and used by architects to this day.

A perfect Golden Mean Rectangle means when You divide the long side by 0.618 and drawing a line across, it forms a perfect square... and You are left with another perfect rectangle. Divide that long side by 0.618 and You create another square... left with another rectangle. On to Infinity... creating a vortex of energy. This vortex is seen in a cross-section of a nautilus shell. Place the Golden Mean Rectangle over a map of Egypt with the Sphinx at the center; pyramids, rather than being in a straight line, are on the arc of the vortex. The Woven Spiral Star facilitates energy in the meridians. {Ch 10: **Secret of the Spheres**}

Before the session clearly explain the procedure because it's easier for them to visualize with their eyes closed... when striking the tuning fork may be startling, so explain: "For each energy center, I bring a fragrance then strike the tuning fork so You can hear and feel the vibration; and I will say affirmations. Finally, as I use the Woven Spiral Star and move over Your meridians, I will ask You to repeat affirmations from Your Heart of Hearts. When we are complete, I will sit for a few minutes in quiet Thanksgiving."

With them face up on the treatment table, pillow under knees relieving pressure at the low back, remind them – as much as possible, gently caress the roof of the mouth, with mindful breathing – to encourage communion between Heart and Pineal centers.

{Adjust the following Script as You see fit.}
Place Your arms at Your sides palms up – this is a receptive position. I Am placing boji stones in the palms of Your hands. The smooth stone goes in the left hand, controlled by the right brain, balancing female energies. The stone with the projectiles goes in the right hand, controlled by the left brain, balancing male energies. Bojis balance those energies; every woman has testosterone; every man has estrogen, produced by the adrenals. Boji stones orchestrate balance.

{As You place the stones:} At the top of Your forehead... amethyst instills the crown energy center with creativity, especially on the spiritual level.
At the third eye energy center... sodalite enhances Your Inner Voice Intuition.

At the throat energy center... blue lace agate encourages honesty and integrity in communication.
Rose quartz and green aventurine soothe the heart, especially in the face of adversity. We have 2 heart centers: personal love, and universal love.

Between the navel and the rib cage... citrine energizes the solar plexus center – enhancing the liver, gall bladder, pancreas, stomach and spleen – facilitating digestion and assimilation on the physical level.

Between the navel and the pubic bone... peach aventurine facilitates digestion and assimilation on the emotional level.

At the pubic bone... red jasper stabilizes and grounds the root center.

The Practice of Vibrational Energy Medicine
Now, take in a deep, caressing breath... (as the person exhales, surrounding Yourselves with Golden Light and Love, say:)

Great Spirit... Creator of All Life Everywhere,
Thank You for the Love that flows
through Our Hearts,
for it is with this Love that We are able to see You
in the eyes of every Being before Us
and as the Essence of All that Is.
Thank You for sending all those Angels
who stand firm in Love, Truth and Beauty,
Trust, Harmony and Peace
throughout the Cosmos,
Those who work with Us
and are here with Us now.
Thank You for opening Our minds and Our hearts
as We manifest Love upon the Earth.
And Thank You for blessing, cleansing and purifying
these stones and tools of healing,
that the Radiant Energy of Eternal Life
shine brightly through them, and through Us.
We are grateful to be One with You, Great Spirit...
Here and Now...
now is forever.
So Be It!
And So, It Is!

~~~~~~~~PITUITARY ENERGY CENTER~~~~~~~~

Now take in a deep, caressing breath... bringing in the fragrance of lavender.

(Bring the cap of the scent to the nose, gently moving from one nostril to the other as the person breathes in and out 3X. Recap the bottle; pick up the B tuning fork. Strike it gently holding the stem and bring the open end to the person's left ear, saying:)

Now visualize violet light coming in through the crown of Your head.

(Pause for 20-30 seconds allowing the sound to register in both conscious and subconscious minds. Then gently strike it again placing the stem of the tuning fork on the amethyst, saying:)

The vibration of the violet light fills every fiber of Your being, as You mature in love and devotion.

(Strike the tuning fork a 2nd time, placing stem on stone:)

With Truth and Love, You respect Yourself and Others.

(Strike the tuning fork a 3rd time placing stem on stone in silence, until vibrations begin to diminish.)

~~~~~~~~PINEAL ENERGY CENTER~~~~~~~~

Now take in a deep, caressing breath... bringing in the fragrance of cedarwood.

(Then strike the A tuning fork bringing it to the person's ear, saying:)

Now visualize indigo light coming in through the crown of Your head, bathing Your eyes and ears, Your nose and mouth.

(Pause, then strike it again, placing the stem on the sodalite, saying:)

The vibration of the indigo light helps Your Intellect to understand that, as You see through loving and thankful eyes, as You hear through loving and receptive ears, and as You speak with words of Love and Wisdom...

(Strike the tuning fork a 2nd time, placing stem on stone:)

You radiate the Harmony and the Glory of Great Spirit, the Creator of All. You perceive, intuit, and express Your Highest Choices.

(Strike the tuning fork a 3rd time placing stem on stone in silence, until vibrations begin to diminish.)

~~~~~~~~THYROID ENERGY CENTER~~~~~~~~

Now take in a deep, caressing breath... bringing in the fragrance of blue chamomile.

(Then strike the G tuning fork bringing it to the person's ear, saying:)

Now visualize soft blue light coming in through the crown of Your head, bringing it down to Your neck and shoulders, Your arms and hands.

(Pause, then strike it again, placing the stem on the blue lace agate, saying:)

As You use these parts of Your body in communication, the vibration of the blue light is soothing, and empowers Your ambitions to be gentle and loving with Our Mother Earth and All Her Children, including Yourself.

(Strike the tuning fork a 2nd time, placing stem on stone:)

With tenderness and vitality, You express Love and Wisdom.

(Strike the tuning fork 3rd time placing stem on stone in silence, until vibrations begin to diminish.)

~~~~~HEART & THYMUS ENERGY CENTER~~~~~

Now take in a deep, caressing breath... bringing in the fragrance of eucalyptus and rose.

(Then strike the F tuning fork bringing it to the person's ear, saying:)

Now visualize green light coming in directly through Your chest, filling every chamber of Your heart and lungs.

(Pause, then strike it again, placing the stem on the green aventurine, saying:)

The vibration of the green light transmutes all forms of anguish, grief and jealousy. The green light empowers You to be willing to benefit from positive change.

(Strike the tuning fork a 2nd time, placing stem on stone:)

Protected by the green light, You are daring and brave. It gives You the experience of Being One, with the Infinite Power of Love.

(Strike the tuning fork a 3rd time placing stem on stone in silence, until vibrations begin to diminish.)

~~~~~~~~PANCREAS ENERGY CENTER~~~~~~~~

Now take in a deep, caressing breath... bringing in the fragrance of lemon.

(Then strike the E tuning fork bringing it to the person's ear, saying:)

Now visualize yellow light coming in through the bottoms of Your feet, going up Your legs, bathing the area above Your navel.

(Pause, then strike it again, placing the stem on the citrine, saying:)

The vibration of the yellow light transmutes all forms of anger and fear, and empowers You with a willing attitude.

(Strike the tuning fork a 2nd time, placing stem on stone:)

The vibration of the yellow light coordinates all messages between Your mind, Your body and Your surroundings. You are strong, tranquil and responsible.

(Strike the tuning fork a 3rd time placing stem on stone in silence, until vibrations begin to diminish.)

~~~~~~~~ADRENAL ENERGY CENTER~~~~~~~~

Now take in a deep, caressing breath... bringing in the fragrance of ylang-ylang, the flower-of-flowers.

(Then strike the D tuning fork bringing it to the person's ear, saying:)

Now visualize orange light coming in through the bottoms of Your feet, going up Your legs, bathing the area below Your navel.

(Pause, then strike it again, placing the stem on the peach aventurine, saying:)

The vibration of the orange light brings awareness and stability to Your emotions and balances Your sentiments with the light of reason.

(Strike the tuning fork a 2nd time, placing stem on stone:)

The vibration of the orange light enhances Your faithfulness. You are confident and assured within Yourself.

(Strike the tuning fork a 3rd time placing stem on stone in silence, until vibrations begin to diminish.)

~~~~~~~~GONADAL ENERGY CENTER~~~~~~~~

Now take in a deep, caressing breath... bringing in the fragrance of vetiver.

(Then strike the C tuning fork bringing it to the person's ear, saying:)
Now visualize red light coming in through the bottoms of Your feet, going up Your legs, bathing Your hips and Your pelvis.

(Pause, then strike it again placing the stem on the red jasper, saying:)

The vibration of the red light invigorates Your life force and restores physical... emotional... mental... and spiritual balance.

(Strike the tuning fork a 2nd time, placing stem on stone:)

With love... You appreciate and assimilate the vibration of the red light, as it stimulates Your creativity and originality.

(Strike the tuning fork a 3rd time placing stem on stone in silence, until vibrations begin to diminish.)

~~AURAL / HYPOTHALAMUS ENERGY CENTER~~

Now take in a deep, caressing breath... bringing in the fragrance of angelica and frankincense.

(Then strike the C# tuning fork bringing it to the person's ear, saying:)

Now visualize white light all around You.

(Pause, then strike it again placing the stem at the crown, saying:)

You are in total balance. Your system is in order.

(Strike the tuning fork a second time, placing the stem at the crown:)

You are a pure being of radiant energy... You are Pure Awareness exploring human consciousness.

(Strike the tuning fork a third time placing the stem at the crown in silence, until vibrations begin to diminish.)

(Then hold the Woven Spiral Star magnet side away from the person, to direct the affirmations into the person's etheric body. If using a crystal, hold cloudy end away. Begin at the top of the head and *slowly* move to the base of the spine while saying:)

Surround Yourself with Golden Light... and please repeat after me.

Life Itself supports me.
I trust the Power that sustains the Universe.
I freely give Love and Trust.
I trust the process of life.
I Am now safe.
I bring my life into balance by loving myself.
I live in the moment and love who I am.
It is easy for me to expand my consciousness.

(Beginning at the right foot, moving to the pelvis:)

Life is change and I Am always new.
I Am the loving operator of my mind.
Communication is easy and instantaneous.

(Clockwise at the pelvis:)

I Am now in total balance.

(Magnet side down, or cloudy end of the crystal down, and moving slowly counterclockwise around the pelvis, directing energy from the person's etheric body:)

I release the patterns in my consciousness
that create any condition of imbalance.

(Resuming magnet side up, or cloudy end up, moving slowly clockwise around the pelvis:)

I Am now willing to change.

(Moving up the right side:)

I love and approve of myself.

(Moving from right shoulder to right hand:)

My life is Divinely guided
and I Am always going in the optimal direction.

(Beginning at the left foot, moving to the pelvis:)

I assimilate new ideas easily. Life agrees with me.

(Clockwise around the pelvis:)

I perfectly reflect the rhythm and flow of life.
I Am now safe. All is well.
(Moving up the left side:)

I choose to enjoy Life
through the Sacred Space of my Heart.

(Moving from left shoulder to left hand:)

I look for Love, and find it everywhere.

(Moving from both feet to the head:)

I welcome what is useful in my Life.

(Magnet side down, moving from the head to the feet:)

I now comfortably and easily release the rest.

(Magnet side up, forming a clockwise ellipse between the right hemisphere of the brain and the left side of the pelvis:)

I heal my feminine energies.

(Between the left hemisphere and the right side of the pelvis:)

I heal my masculine energies.

(Circling the entire head and pelvis clockwise:)

I Am now one.
I Am whole and complete.

(Circling the person from head to feet:)

I Am Pure Consciousness...
Creating Pure Awareness
exploring human consciousness.
I Am the Delightful Expression
of the I Am Presence that I Am!
I Am So Blessed!

(Then draw the star toward Your mouth and blow 3X through the central portion of the Golden Mean Rectangle – or cloudy end of the crystal – toward the person's head, saying *silently*: Thank You, Great Spirit, for creating all that is.)

(At this point, music still playing, Meditate in Thanksgiving. The person subconsciously indicates Energies have been assimilated with a sigh... a deep breath... or clearly the person may be in a relaxed state, perhaps even asleep... then in a soft voice:)

And now...
take in a deep breath...
gently come back.

(Then gently remove the stones. This completes the re-calibration of the endocrine energy centers.) ~.~*

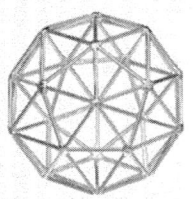

Addressing Emotional Balance

Check the physical and emotional heart energies: with Your left hand hold the person's left hand, palm up. Using pressure of about 5 lbs... with Your right thumb press against their thenar pad; there are two areas, one toward the wrist – tenderness indicating challenges with the physical heart; the other toward the thumb – tenderness indicating challenges with the emotional heart. If the first point shows tenderness, aerobic cardiovascular exercise and lifestyle changes {M.E.D.S.} strengthen the physical heart. If the second point shows tenderness, check for the thought-form presenting the emotional challenge... and make a positive affirmation as a correction.

Hold the person's left hand with Your left hand – as though engaged in a handshake – and mentally divide the underside of their forearm into twelve equal spaces... between the creases at the elbow (#1) and the wrist (#12). Then supporting the arm underneath with the fingers of Your right hand... with Your right thumb, count out loud from 1 to 12 as you press on the underside of the forearm – which is facing upward. Ask them to tell You the number... or numbers... that are sensitive, ticklish, or different feeling.

Many emotional issues go from one layer to another before reaching the core. Each number relates to a specific Challenge / Affirmation. If none are tender... do #12, saying to the person: Surround Yourself with the Golden Light of Love. Please repeat after me.

1 – Suspicion / Faith

I Am a reliable, trustworthy person full of confidence in my future. I believe now with all my being that everything is for the best.

2 – Disorganization / Order

I Am poised and balanced. I Am systematic in my life plan. I now express peace and harmony in my new organized life order.

3 – Hate / Love

My Heart of Hearts now freely expresses love for all.

4 – Excess or Misjudgment / Freedom

I have loving perceptions. I encourage and bless every person in my life. I Am a reasonable, thoughtful, understanding person full of inspirational wisdom.

5 – Misunderstanding / Understanding

The light of understanding permeates my being. I always interpret Life's plan with the light of Love. I intuitively comprehend what the Source of All has for me to accomplish.

6 – Despair / Life

I Am full of endurance and animation. I fill my memories with love. I Am now full of hope and vitality.

7 – Destruction / Creative Image

I realize what I picture in my mind with feelings.... I cause to come to pass. I use this image power to see only wonderful things.

8 – Antagonism / Will

I Am always ready to follow my Inner Voice Intuition. I have spiritual knowing of when to act. I Am always flexible, and lovingly do what gets to be done.

9 – Criticism / Power

I Am a person who uses my voice to speak only of wonderful things. I always speak about the Love in everyone. I know whatever I voice out loud... I will cause to happen.

10 – Lethargy / Enthusiasm

I Am eager and dynamic in doing those things that are mine to do. I Am enthusiastic about Life... and what it is all about.

11 – Hesitation / Strength

I Am a courageous person, strong and determined. I do things well that are mine to accomplish in this Life. I have the strength and the voice power to create all my wishes.

12 – Procrastination / Elimination

I transmute all my pent-up emotions... and empower all thoughts, feelings and experiences... to be One with Divine Love. I now purge my entire being from all things that interfere with my healing. I recognize myself now as a pure being of radiant Energy – One, with Infinite Source... explOring Infinity through Me!

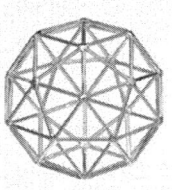

Affirmations for the Lessons of Life

Repetition helps re-program the subconscious. Affirmations consciously acknowledge Life's Purpose. Your Intention sets the stage for expansive, creative flow as You manifest Your highest choices. Always begin with Gratitude:

> I Am Grateful for the experiences of the past.
> I generously allow Life to flow through me.
> Giving thanks for the present moment,
> I look forward to a joyful future.

For those whose challenge may be **stability** at any level of Life – physical, emotional, mental or spiritual – for a feeling of security and grounding, we claim pelvic balance:

Life Itself supports me. I trust the Power that sustains the Universe. I freely give Love and Trust. I Trust the process of Life. I Am now safe. I bring my Life into balance by loving myself. I live in the moment and Love who I am.

For those whose challenge may be **self-esteem**, we claim sexual balance:

It is safe to be who I am. I rejoice in my own expression of Life. I Am perfect exactly as I am. I love and approve of myself as a powerful, capable person.

For those whose challenge may be **procrastination**, we claim glandular balance:

I Am the creative power in my world. Divine Order guides my ideas and activities. I Am enthusiastic and joyful.

For those whose challenge may be **digestion** and **assimilation** of food… emotions… or ideas, we claim digestive balance:

I assimilate new ideas easily. Life agrees with me. I absorb all that is useful… and release the rest with joy. I perfectly reflect the rhythm and flow of life.

For those whose challenge may be **sorting things out** on the physical, emotional or mental level, we claim kidney balance:

Perfect Divine Order takes place in my life all-ways. Only growth comes from each experience. It is safe to grow and mature; growth means life. I welcome what is useful in my life; comfortably and easily, I release the rest.

For those whose challenge may be **anxiety** and **stress** in Life, we claim adrenal balance:

I love and approve of myself. It is safe for me to care for myself. I Am energetic and enthusiastic about Life.

For those whose challenge may be **anger** or **resentment**, we claim liver balance:

I cherish Love… Peace… and Joy. I now choose to enjoy Life through the Sacred Space in my Heart. I look for Love and find it everywhere.

For those whose challenge may be aligning with **Life's Purpose**, we claim lymph balance:

I Am totally centered in the Love and Joy of being here on planet Earth. I love and approve of myself. I flow with Life. I Am now safe. All is well within me and around me.

For those whose challenge may be experiencing **frustration** in life, we claim pancreatic balance:

Life is sweet and so am I. I Am in total balance. My system is in order. I create the Sweetness and Joy that is my Life.

For those whose challenge may be **giving** and/or **receiving**, we claim respiratory balance:

The Breath of Life flows easily through me. I have the capacity to take in the fullness of Life. I have the courage to give of myself freely… and to receive graciously. I Am now safe. I Love my Life.

For those whose challenge may be **insecurity** and **fear** in matters of personal Love, we claim heart balance:

I joyfully accept all of Life. I lovingly allow Joy to enter my mind, my body and my experience. I bring Joy to the Sacred Space in my Heart. I Am free to Love. I now express Love with ease. I look for Love and find it everywhere.

For those whose challenge may be **inflexibility**, we claim neck balance:

I see all sides of an issue with flexibility and ease. There are numerous ways of doing things… and seeing things. I Am now safe. I Am peaceful. I feel relaxed and confident with my Life's Purpose… allowing others complete freedom to choose as they see fit.

For those whose challenge may be **integrating right brain / left brain activities**, we claim cerebral balance:

It is easy for me to expand my consciousness. Life is change and I Am all-ways new. I Am the loving operator of my mind. Communication is easy and instantaneous. I Am now in total balance.

With **Gratitude** for all Your blessings, **Praise** Yourself for each success. **Congratulate** Yourself for all the progress You are making. Enjoy the Infinite Possibilities on the path of Love and Compassion!

I choose to create my physical form in the highest possible perfection. My body remembers the natural

Order and Harmony, and brings forth normal healthy cells, normal productions. My glands and my organs are happy, doing an excellent job keeping me healthy.

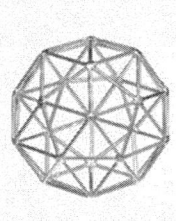

DAILY VIBRATIONAL ENERGY MEDICINE

4 – VIBRATIONAL ENERGY MEDICINE AS FOUND IN MEDITATION AND MAKING LOVE

How can You speak of others?
Rather, speak of Yourself,
in other places, with other faces!
Can You see how You are linked?
The light of Your heart complements the other.
Be the Other, and You will be everywhere
at once… in all minds…
You will be what I Am… which is Yourself.
(The Essene Master Jesus or Issa)

While at first blush meditation and making love seem worlds apart… in reality, they are One and the same. When totally focused in meditation, we make love with our true Self. When totally focused in making love, it is truly a meditation. Both are Energy Medicine… raising frequencies and celebrating wholeness – they both are explorations in human consciousness.

The definition of meditation is a devotional exercise of contemplation, or spiritual, uplifting thoughts. Meditation, however, means more than "to reflect upon or ponder." Ancient Wisdom says "virtus stat in medio" translated usually: "virtue stands in the middle" more completely: "rather than being in extremes, such as prudery or lasciviousness, virtue is found in the center… *in medio.*" Meditation is a state of being *in medio,* in Your center.

Finding Our Center
We spend the majority of our time letting our senses draw us outward… to the world of transition, where things are always wearing out, rusting, chipping, cracking, breaking and/or dying… with "oooh's" and "aaah's" we point to our stately homes and our proud possessions, of which we say, "Isn't this gorgeous?" We can show our friends around the home. "Oh, look

at this" and "Oh, look at that" and "Listen to these speakers… the finest resonance, free from distortion… have a seat. These cushions are made from Egyptian cotton! And how do You like my antique Persian rugs?" Then, to complete the full spectrum of our senses, "Have a whiff of these organic desserts. Here. Have a taste!" Our physical senses tend to draw us outward.

While it is wonderful to enjoy the finer things in life… all too often these "things" are made to be gods in and of themselves: "graven images" that provide only temporary happiness. Permanent happiness is within. We can bring a high vibration to our possessions by being unattached to them while being attached to our real purpose which is to experience Love. Augustine says "Love God, and do what You will." Jesus says "Love God and love Your neighbor as Yourself." We can enjoy our possessions and have truly wonderful times with our friends when we are in a space of pure love: enthusiastically giving, *equally* enthusiastically receiving. Completing the cycle by graciously receiving is an open invitation for another cycle to begin… as Love continues… giving and receiving… again and again. Letting our senses draw us outward is appropriate to an extent, since we find ourselves as spiritual / conscious beings in physical bodies, in a physical world. Harmonious balance lets our senses also draw us inward… where we can truly experience: "The Kingdom of Heaven *is* within You."

Turn Your senses within… to experience… All That Is. In *this* world of constancy, there are manifestations of the Source of All. Fractal geometry shows the intimate dual relationship between microcosm and macrocosm. When scientists split the atom, they find Infinite Being expressing as light, sound, radiation and vibration. According to Raja yoga, turn Your senses within to find Your center – experience Celestial Light, Harmonies, Nectar and the Sacred Vibration that sustains All – experience permanent Blissful Awareness… ready to share… whenever You choose to "tune-in"!

alo Ha…
alo: Being in the Presence of
Ha: The Breath of Life
Many go to Hawai'i for a honeymoon or the vacation of their dreams. They hear Aloha as "hello" "goodbye" and "love." Yet literally, Aloha means: "being in the Presence of the Breath of Life." Experience this; follow the breath: the in-breathings and the out-breathings of the Spirit: in-spiration and ex-spiration. Latin *spiritus* is

a translation of the Greek *pneuma* – air, wind, breath – I breathe: *spiro*. From our first breath until our last, we are said to be alive, although Life begins before that time and Life extends beyond in the next stage of Consciousness Infinite Being chooses to share. Meanwhile, we do well to breathe fully, deeply, bringing in oxygen and Life Force – and then breathing out completely, releasing toxins and wastes.

As much as You may think You have emptied Your lungs, they still retain 30% capacity; nevertheless, when we exhale completely, we are ready for our next deep breath bringing healing oxygen deep into our lungs. Many times, experiencing fear, grief, anger or a confronting situation, breathing becomes shallow or stifled; especially at these times we require deep breathing to nurture Your feeling body, sharpen Your thinking body, and prepare Your acting body.

The Breath of Fire, practiced in yoga, thoroughly energizes every organ and system, leaving one with a tingling feeling – as fresh oxygen courses through our HeartMindBodySpirit!

Standard texts in medical physiology speak of the vital signs – temperature, pulse rate and blood pressure – and mention the normal respiration rate averages about twelve per minute. What may be normal for the average person, allows only 2½ seconds to breathe in, and 2½ seconds to breathe out. This shallow breathing provides minimal exchange of air in the lung fields. At this rate, the air exchanged is mostly in the bronchioles, which lack the capacity to take in oxygen or expel carbon dioxide; bronchioles function as passageways leading to the lungs where the real work, the real exchange, is done.

Eventually, textbooks will add a footnote, as incidental information: the optimal respiration rate is about half of the normal rate. 5 to 6 breaths per minute allow the lungs to fully expand – to exchange fuel for waste. Those who habitually sigh, yawn or feel drowsy can rest assured... deep breathing transforms dullness and lethargy into vitality and enthusiasm.

Geological studies under polar caps reveal 300 years ago our ancestors breathed air containing 38% oxygen; now it is 21%. With practice we connect Breath with Spirit. Indeed, German for breath is atem and to breathe is Atmen. Sanskrit for Spirit is Atman. In Icelandic, to breathe is ad anda, while anda means

Spirit. Sanskrit ananda means bliss. There is a definite connection between Breath and Bliss. The only way to know is follow the breath and see where it leads. The Way Out of any suffocating or confining experience is to go within. Breathe deeply. Exhale completely. Explore, and Enjoy true Freedom!

Creating A New Habit

> To go out of Your mind is important.
> By going out of Your mind, You come to Your senses!
> *Meditation*, Alan Watts

Rather than being an end in itself, taking time to sit in meditation is actually practice for daily living. Meditation, a totally exquisite experience, tunes-in to Your power, the Power that sustains All. Whether meditating for five, fifteen or twenty minutes or an hour or more – You are, for that time, in the Consciousness of the present moment... here and now.

Ram Dass says, when You feel You are going *nowhere*, then make the shift in meditation to be *now here*. That is the reason he named his book *Be Here Now*. When You leave the past behind... and realize the future takes care of itself – especially while remaining fully in the present, planting the seeds for tomorrow's harvest – our focus remains... moment to moment... on blissful Breath.

Neophytes to this experience have an abrupt introduction to Monkey-mind, swinging wildly from one thing to another. The mind, accustomed to being in charge, loves to bring up the pain of the past, haranguing or sentimentalizing – if only this had happened... or, if only this *could* happen – distracting us with fear of the future. Monkey-mind chatter has detailed plans, with constant revisions, and needless worry. Nonsense! Be aware... and once Aware... You are Free from the pain of the past. Free from the fear of the future. Indeed... You are Here and Now... and... nOw is forever. Eternity awaits Your experience... with Your next Conscious Breath. Why wait? Be *there* nOw!

> Yesterday is history... tomorrow is a mystery...
> each day... each moment...
> each Breath... is a Gift...
> that's why it's called the Present!

The words You have read so far... are in the past. Words and concepts You are about to encounter... are in the future. The only thing that's real, the only thing that's really constant is the present mOMENT, the present Sacred Breath. That is the Eternal nOw.

So right now... free Yourself from thoughts of the past. Free Yourself from thoughts of the future. With open eyes take a deep breath, gently exhale. Feel the Gift of the Present Moment... experience Blessings of the Breath. Staying in that space for an extended period is called being in meditation.

Setting aside time to sit and practice *being* in meditation with whichever technique One would like to explOre... beginners may be frustrated by Monkey-mind. Some newbies find it handy to pull in the reins on the gallivanting mind by having pen and paper within reach, as we shall see. First... let's get settled.

Practicing meditation, being comfortable is the priority. Wear loose fitting clothing for a comfortable temperature. Be free from disturbances: phone / devices elsewhere. Create the privacy and space You deserve. Whatever it takes, feel grounded... totally supported and safe. A few may be comfortable with the full lotus position, some prefer a seiza bench to half-kneel, half-sit. Some sit on a cushion, others sit on the edge of a chair with back free and feet flat on the floor. Some prefer to lie flat with knees bent, feet flat on the floor... or legs straight, with a small pillow under the knees taking pressure off the low back. Whatever... be comfortable with spine straight. Perhaps have hands palm up resting on Your legs, or one hand on top of the other – thumbs together. Experiment. Zen Masters say: Everyone can benefit from 20 minutes a day... unless You're too busy – then make it an hour! Practice. In time, meditative Thanksgiving fills the day.

Begin with a moment of Thanksgiving. Gratitude nourishes the Spirit. Surround Yourself with Love and Light. Give thanks for the Presence of Your Angels and Spirit Guides. Empty Your ego self before the One... Source of All... emptying, we experience true Self, open to Gifts of Spirit.

Caressing the bump at the roof of Your mouth helps maintain Your focus. We maintain connection of the microcosmic circuit by simply touching tongue to palate. Taken to the next order of magnitude, tongue gently *caressing* stimulates the palatine nerve connecting to the Pineal Center. The tissue at the root of the tongue and tissue forming the pericardial sac

holding the heart are embryologically One. Caressing, connects Pineal and Heart centers. Gently caressing... with focus on Sacred Breath... slowly breathe in... to the point where You feel comfortably full... focus on that still point... then caressing, with focus on the Breath, slowly breathe out... to the point where You feel comfortably empty... focus on that still point... repeat. Enoch says: "Be still, and know, I Am God!" When we actually take the time to create a daily habit of meditation, we realize: I Am the I Am that I Am - Infinite Being, being finite, exploring Here and Now.

While Monkey-mind may be distracted by focusing on the *breath*, another tradition focuses on the *temperature* at the tip of the nose: cool as we breathe in... warm as we breathe out. Especially when first beginning to meditate, Monkey-mind may be somewhat challenged remaining quiet. Sometimes the mind rebels attempting to resume control with ventures into past and future – attempting to distract from the experience You are choosing in the moment – attempting to be *in charge* once again.

What You Resist Persists!
What You Allow Changes!

Rather than chiding the mind, upset with the interference – which fuels the situation – honor the mind. Thank the mind for being efficient... and take a note, with paper and pen at Your side.

For instance, things may be going quite well. You've already been attentive for 5 or 6 breaths or even 5 or 6 minutes. Monkey-mind chimes in: "Call Mother. You said You'd do her windows this afternoon, and You haven't heard from her... she said she'd confirm and hasn't. Maybe she made other plans, You'd better call her. Who knows she might have something else for You to do and You'll have to go to the store on the way." On and on. Monkey-mind can keep on going. So, nip it in the bud. With the first words "Call Mother..." while still focusing on Sacred Breath, simply honor the mind for being so thoughtful, helping You remember everything; then write on the paper: Call Mother, focusing on Breath... slowly, evenly breathing. After a while the mind may take another route in its attempt to resume control. "Uh-oh, the book was due at the library last Tuesday... get up and put it with the car keys to return it." Nice try, Monkey-mind. Again, while focusing on Sacred Breath, honor the mind with thanks for being so efficient and make a note: Return library book, focusing on Your Breath.

At first, the mind may be obstinate and take any ruse to re-gain control. Simply maintain Your calm. Focus on Your breath even as You make the required notes of things to do. Be sure to spend the whole of the allotted time, whatever You have chosen – 20 minutes or an hour – entirely focused as much as possible. You have made Your point. Monkey-mind will understand You believe there is value in being still, and… You can handle any attempted interference. The most important thing after meditation is to *do everything on the list*! Otherwise, the next time beginning Your list the mind will chime in: "Making a list doesn't matter. Remember last time You did only 3 out of 5 things on Your list. And this is important. Get up now and do it! You can always come back at a later time to meditate… for twice as long, that's a promise… get up now and do it!" Such is the devious nature of Monkey-mind. So, do everything on Your list. That's an additional advantage to meditation – keeping You focused in the mOMent… making sure things get done… builds self-esteem.

Exploring other possibilities of meditation… consider the one quality You choose to create in Your life: Joy, Love, or Peace. Often overlooked… let's use Joy. Slowly, caressing, breathe in… think: "I bring Joy into my life." And as You breathe out, think: "I express Joy to the world." Repeat this as You breathe in and out. Perhaps one word in: Accepting… out: Releasing. Soon words fade. You experience Sacred Breath… as consciousness of Breath fades – You experience Pure Meditation. Bliss covers You like the dewfall… Consciousness is ecstatic; You experience a mOMent of Heaven on Earth.

Once comfortable with meditation… being still, focused, connecting with Self… You are able to direct meditation. Being still, focused - as You breathe in, ask: "Who am I?" As You breathe out, Listen. Repeat 3 minutes. Then breathe in and ask: "Where am I going?" As You breathe out, Listen. Experiment. Explore. Connection with Sacred Breath is a stress-buster preparing for the "stuff" of Life.

Keeping Your New Habits

Time in meditation is required to experience Inner Peace. The real test comes after. With continued practice, there is no "after" meditation. Eventually, being in the "practice" of meditating, we remain in that focused *space* even as we get up from our meditation *place*… and *move about our day*! That's the promise as well as the reason for practicing. Peace! Finding that peaceful space… with time… we can remain at peace as we live our daily lives… in whatever capacity, with complete integrity.

Caressing the roof of the mouth, focusing on the breath… focusing on the *vibration* that sustains the breath… is habit-forming. Soon You find Yourself focusing on Your breath while driving, rather than focusing on the race that seems to be going on all around…. finding Yourself in a comfortable lane, driving at a comfortable speed, and arriving… quite comfortable, and feeling at Peace. While chopping vegetables rather than focusing on what someone said yesterday or what will happen later – with Sacred Breath… caressing, feeling Love and Peace… the secret ingredient makes food deliciously divine.

You find focus on Sacred Breath while cleaning… rather than letting Monkey-mind complain. Meditation turns housework into an act of love – a real morale booster, building self-esteem. Meditation frees us from judgment and coercion. Meditation can transform every activity into Pure Love. How does it get any better than that? Freedom. Love. Peace. Here & nOw!

Making Love

Consciously loving is the single, most completely holistic, rejuvenating therapy available – cost-effective and enjoyable. A young man asked his father, "How long does it normally take to make love?" The wise man answered, "Well, son, if You are looking to get something, it's a short time; if You are looking to give something, it's a lifetime."

While some physicians say that a session of lovemaking is equivalent to a four-mile walk, research shows it goes far beyond cardiovascular benefits. Rather than merely having aerobic sex, true lovemaking nourishes self-esteem, heals the mind and emotions. There are clear psychological and physical benefits enhanced with the spiritual dimension and, altogether they boost the immune response system.

Exploring consciousness, begin sacred sexual union with a period of yoga, stretching, or foot reflexology – followed by meditation. Maintain focus on Sacred Breath before, during and after lovemaking. Meditative lovemaking can transform both the individual and the couple… exposing the Magical Mystery of Who we are, and what Life is all about… feeling whOleness in HeartMindBodySpirit… feeling One. Be-ing Love.

In the theology of Creation Spirituality, the focus is on Original Blessing, rather than Original Sin. We were created in the state of Grace, and lived as loving beings. Whatever the circumstances, whatever the reason... somehow, things turned from Grace to Greed. The tendency, in the past, has been to shift the blame rather than accept responsibility. Eve said, "The devil made me do it, promising all these wonderful things." And... Adam said, "Eve made me do it." A sad thing for both to say; for someone else to "make us" do something, we must give up our own power... turning our Free Will over to another! This... is the nature of sin. The word *sin* is said to come from an Arabic word that means: "to miss the mark." Instead of hitting one of the center circles, we miss... sometimes, we may miss the target altogether.

Accepting responsibility... we pull ourselves together and once again make the choice to exercise our Free Will. We carefully take aim, setting forth to accomplish our goal: expressing ourselves as a human being, being human... Loving and Joyous... a Blessing to all around us. This is the World Vision we can create, wherever we may be.

In the past, we may have sinned by relating to others from the standpoint of what we can get from them. The original sin *may* have had something to do with sex. Acting in a self-centered way turns it into an *act* of sex. You are on target when You exchange respect and tender love, experiencing sacred sexual commUnion – Infinite Being Gifting and Receiving with Self.

Joyously giving and receiving, the Essence of Love begins to overflow into Life... recognizing Others as equal creations of the Divine Presence. Truth dawns: the main **Lesson of Life: Living = Loving = Giving**. This is the source of Lasting Happiness, Pure Ecstasy. Meditation facilitates the Lesson. With clear Intention... Sacred Sexuality is Vibrational Energy Medicine – the ultimate experience of Holistic Healing.

Beyond Tantra
The Sanskrit word *tantra* means: to weave. The Taoist symbol of yin / yang portrays inter-connectedness of right-brain / left-brain energies feminine and masculine sides of our personalities... receiving and giving in real Life. The symbol is a *clue* how it all weaves together.

Yin is the feminine aspect of Self: softness, compassion, the stillness of soul. Yang is the masculine aspect of Self: taking care of busy-ness, the active expression of soul. At first glance... polar opposites. Yet within the dark recess of the yin, there is a white dot – representing the shining forth and potential of yang energy. Within the white yang, there is a black dot – representing the shining forth and potential of yin energy. Nothing remains all yin or all yang. With fullness, one turns into the other.

Human sexuality extends (yang) and receives (yin). Anatomy reflects these two principles. Yang extends outward, and the Sanskrit word for penis is *lingham*, meaning Wand of Light – focused outward, direct... with a Gift to bestow. Yin receives within, and the Sanskrit word for vagina is *yoni*, meaning Sacred Space or Cosmic Door to Creation – focused inward, mysterious, ready to receive the Gift.

Within the *yoni* is a woman's powerhouse of sexuality. Stimulation of a glandular area known as the g-spot can cause a woman to experience a yang-like gushing forth of energy accompanied by fluid release. The possibility of this orgasmic transformation from yin to yang is predicted by the seminal white dot on the dark side of the yin / yang symbol.

The male correlation to the g-spot is at the perineum, between the scrotum and the anus. This area allows stimulation of the prostate gland, a sexual organ that is interior, concealed, yin-like; pressing against this spot facilitates control of ejaculation – retaining the seed. Rather than mere genital orgasm culminating in outward ejaculation, manual pressure at the perineum allows him to go within, and experience total body orgasm. The possibility of this orgasmic transformation from yang to yin is predicted by the seminal black dot on the white side of the yin / yang symbol.

Ancient Wisdom says, change is the only constant. Human Wisdom says, entrenched in either extreme we are incomplete – missing an integral part of ourselves. Sacred Sexuality charges the dynamic forces of yin and yang in a conscious and interactive way. No man is all yang. No woman all yin. There is no perfect partner who magically makes us whole. We each have the desire to give. We each have the ability to receive. We find balance when we recognize beneficial qualities on both sides of the scale. Being complete, we offer our complete self to our Beloved. With two complete individuals joined in sacred sexual union, the perfect partners melt in a sphere of ecstasy – Sacred

Communion. From this experience of Love, with Divine Consciousness and Harmony flowing we can live our lives en-Joying each mOMent with each Other... in the Here & nOw... with every Sacred Breath.

Caution: many a book or video purports to espouse Tantra Yoga. Most really deceive, and are clear-cut pornography, the climax being ejaculation. Tantra, like *Karrezza*, focuses on retaining the seed whenever possible... feeling the energy of Sacred Sexual Union – Giving – Receiving – Being – a Gift of Infinite Love. Retaining the seed, man retains strength and vitality – thoroughly energized and satisfied – he is ever ready to care for his Beloved Goddess – perhaps even multiple times a day!

New Age Tantra Yoga: The Cybernetics of Sex and Love, by Howard John Zitko (1975), from the holistic, Essene perspective, is written in dialogue format – easy for a couple to read together.

Gary M Douglas & Dain C Heer have some interesting points of view to explore as well: *Sex Is Not a Four-Letter Word but Relationship Often Times Is*.

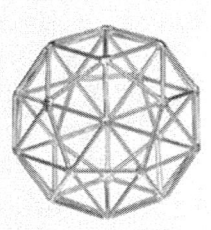

5 – ENERGY MEDICINE AS FOUND IN CLEANLINESS, EXERCISE AND REST

Soap: Dirtier than Dirt?
One square inch of skin = 19 million cells, including 650 sweat glands, 100 sebum or oil glands, 65 hair follicles, 19,000 sensory cells and 13 feet of microscopic blood vessels. The skin of an adult weighs around 8 lbs, and measures 20 square feet stretched out. Over an average lifetime 40 pounds of skin are shed!

The thickness of skin measures from 1/25th of an inch – at the eyelids, to 1/8th of an inch – at the soles of the feet. Skin functions as a nutritional factory, producing Vitamin D-3, a necessary ingredient in the formation of bone, helps metabolize carbohydrates and amino acids. Skin is our defense against foreign invaders, part of our immune response system; it identifies and neutralizes foreign matter entering through the epidermis, and protects the body from infection. Your skin is a living part of Your body with well-developed, interrelated circulating systems – blood, sweat, sebum, nerve and lymph – all can be damaged by absorption of chemicals, and enhanced by proper skin care.

Myths about hygiene are rampant. We have been cajoled by the soap and cosmetic industry; they tell us that "really fresh feeling" comes with their brand of soap, and it is better to smell like their perfume or cologne than to rely on Your own pheromones. Having been soft-soaped by advertising, we regularly buy and use their products, free from doubt or hesitation. The origin of the expression to "soft-soap" someone, derives from the fact that soft soap is 95% lye – an example is to convince an Eskimo that a freezer is both convenient and necessary for any well-appointed igloo. The facts about soap are simple. Soap is a wonderful agent when washing away grimy oil and grit. A little soap goes a long way to clean our clothes. We typically use twice as much as required to get natural body oils from our clothing.

While it is quite appropriate to use some soap, even a scouring pad, on our hands after working on mechanical, greasy things... to wash our whole body with soap every day is a waste of soap and a waste of energy, in more ways than one. While soap is basically an alkali, skin prefers to be *slightly acid* to ward off unfriendly, toxic microbes efficiently. This is one of the paradoxes of life: the body likes to be slightly alkaline inside and slightly acid outside. When we soap up, we wash our natural protection down the drain – then the body spends energy reconstructing an acid environment so colonies – millions of microbes – can re-establish themselves for our protection, for survival.

Microbial flora can be found in the *stratum corneum* – porous tissue that is actually renewed constantly, as older parts are washed away or rubbed off. Skin is covered with life. The major tribes of microbes are: Micrococci – living near the surface, they like an airy environment... Diphtheroids – living deeper, like a moist environment, close to oil glands that produce their food. Gram-positive and gram-negative bacteria are found in children and adults to some degree – while entirely free from causing disease.

Like all living creatures, microbes must eat. Your skin is a large farm, where the food supply is drawn from below the surface. Like all good farmers, the microbes tend the land that feeds them. This good husbandry requires protecting the skin and the body from harmful bacterial invaders that may try to colonize. The "skin farm" contains nutrients and natural selective bactericides that inhibit or kill harmful bacteria.

Sweat is a rich source of sodium chloride and water, essential nutrients for healthy microbes. The friendly skin microbes benefit from trace minerals, lactic acid, and urea – found in sweat. Apocrine sweat, found mostly in the armpits, contains ammonia, carbohydrates, iron and protein, particularly attractive to dyphtheroids. Oils are secreted by the sebaceous glands of the skin. The dyphtheroids metabolize this oil producing oleic acid, which inhibits the growth of many unfriendly bacteria.

As a sustainable farm, the skin is guided by permaculture – a self-sufficient ecosystem where the surface and its vegetable and mineral constituents co-exist in the proportions that most effectively sustain each other's health and well-being. As a result, any foreign microbe or fungus that finds its way to Your skin finds the defenses are strong and resisting attack. With soap, Your defense system suffers upheaval.

Soap and water have the immediate effect of removing the skin's protective flora – micrococci, and gram-positive and gram-negative bacteria. The soap breaks down and removes skin oils that feed the diphtheroids, and large numbers of the latter are washed away. Nutrients from sweat are also removed. The skin's natural defenses against unfriendly bacteria are weakened, and the immune response is compromised. The skin is left with a few scattered colonies of surviving microbial flora and a reduced supply of nutrients, which hampers their effort to re-establish themselves promoting our well-being.

Skin responds by secreting oil to feed the survivors. Over-agitated, the oil glands tend to over-produce. Excess oil, combined with humidity caused by washing, enables a rapid expansion of the diphtheroid population, and a large amount of their by-product: oleic acid. Although oleic acid is a natural germicide – one variety of microbe *Corynebacterium acne* actually thrives on the skin *only* when oleic acid levels are unnaturally high. There are some *C. acne* microbes normally present on the skin surface at all times. They form dense colonies only when the oleic acid levels

become high enough to support them. Repeated washings *intensify* the situation.

Skin surface can also dry out and become lifeless. The resident microbes move deeper into the skin where oil levels are normal, and conditions are friendly; the dry skin falls away. On the scalp, this is particularly marked after frequent shampooing and within a day, once the moisture level has returned to normal, skin particles fall off in large quantities… appearing as dandruff.

When the thin layer of oil secreted by our sebaceous glands is washed away with soap, it becomes easier for particles to adhere to the skin – sulfur compounds from the atmosphere, lead particles, dust, grease and grime. This opens the way for harmful microbes to move in. These unfriendly bacteria may appear as a rash or sore and lead to deeper infection.

The following has taken place more times than doctors care to admit: a patient regularly washes away the friendly microbes with soap, and eventually develops a colony of harmful microbes – causing a skin infection. The doctor prescribes an antibiotic salve, completely wiping out the skin's remaining microbial flora; the infection-causing bacteria turn out to be antibiotic resistant. More and stronger antibiotics are administered that only exacerbate the situation. Natural physicians say: "Simply leave it alone; cover with a light bandage if anything, and let the skin's flora become re-established." The best advice to the patient is… be patient… Breathe… Hydrate… Visualize.

Some areas of the skin have higher concentrations of microbial flora where the skin is most active removing body wastes… armpits, feet and crotch are areas with the greatest amount of damage from soap and water. The armpits in particular exude most of the body's apocrine sweat, which is metabolized by the normal dyphtheroid microbes – usually an odorless process. When the dyphtheroid population is at a sub-normal level, that is – after washing with soap – other bacteria begin to metabolize the apocrine sweat with the by-product being a variety of unpleasant-smelling alkaline substances. Regular washing with soap and the use of anti-perspirant chemicals contribute to this imbalance in the armpits and creates a greater tendency to body odor. Showering with a loofa sponge is sufficient.

The benefits of soap are greatly exaggerated. The dirt that collects on healthy skin can usually be removed by gentle abrasion with wet hands or a natural sponge; a wet loofa sponge has a mild abrasive effect, and removes surface dirt, leaving behind the healthy constituents of the skin's environment. Moisture is as beneficial to the maintenance of healthy microbial flora, as the occasional rainfall is to the health of a meadow. Heavy rubbing with soaps disturbs the balance of the skin's ecosystem.

To encourage the normal ecosystem, regular exercise and loose-fitting clothing stimulate secretions of sweat and oil required by the flora. Massage has a beneficial effect in stimulating the oil glands. Sesame or olive oil is traditional for newborns and children of all ages, including those in their second childhood. Coconut oil has medium-chain fatty acids. Hemp seed oil has the complete family of Omegas.

Your original microbial flora population was a birthday present from mother. Microbes from the walls of the vagina colonized Your eyes, mouth and skin as You passed through into the outside world. The protective coating of flora is the birthright of every newborn, yet hospitals still attack it immediately with disinfectants. Rather than wiping it off, wise midwives rub in the *vernix caseosa* – the cheesy coating covering the newborn. If it is a full-term pregnancy or overdue and the vernix has already absorbed, they rub some warm olive oil into the skin. There is simply no medical reason to wipe away this protective coating. Even if there is a little neo-natal blood mixed in, what harm could it do to rub in the vernix?

Why persist in the practice if soap has harmful effects? At Unilever – the major soap-manufacturing company in Britain – market researchers sought to answer this question to effectively aim their selling pitch. They found "freshness" – rather than "cleanliness" – was desired. Freshness, associated with coolness, equals self-control the root condition of Puritanism. The word "dirty" is interchangeable with "sexy" in the Puritan vocabulary, as in dirty mind or dirty joke. Psychiatrists are familiar with the obsessive hygiene of the anal-retentive mentality, which may even extend to wiping doorknobs. This deep-seated anxiety – often connected with guilt feelings from early toilet training – is reinforced by over-anxious parental training, and leads to compulsive washing. Some people lather up and shower several times daily. Mickey Cohn, retired gangster, was notorious for his habit of washing his hands several times per hour. An understanding of the importance of microbial flora to the skin's true health reveals the contraindications in this attitude. In fact, when defined by the effect it has upon normal skin surfaces, soap is dirtier than dirt!

For those who would like to break the soap addiction, simply confine Your use of soap to appropriate times: after the toilet, simply rinsing with water is sufficient! When removing grease or oily dirt... after working with compost or in the garden... before preparing food... before tending open wounds... these are appropriate times to wash hands with simple soap. Antibacterial soaps are overrated and overused, making a mountain out of a molehill finally banned by the FDA because there was no evidence they improved on plain soap and water! That was the given reason. Of course, they are beholden to industry and would never admit the first ingredient in antibacterial soaps is triclosan, and studies have shown for years that this chemical interferes with the function of the thyroid gland! Be cautious... anti-bacterial agents such as triclosan are ubiquitous. For everyday cleansing of the skin, use simple castile soap derived from olive oil, such as Dr Bronner's. Read the label; always dilute!

Hair is another issue; actually, another tissue. Hair is like fabric; it picks up smoke and air-borne grease and dirt. Commercial shampoos and conditioners are loaded with chemicals that are harmful and absorb through the skin. Natural shampoos and conditioners are available at health food stores, yet be wise... some "known and trusted" brands have copious synthetics such as sodium lauryl (laureth) sulfate in their soap and toothpaste. Always read labels!

After a warm bath or shower, it is stimulating to finish with a brisk, cold rinse to close the pores and energize – stimulating blood flow. Freshen skin and hair with a splash of apple cider vinegar to bring out radiance, luster and sheen, creating a slightly acidic environment to benefit the friendly skin microbes. In a few minutes the aroma dissipates; it's worth it. You can also enhance Your natural pheromones with a drop or two of pure essential oil in 1 oz coconut oil – ladies, ylang-ylang; gentlemen, pine. Most perfumed soaps, perfumes and colognes are laden with synthetic chemicals people literally splash on to cover body odor. While they think offensive odor is caused by nerves or poor hygiene – leading them to use more soap – it is caused by poor dietary habits, as well as using too much soap too frequently, as we have already noted. Skin – the largest organ – acts as a third kidney. When the body is underhydrated, the kidneys become overloaded with toxins; for survival, the body eliminates acids and whatever else it can via the skin.

A diet filled with an indiscriminate mixture of animal proteins, starches, refined flour and sugar, caffeine, alcohol, nicotine, sodas, etc., results in acid indigestion, flatulence, gas, acidic burps, and halitosis, with gases and acids also eliminated through the skin. The pores on the soles of the feet are twice as big as the pores on the rest of the body, so expect foot odor. The pores and lymphatic glands are plentiful in the axillary region, so expect underarm body odor. The body simply responds to this overload of dietary indiscretions. To keep the pH within limits for survival, acids and toxins are cast off through the skin. Meanwhile some people continue to consume a wild mixture of junk food laden with synthetic additives, and splash on whatever fragrance catches their attention as being in vogue. Hydrate instead!

Those who begin to choose their foods wisely and eat reasonable amounts in proper combination – especially those who eliminate flesh and dairy products – may initially go through cleansing that results in offensive odors. The good news is that after this brief initial cleansing, they exude the sweet fragrance of a natural human being. And ladies changing to 100% vegan will notice diminished clots and cramps once going through a complete moon cycle as vegan – the next cycle will be quite different.

Great yogis have the fragrance of flowers. They all say they are average and everyone can attain true bliss and consciousness. You have the power. You are the Power. Go for Your highest choice. Experience the wonder-filled possibilities waiting for You. This is the Miracle only You can perform!

Cleaning the Nose, Teeth and Tongue
Cleansing the nose with lukewarm salt water is an ancient practice. Some put a pinch of salt in their hand with a few drops of warm water to snort through each nostril, spitting the water out the mouth. Others find a neti pot convenient, from health food store or Indian shop – *neti* means cleansing. In India it is more common to cleanse the nose and scrape the tongue as good oral hygiene, rather than brush the teeth. After a meal, they snap a small twig from "the toothpick tree"

and suck on it to soften – when fibers separate forming a little brush, they clean their teeth, gums and tongue. Neti refreshes the nose... becoming pleasantly open. The entire nose area is relaxed and cleansed from the inside – mucus, dust, dirt, pollen, smoke, and allergy provoking particles are rinsed away. How does it work? Microscopic hairs, cilia are found in sinuses and mucous membranes and they all vibrate in the same direction. Under a microscope they resemble a field of grain swaying in the breeze. Cilia are coated with a layer of mucus to catch bacteria, dust and pollen and act as a conveyor belt – transporting mucus and particles through the nose, down the throat, to the stomach. Dryness, viruses, and allergy producing substances paralyze the cilia... cleansing with salt water keeps the mucous membranes moist and healthy. For challenges with dry mucous membranes due to heat and a/c, add a drop of almond or other plant oil. The nasal cavity is connected to the sinuses by small orifices. These channels may close leading to sinusitis because of excess mucus in the diet, stress, or overwork; neti cleanses these channels. Regular neti use prevents colds because it moves the pH toward alkaline. If the mucous membrane is too acidic, viruses can survive and attach creating an infection. With a slightly high pH, the virus dies. Neti can relieve psychosomatic ailments, stress-induced asthma.

Add a pinch of salt to warm water in the neti pot. Some experience an allergic reaction when using sea salt because of pollen in the seawater; use less salt. With only a pinch, the water in the pot will be equivalent to the salt concentration of the body (0.9%). Lean over the sink, turn the head to one side breathing through an open mouth, gently fitting the tip of the pot into Your upper nostril, sealing it... tip the pot slightly. Water runs through the nasal cavity and out the other nostril. When half the water has run through, gently blow out any remaining water and mucus. Repeat in the other nostril letting water flow in both directions. Besides a fresher feeling – being awake, and clear in the head – neti can relieve different forms of headaches, and allergies.

Following neti, brush Your teeth. While this may be adequately accomplished with a wet toothbrush, some prefer an alternative to chemical and sugar-laden commercial toothpaste. Be careful of the natural toothpaste at the health food store. Most have sodium lauryl (laureth) sulfate and other carcinogens. While some mix a little baking soda and a pinch of salt... it is quite abrasive. Simply use a moist toothbrush... if You prefer some sort of medium such as toothpaste, use cured clay – see **Ch 10**. The juncture of teeth and gums is the critical area to brush. Floss and / or use a flat wooden toothpick between the teeth after each meal.

After brushing You may enjoy tongue scraping, or at least those You kiss will enjoy Your fresh mouth and breath. In the Orient, doctors and dentists prefer tongue scraping to tooth brushing. The reason is, the tongue traps food particles, especially from cooked, processed foods; they decompose causing bad breath, and combine with saliva and bacteria to form plaque – a major cause of cavities and gum disease. This bacterial plaque settles on teeth while sleeping, and eventually solidifies into tartar.

Tongue scrapers are a flexible band of stainless steel that contours to the tongue. Gently scrape from the back forward rinsing off the mucus and bacteria that collect. Some simply use the edge of a spoon, although immediately after using a spoon, they will be amazed at what is removed with a proper tongue scraper. For further information: "Oral Hygiene: A History of Tongue Scraping and Brushing," by Drs. Christen & Swanson, *Journal of the American Dental Association*, Feb, '78.

Exercise and Movement: One of Life's Essentials

The number one cause of preventable death is smoking. Second is obesity. While death certificates may list high blood pressure or stroke, many of these conditions are linked to obesity, medically defined as 25 lbs over normal weight. Avoiding animal foods and taking algae, enzymes and probiotics, and drinking adequate re-mineralized and re-energized r/o or distilled water all contribute to health. Exercise is an equally important pillar of a holistic lifestyle – simply get out regularly for a brisk walk.

Many were taught jumping jacks, bouncing toe touches, straight leg sit-ups and other exercises seemingly designed to hurt as much as possible. "No pain, no gain" has been the motto. Current knowledge in exercise physiology has changed. With conscious enzyme-rich, diet free from cooked animal protein… even as we sage our joints, muscles and ligaments will retain water content and reasonable elasticity.

When undertaking any form of exercise, begin with a warm-up… stretching muscles this way and that, twisting gently in all directions, bending forward and backward, side to side. Muscles and nerves are alerted, prepared for exertion. Here are conservative alternatives to "normal" dangerous exercises.

The Windmill is a rapid movement that twists the spine, leaning over from the waist and touching opposite fingers and toes. The whole thing is rather dangerous: quick movement, severe spine twisting and leaning over from the waist without back support. As an alternative, do the hamstring stretch. Lie on Your back, raise one leg to the point of tension at the back of the leg, keeping the knee as straight as possible; lower the leg and repeat on the other side. Keep Your hips on the floor; support Your neck with a small pillow.

The Standing Toe Touch tightens hamstrings rather than relaxes; it also strains the back. As an alternative, place the heel of Your right foot on a low step, keeping Your knee straight. With Your hands on Your right thigh, bend forward from the hips until You feel slight tension in the back of Your right leg; change sides.

The Double Leg Lift supposedly works the lower abs, yet tightens the hip flexors attaching thigh muscles to the hips. Alternative: reverse trunk curls. Lie on Your back, bringing knees to Your chest. Cross arms over chest and contract the abs, lifting knees to Your face.

Full Sit-ups strain the hip flexors. Your abs begin the motion and after You lift Your trunk about 45° the hip flexors take over, pulling on the low back adding to the strain. As an alternative, do the crunch. Lie on Your back, feet flat on the floor and cross arms over chest, tightening Your abs. Raise Your chest toward the ceiling. Take two counts to reach 45° and two counts to come back down.

The Bicycle is yet another strain on the hip flexors. Lying on Your back, pumping Your legs also contracts the lower back muscles. As an alternative: twisting trunk curls. Lie on Your back knees bent, feet flat on the floor, cross arms over chest. Tighten Your abs and lift the torso slightly, rotating the trunk to engage the obliques, keeping the opposite hip on the ground. Change sides.

The Yoga Plow puts pressure on vertebrae in the neck and disc spaces – conservatively recommended only for accomplished gymnasts and yogis. As an alternative, lie on Your back and interlace fingers behind Your head. Use Your arms to slowly pull Your head toward Your chest; when You feel tension, pause and hold for a few seconds breathing deeply. Return to the ground; repeat.

Pole Twists have been around for centuries, going back to the Greeks with their javelins, and surely before. As a warm-up, the back muscles are cold and can be injured. The goal of a warm-up is: raise core body temperature, softening the muscles and preparing the body for the work that is to come. As an alternative warm up walk, jog, bicycle, or any easy activity, to develop a light sweat.

Deep Knee Bends are dangerous unless You are accustomed to squatting. As an alternative and to arrive at that point, do a 1/2-squat – forming a 90° angle, as though You are sitting in a chair. Hold for a few seconds, stand, and then repeat. As You become comfortable, move to a 3/4-squat, then a full squat.

The Fire Hydrant finds You on all fours, lifting one leg repeatedly, extending it to the side. This strains the back. As an alternative, lie on Your stomach extending and raising opposite arm and leg a few inches, holding a few seconds, return to the ground; repeat with opposite arm and leg.

These exercises can be done as a warm up and then repeated more vigorously for a half hour of aerobics, or move on to serious aerobics. When complete with warm-up, aerobic or resistance exercises, rather than falling into a chair or elsewhere, take some time to cool down with a brisk five-minute walk with Your arms swinging freely at Your sides. This allows the body to begin eliminating lactic acid and accumulated wastes resulting from strenuous exercise.

Aerobic Exercises

Respiration is the essence of life – bringing nutrients and releasing wastes. While that seems simple, there are blatant incongruities, such as doing aerobic exercise – increasing the heart rate and expanding the lungs – at the side of the road with the attendant fumes! While aerobics are known to stimulate the production of endorphins and enkephalins, part of the "runner's high" could be the body's immune response to the carbon monoxide, lead and other toxins driven deep into the lungs. This is really *negative* Vibrational Medicine, diluting and polluting one's energies.

Aerobics can be positive Vibrational Energy Medicine normalizing blood chemistry, raising levels of awareness and energizing HeartMindBodySpirit. Aerobics tone the cardiovascular system, the skin and muscles. Always wait ½ hour after a meal, longer after animal products. Always exercise after getting up rather than before bed or a nap. Aerobics can loosely be described as any activity involving the whole body, sustained for 20-30 minutes. The reality is… it takes 12 minutes of sustained activity to reach the aerobic stage. The length of time You maintain that activity after those 12 minutes is the actual time that You have done aerobic exercise. Studies show going beyond 45 minutes, You have diminishing returns; if You are attracted to long periods of strenuous exercise, enjoy a 15-minute meditation between 45-minute sets to get the most from Your efforts.

Swimming is at the top of the list because the body is supported by water and the joints are exposed to the least stress. The drawback is swimming in pools with chlorine, which absorbs through the skin as well as the lungs, and weakens the hair. A pool purified with ozone eliminates the danger. Bicycling is also fairly safe, as long as it is away from the fumes of traffic. When possible, ride "no hands" to work Your upper body pumping Your arms. Dancing is safe and easy. Start Your favorite music and get moving. This can be in the form of shaking, jumping up and down… any dance. Keep moving even with a brief pause in music between songs. Enjoy dancing, running, jumping, skipping rope, or simply moving around, having fun on a rebounder… the key word: Enjoy!

Helpful hints with rebounders: before using, take off the rubber or plastic cap from the bottoms of the legs. Go to the hardware store and get flat washers that fit snugly inside. This way when You jump, the edge of the metal legs contacts the washer, rather than cutting through the end cap.

Another helpful hint with any jumping exercise: the lymphatic system is one of our waste removal systems and is stimulated by jumping. The lymphatics are governed by a series of one-way valves and fluid moves most readily when we are in a state of weightlessness, so in that *instant*… between when we stop going up, and we start coming down… lymph flows easily. Rebounders and trampolines are powerful and energizing.

Interestingly, the profession with the longest average life span is the orchestra conductor. Many lymphatic vessels are under our arms and in our groin. Constant movement side to side, slightly bouncing up and down, arms vigorously waving overhead... stimulates the lymph system. So, put on Your favorite music and be the conductor... 20 minutes every other day.

DIY rebounder! Create Your own bouncing rhythm on the balls of Your feet. Jumping rope also has up and down motion, moving Your arms. When lymphatics remove waste efficiently, You feel and look radiant. For the **Control Group** preferring passive lymphatic exercise, a Chi machine gently moving Your legs back & forth, can create miracles – especially when incorporating strategic placement of Your arms, Sacred Breath, and Humming for Cranial Health. 15 minutes, 3X/day. Also, these dedicated Minimalists are wise to begin the day with at least the 1st of the 5 Tibetan Rites of Rejuvenation: turning clockwise 21X – at whatever speed. EnJoy!

Loved by many, running has serious dangers to consider in the 2020s with Weather as Warfare graphene oxide particulates rushing down our throats! Running on the sidewalk also puts You in proximity to the fumes of the road, and the joints of Your ankles, knees and hips are under tremendous strain. Run at the beach, on grass at the park, or on an earthen path such as natural wood chips. This way Your joints suffer less. When You run on the balls of Your feet, there is more spring to Your step and Your joints suffer less.

Barefoot is Best! Mother Earth is charged with negative ions – free electrons reducing inflammation, neutralizing wandering free radicals promoting normal functions and hormone production. We inhale Mother Earth's energy through our feet, and exhale as well. The pores on the soles of our feet and the palms of our hands are twice as big as the pores on the rest of the body. Running or walking on wet sand or wet grass helps rid the body of toxins, pulling negative ion energy through the soles of our feet. Walking barefoot experiencing the cool morning dew is energizing – if the early morning grass is dry, sprinkle it first and walk on it while You spray the vegetables and flowers. Critics doing the **30-day test** become converts. Improvements are reported with conditions as diverse as arthritis, allergies and general malaise. Be One with Mother Nature. She nurtures You.

Exer-cleaning is a way to get housework done exercising at the same time: moving quickly around the house doing chores; simply exaggerate Your movements, stretch and move energetically. Vacuuming, washing the car, bringing in groceries and putting them away, all can be done with a swiftness underfoot that can be likened to a dance. When unloading the dishwasher, squat keeping back straight, rather than bend from the waist.

During this... or any exercise... when there is pain, take a breather... along with slow, deep, caressing breaths. With **chest pain**, deeply massage the left thenar pad with fingertips and nails of the right hand... then vigorously massage index finger and pinky of the left hand; squeeze them at the tips. Hydrate. Breathe deeply, exhale completely. **Deep chest pain**: the Harvard Ha–Ku Breath is recommended: with open mouth make the sound Ha inhaling, then forcefully exhale saying Ku – repeat until the pain disappears.

Walking is easy exercise for most. Whenever possible walk outside in the fresh morning air or late afternoon sun. Asphalt walkways in many parks have deleterious effects – both for runners and for the aerobic walker. Avoid the pounding of the ankles, knees and hip joints. Simply walk alongside the asphalt or walk through the woods at a brisk pace. Walking on Mother Earth we re-connect on many levels, especially when barefoot. If conditions are muddy, keep an extra pair of walking shoes in a plastic bag in the trunk. Walking sticks are helpful at a brisk pace on uneven surfaces; the optimal height is the crest of Your hips; use branches of a tree; feel Mother Nature in Your hands. Involving the upper body maximizes benefits similar to cross-country skiing.

Aerobic walking is walking with determination – arms swinging freely at Your side. **Strict aerobic walking** brings each step to the mid-line, like walking the white line – hold the arms bent at 90°... and as You step forward with Your right foot, Your left elbow comes in line with Your left hip and Your right wrist comes in line with Your right hip. As You step forward with Your left foot, Your right elbow comes in line with Your right hip and Your left wrist comes in line with Your left hip. Create Your own rhythm and speed. You will know You went for a walk, raising Your vibrations. The next level? Add 1lb weight to each wrist and ankle. More than this... and You enter another world – the world of resistance exercises.

Resistance Exercises

Using weights, resistance exercise, builds muscle mass and strong bones. This can be fancy, getting the latest from the local pro shop, or simply fill plastic jugs with water or wet sand. Lift with the legs as much as You can; the muscles in the legs are the largest in the body. While muscles in the back are many, they are small and prone to strain and possible tearing. People who enjoy resistance exercises like to do it every day. Since it takes a day to recover, work the lower body one day, upper body the next. Many repetitions with light weights bring more results than a few repetitions with lots of weight.

If You enjoy body building and working out 2-4 hours a day, resistance exercises provide bulges and ripples. Resistance exercises are also a commitment. Once You stop, You look out of shape for quite a while before Your body re-adjusts. If You enjoy working out and are committed – great. If it is a *chore*, consider other means to get in shape and tone Your body.

T-TAPP Exercises address body toning, bone-building, cardiovascular fitness, pain relief and rehabilitation. In her video, Teresa Tapp does the entire Total Workout standing in an area with just enough room to fully extend arms and legs to the sides, front and back. Only supportive shoes and flexible clothing are required, making it attractive for busy executives, traveling models and others looking to create these qualities in their lives.

Teresa has always had an ardent interest in health and fitness, specializing in Exercise Physiology, Public Health and Nutrition – her Master's thesis is *Metabolisms in Women Over the Age of 30*. Her original plan was to pursue a medical degree; tuition money was a challenge, and the fashion industry called. Combining the French philosophy of gustatory delights and exercising in secret... along with the fact that models are constantly on the go, living in hotel rooms unable to spend hours slaving away at the gym... led this cutting-edge fitness expert to develop a novel approach. Done free from weights or body-jarring aerobics, anyone can work out for less than an hour in the privacy of their home or hotel room.

Movement gives maximum results with minimum effort, keeping the body in alignment. While Teresa's movements are rehabilitative and look easy, they provide a workout that removes inches from the waist and thighs. Her SitFit program is perfect for all, **even if confined to a wheelchair**. Michael E. Mcivor, MD, of Foundation Research in St. Petersburg, FL was so impressed with her data from the last 20 years he began a study: *The Role of Exercise in the Treatment of Chronic Heart Failure: The Sit Down for Cardiac Fitness (SitFit)*. Sloan-Kettering confirms the data and benefits. https://www.t-tapp.com

Building muscle mass and strong bones is vital. Since we are 80% water, drink at least two quarts of re-mineralized and re-energized r/o or distilled water a day in addition to earth milks. Green foods such as broccoli, celery, collards and cucumber, seaweed and other forms of algae, as well as yellow and orange fruits and vegetables bring minerals and muscle tone.

Alfalfa, *Medicago Sativa*, builds tissue and helps put on weight. Too much green alfalfa can kill a cow or a horse, yet dried hay is their greatest food – one of Life's mysteries. You can eat alfalfa as green sprouts, juiced, or dried in tablet form... or take the homeopathic **Mother Tincture of alfalfa *Medicago Sativa***: 1tsp in 1 oz water 3x/day, between meals.

Also, **Mother Tincture of oats *Avena Sativa***: 5 drops in 1 oz water 3x/day, between meals. This is a natural stimulant and body builder that nurtures the nerves acting as a restorative for nervous exhaustion and general debility. When taking more than one homeopathic remedy, take 15 minutes apart and 15 minutes away from any other tastes, before and after.

Taking homeopathic remedies: avoid basil, camphor, and eucalyptus altogether. Avoid peppermint a half-hour before and after remedies. {Ch 9: **Vibrational Energy Medicine as Found in Homeopathy**.}

Tibetan Rites of Rejuvenation

Raising vibrational energies and increasing vitality, these exercises have transformed many lives. Peter Kelder tells Colonel Bradford's complete story in *Ancient Secret of the Fountain of Youth*, first published in 1939... called *The Tibetan Rites of Rejuvenation*. The Colonel, a British officer stationed in India, repeatedly heard stories of a remote lamasery in the Himalayas where people seemed to avoid growing old. Men over 100 retained the strength, vigor and appearance they had when 30... and old men who went to live in the lamasery reportedly began looking and acting dramatically younger within a few months.

Colonel Bradford found himself aging rapidly after retirement – growing feeble, using a cane. Remembering the stories of the lamasery in India and, having nothing to lose, he thought to return to India, and find it. He asked his friend Peter Kelder to join him, and Peter – seeing a senile man on a wild goose chase – refused. Determined, the Colonel set out alone.

After months, the Colonel found the lamasery and began their way of life. Within a few weeks he began to feel younger and stronger; he left his cane behind and began hard work in the garden. He spent two years at the lamasery and then a couple of months in India sharing his newfound knowledge. The lamas made no effort to conceal their wisdom. Their remote location, human skepticism and laziness kept their rejuvenating Way of Life from being known and practiced.

At the lamasery Colonel Bradford learned the secrets of a simple life: clean air and water, working outdoors, eating whole grains and vegetables, positive thoughts and a spiritual focus. He also learned the simple exercises known as *The Tibetan Rites of Rejuvenation*. When he returned to New York, the Colonel went to see his friend Peter Kelder who was expecting to see a 70-year-old man, and instead opened the door to someone who appeared to be 40ish. At first, he thought it was the Colonel's son. When the Colonel shared his experiences, Peter began practicing the Five Rites and found them invigorating. He organized classes for the Colonel; others began to benefit.

While resistance exercises build muscular strength… and yoga promotes flexibility… these Rites increase energy and vitality. According to ancient teachings learned by the Colonel, the Rites restore balance and spin to the chakras – endocrine energy centers – spinning equally at high speed as in a young and vigorous person. This may be checked with a pendulum. When congested – physically, emotionally, mentally or spiritually – the vortex begins to slow in one or more energy center, out of harmonious synchrony… slowing the energy flow, weakening the body, leading to depression, nervousness, disease and decay.

Daily practice of the Five Rites restores the spin of the vortex found at each endocrine energy center, facilitating the regulation of our hormone output. Most feel the difference within a few days. 1st week, the Colonel recommends each of the Five Rites repeated 3X. 2nd week, 5. 3rd week, 7. Add two reps per week until 21X, then maintain that level. As with yoga, focused in meditation creates optimal results.

1st Rite is so ingrained children do it for sheer joy. Some say it is so profoundly effective that – if time or circumstances prevail – it is sufficient to do this one alone. Simply stand with arms horizontally outstretched, left palm up, right palm down. Focus on Your thumb to allay any dizziness. Slowly breathing… caressing… turn clockwise 21X – looking at Your right thumb and begin spinning: bring Your right arm behind, left arm forward as You turn. Speed is inconsequential. Go slowly, or briskly if You are up to it. Spinning several times briskly, You may feel dizzy for a few seconds when You stop – even though Your focus is on Your thumb. Why? Your eyes are filled with water & spinning, the water forms a vortex. When You stop, it continues to move momentarily. To avert feeling dizzy when You stop, simply close Your eyes. Unstable? Bend over slightly, grab Your thighs for 3 seconds. Then stand with hands on hips for 3 Sacred Breaths.

Doing bending exercises – such as the following rites, or with yoga – it makes physiological sense to breathe in arching backward, making room for our expanding lungs… and breathe out bending forward, compressing our lung field as we exhale completely.

2nd Rite is performed lying on Your back, hands flat on the floor, thumbs under buttocks. Take a deep, caressing breath… as You exhale bring Your chin to Your chest and, keeping Your knees as straight as possible, raise Your legs to a vertical position… possibly extending over Your head. Hold for 3 seconds. Then inhale as You slowly bring head and legs to the floor again 21X. Then stand with hands on hips for 3 Sacred Breaths.

3rd Rite is performed on Your knees, hands on backs of thighs – fingers at back, thumbs at sides – tops of Your toes on the floor. Take in a deep, caressing breath… exhaling, touch Your chin to Your chest bending forward so Your toes lift *slightly* from the floor. {If You bend too far forward, bring Your arms straight out to maintain balance.} Then take in a deep, caressing breath as You arch back, extending Your chin to the ceiling. Hold for 3 seconds, return to neutral… 21X. Then stand with hands on hips for 3 Sacred Breaths.

4th Rite is performed sitting on the floor with legs straight out front, hands at Your side pointing out from the hips. Take in a deep, caressing breath and exhale. Taking in Your next deep breath, bend Your knees and push with Your arms, bringing Your pelvis upward, forming a table – with Your arms and calves as the legs and Your torso and thighs as the top. Pointing head toward the floor, gently stretch Your neck backward. As You exhale, return to the sitting position, touching chin to chest... 21X. Then stand with hands on hips for 3 Sacred Breaths.

The Fifth Rite is a modified push-up. Begin face down on the floor, with hands and feet shoulder width apart. Take in a deep, caressing breath and exhaling, bring Your pelvis in the air forming an inverted V... and gently stretch chin to chest and heels to floor, tensing the body for 3 seconds. Then inhaling, bring Your pelvis down to barely touch the floor... keeping the weight on hands and toes, arching Your neck back, tensing the body for 3 seconds... 21X. Then stand with hands on hips for 3 Sacred Breaths.

The Five Rites can set the stage for Tantra Yoga and Sacred Sexuality. Colonel Bradford also taught a 6th Rite for those who have practiced for at least 9 weeks and feel "sexually complete" – committed to a life of celibacy. This rite is performed standing. Bend over, bracing hands on knees and force as much air as possible from the lungs. Then straighten up with Your hands on Your hips and push down, effectively raising the shoulders. Pull in the stomach as much as possible; hold the breath as long as possible. Exhaling, relax. When You feel energy rise from the root of Your being to the crown, You will have accomplished Your goal. Repeat as desired.

Those thinking it would be a profound challenge to do the Five Rites 21X are the ones who derive the most benefit. For those who think it would be ludicrous to even attempt... *visualize* **doing it perfectly and easily 21X.** Simply lie on Your back in the receptive pose of yoga: head pointing north, feet shoulder width apart, arms going out at the same angle as the feet, hands palm up. Close Your eyes and see Yourself doing each step... breathing in and out at appropriate times... and visualize each Rite 21X. You will be amazed at how quickly... You are actually *doing it* with ease! A study measured performance, speed and agility of professional teams. One team spent a month watching videos of championship teams. Another team spent the month practicing. A third team spent the month practicing half the time and watching videos the other half. The team showing most improvement in performance, speed and agility only watched videos of champions! Visualization: a powerful, creative force!

The Polarity Squat

Randolph Stone, Doctor of Chiropractic and Doctor of Osteopathy founded the system of Polarity Therapy, actually an ancient form of Vibrational Energy Medicine. Drawing on centuries of tradition, his simple teachings prepared for the renaissance known as: Healing Touch. Various types of hands-on healing – hands on the body, hands on the aura: inches, or a foot away from the body – exhibit the inherent understanding: subtle energies exist and can get congested. Through the power of thought and through energy transfer based on the power of Love... we assist free flow of energy, relieving pain and bringing balance to HeartMindBodySpirit.

Polarity Therapy is based on ancient wisdom that energy travels from the South to the North Pole. Many cultures sleep with their head pointing north including many Native Americans and others from India and the Orient. Feet are the south pole and the head is the north pole of our body; sleeping in such a fashion aligns us with the energy flow on Mother Earth. Beneficial also for the treatment table.

Polarity Therapy recognizes the right brain, our feminine receptive self, controls the left side of the body; the left brain, our masculine outgoing self, controls the right side of the body. As the right-hand projects energy, the left-hand receives energy. Where we place our hands – on or above the body – influences energy flow relieving pain and blockages. As a preliminary, rub hands briskly together, including the tops warming the hands, stimulating energy flow. Briskly rub fingernails against each other, to stimulate flow of Chi in the meridians. With the right hand on the sacrum and left hand on the head, visualize energy flowing with 3 Sacred Breaths. This assists spiritual awakening of kundalini, freeing the coiled energy at the sacrum harmonizing HeartMindBodySpirit. With hands making contact, held in position for a few minutes or for several minutes, follow Inner Guidance: the right hand may jiggle gently, as though saying "Wake up, now..."

Polarity Therapy recognizes connections between our energy centers, the five elements, and our fingers /

toes. 1st Root - Earth - Little finger. 2nd Emotional - Water - Ring. 3rd Solar Plexus - Fire - Middle. 4th Heart - Air - Index. 5th Throat - Ether - Thumb / Large toe. Dr Stone says the Polarity Squat makes holistic connections. While a universal posture for children around the world, in the West we are accustomed to civilized chairs offering little support for the human anatomy. To build strength, practice squatting.

For beginners: stand with feet 6" apart at the heels and 12" apart at the toes – arms straight in front, palms down. Gently move downward, as though going to sit in a chair. Going all the way, buttocks touching the backs of Your calves, You are ready for the next step. If You get part way and have second thoughts, return to the standing position. Wonderful! Do it again... gently... then add a few stretching bounces before returning to the standing position. Feel Yourself stretch with each bounce. Repeat, stretching as You go... until You are in full squat position. Whatever it takes, You can do it. Visualize.

Once You achieve the full squat, take 3 deep, caressing breaths and feel the actual comfort of this position. If at first less than comfortable, be confident... this exercise brings wonderful benefits. Focus on the breath... caressing... place Your armpits over the knees: gently rock back and forth a few times and then sideways a few times. Then wrap Your arms around the knees and join hands: gently push toward the center with Your arms, resisting with Your legs; then gently push Your legs apart while resisting with Your arms. Then take a deep, caressing breath and let it out with a **grunt** – promoting relaxation.

This prepares for Dr Stone's Youth Posture. Spread Your feet about 6" further apart. Above all... be comfortable. As You settle into the squat, bring Your hands together fingertips touching, thumbs at the bridge of Your nose... and bring Your elbows inside Your knees. Gently rock back and forth a few times and then sideways a few times. Gently push legs together while resisting with the elbows. Then push elbows apart, resisting with the legs. Take a deep, caressing breath and let it out with a **grunt**.

Completing Dr Stone's re-wiring of the electrical circuits for free flow of Chi: place elbows on Your knees doing a full squat with fingertips together from hand to hand keeping them apart, with thumbs on the bridge of Your nose.

Gently rock back and forth for 3 Sacred Breaths. Sideways for 3 Sacred Breaths. Sway in a circular fashion, first counterclockwise for 3 Sacred Breaths. Then clockwise for 3 Sacred Breaths. Take in a deep, caressing breath. **Grunt!**

Kegel Exercises
Primarily taught as a preliminary to childbirth, this relatively easy exercise can be done almost any time, any place: simply tightening both sphincters, anal and urethral, for several seconds during inhalation, or exhalation; then 30 seconds, 60 & 90 seconds. Deep, caressing breathing is the key. Strengthening muscles at the floor of the pelvis... facilitates control over pelvic movements during childbirth. Some do these exercises 200X/day. For both women and men, it is a sexual tonic facilitating prolonged lovemaking – even facilitating orgasm free from ejaculation, preserving male energy and vitality. This is also used in meditation to facilitate coiled energy rising from the sacrum to the crown.

Low Back Stretch
Stretching the piriformis and muscles of the low back brings relief, even for pain running down the leg. On all fours, doggy-style: cross one knee over the opposite leg, and with both knees on the floor, **drop Your elbows** to the floor as well – this changes Your line-of-drive, and isolates the piriformis. Gently push buttocks toward the feet, bringing chin to the chest. Hold this stretch for a few seconds... then take a deep, caressing breath and... exhaling, go back even further... then, a third time, going back further. Return to all fours. Switch knees and stretch again. Always do both sides 3X for pelvic balance.

The Salutation to the Sun
Salutation to the Sun: an orchestration of twelve graceful movements... raises vibrational energies, increasing awareness. Each movement flows smoothly into the next... as body... mind... breath... join to experience liberation of spirit. The movements bend the body alternately forward and backward, loosening and stretching from head to toe. As part of the flow, deep rhythmic breathing effectively massages internal organs, the spine is charged with energy. Circulation increased, the body pulses with vitality; mind is calmed, focused on the inner core, the center of Your being. This exercise can serve as preparation for yoga postures, or by itself.

In Hindu mythology, sun is the sustainer of life and health... and guardian of immortality. Sun represents the highest form of altruism, giving free from question or judgment. Sunshine is for everyone and everything. Although practiced any time... traditionally it is performed in the serenity of early morning with an attitude of Gratitude, a spirit of Thankfulness.

At first... one is mindful of precision with each step of this dance. Practice deepens the flow of consciousness and energy. The influx of prana may bring spontaneous movements, radiating from the twelve basic positions.

Gradually it becomes a meditative flow. Benefits soon begin: body, mind and emotions become harmonized... the mind becomes relaxed... the nervous system strengthened... internal organs massaged... circulation increased, joints are free, muscles and ligaments toned. With a challenge to do a particular movement exactly as described, relax... gently stretch and moderate Your motions. With faithful practice flexibility develops, amazing suppleness being the wonderful side-effect.

On Your Mark... Get Set...
Beginners find it convenient to record the Sun Salutation... slowly... allowing ample time to feel... each position... each movement.

First, face the sun with palms together at the Heart – fingers touching, pointing up. Take slow, deep breaths... feel Gratitude, Joy and Humility.

Stand erect... feet together... with toes spread apart... feel them. Distribute Your weight evenly with arms freely at Your side... pull up Your kneecaps, tuck in Your buttocks, pull in Your abdomen, chest up and chin up. Breathe... *feel* this posture... the weightlessness, confidence and poise. Breathe in... as You breathe out, bring palms together at the Heart – fingers touching, pointing up.

Breathe in... keeping thumbs locked together with index fingers touching at the sides, while spreading both hands flat and stretching arms overhead. Keep Your arms by Your ears and keep Your buttocks firm. Arch the spine backward one vertebra at a time, top down.

Caution: pushing hips forward or bending the knees, creates tremendous pressure on the low back. Experiment: pushing the buttocks back, the chest forward, and the arms back in a spring-like motion. Exhaling fold Your body forward, keeping Your arms by Your ears. Folding from the hips, touch Your palms flat on the floor... fingers in line with toes. If required, bend Your knees to accomplish this position; if possible, bring Your head to Your knees.

Inhaling, stretch Your right leg all the way back, with Your knee on the floor... keeping Your head and chin up. Hold the breath as You bring the other leg back; support Your weight on Your toes and the palms of Your hands... head, neck and body in a straight line.

Drop Your knees to the floor, resting the tops of Your feet on the floor. Push Your hips up and raise Your head, arching the spine. Lower Your chest and chin to the floor. Inhale bringing Your hips to the floor, sliding forward, arching Your back, with chin pointed up.

Curl Your toes to support Yourself, bringing Your hips in the air – forming an inverted V – as You exhale. Press heels toward the floor, and head to Your chest... gently stretching the hamstrings and shoulder muscles. Inhale bringing the right foot forward between Your hands... hips down and head up. (The opposite the fourth position.) Exhaling, bring the other leg forward, fingers in line with the toes, head to the knees. Inhaling, reach forward, up and back in one smooth movement, interlocking the thumbs as in the second position.

Exhaling gracefully, bring Your palms together at the Heart – fingers touching, pointing up, standing erect. Lower Your hands to Your sides returning to the original standing position, ready to begin again – alternating sides, beginning with the fourth position. Traditionally 6-12 rounds are done.

Exercises to Reprogram the Subconscious
Integrating left and right brain – logical and creative forces – with Your extremities crossing the midline, the subconscious pays attention and access may be made... an effective and powerful way to change beliefs; repetition drives the conditioning process deeply into the subconscious. First re-create Your beliefs and highest choices *inwardly* – to re-create Your *outward* experience of Reality. These exercises summon powerful forces, and require preparation.

With holistic lifestyles... affirmations flow naturally in conversations and throughout the day as situations arise. When creating time and space for intentional work with affirmations – warm-ups are as important as with physical exercise. Here You are exercising the mind – engaging in the task of reprogramming Your subconscious to Rehabilitate Your Inner Child and... Recreate Your Life. Perhaps set the stage with soft acoustics, such as Tom Kenyon's *The Ultimate Brain: Opening the Heart* – written in the Key of F to facilitate communication between the right & left hemispheres – soothing the cerebellum – nurturing Heart energy.

With love, honor and respect for the various levels of Your Being... HeartMindBodySpirit... approach with Joy, Thanksgiving. The cranial vault has the Motherboard, the complex neuro-vascular network which is directed by the hypothalamus, taking cues from the Heart. Facial bones have several sinuses. Through breath and vibration, we can project the voice through the maxillary and sphenoid sinuses, creating resonant tones. Breathing deeply, each exhale is prolonged... ending with a vibrating hummm: Haaame...Heeeme...Haaahm...Hooome...Huuum... again and again, until Your voice is felt coming from Your face, rather than from Your throat. Opening the resonant sphenoid sinuses, vibrations eventually can be felt at the top of Your head!

Cranial neurovascular system now fully alert, making subtle energetic connections Your warm-up to reprogram Your subconscious continues. While it is recommended generally to caress the bump at the roof of Your mouth connecting Heart and Pineal centers... as this Cranial Awakening begins the tongue rests at the lower jaw, teeth apart, lips lightly closed. Breathe in as much as possible, and exhale humming with closed lips with Your deepest, most resonant voice... feel the vibrations... exhaling completely, bring Your teeth together and swallow... then separate teeth and tongue for the next round – do this 3X.

Then another 3X using the same protocol with lips closed now teeth touching, and smiling throughout... with the tongue caressing the roof of the mouth... swallowing after every exhale.

Finally, 3X as above, with eyes focused center and up... thumbs firmly fixed in Your ears, fingernails facing posterior humming... swallow after every exhale. Any fragrance or taste summons the olfactory nerve.

Through breath, vibration and energetic contacts, all levels of Your HeartMindBodySpirit are now fully awake and aware. Your subconscious is fully alert. Attentive. Receptive.

Now with 3 Sacred Breaths: feel Gratitude... Humility... Joy... approach Your subconscious through Your Heart of Hearts. With closed eyes, touch Your Heart center, feel the warmth under Your fingertips, under Your hand. Breathing slowly, a signal is sent: I Am now safe. The sympathetic system: at rest; the immune response: alert.

For 3 minutes while briskly rubbing Your fingernails together... nurture feelings of Appreciation... Gratitude... Compassion... and Care... for Mother Earth and All her children, including Yourself. Now, energy freely flowing through Your energy body, with Your Intention set, You are ready to exercise.

Visual Stimulation – extend Your arms in front, clasping hands together fingers interlocked, thumbs crossed, index fingers pointing straight. You will be making motions of a figure eight on its side – ∞ – tapping into Infinity. Move Your arms first to the top left, then down the side, making sure You come up through the middle of the figure – eyes following Your thumbs through the motions – with head straight, move only Your eyes.

Doing so, Voice the statement of Your highest Choice to re-program Your subconscious. Repeat the motions, saying Your statement aloud with a smile on Your face. Your statement may be general: I Am Love in Service! or: I Am a courageous person, and speak before large groups with confidence and ease! Repeat 3X.

Auditory Stimulation – massage the outer rim of both ears simultaneously with opposite thumbs and index fingers. Start at the top of Your ears and gently roll and pull outward and back all the way down to the bottom. Repeat this motion with a smile on Your face, affirming Your statement 3X.

Motion Stimulation – standing with feet shoulder-width apart, arms raised bent at the elbows bring left knee and right elbow together. Return to Your original position, and repeat with opposite knee and elbow. This soon becomes a smooth flowing motion. Repeat smiling, affirming Your statement 3X.

Spiritual Stimulation – standing with feet shoulder width apart, place one hand on top of the other over the sternum; *feel* Your happy, smiling, voice vibrations as You affirm Your statement aloud 3X. Then, in the receptive pose of yoga, with 3 Sacred Breaths, repeat Your statement to Yourself. Give Thanks! Feel Joy! Feel the Pineal and Heart Center as One. Be Love!

Rest on the 7th day
With speculation about the Creation account in the Book of Genesis… Creationists literally interpret: the world was created in six 24-hour periods. Evolutionists believe it was created in several eras of indeterminate time. Whichever… one important message of *Genesis* is, after the work was done – "on the seventh day – God rested." The lesson: if God took a rest… it is important for us to have a day of rest! Some take one day a week and completely rest from everything: exercise, work, chores around the house, superfoods and supplements, and even food. They use the time to enjoy a luxurious bath – 2lbs Epsom salts and 2lbs baking soda – followed by a cool rinse, and an apple cider vinegar splash and relax with a tall glass of re-mineralized and re-energized r/o or distilled water. Observe. Count Your Blessings. On this special day of rest, do something special… receive a massage, or other energy work… have extra water… lay in the sun, walk in the woods, listen to the birds, have more water… sit outdoors by the water or by a fire, read a book, write letters. Create time and space for private reflection… You deserve it. You'll be much more efficient and satisfied with Life… explOring Your Spirit's Quest. Blessings on Your Sacred Journey!

Yoga Nidra: The Inner Communion of Sleep
A relaxing way to end the day – *Yoga nidra* (NEE-dra): *Yoga* means inner communion, *nidra* means sleep. Yoga nidra induces deep relaxation of the entire human structure and personality and can eradicate deep-rooted psychological complexes, neuroses and inhibitions. Yoga nidra as a tranquilizer relieves insomnia… opens potentials of the mind… awakens intuition… normalizes blood pressure… and can improve absorption and retention of information.

For someone who physically requires rest, yoga nidra offers the benefits of deep, refreshing sleep. The student is generally asked to remain wakeful. Observing.

For students practicing yoga… yoga nidra offers psychic sleep – a state of conscious dreaming, where one can see visions of the subconscious mind. As the person hovers between sleep and wakefulness, challenges of the subconscious may surface such as fear, resentment and suppression. Regular practice cleanses these from the mind.

Practicing yoga nidra for some time, we can achieve the state of sleepless sleep balancing between introversion and extroversion… awakening the kundalini – a mystical state, and the ultimate achievement of yoga; with desires and imaginations rooted out, we are free from karma.

Yoga nidra induces physical and emotional tranquility… releases tension from the mind… induces inner knowledge and meditation – bringing the experience of Inner Peace. Yoga nidra goes beyond the conscious mind, with its surface thoughts and perceptions of the outside world… goes beyond the subconscious mind, experienced in the dream-state as individual memory and thought-forms… and even goes beyond the unconscious mind, experienced in deep sleep as collective memory and thought-forms.

Yoga nidra explores and transcends different states of mind. Transcending the mind, we can enter the vibration of super consciousness – pure, illumined consciousness of Infinite Being.

Sound Vibrations and Yoga Nidra While one may go through the stages of yoga nidra on an individual or internal basis, it is beneficial to hear the vibrations of the words. Record it, or ask someone whose voice You find soothing. Keep the voice calm and clear, allowing time… slow enough to follow, fast enough to keep attention from wandering. With deeper relaxation, instructions can be recorded again, slower. The advantage of recording is the central nervous system responds to repetition and consistency… the same voice… same words… same tonal inflections… bring the desired result: either deep sleep or deep awareness. The sound of the voice is the link enabling explorations of deeper layers of the mind. Without a guiding voice You slowly lapse into sleep. While this is acceptable when one requires rest or with insomnia, the student of yoga nidra goes beyond sleep… achieving high states of awareness. Rather than thinking about the words, remembering or anticipating… simply relax with the sound of the voice.

Preparing for Yoga Nidra Light, loose clothing is appropriate. In cold climates wear enough to remain warm throughout the practice, or cover with a blanket. When it is hot, use a fan on the low setting avoiding direct blasts of air... use a mosquito net if appropriate. Tradition recommends practicing in the confines of a quiet, dark, clean room, rather than open air. Remove any wristwatch, jewelry and ornaments. To remain in one position for a period of time, prepare by doing stretching, bending and twisting; perhaps the Tibetan Rejuvenation Rites or Sun Salutation. Wait at least one hour after eating. Practice any time You require rest.

A Resolution for Life An integral part of yoga nidra is creating a resolution regarding some aspect of Your life. I Am positive and dynamic. I Am successful in my work. I Am perfectly healthy. Inner Communion is part of my everyday life. Choose a resolution with which You resonate and keep it – until it bears fruit in Your Life. Then create another resolution. Someone choosing to be in service to Infinite Being, may say: Make me useful.

Rotating Awareness from One Body Part to Another When Your perception is directed to each physical center, feel the sensation rising from that particular part and mentally pronounce the name of that part once. Visualize that part being relaxed, healthy and whole. Focus awareness on the sound of the voice and the body part named. Rather than dwelling on a particular body part, allow the rotation of awareness from one body part to the next. At first instructions can be somewhat brisk to avoid distraction or dwelling on one or another part. With practice another recording may be made at a slower speed.

The Completion of Yoga Nidra The final statement is: Yoga nidra is complete. If You are using yoga nidra to fall asleep, breathe and be there. To deepen awareness, keep the eyes closed for a few moments being One with the experience. Take in a deep, caressing breath and slowly come back... slowly move Your hands and feet... be aware of external sounds... open Your eyes... slowly move into the squatting position... then slowly stand tall. Look out a window; pulsate with the Vibrations of Life.

The Posture of Yoga Nidra Choose a posture to be comfortable for an hour. Traditionally recommended is the receptive pose of yoga. Spread out a sheet or a large towel; if necessary, a pillow under Your neck or under the knees to relieve pressure on Your low back. Lie with feet shoulder width apart... arms palm up at the same angle as the legs. Relax; then tense all Your muscles and *relax* them. When ready to lie perfectly still, begin yoga nidra affirming: **I relax completely and maintain awareness**.

The Script for Yoga Nidra (spoken by the facilitator, or recorded) Now take in a deep, caressing breath and hold it while raising Your arms, legs, head and shoulders off the ground. Stretch and tense Your whole body as much as possible. Stay in this raised, tensed position as long as You can comfortably hold the breath.// Then lower Your body, breathe out and completely relax.// (This is one round; do 3.)

Now adjust Your body so You feel really comfortable. Adjust Your clothing, adjust Your pillows... be comfortable so You can remain motionless during the practice of yoga nidra. Have Your legs straight and slightly apart; have Your arms straight, slightly apart from Your body palms up. Close Your eyes and remain in this position until we are complete. The rest of the practice is entirely mental.

Be aware of Your whole body.// Visualize Your body, as though You are above looking down.// Feel heaviness in Your whole body.// Imagine that Your whole body is heavy.// Feel heaviness in Your right leg// left leg// right arm// left arm// feel heaviness in Your whole body.// (Repeat this process.)

Be aware with natural breathing.// As You breathe in, know that You are breathing in.// As You breathe out, know that You are breathing out.// Be completely aware of one thing, the process of breathing.// As You breathe in, count 1./// As You breathe out, count 2./// Continue in this manner until You reach a count of 50./////

At this point, please repeat Your resolution silently with intensity, with feeling.// Feel Your whole body and mind vibrate with the mental repetition of Your resolution.// Speak it mentally and wholeheartedly 3X.//

**We will now rotate awareness through the different parts of the body.// We will take a trip through the body.// Remember to be aware of each part of the body in turn.// You can either *feel* the sensation from each part of the body/ or You can create a mental *picture* of that part of the body/ or You can mentally *name* that part of the body once./ Choose for Yourself./ Please remain alert and aware of instructions./ Choose to make this easy… it truly is an easy process.//

First be aware of Your right hand.// Then right hand thumb/ index finger/ middle finger/ ring finger/ little finger/ all fingers together/ the palm and back of the right hand/ be aware of Your right hand.// Now Your right wrist/ forearm and elbow/ Your arm and right shoulder/ armpit/ right side of Your waist/ right buttocks/ right thigh/ knee/ calf/ ankle/ heel/ sole/ top of right foot/ big toe/ second toe/ third toe/ fourth toe/ fifth toe/ all toes together.// Be aware.//

Now the left side./ Be aware of Your left hand.// Then left hand thumb/ index finger/ middle finger/ ring finger/ little finger/ all fingers together/ the palm and back of the left hand/ be aware of Your left hand.// Now Your left wrist/ forearm and elbow/ Your arm and left shoulder/ armpit/ left side of Your waist/ left buttocks/ left thigh/ knee/ calf/ ankle/ heel/ sole/ top of left foot/ big toe/ second toe/ third toe/ fourth toe/ fifth toe/ all toes together.// Be aware.//

Now the back.// Right buttocks/ left buttocks/ both buttocks together.// Right shoulder blade/ left shoulder blade/ both shoulder blades together.// Be aware of the spine from top to bottom.// The back of the head/ top of the head/ forehead// right eyebrow/ left eyebrow/ the center of the eyebrows.// Be aware of the right eye/ left eye// right ear/ left ear// right cheek/ left cheek// nose/ upper lip/ lower lip/ both lips together.// The chin/ throat/ right side of the chest/ left side of the chest/ the whole chest// The navel/ right side of the abdomen/ left side of the abdomen/ the whole abdomen.// Be aware.// Now the major limbs/ the whole right leg/ the whole left leg/ both legs together.// Right arm/ left arm/ both arms together.// Be aware of Your head.// Be aware of Your whole body.// Your whole body.// Whole body.//

Please maintain awareness.// Please remain still.// Simply be aware.///

Repeat Your resolution silently, with intensity and feeling.// Feel Your whole body and mind vibrate with the mental repetition of Your resolution.// Speak it mentally, wholeheartedly 3X.// Remain still.// Be aware.///

{If time permits – repeat 3X; begin with **We will now rotate awareness…}

Visualize Yourself now at peace with Mother Earth.// In a peaceful protected part of the woods/// on the porch in a peaceful rain/// by a peaceful waterfall resplendent with flowers and the sounds of birds/// stroking a dog or a cat/// in a flower garden/// in front of a fireplace on a cold night/// at the ocean with the waves breaking on the beach/// hear the pounding of the waves/// be aware of the immensity of the ocean/// be aware of the calm ocean on a warm summer day/// feel the calmness and hidden power within the ocean.// This is like Your mind.///

Repeat Your resolution silently, with intensity and feeling.// Feel Your whole body and mind vibrate with the mental repetition of Your resolution.// Speak it mentally, wholeheartedly 3X.// Remain still.// Be aware.///

You are complete with the practice of yoga nidra.// Be aware of Your mind.// Say to Yourself "Yoga nidra is complete."//// Take in a deep, caressing breath.// Gently come back.// Slowly move Your hands.// Slowly move Your feet.// Be aware of outside sounds.// Open Your eyes.// If You feel relaxed and have time available, remain in the lying position.// Otherwise, gently raise Your body upright.// Be aware.////

Yoga nidra is an excellent way to re-program the subconscious. With Your resolution, You continue to Voice Your Choice – creating Your New Reality!

"…And to All a Good Night!"
With challenges getting a good night's rest, yoga nidra is a wonderful exercise before retiring. Wisdom of the Ages gives other sound principles: subtle, yet profound. Finish Your last meal or snack at least 3 hours before bed. Every hour's rest before midnight = two hours rest after. Going to sleep at 10 o'clock and getting up at dawn provides restful sleep and rejuvenates the immune response system. Sleeping with Your head pointing north puts the polarity of Your body in alignment with the polarity of the planet. Energy travels south to north. Your feet, the south pole of the body, receive energy and allow it to flow to Your head, the north pole of the body, providing restful sleep. The Vastu school of thought says opposite poles attract and similar poles repel. They suggest sleeping with the head pointing south. Experiment.

Placing furniture, some practices have been around for centuries known in different cultures by different names. Feng Shui (pronounced fung shway) means wind and water, two elements that are primary factors to move chi (pronounced variously: chee, shee or kee) energy... prana... soul / spirit. Feng Shui, an ancient Chinese art form, is rooted in Taoist and Buddhist philosophies. According to Feng Shui – if You are born in the summer, point the head of Your bed north to cool the spirits; if You are born in the winter, point the head of Your bed south to warm them; to encourage relationships point Your head to the northeast corner of the room – with the doorway being the south end, regardless of the compass. Point Your head to the northwest corner to encourage wealth and blessings.

Among things that interfere with our subtle energy fields and sleep patterns are quartz numerical display clocks, whether on Your wrist or on the bed stand next to Your head. If a clock radio is how You get up in the morning, keep it as far away as possible; this also applies to other electrical appliances such as IT devices, TVs, computers, electric heaters and clocks.

Cell phones and wireless devices have been seriously incriminated. *Cell Phones: Invisible Hazards in the Wireless Age*, by Dr George Carlo advises using the speakerphone, keeping them away from Your body, especially Your lap – these admonitions are in small print which people rarely read. Radiation plumes are most intense during ringing and dialing; avoid keeping it attached to Your waist. Children under 10 should be kept away altogether. Some advanced countries outlaw use of cellphones by children under seventeen. Why? Children have thin skulls. The human skull matures reaching full thickness and, more significantly, reaching neurological maturity... after the age of **25**.

If it runs, it produces electromagnetic fields (EMFs) linked to serious health issues, brain tumors and breast cancer. Keep these appliances at least 3' from Your bed; after that the EMFs rapidly decline. While our houses surround us with a grid of electrical current, it is quite another thing to lie all night on a waterbed that is warmed by an electric heater. Water conducts electricity, and the waterbed becomes charged, interfering with our subtle energy fields. The majority of chiropractors see waterbeds and recliner chairs as good for business. Another offender is the electric blanket; remaining plugged in, it carries a steady stream of EMFs all night long. These blankets are made from polyester... irritating to the skin, emitting formaldehyde gas. Some are hyper-sensitive, so to avoid the EMFs they turn off all circuit breakers, except the refrigerator, and notice a more restful night's sleep, awakening more refreshed. At least turn off Your router! Explore EMF dangers, as well as protection: https://www.giawellness.com/23215/products/energy/

97% of carpets are made from synthetics emitting over 100 chemical gases including benzene, formaldehyde and xylene. The new carpet smell is a special chemical that can burn eyes, blur vision, produce chills and fevers, memory loss and depression. The healthy option is tile, cork or hardwood floors covered with jute or natural cotton coil rugs. Use natural primers, sealers, varnishes, stains, paints and flooring when building or refurbishing.

Bedroom furniture can pose a serious hazard. Modern furniture is mostly particleboard: wood chips, sawdust and glue: urea-formaldehyde resin. Most furniture gases are emitted the first ten years. Antiques and modern hardwood furniture are safe, adding a feeling of warmth.

Avoid reading papers, watching TV, or listening to radio news before bed... bringing negative consciousness to bed begs for a stressful night's "rest." Instead... spiritual reading will raise consciousness. Meditation and "Standing in Your Wish Fulfilled" provide seeds for the subconscious to sprout Your creative energies.

Avoid mirrors and lights in the bedroom; block out glaring outdoor lights. Even nightlights can disrupt the brain's sleeping mechanism. The pineal gland only produces melatonin in the dark. Rather than a nightlight in a child's room, leave the door slightly ajar to keep the room dark, yet offering the solace of a red light in the hallway. For sleep-challenged individuals or those who work nights, a sleep mask is a good investment blocking light and allowing Your pineal gland to regulate its own rhythm. Be sure it is natural fiber or, sweating You become uncomfortable and it comes off. Some airlines offer masks on long flights. They are synthetic and irritating, yet can be made suitable by using a soft paper towel or a handkerchief between Your eyes and the mask.

Synthetics are soft thermoplastics made from petrochemicals. Restricting the skin's ability to breathe, they are irritating... and are loaded with other chemicals such as formaldehyde... found in pajamas, sheets, pillowcases, curtains, drapes and carpeting. Sheets, pillowcases and pajamas may be treated to resist wrinkling. This finish is permanent remaining in the fiber releasing gases for life. Symptoms of formaldehyde sensitivity are insomnia, fatigue, headaches, irritation of eyes, nose, and throat, coughing and rashes. There is a solution. Avoid polyester, even blends. Learn to live with wrinkled sheets. A 50/50 sweatshirt is tolerable when worn over a long sleeve cotton shirt – which allows the skin to breathe. There are healthy options, including combed-cotton percale sheets, with >200 threads per square inch, they provide a tight weave with soft, smooth texture. Organic cotton sheets are chemical free and have a silky feel that grows softer with age. Cotton flannel sheets may be less durable than percale, yet they provide their own comfort throughout the year. Organic linen and bamboo sheets are also available. Always wash residues from new material first.

Mattresses and pillows are big offenders... being filled with polyurethane releasing a chemical associated with respiratory challenges, skin and eye irritation. Highest concentrations are released in the first few years. There are cotton mattresses and box springs that have cotton batting (stuffing) and ticking (fabric covering). The most economic and healthy option is an organic cotton futon, avoiding the metal grid found in conventional mattress and box springs interfering with our subtle energy fields. Futons can be ordered extra thick. A wooden frame keeps them off the floor, allowing air to circulate. There are options to choose: a standard bed or fold-out couch.

You spend 1/3 of Your Life at rest, and other times are spent in bed. For optimal health, avoid the glitz and glitter of Madison Av leading You down the Primrose Path with "wrinkle-free" synthetic sheets. Avoid synthetic clothing. Avoid synthetic foods! Invest in Yourself with organic bedding, clothing, and foods. Get the Best. Treat with Care. Would You drive a Rolls Royce through a car wash?! Maintain quality. Avoid heat & spinning in the dryer. Lint that collects is the "body" of the fabric, getting less with repetition, hence shorter lifespan with less comfort – leading One to wonder about perceived value. Preserving integrity is easy. Always hang to dry. Learn to appreciate the soft, luxurious feel of organic wrinkles. Love, honor and respect Yourself... and Your Beloved!

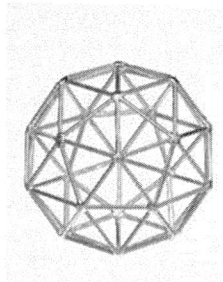

6 – ENERGY MEDICINE WITH FENG SHUI

Feng means Wind... Shui means Water... two primary movers of energy. Pronounced fung shway, Feng Shui is an artform: profound history based on profound results. While members of boardrooms may spend hundreds of thousands for the best advice to interfere with an opponent... advance their bottom line... and design their lobbies and offices – our considerations are simple and practical, beginning in the bedroom where Life begins, and often ends.

Healing vibrations are essential for proper rest in the bedroom... look at the house as a whole. Ancient Wisdom, *Innate* Wisdom, realizes our environment profoundly affects us. Some surroundings actually can be more *fortunate* than others. The goal of Feng Shui – known as geomancy in the West – is altering and harmonizing the environment to improve one's health, happiness and good fortune. Feng Shui – wind, water – utilizes elements that bring movement and vitality. The Feng Shui consultant or geomancer discerns congested or inappropriate areas of energy, such as a toilet in the wealth and blessings corner, symbolically allowing Your finances to be flushed away.

If that happens to be the situation, the solution is: always keep the lid down when not in use. As an extrapolation from that one example, keep the lid down wherever Your toilet may be, to prevent energies from being drained. If there is no lid on the toilet, place a mirror on the outside of the door and keep it closed. In fact, it is beneficial to always keep bathroom doors closed to neutralize the energy of the drains, which represent elimination.

One of the first written symbols of Feng Shui shows an arc with a dot in the middle... meaning it is proper to have backing with Your front open and Your associates to Your side, rather than across from You. When the Chinese build a house, the mountain is behind and the valley in front. We can have backing of a chair with a commanding view of the door – proper Feng Shui.

As for the front door – the entrance point of energy – place a red flowering plant inviting abundance and prosperity on the left side.

If it faces south, Fire energy – which creates Earth: place a plant on either side of the door, or paint the door yellow.

If it faces west, Metal energy – which creates Water: place a bowl of water, or paint the door dark blue or black.

If it faces north, Water energy – which creates Wood: place some wooden décor, or paint the door green.

If it faces east, Wood energy – which creates Fire: place a lantern or lamp; paint the door red.

When stairs are inside the front door, or if there is a clear visual route from front to back door, the energy can swiftly drain away. Certain things cancel the energy-draining aspects of homes or offices. Paint the back of the front door a strong color, or put a mirror on it. A sparkling object at the stairs attracts forces that otherwise might run away: a piece of cut glass, crystal, or hanging glass ball... perhaps a chandelier.

When there is a notch out of the far-right corner of the house plan, opposite the front door, there is a negative space in the area of relationships and marriage. To rectify this anomaly before finding that special someone or experiencing challenges... place mirrors to create an illusion of space at that point.

Plants serve a useful function in Feng Shui cleaning the air and filling space between furniture. They bring living, vital energy keeping us tuned to Mother Nature. Plants and flowers enhance any area. A splash of green from leaves or fern along with some yellow and pink flowers can stimulate the energies in Your relationship corner: opening the doors for new ones, embellishing what You have. Round leafed plants are preferred. Pointed ones, especially spiky leafed plants – aloe included – are like sharp knives and are generally kept outside – although these plants may be useful to correct oppressively low ceilings, this would be an unusual situation. Similarly, high rooms benefit from horizontal elements, such as a long, low sofa. Mirrors and pictures of seascapes or landscapes can give the appearance of depth to confined spaces.

Bright colors are preferred over dark, curves and softness over sharp angles... order over clutter.

Sometimes the house is out of alignment! A writer spent a fortune buying / remodeling a cottage on Long Island. And it simply "felt wrong." Unable to write or sleep well, let alone invite guests... a Feng Shui consultant noted the house was built in the U-shape. The front door was recessed at the center and the two projecting wings contained the bedroom area and kitchen / dining area. According to Feng Shui principles, the line of the front door is where the house starts, so the two wings were "outside the house" so to speak. Energy-wise it was as if the owner were sleeping... cooking... and entertaining... "out in the open." Simple solution: building a short brick fence connecting the wings, the gate at the fence became the "front door" and the bedrooms and kitchen were "reconnected" to the main house – beautifying the garden, now the foyer of the house, the Career path received a huge boost of energy.

There are simple remedies for common problems. Place a convex mirror to scatter the energies of an overpowering presence, such as a larger building or a larger house – even a brass door knocker with convex center scatters inauspicious energy. If possible, have the front door facing east or south.

When the path to the front door is curved, You have an auspicious entranceway for energies to flow. To correct a straight path, change the texture of the walkway by lining both sides of the sidewalk with a variety of bricks. Plant flowers along each side – perhaps alternating colors, allowing the eyes to flow energetically... inviting chi. Once inside, keep the energies flowing. Traditionally, crystals hung with red string or ribbon in 9" increments, wind chimes, mobiles, round and soft plants, water or pictures of water, help activate beneficial forces. Major structural reconstruction can be avoided by the clever use of mirrors or pictures, creating the appearance of space.

When the desk is on the east side of the house, the brightness of the new day energizes that vital area. When at Your desk paying bills, always have Gratitude in Your heart. Rather than grumble, "There goes another $100 to Ma Bell" (whoever)... always be grateful: "I give thanks I Am able to pay my bills in a timely manner." Abundance flows. You can even write Thank You! on the check, or Blessings! Paying bills at the kitchen table, dining room table or even in the bedroom, confuses the energies – these places are associated with pleasure, relaxation and enjoyment. Tacking bills to the refrigerator is exactly that: tacky. It can make You lose Your appetite, especially if bills are a challenge. With space or furniture factors, simply have a small table or counter space... with bills organized in a folder. Remember, clutter is the opposite of simplicity – essential for Feng Shui. Organize; clear clutter; enjoy the flow of energy.

Your birthday, numerology reveals the energy of the year You are beginning. Simply add the numbers of the month, date and year (using all four numbers of the year) reducing to a single digit. **1** indicates new beginnings – a powerful position to be in. **2** focuses on relationships and partnerships. **3** evokes creativity, expressing oneself. **4** opens expansion in every direction. **5** calls for communication and change. **6** focuses on heart, home and hearth. **7** calls for inner work and spiritual perfection. **8** brings wealth and abundance. **9** brings things to completion... ready to begin another cycle.

The Grid of Feng Shui

The grid of Feng Shui known as *Ba-Gua* – meaning eight areas – may be used properly by visualizing the position of Your driveway, Your sidewalk, or Your doorway to Your office... Your home... and each individual room. When the driveway to the property or door to the home is in the center, You enter through Your Career Path... to the right, You enter through the area of Helpful Friends... to the left, You enter through the area of Inner Knowledge and Meditation. According to ancient interpretation of Feng Shui, these are the only 3 possibilities.

There are practical applications. A widow, having gone through a year's mourning period, felt it was time to get on with her Life and nurture a new relationship. She told her friends and "put it out to the Universe." Over a year went by; possibilities went from bleak to none. Beginning to feel she was meant to be alone, hearing of Feng Shui she thought: there's little to lose... perhaps much to gain. At the relationship corner of her property, she planted a tree. The relationship corners of her house, and each room of the house were enhanced with mobiles, mirrors, water, brass chimes, plants with rounded leaves, along with pictures of landscapes and moving water. Within 2½ months she met her man and they eventually married. While the

skeptic might say: anecdotal... what would it take to be open to the possibilities? Experiment!

The grid of Ba-Gua has 8 areas. The central area is aka the Sacred Space of Tai Chi: Balance and Peace.

WEALTH AND BLESSINGS	FAME AND ENLIGHTEN- MENT	MARRIAGE AND RELATION- SHIPS
ELDERS AND FAMILY	TAI-CHI: BALANCE HEALTH PEACE	CREATIVITY AND NEW PROJECTS
INNER KNOWLEDGE AND MEDITATION	CAREER PATH	HELPFUL FRIENDS

Cartographers... those who create, read and interpret maps... have North at the top of the page. Some interpret Feng Shui using a compass for the property, house or building, *and* each individual room. While both systems work, the interpretation given here is the most ancient, and simplest to decipher and utilize.

Enhancing the Energies
"Form follows function."
Frank Lloyd Wright

Stimulating, delighting the senses with pleasant surroundings invites chi... Energies Flow: bright colors and abundance of light elevate Your mood and energize Your space. Natural sunlight is optimal, or full-spectrum lighting. Both have healing effects on Seasonal Affective Disorder: dark days of winter bring depression to some. Light support the liver clearing jaundice, whether in a newborn or someone with a liver challenge. DC is preferred over AC, incandescent light over fluorescent light – which flickers on and off 100X per second... upsetting our subtle energy fields.

Abundance of light promotes happiness. The vast majority of energy required to maintain our systemic equilibrium comes from environmental infrared light exposure. Near-infrared primes the cells in Your retina for repair and regeneration. LEDs have zerO infra-red and sabotage health, promoting blindness. Swap LEDs for incandescent or low-voltage incandescent halogen lights. Limit Your exposure to blue light during the day by wearing protective glasses while on all devices. Avoid all devices and screens for **2** hours before sleep.

A silent home or office is a sad place. Silence is unnatural. Nature abounds with sounds – if only wind blowing through trees... birds and other animals. Bring natural sounds indoors. With the flip of a switch... sounds from Mother Nature... such as a 10-gallon aquarium with a layer of colorful rocks and a tank pump... decorated with leaves and flowers... pleasant sounds of a waterfall for pennies a day. Water is our first connection to Life as we floated in the womb; sound is comforting... even pictures of moving water are comforting. Since all life comes from water, it is vital to fix leaky faucets or toilets, conserving this commodity – leaky faucets in Feng Shui indicate a lack of capacity to plan for the future. Also fix squeaks. These sounds irritate, and interfere with the free flow of energy. Slamming doors because they "stick" – take a pencil and scribble lead on both door latch and plate. Graphite assures smooth, quiet closure... maintaining smooth flow of chi.

Color enhances Ba-Gua: Wealth and Blessings – purple or burgundy. Fame and Enlightenment – red. Marriage and Relationships – pink, or white and red. Elders and Family {Friends} – green. Tai Chi, Balance, Health and Peace – yellow. Creativity {Children} and New Projects – white. Inner Knowledge and Meditation – dark blue. Career Path – black. Helpful Friends {Travel} – gray, or black and white.

Color has fascinating factors to consider. Red, orange and yellow are warming and energizing, green is neutral, while blue, purple and violet are cooling and soothing. The latter colors are appropriate for the bedroom. Reds and oranges in the kitchen or dining area encourage fast eating and great thirst – both interfere with proper digestion. Fast-food restaurants use these colors to hurry the customers along... high turnover means less waiting line, ultimately, more profits. Drinks in restaurants are a high profit item, easy to bring to the table along with a high bill... and high tips. This is the nature of business. Around hOMe – create a wholesome atmosphere. Yellow is still a warming color, yet on the neutral side of the spectrum and, the color for the solar plexus, it activates organs of digestion: gallbladder, liver, pancreas, stomach and spleen. A green, leafy plant near or above the sink alleviates energy drainage, providing a clear pathway to healthy living. Green as a neutral color enhances conviviality, beneficial for every room.

The Five Elements have associated body influences in the Ba-Gua: Wealth and Blessings – **Wood**, hipbones. Fame and Enlightenment – **Fire**, eyes. Marriage and Relationships – **Earth**, internal organs. Elders and Family – **Wood**, feet. Tai Chi Balance, Health, Peace: – **Earth**, HeartMindBodySpirit. Creativity and New Projects – **Metal**, mouth. Inner Knowledge and Meditation – **Earth**, hands. Career Path – **Water**, ears. Helpful Friends – **Metal**, head.

Besides color and the elements, further enhance these areas: Wealth and Blessings: a fountain, or picture of moving water... symbolizes money, abundance, peace. Fame and Enlightenment: hang 9 firecrackers to promote fame, success and wealth. Marriage and Relationships: place two ceramic candlesticks with two pink candles; light them frequently. Elders and Family: 3 family photos in antique frames, along with other antique pieces. Tai Chi Balance: remains open, free. Creativity and New Projects: sound system or musical instruments to enhance creativity. Inner Knowledge and Meditation: eight small crystals, preferably round and faceted, on a bookcase with books that relate to Your Wish Fulfilled – where You see Yourself Going. Career Path: an aquarium with eight black and one goldfish, or vice versa. Helpful Friends: an empty crystal bowl symbolizing receptivity to beneficial connections; place business cards of benefactors or potential benefactors nearby.

Feng Shui for the Workplace
Feng Shui transforms the workspace allowing energetic forces to soothe frazzled nerves. Certain things avoided; other things can be compensated. Avoid a home or office next to telephone poles or transformers. Stay at least ½ mile from heavy electric power lines. They bring physical, mental, emotional stress, diseases, frequent quarreling.

As Feng Shui requires seeing the door from Your bed and favorite chair, the same is true at the office. Make sure You see the door or entrance to a work cubicle from Your desk. When You can be surprised from behind, it is a challenge to be focused and present with Your work. If factors prohibit moving the desk, position a mirror on a wall or desk to reflect the doorway. Sitting with a solid wall behind is preferred. Sitting under high shelving can deplete energies... feeling everything is getting on top of You. With a bookshelf behind You, put heavy books on the bottom shelves (common sense) keeping the spaces above open – for plants, seashells or mobile whatnots.

Light on the work surface is essential... a powerful motivational force making us happy to be there, happy to perform. Let light from a window feed into Your dominant hand avoiding shadows on Your work, diminishing concentration for the task at hand. If You are right-handed and have a window on the right side of Your desk, turn the desk around – otherwise place a full-spectrum lamp on the left side of the desk.

Chi-enhancing objects on the work surface vitalize quiet, creative times – anything that can be spun, rotated or moved, electrically or mechanically. Nature is equally enhancing: seashells, rock, driftwood, a small fountain, plants, a picture of Your favorite place outdoors... lift Your creative spirit. UV light can bring the subtle smell of the great outdoors into the workspace benefiting mood and the bottom line. https://www.airoasis.com/

Doorways always must remain clear to allow free flow of energy. Red and black rugs and carpets attract wealth. Wearing yellow is discouraged as it is considered too peaceful and relaxing. Red, green or black are preferred. Plant vitality brings energy, countering negative effects of office equipment. Rounded leaves are inviting and avoid a "prickly" atmosphere. Since 3 is a lucky number for the Chinese, a clock always must have 3 hands, ideally... an octagonal clock. An octagonal mirror moves energy around the room. Pictures give visitors focus when entering, to feel relaxed and comfortable. Goldfish boost positive forces signifying prosperity and money. 3, 9 or 13 fish are recommended... one gold, the rest black... or vice versa – placed in the wealth and blessings corner. Sounds of water attract energy.

With a home or office having an L shape, plant a tree, or shrub in a large terracotta pot at the point of the missing corner. Having doors that open in a straight line allows energy to rush through creating havoc and chaos. Hang a brass wind chime, a mobile or a crystal somewhere in between to circulate energy.

Remove all clutter, allowing rooms to be clean, bright and clear. A blocked door symbolizes something blocked in Life... or Health. Mirrors are useful if untarnished or uncracked: a wall of square mirrors has many breaking lines creating chaos in Your energy field. A solid mirror reflects energy clearly – round, oval and octagonal preferred. Some feel uncomfortable when a mirror is hung too high... or too low, they can cause headaches. A hallway ending with a wall or a closed door creates a dead end, blocking career opportunities – a mirror there reflects chi. Always make sure basics are working well. Replace a burned-out bulb even if rarely or never used. Clogged or dripping plumbing affects health and energy.

Because of the public perception this is a lot of hocus-pocus, some big corporations are reluctant to come forward and admit they adopt the principles of Feng Shui. Corporations using these principles see the difference in the atmosphere and productivity of their workplaces, thus the bottom line. They find it worth spending thousands – sometimes hundreds of thousands – for an expert Feng Shui consultant to resolve a difficult situation.

Feng Shui, known as geomancy in the West, sees a correlation between where and how we live and work. Geomancy understands and resolves situations arising from an unhealthy environment. With a metaphysical eye, geomancers find underlying patterns in the environment; with pendulum, dowsing rods or intuition they may detect underground stressors such as an underground stream. These can cause illness, and accident clusters. Hammering copper stakes as interrupters into the ground disperses those energies. Ancient Wisdom provides guidelines for the optimum space within which to flourish. In balance and harmony with Cosmic Order... Prosperity and Vitality flow freely – Happiness prevails.

Other Cultural Influences

Various cultures have their own version of geomantic design. Madagascar calls it Vitana. Hindus speak of Vastuvidya. Bilkis Whelan, *Vastu in 10 Simple Lessons*, sets forth basic rules:

For free-flowing energy – the center of a room is clear, free from furniture. Positive energies lie in the N, NE and E sides of both home and room. Keep these areas sparsely furnished. The west, south, southwest and northwest are suited for furniture, holding energies.

In both home and room, north is the region of health and wealth: the color is blue... an area rug or throw pillows here are appropriate. This area is for money, jewelry, documents, or a medicine cabinet of healing herbs.

The northeast is governed by purity: the color is black... excellent for visualization or meditating.

The east is where power lies: the color is red. Face this way while sleeping, at work, bathing or in benediction.

The southeast is the region of physical and worldly pleasures: the color is yellow. This is a place to burn candles and incense.

The south is the region of justice: the color is also yellow. Work with Your back to the south, building Wisdom... excellent for siestas.

The southwest is ruled by misery, and the color is black. Do activities here that dispel fears... great for reading.

The west is a region for prosperity: the color is also black. This is a place for eating and feasting.

The northwest is governed by economics and public relations: the color is white. Starting a project... face northwest to bring fortune.

Vastu... Feng Shui... Geomancy... whichever system You are attracted to, even the system of common sense: be cognizant of Your surroundings. Keep things simple. Select colors discreetly. Allow free flow of energy.

Made in the image and likeness of the Creator...
Breath by Sacred Breath...
Wisely Create Your Reality!

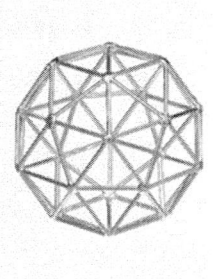

7 – RESTING THE DIGESTIVE ORGANS: GUIDE TO FASTING

A good therapy is one that stimulates the healer within.
Albert Schweitzer

One of Life's greatest challenges is knowing enough about a subject to think You're right... yet not knowing enough about it, to know You're wrong!
Neil deGrasse Tyson

Thank You, Mr Dyson for the sage words. Here I Am 80 – Sweet 16 + 64 years of experience – thinking I was right about fasting and, therefore, sharing... and now, I know: I was wrong – at the very least, ignorant – to teach before being fully infOrmed by explOring Other pOssibilities! After experiencing 3 days (84 hrs) **dry fasting** at the Full Moon of Spring 2021 – without a drop to drink, or even licking my wet lips in the shower – gave new perspective to holistic healing for HeartMindBodySpirit... indeed, we live "in interesting times"!

AnyOne can do *any* kind of 3-day fast... even a dry fast... confidently, feeling totally "care-free" from any adverse effects! Guaranteed... You will feel and think differently. Once they have their adult teeth, even children will benefit, especially with iatrogenic afflictions such as Autism, directly related to vaccinations. From the perspective of a Natural Primary Care Physician following Mother Nature's Ways, there are options to the dry fast already mentioned. Lemon / lime in water with cayenne will cleanse. Green juices with cayenne will strengthen. A water fast for 3 days allows time to be free – from busy-ness in the kitchen – and the opportunity to Go Within – hopefully being Out... with Mother Nature!

Caution: With a strict water fast... avoid plasticized water in jugs. Given environmental toxins, Distilled or Reverse Osmosis water – the former if You are single and on-the-go, the latter if You rent or own Your hOMe – are of equal value. Distilled and R/O water, stripped naked of hormones, pollutants, toxins, *as well as* minerals is looking for electrons, ready for action. **Re-mineralize** dead, Distilled or R/O water with a pinch of whole salt – black, gray, pink or white (unbleached). **Re-energize** by spinning or stirring creating a vortex... à la Rudolf Steiner, or continuous in One direction... while Consciously breathing Love &

Energy into the Process for 3, 6 or 9 Sacred Breaths... or minutes – depending on volume.

Fasting is easy and natural. We do it every day, and we break our fast every day with break-fast. Our ancestors often went a day or two looking for something edible... and thought little of it. The trick is to extend the fast. Every night when we sleep – especially with our last meal or snack 3 hrs before bedtime – our digestive system rests while the body cleanses accumulated toxins and wastes. Water or juice for breakfast recognizes the body's cycle and rides with it; flow with a liquid breakfast: microalgae, power powders, probiotics... with re-mineralized, re-energized distilled or r/o water to facilitate the process.

Some start the day with water and have only fresh juice mid-day, then an afternoon of exercise... feeling alive... followed by water... leisurely pursuing positive reading, artwork, or other R&R... observing how much gets done... and how much time is consumed thinking about, preparing and cleaning up from food! Realizing how easily we can get along without food is totally liberating. Time and Energy spark creativity and originality. As we sage, we require less food and sleep... and more water. Choose wisely and be energized... You will accomplish wonderful things.

Experiments with Eating
Determining the optimal eating regimen has been well researched. Experiments varied from unlimited portions, to moderate and meager... while others were placed on various fasting programs. Results showed: animals **eating two days then fasting the next** had the shiniest coats and the brightest eyes, living almost a third again as long as the average for their species! That is serious Food for Thought! Having done considerable fasting, these experiments were fascinating. 3 days fasting or more... once a month or quarterly at the change of season, is invigorating. Over the years, the routine of fasting on Wednesdays became a vitalizing habit. How would it feel – eating two days and fasting the next?

Considering we are creatures of habit living in a 7-day cycle, fasting two days a week seems adequate. Weekends are known for parties and picnics; that makes Monday a great day to fast. Eating on Tuesday and Wednesday, makes Thursday the second fast day... preparing for weekend parties. Fasting on Mondays and Thursdays habitually will show results

with the acting body, especially with skin and hair, as well as the feeling body and the thinking body... providing clarity and spiritual insight.

The Fear of Fasting
The thought of missing a meal is scary for some. The western diet is "3 squares a day" – a "square meal" having four portions. Breakfast consists of orange juice, bacon and eggs, toast, and coffee; lunch: a hamburger, fries, malted milk and apple pie; dinner: meat and potatoes, vegetables, followed by dessert and coffee... and as a reward, an evening snack while watching TV! Even though research continues to show we are over-proteinized – and even though each of these meals is a combination destined to produce an over-acid condition leading to indigestion, many people feel this is what Life is about. They think their lifestyle makes sense because when missing a meal... they feel a crashing headache... irritability... or tiredness. Little do they realize...

The Standard American Diet (**SAD**) sadly provides more junk than nutrition! The body can filter only a certain amount before burning out fine tubules in the kidneys; after processing what is possible, excess is stored in joints, muscles, organs or tissues... or, excreted through the skin. Feeling any consequences from missing a meal means the body is efficient, using the time and energy for housecleaning – pulling out stored trash, preparing for elimination – leading to cleansing reactions, such as sluggishness or headache. Rather than "getting sick" realize: we are strong – mustering our forces, expelling acidic waste, reclaiming homeostasis... "getting better!" Cleansing reactions are a signal, really a polite request: drink more re-mineralized and re-energized distilled or r/o water to facilitate the cleanse. Enemas and salt-baths encourage the process... as well as Dry Fasting.

What to Do During a Cleansing
With vitality... dietary residual toxins are eliminated through the liver via the blood, intestines and skin... our largest eliminative organ, our third kidney. With lack of vitality due to poor nutrition or insufficient re-mineralized, re-energized distilled or r/o water... the body is hampered flushing out waste. Since residual toxins are stored in the connective tissue – the glue that holds us together – Patience is a virtue!

Over time, antibiotics, anti-inflammatory drugs and synthetics saturate connective tissue with residual toxins, and interfere with organ function. Anti-biotics have been found to effectively interrupt the natural cycle of some bacterial infections. Unfortunately, this suppression of symptoms is far from healing. While antibiotics kill microorganisms that prevail during the illness, and distressing symptoms *may* subside, surviving microbes gather their strength and marshal their forces – becoming Superbugs. The next time anti-biotics are taken, the body is flooded with dead microorganisms, and thriving on this toxic residue, the Superbugs feast. Many times for survival, the body calls a halt to imminent danger by turning up the thermostat and creating a fever. We may experience headaches or other symptoms of toxins released into the system for elimination. Drink extra pure water; keep warm with a cool cloth on the forehead. With a high fever – take an enema.

Sometimes with natural therapies, there is an increase in symptoms. Feelings of tiredness or aching may last a few days and are a good sign indicating the onset of healing. Is it a cleansing crisis, or really a cleansing reaction? Some mistakenly regard the cleansing reaction as an indication to break their fast, or resume their old dietary habits. Eating, their headache or runny nose stops, thinking they really "needed the food to feel better."

Reality is otherwise. The body was in cleansing mode; when taking food, the cleansing was put on hold so the body could focus on digestion. With any cleansing reaction... assist the body by frequently drinking a glass of pure water, facilitating the cleansing process. More than a pint runs the risk of washing out minerals. An 8 oz glass every 30-45 minutes is sufficient, perhaps with a squeeze of fresh lemon.

Rest is appropriate, when possible. An enema will assist elimination. With a rash or itching, add 2lbs Epsom salts and 2lbs baking soda to a warm bath and soak for 30 minutes minimum. Your skin acts as an osmotic membrane, and the alkaline solution pulls acids from Your body. This remedy is excellent for body aches, muscular pain, rashes... even emotional tensions. As the cleansing runs its course, strength returns both physically... along with clarity in the Heart and Head. Give Thanks.

Fasting, You are on Mother Nature's operating table. Knowing whatever is happening is healing... rinse, relax and rest. In Your feeling body and Your thinking body hold the vision of being in balance and harmony as One.

Contraindications

While almost anyone can benefit from fasting one day a week having only pure water... or even fasting on Mondays and Thursdays... someone with a profound challenge, or a gaunt and weak appearance, gets to focus on building strength. Here, even a 1-day water fast is contraindicated, unless under a physician's care.

To help build... fresh organic vegetable juices, especially greens: broccoli, celery, collards, cucumber, parsley and zucchini with some ginger root, provide nutrients and energy. **Chew fresh juice**... 3 or 4 times a day for immediate nutrition; fresh nut and seed milks help build strength; sprouted grain milks build strength and boost the immune response. Chew and see the difference.

Since water fasting – even one day – pulls toxins from the tissues... it is contraindicated in pregnancy and nursing. Be responsible. Focus on nutrients for two.

How to Fast

Almost everyone can drink pure water for a day and continue regular work and activities; some fast longer continuing usual work. Generally, rest and meditation are recommended, perhaps reading books on fasting and spirituality while enjoying a longer fast. An educated individual has the ultimate responsibility. Advice from a doctor or health-care provider is respected, realizing that textbook knowledge is an aspect to consider, and personal experience fine-tunes the perceptions of science. If You feel support would be helpful, find a physician who is knowledgeable about natural healing, a physician who walks the talk. In the end it is the individual who determines what is suitable in the moment for one's own growth and development. Muscle test. {Ch 10: **Muscle Testing, Pendulums and Switched Energies**}

Fasting provides the physical body with rest, allowing organs and tissues time to gather and cleanse congestive trash, refreshing strength and tone. How to do this is simple: rinse out. Drink a glass of re-mineralized and re-energized distilled or r/o water every 45 minutes or so... or caffeine-free and sweetener-free herbal tea. Drink water. Muscle test.

The recommendation of Stanley Burroughs, formerly of Hawai'i is the Master Cleanse – every hour drink 8-10 oz distilled or r/o water with juice from half a lemon, a Tsp of maple syrup and a shake of cayenne pepper. Doing this for 7 weeks in Hawai'i in 1973, unfortunately, I consumed over a gallon of maple syrup! Rather, us a drop of stevia. Nevertheless, it was a cleansing that left me weighing the least in my adult life, 119 lbs. Stanley suggested a bold experiment: fast until the tongue turns pink... a delightful experience. *Healing for the Age of Enlightenment* also includes color therapy and his vitaflex foot reflexology.

Tap water is suitable only for washing... even there use pre-cautions. Whenever taking a long soak in the tub, add two pounds each of Epsom salts (magnesium sulfate) and baking soda creating an alkaline solution. Your skin is an osmotic membrane; the alkaline solution pulls acids from Your body.

In addition to water – teas, lemon or other juices are also appropriate. While this generally requires a juicer, a blender can be utilized. Simply chop Your greens, vegetables, add some water and blend thoroughly... strain through a fine meshed paint strainer bag and wring out the vital nutrients that remain. While a hydraulic press is fitting, strong hands are sufficient.

Energize the organ systems with various juices for support before a serious fast. Liver / gall bladder system: greens, broccoli, lettuce, parsley, green beans and zucchini with ginger root. Heart / small intestine system: chicory, dandelion greens, endive, escarole and okra. Stomach / spleen (pancreas) system: collards, parsnip, sweet potato, pumpkin and any yellow or orange squash – hard winter squash juiced makes a delicious soup. Lung / large intestine system: watercress, cabbage, celery, cucumber, garlic and/or ginger and daikon radish. Kidney / bladder system: beet greens, burdock greens and kale. {Watermelon may be used when available. Wash thoroughly and juice, or blend and strain the whole thing – the skin has chlorophyll, the rind has electrolytes, the red has sweetness and the seeds have their special concentrated vital energy. Watermelon seeds may be dried and stored for a tasty, diuretic tea &/or sprouted.

Flush all endocrine glands by using enzymes to clear congestion, and pre-digested nutrients of AFA as a restorative – Klamath Lake blue-green algae – taken together several times a day. {Ch 10: **AFA** Superior

with PUFAs by virtue of surviving cold winters.} Taking algae a few hours before bed may keep You alert and awake, yet taken immediately before retiring can bring a restful sleep, plus pleasant dreams. See how You feel and think after 7 days. **Enzymes & Algae may be taken sublingually, or chewed... coating gums and cheeks for quick absorption and mental clarity.**

Water fasting a few days at a time is generally safe. Extended water fasting is best in a pure environment with clean air, clean water... when possible, a warm climate to support You... and perhaps with a Kindred Spirit. On a prolonged fast, mucus is cleared from the basement membrane of our cells which becomes thin; pollution in cities has adverse effects entering our cells, poisoning our system. A certain amount of mucus clearly is normal, acting as a barrier from pollutants. After cleansing, juices then juices and whole fruits if sweets are tolerated, then juices and salads. Nut and seed milks re-build basement membranes. If something warm is desired after a few days of juices, germinated, cooked whole grains: = parts quinoa and amaranth or buckwheat provide high quality protein, leave an alkaline residue, and build our Alkaline Reserve, mentioned in Guyton's *Medical Physiology*.

The Ultimate Fast – Dry Fasting. We all know of animals severely injured by a motorcycle or torn apart by a raccoon who refused food and water, only to hide under the porch... emerging buoyant and happy after a week! Dr Sergei Filonov, inspired by his dog, cured his sinusitis in 1 week... inspiring his colleague Dr L Schennikov who investigated, and called the method of Rehabilitation: dry fasting. After several protocols – some reaching 21 days – remarkably even **30** days – both concur: after 11 days benefits diminish. August Dunning, PhD presents details in *The Phoenix Protocol: Dry Fasting for Rapid Healing and Radical Life Extension*. As a former NASA Space Station scientist, he presents a scientifically proven plan to activate... and proliferate... endogenous stem cell production, free! *The Phoenix Protocol* scientifically explains cellular chemistry, and dry fasting for healing and life extension, breaching the quest for functional immortality. Sometimes, it does take a rocket scientist! https://oneradionetwork.com/all-shows/dr-august-dunning-living-longer-in-a-younger-body-through-dry-fasting-may-11-2020/

Dry Fasting requires a meditative space in a pure environment and especially... for more than 3 days...

a salt-water pool &/or jacuzzi for full-body immersion – preferably unheated. Some would like to "ease into the process" of dry fasting, so after a few days of juice fasting to prepare, have only re-mineralized and re-energized distilled or r/o water – drinking as often and as much as You wish. The next day, breathing, caressing, meditating, focusing within, go without anything – 36 hrs. The following day, drink as much water as You wish. The next breathe. 36 hrs. Alternate. Experiment. Muscle test. Follow with several days of green juices. This is obviously for the experienced faster, or someone wishing to become experienced fast. The casual dry fast can clarify consciousness in HeartMindBodySpirit.

During any fast, keep Your focus within… as much as possible, also fast from talking. Explore consciousness and spirituality. As scriptures advise: fast in secret. This avoids negative energies and comments, unintentional though they may be… as we focus our intention within. If required, tell only those who offer encouragement or professional support.

What to do When Peristalsis Stops

The first day or two of a fast, bowel movements continue; then peristalsis – the normal wave-like contractions that begin with the esophagus, swallowing food, churning the stomach – suddenly ceases. While food reaches our stomach by gravity, the esophagus contracts squeezing food through its length into the stomach, which secretes digestive juices and functions optimally at 101°! This initiates even more contractions mixing food with digestive fluids, and as the stomach empties into the small intestines – the peristaltic wave continues, moving slowly through >20 feet of small intestines, where the body extracts nutrients. The ileocecal valve opens allowing peristalsis to begin movement through the large intestine, which functions optimally at 105°! The first third of the large intestine is able to absorb liquids, and the body conserves water. When the peristaltic wave arrives at the cecum and the rectum, our brain is alerted… it is time to allow that peristaltic movement to pass through as we move our bowels. Typically, a bowel movement will follow a meal after an hour or so… or after awakening and having a large glass of water. A baby or healthy pet is on that schedule. If we are healthy, we probably have 2 or 3 movements a day from yesterday's meals.

When we fast, however, the process of peristalsis gradually ceases. Rather than expending energies on digestion, the body takes advantage during a fast… expending energies on cleansing and rejuvenation, bringing wastes and toxins to the colon for elimination. As peristaltic waves cease… toxins sit… and we feel weak… headache or gas may occur. As things accumulate and sit our cleansing reaction continues. Drink warm lemon water to help. **On a Dry Fast, take an enema** bringing in 2 quarts of warm lemon water, as instructed below.

Hawaiians mix 1 Tbs sea salt in a quart of warm water as an effective constitutional & purgative. <u>Caution</u>: common salt is bleached, has aluminum added to keep it free flowing, and some have dextrose – sugar – to hide the bitter aluminum. Use unrefined sea salt, such as gray Celtic Salt or Brittany Salt, or Himalayan Pink Salt. Epsom salt (magnesium sulfate) or Glauber's salt (sodium sulfate) are recommended only for occasional use internally. They may be used freely in a proper bath, a sitz-bath, footbath, or in solution as a poultice to relieve inflammation and pain.

Enemas to the Rescue

The answer to cleaning out the colon is also Grandma's remedy for fever. Actually, an enema does more than control fever. Enemas can relieve symptoms of allergies, headaches, respiratory challenges and skin rashes. These symptoms indicate the body's elimination efforts are congested. When fasting, enemas keep toxins moving out of the body. While taking an enema may seem straightforward… there are considerations.

Disposable enema kits with synthetic chemicals are to be avoided. Period. A douche / enema bag is found in the feminine hygiene department and is easy to put together. You have a choice of nozzles. The larger, about the size of one's thumb with several tiny holes is used for a vaginal douche. The other, the size of one's little finger with one small hole at the end is used for enemas. Once assembled with the clip to regulate the flow… rinse it out with tap water, which has sufficient chlorine to sanitize any residuals; then give a second rinse with pure water.

Fill the bag with warm, pure distilled or r/o water and add the strained juice of ½ lemon to act as a detergent breaking down toxins and wastes accumulated on the inner wall of the colon. With towel spread on the floor and oil handy… once the bag is full, hold the nozzle over the toilet and release the clip allowing air in the hose to be expelled. Once a clear stream flows, clip it shut. Hang the bag 3-4' from the floor. With a few drops of oil on Your finger, lubricate the nozzle and Your anus. Lying on Your left side on the towel, gently insert and release the clip, allowing about a pint of water to flow into the colon. Clip it shut & hold it in position. With Your other hand massage Your lower left side for a minute, working from the groin up a few inches. Then let in another pint or so, clip it shut and massage Your lower left side and the area above it. Then another pint or so and massage Your lower left side, the area above it and the area under Your navel. Repeat this procedure until the enema bag is empty and You are massaging from Your lower left side... up, across, and down Your right side. If You must move Your bowels before the process is complete, simply get up and do so... then re-fill the bag with warm water – and repeat until taking in the full amount – almost two quarts.

Once Your colon is full of water, lie on Your back for a moment or stand up and begin tapping Your belly. Percussion vibrates things loose from the colon walls... bouncing up and down while doing so, can be fun... be sure to smile at Yourself in the mirror... the longer You retain the enema, the more time for the lemon water to act as a detergent to rejuvenate.

At the toilet, it helps to have (pardon the pun) a stool underfoot. This mimics the squat, the normal position to evacuate the bowels & the womb. With good balance squat on the toilet; experience smooth, easy movements. Practice to facilitate good bowel habits.

Always follow a warm water enema with a cool water enema, room temperature. Warm water dissolves. Cool water shocks the colon which likes to be 105° and stimulates circulation to bring warmth and... oxygenated blood, strengthening the colon wall. The longer You retain the cool water enema, the longer the colon can experience a rush of oxygen... and rejuvenate. Again, bouncing up and down and slapping the belly to stimulate energy – makes it fun. Smile in the mirror; say: I love You. You are amazing!

Some may consider enemas unnatural, yet yogis wash their colons in the Ganges from time immemorial. Essene writings indicate gourds were hollowed out, dried and used for enemas. Fasting and enemas restore health and rejuvenate HeartMindBodySpirit.

Coffee enemas have proven to be extremely beneficial for many reasons. Dr Max Gerson popularized the idea. The reason is simple. Taken orally, coffee is a stimulant – actually, a central nervous system irritant raising a red flag internally – and bowels empty to facilitate elimination of the toxin. As an enema, however, coffee reaches the liver through the portal vein; cleanses, releases bile, and heals the body.

Regularly taking warm / cool enemas for therapeutic reasons, it is wise to replace friendly intestinal bacteria... 1 capsule probiotic in warm water, or 2 oz of fresh wheatgrass juice – even a piece of dark green such as kale, blended in a little water and strained, may be implanted in the colon with a small bulb syringe after the final release. Holding the implant for even a minute or two is effective... holding it longer assures absorption... moving the healing chlorophyll energy through the portal vein to the liver – a few minutes meditating or doing EFT, perhaps on a slant-board, helps retain the implant. With tongue caressing the roof of Your mouth while tapping Your right lower rib cage further energizes the liver.

How to Complete a Fast
A short water fast of 1-3 days can be completed with fresh juice from fruits or vegetables... or both. Since eating fruits and vegetables require different digestive juices... 20 minutes after having a large glass of re-mineralized and re-energized distilled or r/o water, have a few pieces of fruit... or small salad. Allow 3 hours between meals for optimal digestion.

After a longer water fast – 1 juice day for every 3 days fasting. Fruits and vegetables may be juiced together such as Granny Smith apple, carrot and ginger root. This warming drink is tasty on a winter day as well as during / after a fast. Before throwing vegetable pulp in the compost, add warm water... <120° to preserve enzymes... cover until cool. Strain, adding kelp or herbs... a delicious drink, or soup broth for later.

Then have small meals alternating between fruits and vegetables. If sweets have been a challenge for Your pancreas... or candida, cancer or other situations are a concern... stay with vegetables and their juices, focusing on spinach and celery, cucumber, cilantro, green beans, kale, parsley and zucchini... avoiding beets and carrots, high in sugar. Then have small salads emphasizing sprouts for a few days. For a tasty dressing: lemon juice with a dash of mustard seed, garlic and cayenne to taste.

If You are healthy enough, introduce modest amounts of cooked, whole grains – preferably germinated – the most nutritious and alkalizing: quinoa and amaranth 3:1 ratio; 1-part grains -> 4-parts water. Buckwheat groats (toasted buckwheat = kasha) are fairly neutral and usually well tolerated. For serious issues, rather than cooking grains – sprout them... blend and strain for nutritious milk.

Fasting reboots HeartMindBodySpirit. Cautiously return to Your routine. Only eat when truly hungry; be aware of combinations; be frugal – a suitable portion can be held in 2 hands, about 2 cups. Chew solids until liquid. Chew liquids to activate salivary glands for optimal digestion. "Be still and know... I Am God." Chew. Enjoy. Be Joyful!

Fasting and Urine Therapy

During a fast some may choose to apply fresh urine to tone their skin and/or use as a hair rinse... others actually dare to take a few swallows. While this may seem shocking or ludicrous to some, drinking urine is part of military survival training. Urine was commonly used for healing benefits >4000 years! Rather than a product of *waste* filtration, urine is a product of *blood* filtration: medically called "plasma ultrafiltrate". The primary function of the kidneys, rather than being excretion, is regulating the *concentration* of elements in the blood. Urine may be compared to leftovers from a meal; this metaphor helps explain why the body excretes valuable elements. To understand the full significance, observe a few eye-openers.

Cosmetic companies such as Revlon and Max Factor have paid pregnant and lactating women for their urine, with high content of the hormone HCG: human chorionic gonadotropin. Lotions, creams and conditioners contain urea. Some women at menopause nonchalantly take hormone replacement therapy such as Premarin™ – from **pre**gnant **mar**e's ur**in**e. Pregnant mares are cruelly kept in stalls with barely room to lie down, so their urine is more easily caught. {Ch 10: **Women's Issues**}

Tales are told of miners trapped by cave-ins who survived on urine. Generally thought to be connoisseurs of finer libations, several Frenchmen were trapped by a cave-in, so they sat down and ate their lunch, drank what was in their thermos, and patiently waited. They had experienced such things before and were usually rescued after a few hours. This, however, was massive. It took 30 days to dig them out. They all survived by drinking their urine and, in fact, came out rather pale – for lack of sun – yet radiant and rejuvenated: some had hair color return, skin became soft, and wrinkles melted away. Arthritic and other pains had disappeared. Much to their chagrin, these benefits were lost when they resumed their regular diet of animal and refined foods.

Kyodo News Service, Tokyo, July 90, "A male cook was pulled out of the rubble in the Hyatt Hotel early Monday morning, 14 days after a powerful earthquake devastated the northern Philippines, officials said. Dry, with only minor bruises on his body, he told reporters he survived by drinking his own urine." *NBC Nightly News*, 16 Oct 92, reported: "In Egypt, rescue workers found a 37-year-old man alive in earthquake rubble. He survived almost 82 hours by drinking his own urine. His wife, daughter and mother would not... and they died."

Drinking urine is really old news... being taught for survival in the basic training of special tactical units of armies around the world – for centuries. Martha Christy, author of *Your Own Perfect Medicine*, tells her story: "When I contracted a crippling, incurable disease early in life, I used every available conventional medicine and alternative healing method over the course of many years without success. When an acquaintance suggested 'urine therapy' I thought she'd lost her mind... with no options left, I swallowed my prejudice and decided to give it a go. To my own (and everyone else's) amazement, my healing was so rapid and so profound with urine therapy, no question remained: someone in the medical community *had to know* more than they were telling.

"After many months of haunting university libraries... I had amassed files and findings on the uses of urine in medicine and healing. I discovered among other things that urine, far from being a toxic body waste, was actually a purified derivative of the blood made by the kidneys, which contains, not body wastes... rather an array of critically important nutrients, enzymes, hormones, natural antibodies and immune defense agents.

"For almost the entire course of the 20th century, unknown to the public, doctors and medical researchers have been proving in both laboratory and clinical testing that our own urine is an enormous source of vital nutrients, vitamins, hormones, enzymes and critical antibodies that cannot be duplicated or derived from any other source. They use urine for healing cancer, heart disease, allergies, asthma, auto-immune diseases, diabetes, infertility, infections, wounds, and on and on – yet we're taught that urine is a toxic waste product!

"Why? Maybe they think it's too controversial. Or maybe, more accurately, there isn't any monetary reward for telling people what scientists know about one of the most extraordinary healing elements in the world." After all, who can profit from, or put a patent on, Your own urine? *Your Own Perfect Medicine* references and quotes various studies on the subject, providing worthwhile research for inquiring minds who choose to know.

Uses of Urine from the Past

We learn a lot about the uses of urine from history, recorded from a show on Radio 4 in London, in the Spring of 1994, called *"Now Wash Your Hands,"* presented by Corrine Julius, produced in Manchester by Julia Shaw.

"Before indoor plumbing people would save their urine in a 'slop pail' and save it for 'Piss Joe' – who went about in smock, frock and cap collecting buckets of urine and giving them a penny. He was known as the 'lent man' because lent was another name for urine. He would collect the urine from door to door and put it in wood casks on his cart and take it to the dyers and the woolen mills and sell it to them for their processing. When he died, he left 50,000£ in property, a tidy sum in those days. It is fair to say that British industry could not have developed without the contents of the slop bucket!

"In the 1840's, northern coal towns collected urine in a common barrel from which each family was supplied on wash day. 'Where this practice continues, the state of the atmosphere is altogether unaccountable to those who are not aware of the cause on washing days.' This continued until the 1890's.

"So important was urine to the economy that the Lord Chancellor might well have found himself sitting, not on a wool sack but on a cask of amber fluid. Urine was essential in softening wool, dying cloth, even hardening steel. For generations it was the number one household cleaner, getting floors more gleaming, glass more sparkling, and whites whiter than anything.

"It was used for beauty and the beast, to put a gloss on human hair and animal hides. It made the grass grow and tomatoes thrive:

'It is my firm belief
that feeding through the leaf
will make all crops healthy as can be.
And after careful test,
I find urine is the best,
it feeds the plants and keeps them insect free.
All plants do truly need
a much-diluted feed
and this is how dilution should be done:
to eight pints of water
add urine one quarter
in other words, just thirty-two to one.
Sprayed gently on the leaf,
above and underneath
it kills the pests and checks the mildew too.
The growth it seems to charm
and flowers take no harm
sprayed once each week – with one in thirty-two.'

"The names for urine in its varying states of freshness, 15 in Welsh alone, indicates its importance: lent, sig, strang, chamberlee, chamberlye, wetting, netting, piss, pizzle, piddle, pee, old swill, old pot, scour, slop.

"On Hadrian's Wall lies proof of one of its earliest uses as a dye. 'It may not have been Imperial Purple, but the purple band on the Roman soldier's toga owed its brilliance to urine. Natural dyes have a pleasant but a mute appearance. This purple was almost garish, it was a brilliant purple; it was the sort of purple one would associate with modern synthetic dyes from the chemical industry; it was lichen purple, a dye commonly used throughout Western Europe until the 1860's. Lichens were scraped off the rocks and then soaked in stale urine. They would leave it for 2 or 3 weeks stirring occasionally to let the air in, because that's a necessary part of the chemical process, and a beautiful purple paste develops that can be collected and used as a dye-stuff. Factories were set up to make the dye, starting in Scotland in the late 18th century. There's no doubt the Romans knew about it. It was a cheap and cheerful dye, though it was very fugitive to light, and the Roman, instead of only washing his toga once a week might have re-dipped in the dye, to top it off. The Welsh, too, used urine to make their famous blue-black dye mixing it not with lichens, but with bracken ash. In northern Nigeria, indigo plants are still fermented in huge vats of the stuff to create the special iridescent blue of indigo.'

"In 16th century Venice, red hair was popular. Venetian courtesans would soak their hair in urine and then drape it over the brim of a crownless hat and sit in the sun, and the length of time they were in the sun would make it either bright yellow, bright red or pale blond. And these were Titian red trusses.

"Urine in fact is good for hair. Barbers used old urine as lye, as a shampoo for hair. And in fact, the word lotion is from Latin: *lotium*, meaning urine. Roman barbershops used old urine as a shampoo. The ammonia stripped the grease out of the hair and left the hair in good condition. Urine was also good for removing dandruff because of the slightly anti-bacterial quality in fresh urine.

"The recent use of urine in Sydney, Australia is enough to make Your hair curl. The Society of Matrons of Sydney were all talking about the simply amazing new hair salon that guaranteed longer lasting sets and perms – the secret being a new setting lotion formula. Business slumped when a rival establishment claimed that the wonder formula contained urine. Although some were upset, they did admit they had the most beautiful and long-lasting perm ever.

"It wasn't only human hair that was treated to a dousing. From the Romans onward, it was the key ingredient in getting greasy wool soft and cuddly, and in shrinking the woven cloth. The urine and the wool heated up as they fermented, producing ammonia that combined with the lanolin to make a kind of soap. This washed out in cold water leaving the wool clean and soft. Every medieval cottager had a vat of urine. They lived in the same room in which they were soaking the wool and the weft, and the cloth in this stinking liquid often had pig dung mixed with it as well. One of the smelliest processes was to soak the finished cloth in old urine and then cuttle it on the floor, putting it in folds, one on top of the other – pouring urine on it and leaving it overnight; then in the morning the whole family would trample it, and take it down to the fulling mill where it was put in a falling stock and then washed. But the clothier had to carry it to the mill, sopping over his shoulder. 'Cloth that cometh for the weaving, is

naught comely to wear until it be fulled underfoot.' *Pier's Plowman*, 14th century.

"In a West Reading Mill in the 1950's, 'they were still using fresh urine to put an expensive finish on a cheap blazer cloth. And so, by spraying fresh urine on and giving a final pressing, they gave it a lovely, superior handle and soft feel. And I was at school in the 1950's wearing a navy-blue blazer cloth that probably came from this mill, and when I dropped custard on my blazer and sucked it off – I was getting more than I bargained for!'

"It was more than the woolen industry that found urine to be a magic formula. It softened leather and hardened steel; it was used in wire-making, cleansing copper, toughening tools, and mending machinery.

When I was about 16 and first went into the mill, I worked with a very old mill engineer. We had one particular problem with a machine in which a rather large driving wheel kept coming loose. He repaired this on a number of occasions and it still worked loose. So finally, he says to me 'Clear the area of all the women operatives, please.' And I asked, 'What You going to do?' And he said to me, 'I'm going to pumice it down and pee on it.' And that's exactly what he did, and I said to him afterwards, 'Why did You do that?' 'That wheel won't come loose now, because the acid in the urine actually binds the two pieces of metal together.' And it never, ever did come loose again to my knowledge.

"'They used to call it rust-jointing, to fix a slack joint, say in a fly wheel, where the spokes of the wheel went to the rim. They would collect some iron filings and mix it with some ammoniac and then they made it into a paste with urine. It was like glue; it dried rock hard.'

"While the acid in urine cemented metal joints, it also soothed inflamed skin. When Nancy Cooper reached desperation with the pain from her chilblains, she recalled a remedy that the kitchen maids used in her childhood. 'I had an old chamber pot without a handle that I kept a plant in and I decided that would be OK to put my feet in. I kept it up for 10 days or a fortnight, enough to cover my feet, and it did the trick!' Some think she's slightly potty. 'For chapped lips or dry skin, take Your own water and boil it to a syrup with some double refined loose sugar, and keep it for Your use.'

"Midwives and mothers all over England, at least until the mid-1930's, and in my district until the 1960's or 70's, would take off the baby's wet nappy and immediately wipe the baby's face with it; they said it gave the baby a lovely skin. There are those who wash their face in it to prevent wrinkles. And if You look carefully at labels on some expensive face creams, they contain a similar compound. A mild astringent, urine closes large pores and discourages blackheads. Front line soldiers have bathed their wounds in it.

"Robert Boyle: *Some Considerations Touching the Usefulness of Experimental Natural Philosophies*, 1663: 'An ancient gentlewoman who'd been almost hopeless to recover from diverse chronic distempers was advised to take her morning draughts of her own water, by the use of which she strangely recovered. A friend of mine that hath tried it in the jaundice affirms it to deserve the commendation he gives it.'

"The Bible too recommends it in the Book of Proverbs providing You stick to Your own, like former Indian Prime Minister Morarji Desai who's chalked up more than a century on a daily dose. {Actually, he passed on a year later in 1995 – at 99 years of age.} It may seem bizarre to drink what is the body's way of getting rid of what it doesn't want. 'The average human puts out about a liter and a half a day and its about 96% water so it's only about 4% solids and of that the bulk is urea and sodium chloride. We end up with only .2% of everything else. According to one company in America, specializing in enzymes, they claim there are 40,000 urinary proteins in there of which they claim to have characterized 400. Sounds like an awfully large number, particularly when it's such a small quantity.'

Research chemist Dr John Gwilt spent a lifetime investigating compounds in urine that may be medically useful, compounds like urokinase. 'After very careful purification so that we've got a virtually crystalline form, it's used to stimulate the lysis, the dissolution, of blood clots in the body. It's used in this country; the first use was for blood clots in the eye. It is also approved now for use with blood clots in the pulmonary artery and coronary artery. The big value of using products that have come from human urine is that the side effects are likely to be absolutely minimal. There is no antigenic response, no intolerance; and none of the side effects that one may get with products from another species.' 'Are they still studying urine?'

'Oh, I think there's an enormous potential for new compounds there. We've barely begun.'

But what matters to chemical pathologists, like Dr Alistair Hay at Leeds University, is the vital clues that urine gives about a patient's health. 'Urine, for us, is an accessible way into the body. A lot of the products that are produced in the body or that get into the body deliberately or through eating food end up in the urine in one form or another. We have a major screening program here for those who take drugs of abuse: heroin, cocaine, amphetamines are in the urine 10 days after someone has taken it. So, we can find it. Drug screening is becoming an increasing feature of pre-employment practices. Most want to make sure that the person they are taking on doesn't drink excessively and certainly doesn't take drugs.' And that's a real money-spinner.

"There are other practical but perhaps forgotten uses. Until the late 19th century urine was the only source of ammonia. It was the Thousand-In-One of its age, a cleaner for floors, ovens and ranges; both a bleach and a detergent. Heartlib, 1650: 'A way to cleanse glasses that washes them more clearly than with salt or ashes, is the washing of them with one's urine.' And it washes canvases as well as glass. It mixes well with pigments, inks and even plaster. A sculptor, Quentin Bell, found it useful when he ran out of ammonia. 'I had made my plaster, and I suddenly discovered the job was going to take much longer than I had supposed. So, I wondered... have I got a retarding agent? I hadn't. And then it occurred to me that I had a good store of ammonia in my bladder; so, I pissed into the plaster. I had quite a fair store in hand, so to speak; and it worked a treat. I was able to go on working for an hour and a half when the plaster would have been dry without it in 10 minutes.'

"The superstition is still strong that Your own urine attracts the lover that You want or increases Your husband's or Your lover's ardor. For instance, You could, after washing his socks, rinse them in Your urine so that he would wear the socks and – unknown to himself – fall more and more in love with You. Or You could take a piece of Your intimate underwear and soak it in urine and put this between two halves of lemon and stick it full of pins and bury it in the garden, increasing the ardor of Your lover, too!

"In the early days on the Western Front (WWI) urine was the only protection against the effects of gas. The idea came filtering through the lines that the solution was to urinate into a handkerchief and use it as a face mask.

"Urine has been a precious commodity, so could it find its place in one of its oldest and down to earth applications: in the garden? On *Gardeners' Question Time* {excerpted from another Radio 4 program}: 'In these days of concern about the environment, have the panel any ideas on how we can use our own waste products, such as urine in the garden?' 'Well, now,' (the announcer, Clay Jones) 'that's a new one; it is indeed. Stephan, could we have a wee word from You?' (Laughter from the audience.) 'Certainly, I don't see why we shouldn't use our own urine in the garden, after all most of the local felines come and deposit theirs in the garden, so why shouldn't we? Absolutely, no reason at all. It's actually a good source of nitrogen for plants to grow, because one of the forms that plants use nitrogen is ammonia, and urine, we all know, is rich in ammonia. One of the best uses I've seen made of this was two chaps that I know down in Kent who ran an efficient *allotment*. {These are British leftovers from the middle-ages, known as the Victory Gardens of WWII. Vacant land is divided among those in the neighborhood without yards to grow gardens. These spaces are highly coveted.} They have a series of containers at the entrance to their allotment that comprise several gallons of urine in varying stages of fermentation. And when the stuff has been there for about 6 months, You then use it as fertilizer, especially on a plant called comfrey; and excellent stuff it is; very good indeed.' 'This reminds me actually,' (chimes in the announcer,) 'of not a use in the garden, but when I was a little boy, and if I had earache, Grandmother's remedy was to pour a thimble full of my own urine into my ear and plugged with cotton wool, and I assure You ladies and gentlemen, it worked; within half an hour – no more earache. Sometimes difficult to get it into the thimble! (laughter) How do You manage it, Fred?' 'You must have been a very good shot, Clay. I have trouble getting it into a bottle, never mind a thimble!'

"(Interviewing another gardener:) 'Now, if You can imagine the back of this shed, with about half a dozen or maybe eight cowboys and those big bottles all full of a foul liquid or maybe partly full, and especially on a Monday morning when they've been out on the booze; the one on the end was the special container because my grandfather always reckoned that one was the best brew, it was the strongest and the ferns grew best off that than any of the other bottles. He said it was the Stout that he drunk on a Saturday night, but I didn't fully believe him. We use it mainly to feed asparagus fern that You usually find in wedding bouquets, because wedding bouquets in those days were great big bulky things and the trails of them, the fern went almost down to the ground. We tried all sorts of things to produce a longer strand. But it was the urine that always came out on top. I would think there's all the nutrients the plants needed and there was plenty of nitrogen, and it's truly organic, isn't it?'

"And it starts off the compost heap with a treat. Urine is sterile when it first leaves the body. There can be a risk of infection; so, it's wise to know Your sources.

"Every day we flush away millions of gallons of this once valuable commodity; and it ends up in sewage works. Disposing of urine is a costly business. It can't be separated from feces or industrial waste. Breaking down the ammonia into acceptable levels is a problem facing technical assistant Chris Nurienen: 'We are currently using quite a lot of energy in our aeration processes, and all our treatment processes elsewhere. We utilize a lot of energy in the oxidation and breakdown of urine components, such as uric acid, ammonia, etc. It would be ideal if we could find a way of disposing of, or utilizing ammonia in the future.'

"That solution has to be found quickly as a new EC directive severely restricts the amount of ammonia that can be discharged back into our rivers and into the water cycle. At the Centre for Alternative Technology in Aberystwyth, Dr Jeremy Light is one of a handful of scientists trying to attack the problem at source. 'You need a modification to the toilet, to an ordinary flush toilet, so that the urine is collected separately, and that could be run via small waste pipes down to a tank underground outside. And then it could be collected by a tanker and go through minimal treatment before selling to the farmer."

"And need collection in bulk be such an insuperable problem? After all they managed it for the alum industry in Whitby in the 17th century. 'The use of urine in the alum industry began about 1607 when the alum shales in Sound's End near Whitby were discovered by Thomas Challinger. The processing of the alum required thousands of gallons of urine that would be impossible to get from the surrounding countryside. And so, the ships that took the alum to London, say 23 tons, would come back with a similar amount of urine. That would be about four thousand wine gallons of London urine that was bought cheaply, transported cheaply by ship, and taken to the works. And if they had to collect this urine from the villagers around Whitby, the cost of land transport would have been so high that they simply couldn't have carried on their works. London urine was essential from 1607.'

So, it's conceivable that if we overcome our distaste of urine... we, like the Victorians, could put a price on spending a penny.

"*A Treatise on Hygiene and Public Health*, (1892): 'Average amount of ammonia voided per annum by the average person 11.32 pounds in urine and 1.64 pounds in feces. The money value of the total constituent ammonia, phosphates and potash in urine is 7 shillings and thruppence, in feces 1 and tuppence, 3 farthings: total 8 shillings, 5 pence and 3 farthings. But in calculating the value of sewage, it is better to take the annual excretion of the individual as being equivalent to 10 pounds of ammonia, worth 6 shillings and 8 pence'."

Thus, ends an impressive history lesson! After using urine therapeutically for over 20 years, I heard the promo for *Now Wash Your Hands* and knew I *had* to tape the show; everything truly *is* Perfect Divine Order!

Urine Used in Healing
Ancient cultures have used urine therapy for ages. Mahatma Gandhi among others took a daily dose. While most generally view urine as a waste product, it is 95% water, 2.5% urea and 2.5% enzymes (proteins), hormones, minerals and salt. *Toxins and wastes are eliminated through the intestines, lungs and the skin... rather than through the kidneys!* There are more toxins in the person's out-breath than in their urine! Drinking one's urine activates the lymphatic system and stimulates the production of anti-bodies and Natural Killer cells. Recently, Yoshinori Ohsumi, a cellular biologist from Japan, became a 2016 Nobel Prize winner in physiology and medicine "for discovering the mechanisms of autophagy." The Japanese scientist has scientifically substantiated that fasting is beneficial for one's health. Autophagy – literally: self-eating – is a rather indelicate medical term for a spiritual experience... autophagy protects from premature

senility, rejuvenates by creating new cells and by removing defective proteins and damaged intracellular organelles.

Traditionally, it is recommended to drink the middle catch. First let a stream flow for a few seconds; contract the urethral sphincter to stop the flow; let the next bit flow into a cup or glass; toward the end, contract again, and let the last part flow into the toilet. This fluid is absolutely sterile first leaving the body, so drink it right away. Energetically... 3, 6 or 9 sips. It may also be used as a skin softener, gradually melting away wrinkles. If allowed to sit and ferment, it is a conditioner making hair soft and lustrous, enriching the skin.

Although skeptical one woman, a model, thought to experiment – keeping the secret from her husband. Surprisingly, achieving her goals with her hair and skin after only a month of daily drinking, and using the rest as skin lotion... her husband nuzzled up to her neck in bed one night saying: "Sweetheart, I've really gotta say: You smell... sooo... good!" Relieved... she kept up with her beauty secret.

Some people are turned off by the thought of drinking urine, yet their intuition and curiosity are intrigued by the results that may accrue. They adjust their left-brain objections with some right-brain creativity by adding a tablespoon of the middle catch to a glass of water. Next day they take two tablespoons and keep increasing until they get to the point where they feel they may as well drink it straight – it's different from what they assumed. People who know You are Your own best medicine take their daily dose. Some object because of the strong aroma, and the supposed flavor. This merely indicates a **die**t, filled with pollutants: alcohol, caffeine, nicotine, animal foods, refined, fried and processed foods, salt, sugars and synthetics. When excluded, urine loses the pungent aroma and flavor.

This is definitely for the adventuresome... or the desperate. J.W. Armstrong in his classic *The Water of Life* recounts many experiences, some being ghastly situations. One person with terminal challenges and a minimal discharge of thick, foul urine began regular drinking, and over a period of time regained strength, and returned to health! One use of urine in healing already mentioned can be expanded. Using a thimbleful of urine to ease a child's earache has proven successful time and again. In the case of a young child still in diapers, what are we to do? If the child cries in the middle of the night with digging or pulling at the ears, You can use Your own fresh middle catch... plug the ear with a cotton ball and settle down for a restful night; perfectly safe, presuming the eardrum is intact.

Another handy use for urine is on insect bites. Out in nature, You carry Your own remedy. One thing to be aware of, if You apply Your urine right away the stinging goes; if You wait ten minutes or so, it will do little good. The proteins exuded by the offending insect are fairly rapidly absorbed through the skin. Quickly applied, urine neutralizes irritants close to the surface.

Old-time homeopaths, asking for a sample supposedly to analyze, dilute the "middle catch" the "mother tincture." Taking it in another room, making the remedy into 1X, 2X, all the way to 30C, as appropriate.

Urine Enemas

Some people are born experimenters. Hearing about something, they wonder what effect it might have on them and on others. Natural healers explore, and often discover methods appearing to be a contradiction or foolish to the rational mind... yet when applied, they bring results. It is easy to experiment with some things; and other things require a stretch of one's imagination and commitment. It is easy to understand that chemical enemas are harsh and counterproductive to well-being. For many it is a leap of faith to buy an enema bag and put it to use. Some may experiment with warm and cold enemas. It certainly is reasonable.

Talking to a polarity therapist, the subject of enemas came up – is there therapeutic value in a beer enema? While double blind studies have yet to be financed by the brewing industry, anecdotal information must suffice. Of course, the beer is to be opened and left out to ensure it is flat. After all, carbon dioxide is a waste product – let it escape in the air. Dilute the 12 ounces of beer with warm water for a normal enema, described above. Diluted it acts as a homeopathic remedy and could draw out alcohol-related toxins stored in the body. Being of German heritage it was imperative. Actually, it was a fairly normal enema. Follow Your Inner Voice Intuition. Explore. What else is possible?

A thorough cleanse is available during watermelon season: get 9 organic watermelons to eat, juicing the whole thing – the skin has chlorophyll; the rind, electrolytes; seeds, a special charge of energy, and the red, sweetness. Juiced together they make a tasty and cleansing drink, supporting kidneys and liver... the whole body. An excellent time to see the therapeutic value of urine therapy – it tastes like watermelon!

Sergey Maryanovskiy, a born explorer and healer from Ukraine, shares the following information based on the works of Gennady Malakhov, a Russian athlete who, like so many, took steroids and otherwise abused his body for many years, eventually causing degenerative disease. He wrote four books detailing his journey and healing work. Information on urine enemas comes from the book entitled, *Healing Forces*. The theory is similar to the beer enema. Urine, being a part of who we are, acts as a homeopathic remedy – known as a nosode – flushing out disease processes present in our body. Russians and many Europeans are steeped in traditions using simple means to resolve complex issues. While British and Europeans in general, appear conservative – they are open to natural healing and innovative, natural experiments. Americans, on the other hand, appear to be open and receptive, especially to technological advances and drugs yet to be thoroughly tested – yet many are narrow-minded or shy with natural healing and natural experiments.

Mr Malakhov says urine enemas are quite healing if done properly. To prepare, warm the body. One way to get blood circulating is with a sauna. Those who are slim or normal can use a moist sauna; those who are overweight can use a dry sauna. The option is a hot bath (106°) to get blood moving to the muscles and skin. To drive the blood back to the body core, including the intestines, take a cold rinse for 10-20 seconds; a period of aerobic exercise is also warming. To ensure plenty of urine eat fruits &/or drink plenty of re-mineralized and re-energized distilled or r/o water the day before. Collect two quarts in a container with a tight lid stored in the refrigerator. Then bring it to room temperature – place in hot water to speed the process.

If possible, do the enema after sunset, preferably after a bowel movement. Let air out of the hose, lubricate the tip of the nozzle and the anus with oil; spread out a towel on the floor; get on Your hands and knees; insert the nozzle and allow the liter of urine to enter Your colon. Then lie on Your back for 30-60 seconds, massaging Your intestines. Then bend Your knees with Your feet flat on the floor, and lift Your pelvis off the floor. If You can, do a shoulder stand, or bring Your legs over Your head for a few moments. Then lie on Your back and turn on Your right side. These movements ensure that the liquid gets to the entire large intestine. Hold the enema as long as You feel comfortable (5-15 minutes) then release. Mr Malakhov says Your body intuitively knows how long to retain the urine enema, and releases it at the appropriate time; Your innate intelligence knows everything necessary for healing; follow Your Inner Voice Intuition!

The first time or two this enema is taken, some experience minimal discomfort likened to the experience one has when taking a healing dose of cayenne pepper. When we use cayenne on our food, we notice a burning in our mouth, and sometimes at the other end. When we take cayenne for therapeutic purposes, healing the heart and circulation for instance, it can be taken ¼ tsp in an ounce of water, with a glass of water as a chaser, between meals. This gives a sensation of burning in the abdomen for about 10-15 minutes... actually, it is healing and soothing to the abdominal wall, although we may experience slight discomfort at the very, *very* end.

Mr Malakhov says likewise, the urine enema may give the sensation of burning, yet it is beneficial for the wall of the large intestine, healing lesions, and dispelling worms. Follow this procedure every day during the first week; every other day the second week; every third day the third week; then once a week for a month; then every other week for four months.

Doing this routine and feeling adventurous, You may choose to experiment with boiled urine enemas. If You already were in fair health, You may choose to do the boiled version after 3 months. With serious health challenges, follow instructions for the full 6 months before embarking on the boiled variety.

The collection of urine and taking enemas are the same, except: boil a quart of urine down to a pint. Use an old pan *only* for this purpose; salts crystallizing on the bottom are a challenge to scrub clean. Let it cool to warm before using; take the pint full strength.

Repeat 2-4 times a week for two weeks. Then boil the quart of urine down to four ounces, making it even more concentrated. Repeat once a week for 2-4 weeks. Sergey assures me he has done this whole routine – and reports rejuvenating benefits. {https://urine-therapy.org/}

A Case of Cataracts

As a young chiropractor, I exchanged treatments with a polarity therapist in Coconut Grove, FL. I had studied the works of Major Bertrand DeJarnette, DO, DC for my doctorate specializing in Sacral-Occipital-Technique – he had studied the works of Randolph Stone, DO, DC, ND to qualify as a practitioner in Polarity Therapy; these two pioneers in Energy Medicine had similar applications.

Among his regular clients was a woman in the community who operated *The Garden*, a living foods restaurant, in Coral Gables. One day she asked if he would be so kind, to use her urine as a lotion for her weekly massage. He knew she had been drinking it, and regained 80% of her hair color and thickness... and so, he obliged; the next morning he was amazed; his hands felt – in his words – "soft as a baby's butt." She gave him *The Water of Life*, by J.W. Armstrong, which he read and gave to me... truly fascinating reading, I finished it that night.

And, as Perfect Divine Order would have it, the next day a woman named Rheta came to see me. She said, "Doctor, I'm here to get checked out. A month ago, I buried my mother who died at 97. I'm 67, and I'd like to be in shape for the next 30 years or so." We talked about nutrition, & lifestyle; she mentioned her major concern. "I like to go to my evening meetings, and with my cataracts, there are scary haloes around the headlights coming at me, as well as the headlights in my mirror. How can I get rid of cataracts without surgery? I'd rather drive myself to the meetings, than rely on others. What can I do?" One of the case histories from the book, finished the night before, mentioned the dissolution of cataracts! Wondering... do I dare mention it to her? She was an open person, and explaining the episode with my friend, asked if she cared to borrow the book. She said, with doubtful yet smiling eyes, "I'll give it a look."

She arrived a week later with a gleam in her eye and a tale to tell. She "devoured the book that evening and found it thoroughly fascinating." She decided there was nothing to lose, and the next morning drank a few ounces of her middle catch. Her plans were to stay home and do a little work in the garden. Instead, she spent most of the day on the toilet. She was amazed that although her morning water was the normal volume, about an hour after drinking the few ounces of her middle catch, she found herself on the toilet and...

"out came over a quart." Being totally spunky and serendipitous, drinking more middle catch... the process repeated itself regularly through the day "voiding what seemed like gallons!"

The next few days were a repeat; eventually it mellowed. We continued weekly treatments for a couple of months. She was *committed* to her outcome. She called about 3 months later. Her doctor wanted to know what happened to her cataracts. Rather than risk *really* being <u>committed</u>, she simply smiled and said, "All gone!" She knew already, driving at night free from the nuisance of haloes. Some deny it had anything to do with urine – attesting to the power of the mind. Whatever it may be: recognize the truth. Drink up, my friend, and create *Your* Reality!

Holistic healing is a Journey, with us as Captain at the helm of the ship; we have helpmates and, ultimately, it is up to us – where to tack, when to raise or lower the sails. We learn as we go... and from our observations of others... and their experiences. Whatever happens is our Life's Lessons; going beyond the superficial... we find our Life's Purpose. Trusting the Source of All, we trust all things are in Perfect Divine Order.

Our experience of the Journey depends to a large extent on what we consume as fuel. We are wise enough to put kerosene and fuel oil into heaters designed for them... unleaded gas for internal combustion engines, diesel fuel for diesel motors, and jet fuel for planes. Using any other fuel runs the risk of congesting the engine, or burning it up. In the following chapter we explore optimal fuels for HeartMindBodySpirit as support for our Sacred Journey.

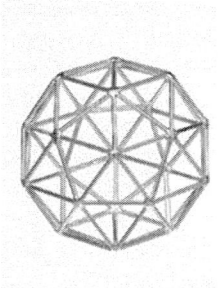

8 – ENERGY MEDICINE AS FOUND IN OUR AIR, WATER AND FOOD

Vibrations in the Air: The Essence of Life

We can go weeks without food... days without water... yet only a few minutes without air. We get **56%** of our energy from the air we breathe... we breathe 400 gallons an hour! Health-conscious individuals have concern for foods they eat, liquids they drink, *and* the air they breathe with >70 years of geoengineering using weather as warfare, there are profound issues and consequences for our environment as well as for ourselves. What to do? Think Global – Act Local.

The first place to start: avoid noxious fumes. Freedom from smoking continues to be a challenge for many, and there are tips to share. I feel eminently qualified, along with Mark Twain: "Quitting smoking is the easiest thing to do; I ought to know, I've done it hundreds of times!" With proper Verbal Diet, remember: *trying* is self-sabotage; *quitting* is a negative image: giving up, doing without. To say "This time I'm really going to try to quit smoking" invites failure. Feeling: "I simply can't do it" or "It's bigger than me" damages self-esteem.

Positively affirm: "I choose fresh air for my lungs!" When an urge to smoke arises, use this affirmation and take a deep, caressing breath, holding it as long as comfortable and then, exhale slowly – *forcibly* through *pursed* lips. This creates **backpressure** forcing more oxygen into the blood stream. After 3X, the desire to smoke is greatly diminished. Rhythmic breathing: inhale fully and exhale completely to relieve the urge.

When exercising, avoid fumes... choose fresh air away from traffic and pollutants, in a wooded park or at the water's edge, or in Your home during inclement weather – turn on Your favorite music and dance for 20-30 minutes continuously – even between songs, keep moving to keep the aerobic flow happening. Breathe deeply and exhale completely. Slow, rhythmic.

Cleaning Indoor Air

Air is free and psychologically of less value; yet it is the essential requirement of life, especially for mammals, whether bats or belugas, hamsters or humans. Actually, clean air is costly, especially when "the most endangered species" continues to create toxins of such magnitude. Subtle as it may be, pollutants of the land and the water have an effect on air quality, affecting indoor air. Fortunately cleaning indoor air is far less costly than cleaning outdoor air. Most of us spend 90% of time indoors; the EPA ranks indoor air pollution as the top environmental risk we face!

Sources of Pollution

Some indoor pollutants are easy to see and smell: smoke, odors, mildew, mold and dust. Tobacco smoke in its particulate phase for the smoker contains nicotine and tars, and a host of chemicals; second hand smoke is ingested by the unfortunate individuals who live in the same house; third hand smoke is ingested by unsuspecting visitors who – even though the smoker may be away – inhale residues from the drapes and upholstery. Clearly smoking is deadly. Science is in.

Pollutants are subtle: bacteria, chemicals, gases, pollen, static electricity. Formaldehyde is an invisible pollutant entering the air from synthetic materials along with benzene, chloroform, trichloroethylene and carbon tetrachloride. Formaldehyde gas by itself can provoke allergies, asthma attacks, depression, memory loss, and gynecological problems. Formaldehyde, a *known* human carcinogen, is commonly used as a bonding agent in thousands of products: car interiors, counter tops, deodorants, electronics, plywood, particleboard and fiberboard, leaching into the air from furniture, drapes, carpeting and some clothing, especially when new; always wash new clothes before wearing. The EPA studied 10 office buildings, schools and nursing homes for 5 years. At least 500 chemicals turned up in each of the buildings: fumes from room dividers... telephone & computer cables... paint and carpeting.

Organic volatile gases are found in most household products, including dry-cleaned clothing, paint solvents such as cleaners and degreasers, wood preservatives, artificial air fresheners, aerosol sprays, hobby supplies, disinfectants, repellents, stored fuels and automotive products. As an example, methylene chloride – known carcinogen – is widely used in paint removers and, as a propellant in aerosol spray paint: 500**m**/ lbs per year! Asbestos was used in ceilings from 1945 to 1975, as insulation on hot water and steam pipes from 1920 to 1972, wall and ceiling insulation from 1930 to 1950. Inhaled loose asbestos fibers cause cancer. Biological pollutants as mold, pollen, dust mites and animal dander affect 25 million of us, contributing to asthma, hay fever and headaches. Air conditioners and humidifiers provide breeding grounds; regular maintenance is essential.

The average home collects 40 pounds of dust a year, and hosts 15 species of mites that live in beds, pillows and stuffed furniture. Some mites fly through the air, leaving their droppings. When we take in a deep breath... sometimes we get more than we expect. These invisible pests live about 45 days; 42,000 can survive on a single ounce of mattress dust; mites alone send asthmatics to emergency rooms >200K times a year with allergies.

Once upon a time... when things worked, as they say... houses were drafty; carpets, cushions and pillows were beaten regularly, and aired or cured in the sun. Before 1970 the air flow standards required 15 cubic feet per minute, per person. The perceived energy crisis changed that. We began to insulate and seal our buildings more thoroughly – lowering the airflow by 2/3, decreasing a building's ability to diffuse chemicals. This saved energy and trapped pollutants, leaving little fresh air in our structures. Although the airflow standards were raised to 20 cubic feet per minute per person in 1989, our sealed-up homes and offices concentrate pollutants.

We pollute indoor air with chemicals used in modern building materials as well as toxins in household furnishings and products. Carpeting as well as furniture is advertised with protection from dirt, stains, wear and tear, and even crushing. Led down the Primrose Path, people breathe in profound pollutants every day, every night... to ward off a *possible* spill.

Dust mites live on skin fragments which are sometimes seen floating in the air as sunlight penetrates our windows. Mites also flourish in the humid environment of beds unless properly aired or cleaned. The feces of the mite in the air, a protein, can trigger asthma attacks. In humid houses, the mites can flourish anywhere; the drier the house, the fewer breeding places. The bed remains a favorite place for mites... humid, because we lose a pint of moisture overnight... and the bed has skin fragments as food. Daily air bedding before making Your bed. Rather than using this as an excuse to leave the bed unmade – poor Feng Shui – those who are organized and prosperous make their bed daily!

People are keen to keep the vibrations around their home pure and simple, assuring health and balance for them and their loved ones. Most vulnerable are children and the elderly, and anyone occupying a new or renovated home, apartment or office. Eliminate the cause by using non-toxic building materials, and paints and sealants to seal in toxic vapors from walls, floors, particleboard and linoleum. Ensure adequate ventilation.

Charging Home and Office with the Great Outdoors

Those who have experienced its effects know the feeling of being in the great outdoors in an unpolluted part of the world. It's a blessing if You can work outdoors, spending as much time as possible with bare feet on Mother Earth. Reality for most dictates otherwise.

The EPA says the average worker's (student's) output is 18% less than what it could be – due to poor indoor air. The EPA, the American Society of Heating, Refrigeration and Air-conditioning Engineers (ASHRAE), and the Occupational Safety and Health Administration (OSHA) all say the average worker loses 12 work days a year due to poor indoor air quality. Whenever possible, open Your windows. If Your windows are closed much of the time, find a purification system using medical-grade ultraviolet light to kill viruses, bacteria, molds, fungi, spores, VOCs and more. https://www.airoasis.com/

Vibrations in Water: The Channel of Life

From time immemorial, the recommendation has been eight glasses of water per day… at least two quarts a day for most adults, adding juice of a lemon is an option. This is in addition to the water we take in from raw fruits and vegetables or milks made from germinated grains, seeds or nuts because these liquids are carrying nutrients. Re-mineralized and re-energized distilled or r/o water taken in between meals rinses out acidic residues from our own physiological processes, and toxins from our polluted environment. While a simple requirement, it has gotten complicated.

Ground water and well water have been contaminated from synthetic fertilizers and battery farms. Lakes and rivers have been attacked by a litany of predators, all having human origins. Cities continue to contaminate their own drinking water. In the name of science and community health, fluoride is added to drinking water! Excess fluoride = mottled teeth. Where is common sense? The National Academy of Sciences has a position against fluoride. Dr John Yiamouyiannis' book *Fluoride: The Aging Factor* clears any confusion in the

debate. He cites multiple studies and agrees with Dr Takeki Tsutsui and co-workers at Nippon Dental College in Japan who "showed fluoride caused genetic damage, and is capable of transforming normal cells into cancer cells"! Dr Y lists possible symptoms of fluoride poisoning: arthritis, recurrent upset stomach, heart & skin problems and general malaise.

Chlorine mixed with organic matter in water forms tri-halo-methanes – THMs – many are carcinogens. The chlorine levels in municipal water supplies are sufficient to pass tests for chlorine levels in the average backyard swimming pool! Fill Your bathtub: note the color / smell. Municipalities measure hormones, anti-biotics, and other pharmaceuticals in their tap water., yet give little recognition to the Fact: chlorine and fluorine **kill** friendly bacteria in the colon. Tap water = Vibrations of Death.

Most municipal water is recycled toilet water with 40,000 carcinogens, known and identified – the most familiar include aluminum – to get feces, leaves and other solid matter to drop to the bottom of the reservoir; chlorine – to kill off all bacteria; and fluoride – to counteract the ill effects of chlorine! Aluminum is associated with mental dysfunction = Alzheimer's disease. Chlorine destroys friendly intestinal bacteria = poor absorption of food, inability to eliminate toxins. Fluoride, a violent poison, is toxic for humans!

Increasingly large areas of the world become deserts; we cut down forests and mine fossil water to irrigate so-called Green Revolution "food" bred to thrive on expensive synthetic fertilizers and abundant irrigation! With worldwide deforestation, it means reduced evaporation / transpiration of high-quality water… *contributing to overheating* and increased atmospheric turbulence, propelling a great amount of water vapor into the upper atmosphere – never to be recovered. There is now a net loss of water from the planet: endangering Life and leading Earth into dehydration.

Bottled Water

Bottled water on occasion is acceptable, preferred over tap water. Considerations regarding daily or frequent use: some bottled waters are carbonated – carbon dioxide is a waste product. Most bottled water is in plastic containers and the soft plastic adsorbs into the water, especially when exposed to heat – water trucked to Your store was probably exposed to some amount of heat along the way. The bluish hard plastic is safer. Get BPA-free plastic when possible. Another consideration: whatever the size of a plastic bottle... it takes 1/3 of the volume in terms of *petroleum* to *create* that synthetic bottle. After brief use, we dispose of that bottle in re-cycle or landfill; glass is preferred.

Besides the container, consider the water itself. It is bottled in a clean manner, yet it is hardly sterile; although it looks clear, microorganisms begin growing after 10 days. Consider the time between water going into the bottle, and using it. And more seriously, consider: local laws governing bottled water, purified **and** distilled, read: "not more than 1/3 of the total water may be from a municipal source" meaning 1/3 may be... and to boost the bottom line, probably is... tap water with chlorine, etc! "Innocent until proven guilty?" Ancient Wisdom says *caveat emptor*... "buyer beware" – Buyer be Aware! GRAS water free from fluoride: Aquafina, Crystal Point, Dannon, Deja Blue, Evian, Fresh Market, Great Value, Smart Water, Summit Mountains, and Summit Springs. When buying, check in the Here & Now. Look at what is. Do the Sway Test. Be responsible for Your own water!

Distilled Water

Pure distilled water leaches inorganic minerals *from* the body. This *can be* wonderful; having inorganic minerals in Your body is similar to sand in Your gears. You can buy it in gallon jugs at first. Big stores have neutral-tasting water as they move quantity – small stores tend to taste off... sitting in plastic bottles under fluorescent lights.

A small counter-top distiller, or the family size, with carbon pre-filter is best for most kinds of waters, especially municipal tap water with high amounts of Volatile Organic Compounds (VOC's) having a lower boiling point than water; they actually make it through the distillation process. The carbon filter catches the VOC's before they get to the distiller. While bigger units have a carbon pre-filter, smaller units can have post-filtration. Some waters are free from VOC's; taste and see. If it tastes like plastic after it has been distilled, You are tasting VOC's perhaps requiring pre- and post-filtering. Follow directions changing the post-filter.

Distilled water cleanses; after the inorganic minerals are gone from Your body, add a sprinkle of whole salt for drinking between meals. How long to rinse out inorganic minerals? For every year of indiscriminate living, one month of re-mineralized and re-energized pure water to nurture and restore HeartMindBodySpirit.

Also add whole salt to Your soak water for sprouts; catch this nutritious soak-water to give Your plants or garden. Instead of rinsing sprouts, give them a 30-minute salt bath to help them grow. With herbal tea, explore sun tea; combine re-mineralized and re-energized pure water and tea in a glass jar and leave in the rays of the sun. In lieu of a sunny day, heat water to the point where small bubbles begin to form on the bottom... turn off the heat, add the herbs and steep. Keep temperature <190° to maintain vibrations found in water. This is also true of slow cookers. First set on Hi and set a timer for 1 hr, then Low most are <190°.

R/O Water

Reverse osmosis also known as r/o water is the choice for many; it is literally "washed water" that begins with pre-filtration of municipal water or well water, removing particles of dirt, sand, rust, etc. through a process of mechanical removal. Then activated carbon removes chemicals, especially chlorine, as well as pesticides, herbicides, industrial solvents and by-products of chlorination. The reverse osmosis membrane removes dissolved solids, salts and heavy metals: fluoride, lead, and arsenic, as well as inorganic minerals: calcium, copper, and magnesium. As a secondary process, the membrane is an ultra-fine filter. There is post-filtration for the removal of chemicals. It also provides a one-micron filter. Some r/o units are equipped with UV light at the point where the water leaves the unit. Like distilled water, r/o water is empty water – thirsty water – devoid of minerals, and pulls inorganic minerals from the body to fulfill molecular balance; r/o water is suitable for a healthy lifestyle... a convenient choice.

Being Responsible on the Water Planet

O3, noted for its peculiar odor and oxidizing qualities in late 18th century, was called ozone in 1840 – from the Greek *ozein* to smell. In the late 19th century ozone oxidized organic compounds interacting with double bonds; that's how natural rubber was discovered.

Ozone was discovered to destroy toxic and foul-smelling pollution – as well as bacteria in sewage. Wiesbaden, Germany began using ozone to purify drinking water in 1901. This spread throughout much of Germany and many major cities: Zurich, Florence, Brussels, Marseille, Moscow and Singapore, to name a few. Experiments in various forms led to cleansing tissue and blood due to its bactericidal, fungicidal and virucidal action. Highly reactive gaseous ozone readily oxidizes organic matter and kills bacteria and molds.

Ozone, a 3-atom form of activated oxygen, is a normal trace element in Earth's atmosphere. Nature creates ozone to purify the air by electrical discharges or lightning; ozone is created by electrical energy in air space. Nature also creates ozone where we have moisture and strong sunlight... the fresh smell of a waterfall... or laundry hung outside to dry. The world's renowned vacation spots have some of the highest levels of naturally occurring ozone. Ozone is quite effective in residential pools; with commercial applications, ozone remarkably reduces chemicals.

Whatever Your source of water, unless from a clean stream where the water twists and turns and bounces over rapids, or the water bubbles forth from Mother Earth... if it straight from the pipe, it is stripped of energy. Viktor Schauberger has shown the purifying power of water in motion with water-forms. Energize: gently shake or swirl water with loving rhythm.

You may enjoy "spinning" Your water. Vortex Water Technology™ uses magnets and infrared in their Vitalizer Plus™ to create stable hexagonal micro-clustered water; small water molecule clusters are more easily absorbed at the cellular level. The water molecule HOH has a central oxygen atom with two hydrogen atoms attached at an angle of 104.5° and the Vitalizer stretches that angle to 109.5° affecting surface tension of the water so cells more efficiently absorb nutrients and excrete wastes; dissolving a maximum volume of oxygen, it also makes water "fresh." Scientific analysis of water consumed by villagers in parts of the world known for health and longevity show the water is 67-70 Hz – the Vitalizer is 60.816, while standard tap water is 120-160 Hz! The Vitalizer has an octagonal ring at the base containing minerals; they recommend a new one every 6 months... or simply add Himalayan Pink Salt to provide minerals for micro-clustering. The spinning water is a tornado of bubbles; a silver spoon wedged in the ring adds silver ions!

While the Vitalizer has a two-quart capacity and the "charge" lasts 24 hrs, it's pricey at $600. The option is $15 or less for a frother to spin Your pure water with a pinch of Himalayan pink salt {whole salt is required to restructure the water}. You can create the same vortex in each glass of water as You drink through the day. Simply spin while taking 3 Sacred Breaths... blessing the water. You can actually taste the difference when You do this. The frother is portable, and easy to carry.

Vibrations in Food: The Sustenance of Life
"The person who has beer and franks
with cheer and thanks...
might just happen to live longer
than someone who has pears or sprouts
with fears or doubts."
Mark Matthew Braunstein
Radical Vegetarianism, 1981

At one time if You postulated that food had a connection to health, people would look at You thinking You were a few sandwiches short of a picnic. Today, we know about anti-oxidants, beta-carotene, chlorophyll, cruciferous vegetables, enzymes, probiotics and phytoplankton – we know there is a real connection. All animal foods... especially dairy, and processed, refined animal foods... as well as refined grains and sugars congest us, causing dis-ease. This is well-documented... and now our collective disease has spread to Mother Earth as she is in distress. While fossil fuel emissions are a mere **13%** of our present condition, animal agriculture is **51%**! The answer is clear; the question some ask: how do we adequately address this situation? Our personal and collective experiences have planetary consequences... now is time to heal, to make Gaia whole. Go Vegan!

"Our word *diet* comes from the Greek word *diaita*, meaning 'a way of life.' The ideal diet is more than just eating or avoiding certain foods. It is tied to such things as environmental factors. For example, fresh air and water are actually nutrients and the quality of each relates directly to proper nutrition, these factors affect our ability to digest foods properly. Oxygen 'fires' our biological pistons; water cools the system and regulate metabolism and digestion. The ideal diet also relates to stress in our daily lives, our attitudes about life and ourselves, and our inner life, or spiritual outlook. Diet, especially vegetarianism, relates to ethics and morals as well. It is, therefore, not possible to say that the ideal diet always includes a given set of foods or always excludes certain foods. And there is no prescriptive 'ideal diet' that is right for everyone, although there are basic principles that apply to the ideal." {*Friendly Foods*, by Brother Ron Pickarski, OFM.}

In this section the emphasis is on ancient wisdom – based on writings of the Essenes and ancient scrolls in libraries around the globe. Scientists are beginning to express concern. Physiologically, we are the same as we were 1000s of years ago. The foods we consume today are synthetic, chemicalized, engineered, hybridized, processed, radiated, refined and otherwise altered... virtually 100% different from Nature.

Returning to ancient ways restores our former vitality, and brings longevity. A lot of us think we are living longer than ever. Really, we are lingering in nursing homes and hospitals... with modern medication and technology... somewhat less than vital. Hunzas and ancient cultures eat whole foods and incorporate fasting and exercise into their lifestyle... they live well past 100 and spend their years being active... leading busy lives. It is common for an octogenarian or nonagenarian to hike up and down mountain trails, perhaps twenty miles, to have lunch with a relative... and then return home on the same day! How is this possible? We get to look at some basics.

Anatomy and Physiology: Considerations for Vegetarians

Anatomy refers to form. Physiology refers to function. How we are built. How our systems work. We lack a true health-care-system... instead we are floundering in a disease-management-system that is struggling with the monster of greed, created by industrial interests that replaced the small farmer. Quite intense; we are compelled to take a serious look.

When we carefully explore the "bare-bones" facts, it is evident we are meant to eat a diet based on plant foods. The anatomical or structural indications are compelling. Carnivorous animals have much larger liver and kidneys than we have – *relative to body size*. Their intestines are also much shorter... 3-5 times the length of the torso... because *flesh foods lack fiber* and putrefy quickly... so nutrition must be extracted and the poisonous wastes expelled quickly. Herbivorous animals have an intestinal tract 8-10 times the length of the torso... giving time for nutrition to be extracted from the complex carbohydrates in whole grasses and vegetables; rich in fiber, they serve to clean the tract. Our torso is about two feet long and our intestinal tract is over thirty feet long. We clearly are herbivores.

Carnivorous animals have claws and teeth designed to tear and shred flesh. The first thing a wolf does when it catches a bunny is tear open the belly and eat the stomach. That's where the greens and enzymes are...

then other organs: liver and pancreas, kidneys, the brain and eyes: then the major muscles... and finish by munching on a bone, cleaning teeth and gums. Carnivorous animals eat the whole catch... and are healthy. Can You imagine eating like that? Those who "go against the grain" and ignore whole grains in their diet reap the harvest of degenerative diseases. That's what happens to humans who deny their herbivorous nature. We kill animals and eat them; they kill us in the end. We can engage in this cycle, or disengage.

There are clear anatomical differences. Carnivorous animals have sharp teeth and extended canines designed to tear into tough animal hides, and their jaws only work in an up and down motion; they "wolf down" food. Their saliva is twenty times more acidic than humans, and devoid of enzymes to digest carbohydrates. Lacking pores, these animals cool down by extending their highly vascular tongues and panting. Herbivorous animals have teeth designed to tear into an apple with jaws working up and down and moving side to side, grinding complex carbohydrates found in plants, fruits, whole grains, nuts and seeds. Their saliva tends toward alkaline containing enzymes to digest carbohydrates. Having pores, these animals cool down by sweating. Clearly, we are herbivores.

Profoundly different is how animals drink water. All carnivorous mammals lap their water. All herbivorous mammals sip their water. I have found only one exception. While visiting someone in the country caring for two young cows, I was asked to turn on the hose and follow it to the end to fill the reservoir. Picking up the hose creating an arc of water, one cow came over and started to lick at the water, like drinking from a natural waterfall. Still, this is far different from lapping water like the dog and cat families. When we are at a waterfall, we also open our mouths, extend our tongues and take a drink. The other cow came over and sipped from the reservoir. The question is: walking through the woods, how do we approach a stream? Would we lap at the water, or dip our mouth into the stream, or bring the water to our mouth to sip? We sip our water because, indeed, we are herbivores.

The 8b animals killed each year in the US is disastrous. Anti-biotic-hormone-pesticide-laden wastes pollute our ground water... a major source for rivers, lakes and wells. Water is wasted washing excrement down the drain. **50** gallons of water produce **1** pound of animal protein and **5** gallons of water produce **1** pound of vegetable protein. Simply compare production of protein per acre: cattle=20 lbs, wheat=128 lbs, corn=211, rice=260, and soybeans=356.

Farmed animals raised in unnatural conditions require regular antibiotics to ensure they live long enough to get to market. They are given steroids to hasten growth, and hormones such as DES – banned for humans – to encourage fat deposition. They are sprayed with chemicals in addition to those ingested. All this shows up in our water supplies, and in our bodies – causing 100% preventable diseases.

Enzymes for Health and Vitality: Price-Pottenger
Animals in nature are healthy due to continuous consumption of enzymes found in living or naturally dried greens, as well as roots, nuts and fruits for the herbivores... and their stomach contents and raw, enzyme-rich flesh for the carnivores. Healthy choices for entirely different digestive tracts! Usually, animals that get sick are domesticated ones who eat table scraps, and these animals get the same diseases as their owners: diabetes or cardiovascular stress. Others who eat from a can or a bag usually develop a wide variety of health challenges, similar to their owners: eating their processed, enzyme-depleted foods. This was simply a study waiting to happen for the benefit of humankind.

Weston Price, DDS & Francis M Pottenger, Jr, MD vacationed every August on their yacht exploring the islands of the South Pacific. They were shocked with their observations and performed an interesting experiment, reported in *The American Journal of Orthodontics and Oral Surgery*, August, 1946, entitled: "The effect of heated, processed foods and metabolized Vitamin D milk on the dento-facial structure of experimental animals". These results were from a 10-year experiment with 900 cats. They were in separate outdoor cages, protected by a metal roof. Their droppings fell through to the ground. They were fed equal portions of milk and meat from the same source with one difference: one group received their food raw, full of enzymes; the other group received cooked meat and pasteurized milk, devoid of enzymes. The cats on raw food produced healthy, playful kittens with shiny eyes and coats remaining healthy and frisky, reproducing with vigor from generation to generation, throughout the experiment.

The cats on cooked meat and pasteurized milk, produced kittens showing less radiant eyes and coats... described as somewhat sickly, abnormal. The 2nd generation exhibited beginnings of degenerative diseases in the blood profiles; kittens were nasty to each other; some born dead. The 3rd generation, with many born dead, was sick... actually losing interest in reproducing. Their illnesses reflect modern ailments: heart, kidney, thyroid disease, pneumonia, paralysis, lost teeth, difficult labor, diarrhea, irritability, frigidity, impotence. With cooked animal protein, liver impairment was progressive. The 4th generation: so sick, they were sterile. End of experiment!

Price and Pottenger thought they had computed all their observations when they concluded their 10-year study. Then preparing the cage area for another experiment, they noticed abundant, healthy weeds under the cages of the raw food group... and under the cages of the animals fed cooked and processed foods, the weeds were sparse. Thinking there could have been more seeds in the one area originally; they conducted another experiment: pulling the weeds, planting equal amounts of beans in the two areas, watering them equally. Harvest came, and they could clearly see. Plants growing in soil fertilized by the enzyme-rich excrement produced a vibrant crop. Plants growing in soil fertilized by toxic bile in the urine and acidic stools were sickly... producing a crop that was far from commercially viable – too labor intensive to pick out the off-color and malformed beans!

Contemporary of Price and Pottenger, Edward Howell, MD gained an international reputation for his work in the field of enzymes. Previous to Howell's work, *Enzyme Nutrition*, scientists considered enzymes as catalysts... triggering chemical reactions that can be recycled and re-used. Enzymes are much more than inert substances. Each person is an enzymatically-activated organism with over 5,000 enzymes that function by both chemical and biological action. "Enzymes are protein carriers charged with vital energy factors, as a car battery consists of metal plates charged with electrical energy. As the electrical supply in car batteries can be depleted – eventually producing what we call a dead battery – so our enzyme supply can be exhausted, heralding our demise."

Dr Howell's work has been confirmed by dozens of university laboratories around the world. His Law of Adaptive Secretion of Digestive Enzymes holds that the organism values its enzymes highly, and makes no more than required. If some food is digested by enzymes already present, the body makes less concentrated digestive enzymes. Hence the importance of eating living foods such as sprouts and raw foods, as well as taking enzymes with cooked food. Even if some raw foods are eaten at the same meal... the enzymes in the raw food are busy digesting that food. Taking dietary enzymes with all cooked food – even a snack – promotes longevity and vitality by easing the burden on the pancreas and liver.

Dr Howell's book also teaches traditional enzyme-rich fermented foods bring benefits grounded in scientific fact. Sauerkraut, Kimchee, fermented nuts & seeds, and fermented *raw* dairy support vitality, and freedom from degenerative diseases found in long-lived cultures, such as the Hunzas and people living in Caucasus, Russia. *Eskimo* is from an American Indian language and means: "he eats it raw." The Eskimo eats a lot of fats and protein, yet remains healthy because he eats it raw. An Eskimo cleans excess fish burying them where they will keep from freezing, yet begin to "break down" and ferment; when his sled dogs are weak or exhausted, or when he feels the same, this partially fermented feast refreshes their energies. Interestingly, two musher teams went on a long journey and they experimented. One team of dogs was fed raw fish; the other was fed raw *and* fermented fish. At the end of their ordeal, the first team of dogs lost from 3-5 pounds; the second team *gained* 3-5 pounds! Fermented foods are *key* to health and vitality!

Dr Howell tells his tale: "Wheat germ is known as an excellent source of the B vitamins, and I also knew that it contained various enzymes in a more concentrated form than in other foods. What I did **not** know in 1935 was that raw wheat germ was loaded with enzyme inhibitors; this was not discovered until 1944. At any rate, I began displacing my breakfast cereal with an equal serving of raw wheat germ. The product was rather palatable but... in less than two months I had to discontinue wheat germ because severe gastrointestinal symptoms appeared." {Dr Howell was already aware of the dangers of pasteurized milk.}
For centuries Asians have enhanced soybeans and other seeds for their nutrition by exposing them to the action of enzymes in fungal plants... mainly the aspergillus variety, such as *aspergillus oryzae* from rice. Tempeh and miso are staples in the Far East and are carefully prepared; soup is cooked and then allowed to cool until steam dissipates then miso or tempeh may be added safely, retaining the vitality of

the enzymes. They wisely eat soy, only when fermented or sprouted; growing it for horses.

Dr Howell adds to our understanding of digestion with his discovery of the food-enzyme stomach. "Predigestion by food enzymes occurs in every creature on earth. The only exception is humans on an enzyme-less diet. Many creatures are provided with a separate food-enzyme stomach. In primates and man, the stomach has two parts with separate functions: the first part is the food-enzyme stomach. Current research supports the discovery of the human food-enzyme stomach. My research and physiology texts as well as hundreds of scientific papers have shown that peptic digestion of protein takes place in the lower part of the stomach. The upper part is where the enzymes in food, and the enzymes taken with the food, participate in digestion. I have called this the food-enzyme stomach. Except in the cases of raw, fermented and germinated foods... this is where initial predigestion occurs – the first step in the digestion of protein, fat, and starch, by exogenous enzymes. Enzymes made by the body are endogenous; those in food or digestive supplements are exogenous.

"The lower stomach performs the second step in predigestion, but of protein only. In the upper part of the small intestine the digestive juice of the pancreas continues the digestion of all the nutrients. But even this cannot be acknowledged to be complete digestion, but only an advanced phase of predigestion. The cells lining the small intestine accomplish the final digestion of food. Digestion in the food enzyme stomach is as important as digestion farther along in the alimentary canal." (*Enzyme Nutrition*, Edward Howell, MD)

Paul Kouchakoff, MD, documents the consequences of the lack of enzymes in cooked, and otherwise refined, processed food. These foods produce leukocytosis – an indicator of toxins in the system. Doctors discovered this phenomenon in 1846, and Rudolf Wirchow classified "digestive leukocytosis" as *normal* since it seemed to appear in everyone. Kouchakoff, a contemporary of Price, Pottenger and Howell, thought "normal physiological leukocytosis" made little sense. Why should the body interpret our food as toxic? Kouchakoff's experiments found raw foods actually produced no leukocytosis... while cooked foods did... and pressure-cooked foods produced more... pickled, salted and processed foods even more... imagine how microwaved foods would have tested! He also found a largely raw food diet offsets the adverse effects of small amounts of cooked foods... avoiding leukocytosis. Kouchakoff, neither a vegetarian nor a proponent of raw foods, taught 75% living, sprouted, germinated or raw foods, and 25% cooked foods bring balance for most – although some must do more, perhaps all raw. Keep the dehydrator <120° to maintain enzymes. Keep cooking <200° to avoid acrylamide formation found mostly in starchy foods. Avoid fried and baked potatoes and chips. Steaming is preferred to avoid acrylamides and to maintain nutrients.

What Keeps the Antacid Industry Going?

Acidity of the stomach for proper digestion is another aspect of physiology largely obfuscated. While animal foods are best avoided, consider this: When someone goes to a picnic and eats a big steak, the stomach creates an acidic digestive medium – pH around 2 or 3. Someone else at the same picnic, aware of the chemicals, growth hormones, antibiotics and adrenaline in the cow's muscles, declines the steak... and chooses a plateful of potato salad, cole slaw, marinated vegetables and a slice of garlic bread. For this meal the stomach creates only a slightly acidic digestive medium – pH around 5 or 6. A third person choosing a "balanced" diet takes a small portion of steak, potato salad, cole slaw and marinated vegetables with garlic bread.

With the latter meal the stomach is thrown into confusion... being told to produce a very acid pH to digest the protein and fat in the meat... and a slightly acid pH to digest the starch and the vegetables. Compromising, the stomach produces pH around 4. As a result, the protein begins to putrefy, the starch begins to ferment, and mixed together create acid indigestion: acid burps, flatulence, heartburn, sour breath along with sour body odor.

MatrixMediaMafia say "Why worry? Here's something for Your tummy." "How do You spell R-E-L-I-E-F?" "My doctor says..." While we seem to have freedom of choice, true freedom is knowing how to avoid the cause of indigestion. You can avoid the situation by eating proteins and starches... fruits and vegetables... grains and fruits... at separate meals. Combining foods properly makes a profound difference in smooth digestion – it's easy. Vegetables, either steamed or raw in salads, combine well with a protein meal **or** a starch meal. Have protein with a large vegetable salad and some steamed veggies – keeping potatoes, bread, starchy vegetables, pasta and grains for another meal free from protein.

Avoiding animal foods is critical to optimal health: https://www.pcrm.org/ Free from health challenges, choosing a small portion (4oz) of meat on *occasion*, it is prudent to stay away from commercial varieties. Choose organically raised free-range chicken, sardines or deep-water, small ocean fish, or venison [from the French: to hunt] such as duck, pheasant or other wild game. While it is generally recommended to avoid animal foods, especially from mammals, this is stated for clarity to understand proper food combining. {**Caution:** many herds of wild deer are now infected with tuberculosis. To a large extent this has human origins. Some hunters rather than enjoying peace and quiet with Mother Nature – are ready for their easy chairs, TV or cards in the cabin. They put out a pile of apples to attract deer, and as they come together head-to-head to feed, one infected deer can sneeze and infect several others.}

The common diet is a poor combination at every meal... which is why the Standard American Diet truly is SAD. The typical American has toast and eggs, bagel and cream cheese or cereal and milk for breakfast... then a hamburger, hot dog or pizza for lunch... and for dinner, meat and potatoes, or fish and rice, or chicken and French fries, or a chicken burrito... each a combination of animal protein and starch. To deal with the resulting acid indigestion, some think it logical to take an antacid. Since the stomach prefers acidity, ingesting a heavy dose of antacids sets off an alarm in the brain that whips already exhausted parietal cells of the stomach to produce more hydrochloric acid. The stomach returns to an acid state and begins to cope with the mess. It is simpler and less stress to have 1 Tbs organic, raw apple cider vinegar in a small glass of warm water. Better yet... watch out for food combinations! How simple can it get**?**

Another hint for easy digestion is to keep fruits apart from vegetables and starches. Make fruit a meal by itself, preferably the first one of the day or the last one at night – always eat fruit on a totally empty stomach, and wait 2-3 hours before having anything else. At a starch meal have sprouted garlic bread with whole grain pasta (preferably, germinated and cooked whole grains such as millet or buckwheat) and replace meat sauce with onions, garlic and vegetables lightly sautéed in a little water and Nama Shoyu™!

139

Avoid *acid tastes* with pastas and other starches, including tomato-based sauces, orange or lemon juice as well as apple cider vinegar either in salad dressing or in the vegetable sauce. The acid taste temporarily turns off the mechanism to create starch-digesting enzymes in the saliva... the starches reach the stomach without this vital pre-digestion. The stomach then labors more intensively to deal with complex starches, rather than partially digested starches. Avoid the stress. Learn to be creative in the kitchen. https://www.thehealingcuisine.com/

A Question of Temperature
The innocent-looking glass of ice water with a meal actually wreaks havoc! William Beaumont, MD, Surgeon in the US Army, did extensive research due to a freak accident involving a French-Canadian fur trader named Alexis St. Martin at Fort Mackinac on Michilimackinac, Great Turtle Island, presently known as Mackinac Island – off Michigan's Upper Peninsula. In April 1823, the young man got in the way of an exploding musket tearing out half his side. For two years Beaumont took him into his own home and dressed and fed him. At the end of two years Alexis was able to walk, although incapable of earning a living. A fistula remained in the young man's side which provided direct access to his stomach. Experiments on the digestion of various foods were performed for a couple of years. After a brief hiatus, he resumed his experiments from 1829-31.

Dr Beaumont noted the temperature of the stomach ranged from 99-102° depending on the humidity: 99° when humid... and 102° when dry. After exercise, whether fasting or on a full stomach, the temp would increase 1½°... the average is 101°. Dr Beaumont was surprised to find when a large amount of fats was eaten, pancreatic secretions and liver bile would enter the stomach from the duodenum through the pylorus! Documenting the influence of the psyche on gastric secretions, nervous dyspepsia and gastritis, he also noted the influence of alcohol and unwholesome diet on the digestive juices... slowing the digestive process. {*William Beaumont: A Pioneer American Physiologist*, Jesse S. Meyer.}

A glass of ice water before or during a meal, "shocks" the stomach and interferes with proper digestion. Imagine the stomach... comfortable at 101°... ready to secrete digestive juices for a meal... blasted with several ounces of ice-cold water! It takes a while to regain suitable temperature to begin normal secretions for digestion. Meanwhile protein begins to putrefy, starch begins to ferment and indigestion results – even if the meal is properly combined. Wait an hour after a cold drink before eating. Better yet have a bit of warm peppermint or chamomile tea before or during a meal.

Many times, we have "washed down" our food diluting the digestive juices. The solution is to create juices by thoroughly chewing... mixing salivary enzymes for proper digestion. Complex carbohydrates break down to simple sugars the stomach can easily handle; chewing actually makes starches become sweeter. If we "bolt down" starches, they arrive in the stomach without those essential pre-digesting enzymes – another cause of acid indigestion. 90% pre-digestion of starch is in the mouth, so chew well. There is another benefit. One day watching my niece wolf down a bag of snacks, I suggested: "Chew them slowly and it will actually taste sweeter!" A few minutes later, she said: "Mommy, he's right... they do taste sweeter!" It is wise to eat slowly and enjoy the flavors. And after eating, it is wise to let the stomach rest. While having a swallow to quench the thirst is OK, wait at least an hour after eating to drink a glass of water or herbal tea. Wait at least 3 hours before another meal.

Before a meal shall we begin with a pre-prandial? Instead of having it "on the rocks" we may be tempted to think about something straight up. Think again.

How Much Alcohol is Good for You?
One of the oldest-living Europeans of our time, a French woman named Jeanne Calment, born 21 February 1875, was asked her "secret" for longevity in 1992: "I have a small glass of wine with lunch and supper; I simply adore chocolate and I quit smoking... two years ago!" (115!) We is the rare person who broke the rules and beat the odds. And... she "celebrated" her 122nd birthday blind and virtually deaf, in a nursing home in Arles, barely coherent.

There are conflicting reports about consumption of alcohol. The consensus seems two drinks per day are "good for one's heart." *The Boston Globe* reported a study by Dr Carlos Camargo, Jr., of Massachusetts General, which "refines earlier findings that moderate alcohol consumption by men is good for the heart, but it indicates finding the right balance is delicate work. At anything over 2 or 3 drinks a day, alcohol consumption quickly begins to have a negative effect on health.

Camargo's team found 'a significant, sharp increase in cancer deaths' from consuming 2 or more drinks a day.' This study appears in a recent Archives of Internal Medicine - AMA. Several studies over the years have suggested that moderate drinking, around a drink or two a day, reduces the risks of heart attacks, probably because alcohol helps increase levels of high-density lipoprotein known as 'good' cholesterol.

"But Camargo said many past studies (probably the ones funded by the alcohol industry) have compared healthy people who drink with unhealthy people who do not, exaggerating the apparent benefits of alcohol. 'Usually, people have said one or two drinks a day is where the benefit is,' Camargo said. 'We found the benefit is at about a half a drink a day.' And definitely do not read the study as saying having 6 drinks on Saturday night and drying out all week does anything to help Your health."

This study appears to confirm ancient wisdom: 1 drink is nourishing, perhaps stimulating or inviting. 2 drinks are helpful, perhaps for the timid – however, leading to depression for many. 3 are harmful. More is toxic. Alcohol, being the most pervasive drug in our society, kills more people and pickles more inner organs than any other substance. If addictive, it must be left alone. When we have a cause for celebration, it may be appropriate for those who can drink to have a 12-oz bottle of beer... a 5oz glass of wine... or 1½ oz of alcohol in a cocktail. If this leads to more than a couple – having "a few" – recognize the dependency, and simply leave it alone even on special occasions.

In fact, it is best to leave it alone when drinking to experience "the effect" of alcohol: a numbing sensation leading one away from consciousness to stages of unconsciousness... burying emotional pain, fear, grief or guilt. Those issues are properly addressed by doing "inner child work." Psychologists note emotional growth is stunted when we start to drink, which explains why many remain adolescents in emotional development. Once these issues are addressed, we can drink wisely, moderately, no more than 2 drinks on special occasions.

With the lone exception of the aboriginal Eskimo – who had neither the ingredients, nor proper temperature control – virtually every culture on the planet has some form of traditional fermented drink. In honor of Eleusis, the son of Hermes, Greeks had initiation rites –

Eleusinian Mysteries – where they diluted wine with water... sometimes up to twenty times... for its "proper effect." Since wine in those days reached 11-14% alcohol at most, it is assumed that, to have *any* effect with such a dilution, there must have been another ingredient: most probably *Amanita muscaria*, or possibly *Psilocybe cubensis*, or both. {See: *Food of the Gods: The Search for the Original Tree of Knowledge – A Radical History of Plants, Drugs, and Human Evolution*, by Terence McKenna; as well as *Soma: Divine Mushroom of Immortality* – and... *Persephone's Quest: Entheogens and the Origins of Religion*, both by R. Gordon Wasson.}

Alcohol is at once a stimulant... a depressant... and a mood-altering drug affecting all circuits of the brain. It mimics stimulants such as cocaine and amphetamines, tranquilizers such as valium, and endorphin facilitators such as opium: all these, pleasurable to some extent, are highly addictive. Women are more influenced by alcohol as the alcohol-destroying enzymes in the stomach lining is more efficient in men. For both, a nightcap can disrupt sleep – especially the second half of rest.

Caffeine counteracts some of alcohol's effects to a very limited extent. Give lots of coffee to a drunk, and behold: a wide-awake drunk; unsafe to drive. Caffeine interacts with one chemical in the brain: neutralizing adenosine, normally decreasing the activity of neurotransmitters, a soporific effect. According to Stephen Braun, author of *Buzz: The Science and Lore of Alcohol and Caffeine* (Oxford University Press), caffeine is an indirect stimulant with no real power of its own... by neutralizing adenosine it opens the door for other natural brain stimulants – dopamine and endorphins.

Known to have caffeine... chocolate has recently been found to have a marijuana-like effect on the brain. The various fats in a 1½ oz bar of chocolate have enough anandamide, a fat produced by the brain that activates the same receptors as THC, to produce a short, blissful "buzz" similar to marijuana or hashish.

Study the French Paradox... they eat more fatty food than other countries yet have the second lowest rate of deaths from coronary artery disease, behind only the Japanese. They also consume the greatest amount of wine and alcohol. The study confirmed previous research showing the French also have one of the highest rates of liver cirrhosis. These challenges can be side-stepped by avoiding animal fats and alcohol.

The *New England Journal of Medicine* reported the results of a study by Harvard School of Public Health. Apparently, it is beneficial to have a drink or two a day, or even every other day. As long as this leads to no more than that, a healthy liver can metabolize the alcohol. This reduces risks of coronary heart disease by raising levels of good cholesterol, and reduces chances of forming clots, which could cut off blood flow to heart and brain. Interestingly enough, some benefits have been noted with as little as ½ drink per day. The study also said benefits are with red or white wine as the alcohol of choice – organic when possible – because [cooked] distilled spirits wreak havoc on liver and kidneys, while the carbon dioxide in ale and beer is a waste product for the body to eliminate. Ask Your body – muscle test. Surprise – maybe water is best!

As a substitute for red wine, red and purple grapes, and red grape juice are abundant in bio-flavonoids and antioxidant compounds concentrated in grape skins and seeds. Research shows chemicals in grapes help thin the blood, detoxify LDL cholesterol, strengthen blood vessels, enhance our immune response, ward off allergies and inhibit cancer. Red wine, red grape juice and the grapes themselves all have anti-coagulant activity. 3 glasses of red grape juice and one glass of red wine are equal in blood thinning activity. Health food stores offer grape juice without sugar in a glass bottle. Simply juicing fresh red grapes and/or eating whole red or purple grapes provides a healthy alternative to the purported benefits of alcohol… and acidic bottled fruit juices. Concord grapes offer superior energetics.

If it takes joining AA to avoid excessive consumption of alcohol: Just do it! Warning: some people trade alcohol addiction for nicotine, caffeine and sugar addiction! Seek the support of Your loved ones. Get to know and love Yourself; do Mirror Therapy: look deeply in Your own eyes, saying how much You love and appreciate Yourself. Praise Your wonderful qualities. Encourage Yourself to transmute challenges with compassion, gratitude and love. Read books with Your significant other. David Hawkins, MD, PhD: *Healing and Recovery* is the place to start…as well as books on conscious relationships to facilitate conscious communication. Choosing conscious communion, Your Purpose is realized: enJoy Life. Be Love.

An option to guard against the potentially addictive nature of alcohol is a concept called **DrinkWise**. The following thoughts are from a dear friend who found an unusual answer she said I could share.

Moderation is the Answer
My name is Susan… I am definitely not an alcoholic… nor am I powerless. I had a problem with alcohol, drinking it every night. But I no longer do, thanks to a new moderation program that helped me tame what became a bad habit. I'm confident I won't drink every night anymore… or let any habit control me. Still, I'm glad I can enjoy a fine glass of merlot now and again or a smoky single-malt scotch by choice rather than by compulsion. Am I in denial? I think not. I never denied I had a problem. My problem was this: I would wake up most mornings a little foggy and think: "I'm too old to be drinking 2 or 3 glasses of wine each night. Tonight, no wine for me." But by nightfall my resolve had faded. Driving home from work I would imagine the whole wine-drinking ritual: uncorking the bottle, pouring it in my favorite glass, sipping it while I made dinner. Most nights, I was drinking before I even opened the mail. The next morning, I made a new resolution to do without wine. I resolved 100X to break the nightly habit, failing just as often.

Living with the bottle… did I get slobbering drunk? Never! Did I miss work? Never. Did I hide bottles? Never. Did I black out or drive drunk or suffer debilitating hangovers? Never. But did I buy 3 or 4 bottles of wine a week? Yes. Week after week? Yes. Was there always wine in the house? Sure. Would I go in a thunderstorm for a bottle? Never had to I planned ahead. Did I drink alone? You bet. My favorite pastime: Coming home to an empty house, opening a new bottle, sitting by candlelight with my food and wine… and my book… and reading and drinking. Most nights I faded off into sleep, having accomplished very little. The next evening, I had to reread what I had read the night before. At dinner parties, wine turned the conversation scintillating. But why couldn't I remember details the next day? It seemed so fascinating the night before, insights and witticisms I'd never forget. Finally… I knew I was in trouble when my evenings were filled with other things, but still needed a drink to sleep. One night we drove for many hours, but when we reached our motel at midnight I said, "Let's go out for a scotch." I had fantasized about it for 100s of miles. I didn't always drink this way; in college, I hated beer – still do. I remember drinking over a four-year period blackberry brandy, 2 or 3 Singapore Slings and a glass or 2 of Cold Duck on New Year's Eve. A post-college boyfriend and I drank rum-and-Tabs now and again in bed; one boyfriend and I liked sipping brandy on the roof of my apartment at midnight.

The start of a bad habit: I did not drink nightly until a few years ago, when I began writing professionally. I felt nervous, anxious and afraid: of failure, of criticism, and of Who I was… Naked and revealed by journalism. With every essay I tried to hit a home run, but of course many of my swings resulted in limp grounders. I came home every night with 1000 voices in my head: readers, editors, co-workers, family members plus my own crew of internal critics. To quiet the voices, I'd pour a glass of wine. 1 glass didn't quite shut off the noise, 2 worked better. Anyone who drinks knows the body builds tolerance to alcohol. 2 won't give You the buzz it used to… so, You spill a bit more into Your glass. 2 becomes 3. On bad nights, 3 becomes 4. Soon, drinking most of a bottle of wine, thinking: "This has got to stop." I cried out for help for eight months before taking real action. Confiding in friends who are recovering alcoholics, they said: yes… I had a problem and suggested Alcoholics Anonymous. Speaking with doctors and nurses, they said: 2 or 3 glasses each night was OK. I read articles that said a woman who drinks two glasses of wine each night decreases her risk of a heart attack but increases her risk of breast cancer. Despite the mixed messages, I knew I had to stop. What scared me is: I couldn't break my habit with sheer willpower. Turns out I didn't know how.

Living with shame, in a newspaper, I saw a tiny ad: "DrinkWise: Healthy choices for those who drink." I cut it out. A few days later, I called for information. They sent it to me, and I read it in bed one night, sipping from the wineglass… almost always at my bedside. The problem drinker it described sounded a lot like me. But 6 months passed. I didn't want to spend hundreds of dollars to get help I thought I could give myself for free. In those 6 months I vowed to quit many more times. I drank another 100 bottles… feeling ashamed each week pulling my recycling bin to the curb.

Two last straws fell on my heap: First, I read a memoir by writer and newspaper columnist Pete Hamill called: "A Drinking Life." I chose it deliberately, thinking it would scare me into solving my problem. He drank for decades… and much more than I ever did… but quit cold turkey one New Year's Eve after realizing his Life

had become scripted, rather than spontaneous. His memory – every writer's primary tool – was continually fogged by alcohol. After he quit, he soon realized… "I'd been squeezing my talent out of a toothpaste tube. I'd misused it… and abused it… and failed to replenish it… with deep reading and full consciousness."

Then, at my stepson's wedding, I sat next to his bride's father, a recovering alcoholic for 10 years. As we talked about his past, he sounded strong and in control, and I… 2 or 3 wines into the evening sounded fuzzy, vulnerable. Later that evening, when my brother-in-law suggested we stop by a jazz club for a bedtime scotch, I did not know how to say no, and went along, and drank that scotch, all the while wondering what was wrong with me. The next morning, I said: "I do not want to awaken each morning for the rest of my life disappointed in myself." I called DrinkWise.

My counselor made it clear at our first session that the program wasn't for everyone. "When is the last time You consumed 10 drinks on one occasion?" she asked, and I gasped. Those who regularly drink that much probably had a physical dependence on alcohol that moderation could not temper. She said a third of Americans don't drink at all and those who drink, mostly do so moderately and socially. A small percent are alcoholics – able to save themselves only through abstinence. But many problem drinkers like me can learn to cut back, by analyzing why and when we drink… and devising and practicing new behaviors, such as words to say to ourselves and others. Keeping track of how much You drink also helps, like tracking fat grams in Your diet. I began jotting on my calendar each night how many drinks I had that day. She asked me what I thought triggered my drinking: Certain friends? Certain situations? Without hesitation I said, "Evening triggers my drinking." I sighed… She smiled. Even that habit, she said, can be broken. The first week of the 8-week program, I cut back to one glass of wine each night – a very distinct change made worse because a mere glass could no longer soothe me, I said glumly to my husband: "This is like drinking Kool-Aid… no point."

Then I was asked to go completely free of alcohol for the next two weeks. We made an exception for Thanksgiving and decided on that day I would have one glass of wine in mid-afternoon and one with dinner. I learned that thinking ahead, deciding how to drink and rehearsing ways to succeed helped a lot. But the night before Thanksgiving posed my first and biggest challenge. We arrived at our good friends' home late, after a long drive. We stepped through the back door and our host Bob strolled into the kitchen to welcome us. He held a drink in his hand, a fragrant single-malt scotch. I could smell it. I could hear the tinkle of ice. And I could imagine the ease it gave him. "Can I get You a scotch?" he said, and I summoned all the strength of will I had to speak one of my practiced lines: "No, thanks. I'm cutting back." My habit urged me to say yes; training helped me to say no.

While my husband and our friends drank scotch that night, I sipped soda water with lime. Funny, once I had a glass in hand and something to sip, I felt fine. Strong. Even a little smug. In the 3 months since I began to tame my drinking, my weekly consumption has fallen from about 20 drinks to about 3 or 4, spread over 2 or 3 evenings. Most nights I write a big fat 0 in my date book. I tell myself: "I don't need a drink tonight." Instead, I pour into my old favorite wineglass... some cranberry juice and soda water. When I'm upset or hurt, I remind myself: "You shouldn't drink to cope." A hot cup of Lemon Zinger tea calms me now.

When I drink to be festive... 1 glass gives me the buzz that 3 failed to do before. I savor wine now, and enjoy it more. I calculate that about 200 glasses of wine have gone unconsumed by me since starting the program. That's about 33 bottles. I've lost about 13 pounds and counting, passing up 30,000 wine calories and snacking less in the evening. In the morning I feel brighter. I need less coffee. My complexion and my brain are clearer. My face is less puffy, my nose less often red. Mostly I like myself more. I feel in control again. I wish I had been able to curb my drinking on my own, the way many do as they grow older and wiser. Instead, I required structure and guidelines and goals. I also wish critics of moderation programs like the one I joined understood them better.

DrinkWise would never suggest everyone can have a few on occasion. Some cannot. AA has saved many of those, who dare not touch alcohol again for fear of falling back into the abyss. Why scoff at folks like me who found salvation somewhere else, by different rules? Even a good friend of mine... an AA veteran... told me he thinks I am really fooling myself. No! Just as not every heart patient needs open-heart-surgery, not every drinker needs abstinence. I'm glad I found

DrinkWise. It saved me for the second half of my life. https://susanager.net/ {See Ch 10: **Addictions**}

Foods that Make Glue, Do the Same to You
Besides alcohol and that glass of ice water with a meal, there are other seemingly innocent yet dangerous drinks – perhaps even a glass of milk! We are Blessed to know through experience, the majority of health challenges <u>can</u> be reversed. One simple requirement is to exclude factors contributing to congestion, leading to disease processes. Some persistently think there is little or no connection between what we eat and our health... most of us eat basically the same foods and we have a myriad of health challenges, so where's the connection? Actually, we get to factor-in several things, including our genetic make-up: our strengths and weaknesses. Equally important, our epi-genetics: our environment which nurtures our mental and emotional make-up, our stress levels and how we manage them.

Beyond the vital issue of enzymes, certain so-called foods simply congest our delicate systems. Some think that we are omnivores, like the bear, rat and skunk (unpleasant company, for sure) and that our stomach acids can handle anything. This may be true *if* we eat the "trouble foods" raw as well as sparingly or infrequently, take extra digestive enzymes, rest for an hour after eating, and wait 3 hours before we eat another meal. The truth is, many people eat these troublesome foods 3X a day, stressing both the parietal cells of the stomach to produce hydrochloric acid (HCL) as well as the pancreas and liver to produce their digestive factors, straining kidneys filtering uric acid and other by-products of cooked animal protein.

"The human liver and kidneys combined have a limited capacity to excrete only about 8 grams of uric acid in 24 hours, without destroying the fine tubules of the kidneys. 1 lb of meat can generate 18 grams of uric acid. Some uric acid is left in the body from any meat meal, and accumulates to produce the diseases of rheumatism, gout, or the complications of arthritis. Similar situations occur with some forms of megavitamin-mineral therapy." (*Survival Into the 21st Century*, Viktoras Kulvinskas, MS)

Uric acids get stored in tissues, causing congestion beginning in the **capillaries** of our tissues and organs. Red blood cells are discoid in shape allowing them, as they line up in single file, to bend and squeeze their way from the arteriole system, carrying oxygen for

144

nutrition, through the capillaries – where exchange is made – moving into the venous system, carrying carbon dioxide for elimination. Here we have the beginnings of sclerotic formations, plaque and other maladies leading to various degenerative diseases. Interestingly enough… uric acid, a waste product of protein metabolism, has a chemical structure almost identical to caffeine, which accounts for the stimulating effect after eating animal protein.

Besides uric acid in meat there is an abundance of iron; in men this can lead to certain cancers. Women can thank their monthly periods for the chance to dispose of excess, along with other undesirable factors. Speaking of iron and disposing of it… we can set aside another myth. Many think they are doing themselves and their families a favor by using an iron skillet or an iron pot. This actually gets iron into our food; unfortunately, it is inorganic iron that our bodies cannot use and must eliminate or store, making an extra burden. See articles in medical journals about iron pot toxemia. The optimal use for an iron pot is to take a hammer and break it in several pieces. Bury these pieces in the garden where You grow Your greens. Iron leaches into the soil, and the plants transform it from inorganic into organic iron that may then be utilized.

Back to the question at hand, besides meat – what are the trouble foods that tend to congest our system? Who would be surprised to find the most common foods in our diet? These are also among the top 5 food allergens. An egg by any other name is still an egg. Whether commercial with its anemic yolk or free range with a darker, healthier looking yolk… it is congesting to the system unless eaten raw or semi-raw – white cooked with the yolk runny. A thoroughly cooked egg is congesting, especially fried. Frying any food gives an indigestible coating that interferes with digestion. Further, when an egg is overcooked, such as when it is scrambled, the cholesterol becomes oxidized – rancid – and oxidized cholesterol increases levels of inflammation, leading to health problems and pain.
Cooking animal foods alters the structure of protein and major minerals, such as converting organic calcium into inorganic calcium – which the body cannot utilize. What animal in nature develops an allergy to eggs? The only animals so afflicted – and they have other degenerative diseases as well – are the ones who eat cooked eggs and other congesting foods. Besides the question of cooking eggs, consider the egg. Battery farms where 100K chickens are housed

are sickening; cages are illuminated 20 hours a day… stacked one upon the other, the droppings fall from above. Packed tightly in cages they cannot flap their wings, which is their way of relieving stress or exercising, perhaps simply feeling good about life – they certainly do it often enough in nature. When battery farms first started, the chickens would fight, poke each other's eyes out and kill each other so they could stand on a dead carcass and have room to flap their wings. Farmers saw money lost, and developed a miniature guillotine: stick baby chicks' beak in, **wham**, end of money lost. What they couldn't control is the frustration… still craving room to flap their wings.

Frustration translates into adrenaline – the fight or flight hormone – filling muscle tissue… consumed while eating legs, thighs, wings, breasts, organ meats (heart, liver, gizzards) as well as their eggs. Adrenaline then gets in *our* bodies… and we wonder where our anger or frustration is coming from. "What's come over me?!?" The vibrations found in eggs and meat are congesting physically, emotionally, mentally and, therefore, spiritually. *Diet for A New America* by John Robbins – heir-to-be of the Baskin-Robbins Empire – explains to his father why he can no longer partake in the family fortune: both the way the animals are treated… and the effect these foods have on our health. A real eye-opener, the book is about compassion as well as diet with stories how animals have saved human lives and how we treat them.

Another allergenic, congesting non-food is refined flour. Most of us can recall from our **1st-grade lessons** pasting cut-outs on construction paper using glue that *we* made. Our little eyes lit up when teacher said we could make our own glue – she had some white flour and water. She said: "Mix them together and they make a *lovely paste*." And if we were in Italy, teacher would say the mixture makes "*bella pasta*." White flour products do exactly that to our system over time – they congeal and congest.

Refined flour: bagels, biscuits, breading, breads, cakes, chips, cookies, crackers, croutons, donuts, dumplings, gravies, muffins, pancakes, pastas, pastries, pie or pizza crust, pretzels, rolls, stuffing and waffles. Is there any wonder about allergies to wheat? Any wonder how our society can be so congested? Any wonder why people from other cultures who go on our civilized diet begin to experience diseases of "civilization" – cancers: mouth, stomach, colorectal intestines, respiratory tract, breast, thyroid; obesity, diabetes, gallbladder, heart disease?

What exactly happened is a good question. A reasonable explanation is, to distinguish themselves from the dirty, unwashed masses, the royalty and well-to-do took a liking to such delicacies. Thinking white is supreme, they ate their refined, white flour products with their rich meats and gravies, developing unheard of degenerative diseases. And it turned out to be a Field Day for physicians using their knowledge of Greek and Latin, creating diagnostic nomenclature and having *their* names attached to diseases *they* discovered, diseases with a common origin: congestion and nutritional deficiency.

An early ad for Wonder Bread actually made the claim: "During the 'Wonder Years' – 1 through 12 – Your children develop in many ways, actually growing to 90% of their adult height. To help make the most of their 'Wonder Years' serve them nutritious Wonder Bread. Every slice is carefully enriched for body and mind!" In the early 50s, the package said: "Wonder bread… helps build strong bodies 8 ways." Then in the 60s, they found four more ways: "Wonder bread: helps build strong bodies 12 ways." Today it says, "Wonder bread: helps build strong bodies." It really makes one Wonder what happened to the bread? makes You wonder what's *in* the bread most people buy. It says on the label. The first ingredient is enriched wheat flour. When white flour is produced, the bran and germ are removed along with 26 nutrients, which are added to animal feed to bring them to market quicker. This so-called "wonder food" is missing 62% zinc, 72% magnesium, 95% Vitamin E, 50% folic acid (B9), 72% calcium, 78% B6, and 78% fiber.

After eating large amounts of white flour, pure starch, people began exhibiting diseases such as beriberi: deficiency of thiamin (B1) characterized by polyneuritis, cardiac pathology and edema; pellagra: deficiency of niacin (B3) characterized by dermatitis, inflammation of mucous membranes, diarrhea and psychic disturbances. Common sense recognizes the value of whole foods; yet they continue stripping away the 26 nutrients, adding back the basic *four* (thiamin, niacin, riboflavin and iron) to prevent those diseases. Every school child can do the simple math: negative 26 plus 4 = negative 22. Food manufacturers say "enriched" & the gullible are fooled.

The wheat berry, as a whole food, has several parts. Bran is the epidermis or outer covering of the cereal grain. The germ is the embryo containing tocopherol, thiamin, riboflavin and other vitamins. The starch – the pure white stuff we call refined flour – is meant to be a "sack lunch" a *temporary* food for the growing wheat sprout as it sends out its cotyledons and roots – searching for real food in the sunlight… and minerals in the soil. It grows to a baby green, and later to a tall grass, producing a cluster of wheat berries. Taking an isolated factor – the starch – and making it into a food staple invites trouble. Add to this white flour, water and an egg… oh yes, and a little milk… and that spells trouble with a capital **T** and that rhymes with **P** and that stands for pasteurization as we shall see.

Any physician who sees allergies, dermatitis, and all manner of respiratory challenges as an opportunity to recommend the exclusion of eggs, refined white flour, white rice and sugar, and all dairy products, will be looked upon as a heaven-sent miracle worker! In reality, that physician is simply recommending the Laws of Nature. What makes dairy so troublesome? Pasteurization. On his deathbed, Louis Pasteur admitted Claude Bernard, his ideological opponent, was right when he said disease is found in a weak terrain… a weakened resistance = a weakened immune response system. Pasteur contended germs were causing disease. Germs are ubiquitous! Throat cultures of normal people have combinations of diphtheria, staph, strep and many other pathogenic organisms. With strong resistance, we keep them from multiplying. With compromised resistance, they multiply making us feel "run down" and… eventually we "get sick." Do mosquitoes cause the stagnant pond, or are conditions ripe for them to multiply?

And What of Dairy?

In the name of Pasteur, we heat nutritious, raw, *alkaline*-residue-forming milk to 162° for 15 seconds… destroying enzymes and turning it into an *acid*-forming substance to poison us. Pasteurized milk putrefies in the intestines; raw milk merely ferments. Indeed, pasteurized milk will putrefy in the bottle placed in a warm room, and will be a smelly mess in 4-5 days; raw milk only ferments and is *edible* as clabber. Pasteurization of milk results in deterioration fatal to animals; see Drs Price & Pottenger cat experiments.

John Thomson of Edinburgh reports another test with twin calves, one suckled and the other fed on

146

pasteurized milk. The first was healthy but the second died within 60 days. This experiment was repeated many times with the same results. The statement of Hippocrates, "Thy food shall be thy remedy" is as applicable today as it was centuries ago. Considering milk processors and innovators of new forms of preserving milk by powdering or concentrating it, another aphorism of Hippocrates is equally timely: "For they praise what is outlandish before they know whether it is good, rather than the customary which they already know to be good; the bizarre, rather than the obvious." The fact is: "Most of what we eat is superfluous. We live off 1/4 of what we swallow... doctors live off the other 3/4s." Sound timely? It was inscribed on an ancient Egyptian papyrus!

These are long known facts; we wonder why they have been suppressed. More to the point, why is milk pasteurized? Is the real reason our health... to safeguard against bacteria? Milk is sterile when it leaves the cow, and with refrigeration and proper care stays sterile for a while. Why pasteurize, if we know it has harmful effects? Is the real reason longer shelf life, so the dairy industry loses less money?

Also consider... pasteurized casein releases *opiates* during digestion, and... like fluorine in drinking water... is a convenient, covert way to mollify and control the masses! Treacherous tyrants have done so in the past. Why does it continue? What is more important: health or the bottom-line? The choices have been presented; the answer is clear. We can choose to consume what is harmful, even deadly... or leave it at the store.

And what about out-of-date milk? Brought back to the dairy, it's turned into chocolate milk, sour cream, yogurt, cottage cheese and other cheeses. It takes 7 lbs of milk, **1 gallon, to make 1 lb of cheese**. Since government warehouses are full of surplus cheese – and since cows are pumped with chemicals forcing them to produce gallons instead of quarts – another use had to be found.

Someone had an idea to turn excess milk into glue! Preposterous? Look at the back of a famous household white glue and You find the name of an equally famous milk producing company. {When *Harmonious Healing* was first published in 1998, that last sentence was true. It said: Elmer's Glue on the front label, with the Borden's logo on the back. Revising the book... and checking again, now it simply says: Made in China. Keeping this reference for historical accuracy, re-affirms the premise – dairy protein, like white flour, can be *readily* turned into glue!} Indeed, when out-of-date milk is poured into a vat and moisture is cooked off... what settles is the thick protein of milk: casein, a sticky, glue-like protein!

Marketing problem? The situation was serious! To avoid even a remote possibility connecting milk and glue... implying that Elsie's pasteurized milk could contribute to stickiness... which over time, could lead to congestion... and presuming blatant deceptive practices are beyond business ethics... the reasonable explanation is the glue was named after the inventor, whose name apparently is Elmer... rather than Elmer Fudd... it was someone who fudged the truth! Milk has a glue-like quality... having been used to paste posters on windows or walls – brushing on condensed milk as an adhesive, it weathers away from the outside before peeling away underneath! These are indisputable, historical Facts of Life.

Some say, "I only use 2% milk." The fact is, whole milk is only 3% fat, so it's not much less. Even if only 1% milk, they miss the point. It's not really about the fat... cooking (pasteurizing) animal protein – casein – alters its structure, changing nutritious alkaline food into an acidic burden... and contributes to people living with allergies, heart, and respiratory issues. It is dangerous.

"What about the Bulgarians? They eat yogurt and live to a ripe old age." Tell-lies-with-**V**ision commercials would make it seem they are eating the sponsor's brand of yogurt. In reality, Bulgarians eat yogurt made from raw, unpasteurized *goat* milk and remain healthy until they adopt our civilized ways... then they also adopt our "civilized" degenerative diseases.

"Without milk, where do I get my calcium?" This question opens the door for some fresh air, dispelling many misconceptions. First, consider how the cow *makes* all that milk? Cows eat grasses and plants that are rich in living chlorophyll and carotenes. Second, look at the quality of milk. Mammals have different amounts of proteins and vitamins for the young of their species. Cow's milk is designed to build muscles and bones of the calf – most are born standing and follow mother out to pasture – although few do that anymore due to commercialized animal agriculture. The cow's brain is simple and unsophisticated.

Humans, however, walk when they are 1 year old. Human milk is designed to support the development of the most sophisticated brain on Earth – we like to think. Actually, dolphins and whales nurse their young, have sophisticated brains and communication abilities and may have the last hurrah on our Beloved Planet, if oceans survive our polluting practices.

Differences between human and cow milk are notable. Milk contains two major proteins; humans have a ratio of casein to whey **40:60**; cows have **80:20**! Humans have saturated fat at 1.8g/100g, monounsaturated at 1.6 and polyunsaturated at .5; cows have saturated at 2.5, monounsaturated at 1 and polyunsaturated at .1! DHA absent in cow milk is in our milk at .9g!

Why are we so intent upon large amounts of protein? Human milk has far less protein than cow, even goat milk. In fact, human milk has only 1-2% protein... the amount of protein found in fruit. The newborn calf doubles its birth weight in 6 *weeks*... a newborn child doubles its weight in 6 *months*. The child fed cow's milk has an excess of heat-processed, structurally altered, proteins and fats; the body neither recognizes nor fully utilizes them. Overwhelmed, the excess is stored – accounting for thick thighs and bodies – these fat cells stay with most for the rest of their lives. Faulty nutrition leads to runny noses & exudates from ears and eyes.

Only when all 20 baby teeth are in, do we begin producing salivary amylase to digest starches; children fed starch-based foods before that time may develop skin rashes and acidic, burning urine; sometimes skin ulcers may form, all of which ceases when we avoid two offending foods: pasteurized milk and starchy foods. If baby has symptoms while being breast-fed, mother can exclude the offending foods from *her* diet.

Shortly after the 20 baby teeth come in, we stop producing lactase – the milk digesting enzyme. Undigested lactose, a milk sugar, ferments in the colon causing gas, bloating, even cramps and diarrhea. Most adults and many children are challenged with milk products. Pasteurized dairy tends to absorb hydrochloric acid in the stomach, generating excess mucus in our intestines... and, along with the high phosphorus content of milk, *interferes* with the absorption of calcium.

George Romney lost his chance at a Presidential bid because he was man enough to say he was brainwashed about the Vietnam War. It is time for us to look at some facts and admit we, too, have been brainwashed... actually our brains have been white-washed. We are led to believe through media and commercials it is wise, in vogue, to have a white mustache. We are told "osteoporosis is a natural part of aging, so to ward off this dreaded affliction drink 3 glasses of milk a day... and to make sure, have a glass before bed." In the early years, **T**ell-lies-with-**V**ision had a rather dramatic commercial. As we heard the above pitch, there were 3 women in silhouette profiles. Under a shapely body: "20 years of age," under a portly body: "50 years of age," and under a feeble body, supported by a cane: "80 years of age." Then as the announcer drank a glass of the white stuff, the "voice of authority" said: "The preceding has been brought to You, as a public service by the American Dairy Association" – as though a public service announcement. {Sic!} Yet intelligent individuals, if asked to think about it, would know that every radio and TV station must devote certain times for *free* PSAs, and this is clearly a paid commercial announcement by the local dairy industry. Perhaps they stopped airing this commercial because of its blatant lies. Anyone who thinks "osteoporosis is a natural part of aging" is simply ignorant of the Hunzas and old-world cultures. Evidence is abundantly clear: countries with the highest dairy consumption: US, CA, UK and Northern Europe as well as AU and NZ are the countries with the highest rates of osteoporosis! Countries without dairy in their diet are mystified by the word: osteoporosis – describing the disease as "thin or brittle bones" wondering how that could possibly be!?!

A Harvard University study shows pasteurized milk products from factory farms are linked to hormone-dependent cancers; the concentrated animal feeding operations (CAFO) model of raising cows on factory farms, churns out milk with dangerously high levels of estrone sulfate – an estrogen compound linked to testicular, prostate, and breast cancers. Compared to raw milk, pasteurized factory milk was found to contain up to 33X more estrone sulfate. Remembering 1 gallon of milk condenses to 1 lb of cheese, consider the massive influx of estrogen stressing hormone levels.

Confusion rampant in society reflects confusion within. Cows are given massive amounts of estrogen so they produce gallons instead of quarts; residues are in their milk. How many grew up on cheese & dairy, upsetting their normal hormonal balance? Some find themselves in the LGBTQIA+ issue: **Q**uestioning. They may find clarity by avoiding **all** estrogen-laden dairy products, flax, soy, and congesting refined white flour and rice. In time, see the difference in the mirror, and know Who You truly are. {See Ch 10: **LGBTQIA+... QUESTioning?**}

Fortunately, we have hard-core scientists who believe in researching and reporting facts, saving much emotional anguish... and dreadful disease. Evidence continues to mount against commercial, pasteurized cow's milk. While *The China Study* wholeheartedly advocates a plant-based diet and total removal of dairy and other animal products, we can take a look at the type of casein that may be the biggest problem — genetic variants of beta-casein. Raw goat or sheep milk cheese or yogurt may be tolerated by some on occasion; a goat's body is closer in size to our own than a cow's body, and the milk is different. Although each contains casein – a protein found in all dairy – sheep and goat dairy contain far less A1 beta-casein, the most inflammatory casein found in milk and far more A2 beta-casein, the easier-to-digest form of casein. Check your nutrition labels. Cow casein may be lurking in your protein supplements and non-dairy food, used as a whitener or thickening agent. Be Aware.

The China Health Project:
The Grand Prix of Dietary Studies
The Cornell-China-Oxford Project on Nutrition, Health and the Environment – China Health Project (CHP) – has clearly answered the questions. In the early 80s, a group of doctors at a conference on cancer were debating the possibility of any connection between cancer and diet. A variety of opinions expressed, they realized the only way to settle it would be an in-depth study; so they did a 10-year study. The team of doctors was headed by Dr T. Colin Campbell, a nutritional biochemist at Cornell in Ithaca, NY and Dr Chen Junshi of Beijing's Chinese Academy of Preventive Medicine, with doctors from Oxford University (UK), Richard Peto, an expert on the ecology of cancer and heart disease, and Dr Li Junyao, from Beijing's CAMS.

The study required special circumstances found in China. In America and much of the West, we eat foods from all over the world. Restaurants offer Maine lobster... San Francisco sour dough bread... corn grits from Georgia... and a variety of delicious European pastries.... for tasty dessert. In China... they live and die in one locale. Some live near the ocean; seaweed and other seafood is in their diet. Others live far up the mountain where the growing season is short; they may have more animal foods. Others live in between... mostly vegetarian. The Chinese generally travel only within their own district, and eat foods indigenous to their area. The evidence was so amazing – in the interest of intellectual honesty and academic integrity – they issued a preliminary report 8-years into their project, promising a full report at the end of 10 years.

The CHP "began in 1983 to carefully track the daily living habits of 6,500 Chinese in 65 counties dispersed across rural China. The combination of the large number of participants and the long-term nature of the study (researchers will follow subjects for decades), the wide range of dietary, health and environmental factors studied, and the orderly demographics of the Chinese, makes *this* study one of the most *rigorous* and conclusive in the history of health research: 'the Grand Prix of epidemiology' as some scientists call it, referring to the branch of medicine that studies the *cause* and control of diseases." (*EastWest Journal* – renamed *Natural Health* – September, 1990.) Reports are continually updated. There are skeptics and arguments to disprove the facts, yet *The China Study – Revised and Expanded* (2016) clearly resolves residues of doubt. In a nutshell: If Your diet is based on animal foods, You are headed down the road to degenerative diseases... if based on plant foods, You are headed down the road to vitality and longevity!

Reasonably simple: animal foods = high protein, high fat and low fiber... exactly opposite the optimal diet. They verified what many had suspected: diets high in protein, fat, calories and inorganic calcium promote early growth and maturation, early death as well as high breast cancer rates, among other dis-eases. The study suggests: if industrialized societies such as ours can cure ourselves of the meat addiction, it will ultimately be a greater factor in world health than all the doctors, health insurance policies and drugs together. The statistics from the CHP lead to intriguing questions and give revealing answers.

Clearing the Calcium Confusion
Chinese have an average blood calcium level higher than ours, yet our calcium intake is more than twice theirs! Could it be inorganic calcium in pasteurized milk and supplements made from bone meal are found to be inappropriate and stored as osteoarthritis? Suppose a senior citizen falls and goes for an x-ray to

check for fracture. The doctor may say, "The good news is... there is no fracture. But let's take a look at this x-ray. These dense white areas at the ends of the bone indicate osteoarthritis. And look at the shaft of the bone... much too gray, and that indicates osteoporosis. I'll write You a prescription." How many would ask, "Wait a minute doctor, has my body forgotten how to function? How is there be too much calcium in these areas and not enough in between, so close by? What's going on?" How many doctors could explain the mechanism for this quandary?

The China Health Project verifies the long-suspected answer to the calcium question. Consuming an excess of *inorganic* calcium... an unusable form... the body is forced to filter as much as possible, while saving the fine tubules of the kidneys from destruction; then the body stores most excess in the joints, at the ends of the bones. Yet to carry on, the body requires organic calcium to function, to survive... a ready supply is found in the shafts of the bones. Osteoporosis is a better option than death. Avoid inorganic calcium in pasteurized dairy, bone meal or ground rock... eat organic calcium from plants, as the Chinese do: algae, dark leafy greens, almonds, sesame, forms of calcium easily recognized and utilized.

Consider what washes calcium away: caffeine in coffee, tea, soft drinks and chocolate, as well as sugar. Most OTC drugs have caffeine or sugar. >1000 drugs for allergies, colds and pain flush calcium through the urine. Aluminum depletes calcium: buffered aspirins, antacids, antiperspirants, aluminum cans and pans are the chief violators, upsetting calcium balance and well-being. Vegetables cooked in aluminum produce *hydroxide poison*... neutralizing digestive juices, causing various stomach disorders.

Almonds, hazelnuts, sesame and sunflower seeds raw and germinated, increase bio-availability from 75% to 100%! rich in calcium... plentiful also in green vegetables such as broccoli, cabbage, and dark leafy vegetables: bok choy, collards, kale, mustard and turnip greens. Other sources: apricots, black mission figs, carob, lentils, prunes, tempeh, & omnipresent algae – macroalgae from the ocean, and microalgae from Klamath Lake.

The China Health Project... also gives us considerations in regards to iron. In the past, the tendency has been to think iron is primarily from red meat and animal products; yet the Chinese iron intake is almost twice ours, most coming from plant sources. Chinese are, by and large vegan, yet there is no evidence of anemia. South African scientists in a 1990 issue of *American Journal of Clinical Nutrition* say iron absorption significantly improved with silken tofu, as well as rice miso and barley miso. Vitamin C also boosts iron absorption such as found in raw fruits and salads. Seaweed, algae and other dark greens are a great source of iron, minerals, trace elements.

For clarification: Chinese who include meat in their diets – still showing degenerative diseases compared to the vegetarians – only eat *small* amounts, yet... even these small amounts... are enough to do damage! What most Americans would put on a single plate, a Chinese family would cut in strips to season the vegetables, and everyone at the table would have a small portion – yet, they still have degenerative diseases. Americans have been trained to equate protein with animal products, and that is a myth sold to us by the animal foods industry. They say we require animal foods to build strong muscles and of course meat is a muscle. That is the thinking that brought about "head cheese", sheep's brain made into lunchmeat, supposedly to increase cerebral function! Does this make sense? Where does the cow get protein to make milk and grow so big? Where does an elephant get protein for the biggest body on earth? Protein comes from plants that photosynthesize and make chlorophyll from living green grasses, young plants and leaves. Marine mammals are large, eating algae and plankton!

Choices for Health

Acid-forming diets are constipating, interfering with balance and well-being. Many deny dairy, meat, eggs, or white flour – singly or together – can cause congestion: enzymes and stomach acids will dissolve everything! Empirical evidence proves otherwise. Experience 10 days, 3 weeks, or a month without these foods, and see the difference with allergies, breathing challenges, circulation and energy levels. Explore.

Congestion can happen even in pure circumstances. The Great Lakes, the world's largest fresh water system with 20% of fresh water on the planet, prove the fact. The City of Detroit – with a conduit going out 10 miles into Lake Huron – brings fresh water to the Metropolitan area. Reaching far from shore with pollution, the conduit taps into the closest we might call: glacial water. Lake Huron, fed by Lake Superior, is fed by a huge system of relatively clean underground streams and rivers. After many years the conduit required repair and workers were surprised at the huge layer of corrosion, a buildup of minerals. If relatively pure water flowing 24/7 can leave a deposit, consider what congesting foods do to the fine tubules and machinery of the human body... over the years.

Life is full of choices. We have Free Will. We all live with consequences of yesterday's choices, that create our future experiences. Choosing optimal fuel, proper nutrition for our Temple, has consequences. Free from congesting factors, we have energy and clarity.

We know Truth with experience. We can choose intelligently when we know the options... and then, through experimentation, exploring, and experiencing the various consequences of those choices, we can properly perceive... and achieve... our highest goals. Awareness develops a healthy, conscious lifestyle: free from judgment... free from coercion. Everyone is in the perfect place, at the perfect time, experiencing the perfect opportunity to grow, develop and mature.

Principles of Healthy Eating

Destiny brings us experience. Free Will determines what use we make of the experience in shaping our lives. Destiny knocks at our door; we have the choice to open it, or keep it closed. Dryden tells us:

"Fortune at some hour to all is kind;
the lucky have whole days, which still they choose;
the unlucky have but hours,
and those they lose...
"One ship drives east and another drives west
with the self-same winds that blow;
'tis the set of the sails
and not the gales
which tell us the way to go.
"Like the winds of the sea are the ways of fate,
as we voyage along through life,
'tis the set of the soul
that decides its goal,
and not the calm or the strife."

Having noted the dangers of eating animal products... and even more so at the same meal with starches... the dangers of cold drinks with meals... and the destructive nature of cooking, it is easy to understand why people have digestive distress. Avoiding animal foods is easier than most imagine. Simply explore delicious entrees, and create new habits. It is easier still to avoid cold drinks with meals, and to take enzymes with cooked food. For those with health or digestive challenges... and for those who choose vitality and longevity, ancient wisdom is clear:

Only eat when truly hungry. This allows time for the stomach to process the previous meal, and to be at rest. The fact that so many nibble through the day indicates the brain is searching. Most foods have plenty of calories {*calor*, Latin: heat} so we keep warm; constant cravings are calls for nutrition. When we avoid fractionated, chemicalized and processed foods, and eat organic, whole and natural foods, our cravings are satisfied and we find ourselves in shape... in excellent tone... we experience: HeartMindBodySpirit as One.

When Inner Voice Intuition says have a cup of tea rather than eat, listen. Some mistakenly follow the adage: feed a cold, starve a fever. Originally, it was: if You feed a cold... You will eventually starve a fever. Actually, a "cold" is the body's way of eliminating waste through the mucosal system. To eat a heavy meal at this time, ignoring innate intelligence, going against the outward, eliminative flow adds to the body's burden.

Since the body is focused on survival, fever shifts things into high gear and makes sure You rest the stomach. Fever makes You lose Your appetite; the most You taste for is a few sips of fresh juice, soup broth or simply water. Since the pancreas is the organ responsible for balance, a potassium-rich fresh juice would be soothing; high on the list: celery, parsley, string beans and zucchini. If made into soup rather than fresh juice, chop in small pieces, boil for 3 minutes... and when cool, strain for the broth. Supporting the liver, a sodium rich juice or broth containing celery, cucumber, spinach and zucchini. Supporting kidneys, watermelon juice – whole: skin, rind, seeds and red – or watermelon seed tea. Now the body can cleanse & "get well." Only eat when hungry.

Only eat when emotionally stable. Some ignore their feelings, eating to "keep up their strength." With life-altering situations: hospitalization or loss of a loved one... the end of a deep relationship... loss of a job, it is time to think, feel and act differently. These are opportunities to eat sparingly – some fruit, perhaps a small salad later, with plenty of water in between – allowing the physical body rest... and the emotional body to strengthen. Homeopathy can be helpful at these times. *Ignatia amara* 30C for sudden things; *Gelsemium* 30C when things happen gradually.

Only eat small quantities. Those who have vitality, proper digestion, and live the longest, learn to chew food well, savoring the flavors. There is a connection between frugal eating and longevity. Eating large amounts burdens the stomach as well as liver, pancreas and kidneys. The danger of a Smör-gås-bord goes beyond inappropriate food combinations... when You go for *Smör*... You'll surely have *gås*... and end up *bord*... feeling dull and lethargic! That extra spoonful or two of tasty nut loaf, seed cheese, baked tempeh, Kimchee or Sauerkraut can cause digestive chaos, resulting in flatulence and stress. That small piece of watermelon to top off the meal – guaranteed – wreaks absolute havoc!

Only eat simple combinations. Each type of food requires its own digestive juice. A simple meal of whole grains with steamed veggies and a raw salad with a bit of seaweed is easy for our systems to digest. In our youth, we seem to get away with elaborate feasting... and age catches up. Like the teen who thinks he's "cool" or "hot" – depending on where You are generationally – behind the wheel of a slick car, peeling away from the traffic light, slamming through the gears, leaving rubber behind, racing down the road, cutting in and out of traffic; the car may have only a few thousand miles on it, yet it's burning oil and has a strange knocking; it is actually, exhausted. He gets the short end of the deal when it comes to mileage, maintenance as well as trade in value. He learns to take better care of his next car. While our cars have planned obsolescence... our bodies are for Life. Sometimes our lifetime is shorter than planned; or maintenance entails more than imagined. With simple living we give optimal maintenance, and get easy mileage from our bodies.

Only eat in pleasant surroundings. TV's fear-based programming with its violence, hype and negativity can be left out of the home altogether, especially the dining area. Natural sounds such as the ocean, a waterfall, birds and crickets, or soft and gentle chamber music conducive to pleasant conversation – contribute to easy digestion. For those who may think this is too idealistic... or impossible... say YES... create such an atmosphere. Experience it for 30 days... feel it promoting overall health in HeartMindBodySpirit. Setting the tone for the meal, offer Thanksgiving.

Rather than rote prayer, let it be a spontaneous; each one comfortable to say a few words... or be quiet.

Oriental Wisdom says standing while eating interferes with the flow of digestive juices... with physiological reason. When standing, muscles are engaged; the sympathetic nervous system is alert; calculating, ready to move... with this "fight or flight" posture, the brain directs our blood to our extremities. When sitting, we are relaxed; the parasympathetic nervous system "rest and digest" is activated; the brain directs blood to our core, to digest. Oriental Wisdom also says reading interferes with digestion. Reading is the tonifying activity of the Wood Phase and wood, with its roots, controls the earth – and the Earth Phase nurtures digestion. Sitting is tonifying activity for the Earth Phase. Fine-tuning Your approach to the 5 Phase Energetics, simply explore https://elsonhaasmd.com/ especially his *Staying Healthy with NEW Medicine.* The NEW is an acronym for Natural, Eastern, Western. His first book: *Staying Healthy with the Seasons.*

Only eat an enzyme rich meal. Raw fruit makes a simple and delicious meal. Nut or seed milk makes for an enzyme-rich meal for longer satisfaction, or a salad with enzyme-rich dressing based on germinated seeds, such as almond, sunflower, sesame... or sprouted wheat and rye; these enzyme-rich dressings can also be used on lightly steamed veggies. If cooked food is part of Your meal, simply keep the temperature <200° and take digestive enzymes before the meal to facilitate enzyme-rich, easy and efficient digestion. If You remember the enzymes during or after eating, take them – whenever.

Enzymes are actually nutritious because they support our digestive organs. Taken with cooked food to replace enzymes lost in cooking, they may be taken with raw meals as well. Taken between meals, they clean up debris in the bloodstream and help shed unnecessary stored tissue. This is the time to take charge of Your life. Since You do have Free Will, the next step is Yours. Research is abundant.

"We have over 5000 enzymes in the human body that create perhaps 25,000 different reactions. You could say that every action in our body is controlled by enzymes, but we know very little about them. We create different enzymes out of a base or source enzyme, which is more or less finite in our body. If we exhaust these source enzymes, they are not available in sufficient numbers to properly repair cells, so cancer and other degenerative diseases develop. This, in a nutshell, is the enzyme factor." Dr. Hiromi Shinya, MD – *The Enzyme Factor*

When you eat, the food resides in the upper part of your stomach for about 30 minutes. Eating raw fruits and vegetables, by the time it reaches the acids in the lower part of your stomach, it is substantially digested. Eating *cooked* foods, it begins to putrefy in the upper part of your stomach and it calls upon the pancreas to supply all the enzymes necessary to digest it in the lower part of your stomach! When this food reaches your small intestines, it begins to move into your blood stream, even though only partially digested. The particulate size being too large, Your immune system responds to it as a foreign invader, a pathogen, and begins to produce antigens to combat it. These are white blood cells, leukocytes. To some extent, all of us who eat cooked foods have some measure of leukocytosis, an overabundance of white blood cells. You can avoid this by taking enzymes.

Research conducted at Columbia University through the 1970's by Max Wolf MD, PhD proved definitively – *without doubt* – **enzymes are absorbed rather than digested.** Discovering the body **is** capable of absorbing enzymes without digesting them, provides evidence of the central role enzymes play in health.

The first American book on immune-enzymology came in 1994, *Enzymes – The Fountain of Life*, by DA Lopez, MD, RM Williams, MD PhD, and K Miehlke, MD, tracing the history of the European experience, which found its origins in China and Japan. Whatever the medical condition, digestive and systemic enzymes *are* The Fountain of Life – The Fountain of Youth! Systemic enzymes have *proven* to be anti-aging for HeartMindBodySpirit. The benefits of systemic enzymes are backed by abundant, substantial research. PubMed – providing access to medical research – yields hundreds of entries.

As with all things, You get what You pay for... so when comparing price per capsule, also compare ingredients and potency. The brand, the amount to take and frequency are easily determined using muscle testing; rather than involve 2 people, You can DIY with the Sway Test. {See Chapter 10: **Muscle Testing... Pendulums... Sway Test... and Switched Energies** to explore Your Inner Voice Intuition.} When taken on an empty stomach, have a full glass of distilled or r/o water – re-mineralized with a pinch of whole sea salt, and re-energized – to empower Your immune response system and alleviate inflammatory pain. Take as a digestive aid with meals with warm water.

Bottom Line: For those who suffer from congestion, inflammation and/or pain: these acidic conditions are caused by undigested proteins inappropriately stored somewhere in the system. The best natural medicine for ALL these conditions is clearly Systemic Enzymes because of their multiple forms of protease. For those who are "fit & trim" and would like to remain so – especially after 30, when enzyme-producing begins to decrease – take 1 Digestive Enzyme with all cooked foods, even a snack, and 1 as a preventive am/pm on an empty stomach clearing residual debris in the bloodstream. You will be amazed. Happy as You sage!

Moving through the 2020s and beyond, we can thus easily facilitate homeostasis clearing congestion, inflammation and pain. Those who can... the Survivors... will have returned to Mother Nature's Ways, with their hands in the soil – having **Garden of Eatin' tools**, as well as **tools of technology:**

Benefits of grounding with crystals and far infrared: In the 1970's, NASA developed the first infrared therapy devices to put into America's space shuttles. NASA was looking for something to ensure the astronauts' immune response systems were functioning at their best. Today there are many applications of far infrared. BioMat therapy is backed by 20 years of international, peer-reviewed studies and uses natural light wave technology, derived primarily from Far Infrared light generated by natural amethyst crystals and 21 other components. The Biomat converts electricity from Alternating Current to Direct Current, eliminating concerns of EMFs associated with AC products. You can safely enjoy infrared light energy, healing Your HeartMindBodySpirit.

Negative Ions control the balance in the Autonomic Nervous System regarding *insulin* and *adrenal* functions. This helps us resist disease and sickness. When you wear or sleep on synthetic fabrics, calcium in your blood exits through urine. Your blood becomes more acidic, and neurosis may occur causing an exhausted feeling. Synthetic fabrics decrease negative ions, and**... as our negative ions decrease, the amount of sugar in our blood increases.** Diseases like diabetes occur. Wearing or sleeping on synthetic fabrics also decreases the amount of Vitamin C, the resistance of our body to disease weakens, and this causes stress. Absence of the right amounts of negative ions can result in headaches, insomnia and fatigue.

Amethysts are known for producing very high vibrations and negative ions, as well as their source of far infrared light waves. This combination can penetrate the body up to 6" and reaches areas more traditional heat sources cannot. This broader reach of the ions and light waves creates profound muscle relaxation, and can help relieve pain faster and longer (especially when well-hydrated, taking enzymes am/pm and with meals). This natural, deep penetrating therapy is safe for people of all ages – even pets will often try and share the Biomat. Why? These infrared and negative ion therapy delivery devices, helping boost your immune response system, detoxify your body, relieve pain, and help you sleep and relax.

The **Biomat** is constructed of 17 layers, each with its own purpose. One layer produces infrared rays, one blocks EMF, the top layer is filled with fine amethyst; the controller is by Texas Instruments, America's oldest electronics supply.
https://victorkulvinskas.thebiomat.co

Truthfully... Hippocrates yearned for the Biomat, saying: "If there's a way to heat the bones, then all diseases can be treated." And Einstein wisely said: "Future Medicine will be the Medicine of Frequencies!"

Why wait for MedBeds? The Scalar Wave Wand of Light is Here & Now. Used together, with the Biomat creating infrared heat from underneath – the Wand of Light creating heat from above, You take Charge of Your Health and Well-being. These healing tools of technology support survival. (See Ch 10: **Grounding:** You can design Your own **Med-Bed** as well as Ch10: **Relationships**.)

Eating for Vitality and Longevity

Vibrational energetics in our nutrition determine the vibrational quality of our lives. Given optimal fuel, HeartMindBodySpirit reflect balance, clarity and energy. Peace in our Heart of Hearts – One with Nature, Each Other, One with the Source of All – breeds enthusiasm for Life. Enthusiasm is from the Greek: en Theos... in God. Consciousness says: I Am

Divine Energy. I Am Pure Awareness exploring Human Consciousness. Anything less than utter excitement, anything less than a thrilling experience of Life, reflects loss of consciousness to one degree or another, appearing as sluggishness, depression, aches or other forms of frustration, that are sometimes masked with inordinate attention given to food, drugs, shopping, sex, children, gambling or other activities to distract from discovering our Life's Purpose, which is to remember who we are... and to enjoy Life... by being Love and Compassion with Self and Others.

Food, as our earliest memory, is often used as a pacifier. With a perception of emotional and / or time constraints, in the past, parents have used food to placate and soothe bumps and bruises. When the little one falls off the tricycle or has a run in with a bully... have a cookie... or some candy... a soda... or bottled / canned fruit juice. How much more appropriate to take a few moments and simply hug the child, rocking... soothing... humming... words are really superfluous. Simple contact strengthens the parent / child bond. If words are appropriate, comfort with consciousness... using proper Verbal Diet.

As a memory from childhood, we have soothed physical, emotional and intellectual bumps and bruises with food and drink, adding insult to injury. When we are in stressful states our autonomic nervous system switches from parasympathetic to sympathetic function. Rather than normal blood flow to the digestive organs and the endocrine glands – to "rest and digest" – the blood flow to digestive organs practically shuts down; our skeletal muscles receive the oxygenated blood – this is the "freeze... fight or flight response." Eat only when You feel physically, emotionally and mentally composed. Otherwise, go for the hug... be with Mother Nature; with deep, caressing breaths... smile: Truly, I Am so Blessed! Eat only when at peace.

The late, great Paul Bragg challenged a football team to hike the Mojave Desert. They each had a station wagon and could bring anything they considered necessary. Paul thought a fast would be appropriate for the hike... so he only brought plenty of room temperature, pure distilled water. The team thought he would never make it. They came prepared with plenty of ham sandwiches, potato salad, pickles, chips and other vittles, along with plenty of salt tablets and ice water. Paul was amused rather than surprised when they called for the first rest period. He sipped his water watching them set the stage for their eventual withdrawal from the hike. Their support vehicle picked them up one after the other. Those remaining ate even more to give them strength, and took extra salt tablets because they were sweating so much. Paul smiled; in great spirits... he fasted and sipped his water. Eventually, Paul was the only one to finish.

Perhaps Paul was aware of an experiment that goes back at least to the year 1215... it may have been figured out in another culture before then. Emperor Frederick II of the Holy Roman Empire determined that two convicted felons who were sentenced to death would perform a noble service for all posterity. Their last meal was a banquet. Having their fill, they drew straws; one rested for the next two hours while the other chopped wood. They were then executed and Frederick had both their stomachs opened. The one who rested had an empty stomach, while the other stomach was still full of food.

Physical stress inhibits blood flow to, and functioning of, the digestive organs; the same is true for emotional and mental stress – the brain, which computes everything in a holistic fashion, recognizes they are inter-related. This highlights the importance of a peaceful repast for normal digestion. Rest for a half-hour or so after eating, longer after a feast. After that, a walk in the fresh air energizes the digestive organs. A bath after eating, however, inhibits digestion, because blood is pulled from the digestive organs to cool the skin and muscles. "Wash Your hands before You come to the table" applies to Your body as well. If circumstances are such that You eat before You shower, follow with a **cold** rinse driving blood back within... to energize the digestive organs.

Energetics in Our Food Begin with Energetics in Our Soil: A Guide to Organic and BioDynamic Gardening

The *vibrational quality* of food is paramount when eating for vitality and longevity. Demineralized soils produce devitalized foods. While it is ludicrous to think white flour is "enriched" when removing 26 nutrients and adding back four, it is also myopic to think that we can nourish our soils with only 3 minerals – N-P-K – nitrogen, phosphorus, potassium. The results are indisputable.

"Unhealthy plants from 'sick' poison-fed soil, give off slightly higher ethanol and ammonia infrared signals than healthy plants. This is particularly true of modern farmed, ammonia-drugged plants. Ask any professional entomologist what are two of the most universal attractants of insects, and they all agree on **ethanol** and **ammonia** – both are precursors of fermentation and death. That's why farm crops are best harvested before reaching old age, the attractive state bringing hordes of nature's scavengers & insects, to feed." (*Paramagnetism*, Philip S. Callahan, PhD.)

The plants growing in this malnourished medium require support with herbicides to suppress the weeds that are stronger – as they are wild – rather than hybridized. These sad excuses for plants also require support with pesticides: suppressing Mother Nature's response to sickness – sending insects to devour the weak, letting the strong survive. Continuous chemical spraying devastates the worm population in the fields where we grow our food. Worms aerate the soil and leave their castings, enriching the earth as they move along. Chemical sprays have annihilated most earthworms and a variety of microbes required for healthy plant life. Indeed, "old-timers" remember the flocks of birds that would excitedly follow as farmers plowed their fields... upturned worms and beetles provided a veritable feast! And now we see Rachel Carson was correct: *Silent Spring*. Few birds follow the plow anymore; the pickings are slim. After the harvest, some farmers burn the dried stalks and leaves in the fields. Asked why, farmers say it takes "forever" for the coarse material to break down, so they speed up the process. Why? The chemicals used are deadly for worms, beetles and microbes that normally perform such mundane tasks.

An interesting experiment can be performed by anyone and invariably will produce the same results. Take equal sized containers and fill one with ordinary soil and the other with organic, composted soil. Plant a vine seed, such as from the squash family, in each pot. Set them side-by-side in a window and water them equally, encouraging their growth. They will embrace and intertwine. After a while You will notice one vine shows frailty and the presence of pests, while the other is strong and vibrant – while one immune response system is compromised, the other is healthy. The reason is the soil, their source of nutrition. If the "germ theory" prevailed, both plants would be affected because they are in direct contact with each other. The plant with the nutrient rich food in organic, composted soil is resistant to disease... even when the vines are contacting each other. Likewise, foods we eat create either a compromised or a healthy immune response system depending on the soil.

There is an abundance of fascinating reading, such as: *The Secret Life of Plants* as well as *Secrets of the Soil: New Solutions for Restoring our Planet* by Peter Tompkins and Christopher Bird; the latter book exploring the philosophy of Rudolf Steiner and Bio-Dynamic Agriculture. Peter Tompkins' recent work is an interesting journey: *The Secret Life of Nature: Living in Harmony with the Hidden World of Nature Spirits from Fairies to Quarks.* Communion between plants and nature is a fact: mustard sprouts can pick up signals from Ursa major!

Also explore: *Secrets of the Soil, A Bio-Dynamic Farm: For Growing Wholesome Foods* by Hugh Lovel; *The Enlivened Rock Powders* by Harvey Lisle; *Paramagnetism* by Philip S. Callahan; *Weeds and What They Tell* by Ehrenfried Pfeiffer; *Bio-Dynamic Agriculture Introductory Lectures* by Alex Podolinsky... and the inspiration of it all: *Agriculture: Spiritual Foundations for the Renewal of Agriculture* by Rudolf Steiner, translated by Catherine E. Creeger and Malcolm Gardner. See also: *The Botany of Desire*, by Michael Pollan and *The Ghosts of Evolution: Nonsensical Fruit, Missing Partners, and Other Ecological Anachronisms*, by Connie Barlow.

An early work about energetics, perhaps the precursor to plasma physics: *Psychic Discoveries Behind the Iron Curtain*, by Sheila Ostrander and Lynn Schroeder, explores the paranormal and Kirlian photography – capturing energy fields on film. *The Dark Side of the Brain*, by Drs. Harry Oldfield and Roger Coghill suggests the Kirlian effect results from a high-voltage corona discharge caused by pulsed high-frequency waves. Through the action of high-frequency fields, electrons are emitted from the body of an organism, and this energy gets dissipated in a photographic emulsion in the same way as light.

Photos taken of an organic and commercial seed of the same variety... show an amazing energetic difference. Photos of carrots, both organic and commercial... sliced "on the round" show a corona of energy on the photo; the commercial carrot reveals a minimal energy field; the organic carrot shows a brilliant energy field. Other vegetables and fruits, organic and commercial, have also been photographed with the same results.

While we may pay more for organic foods, we benefit with more than **twice** the energy. Energy fields are subtle; we have much to learn. A leaf has an aura that can be seen on the photo; cut away part of the leaf and take another photo, the auric form of the whole leaf remains, for a day or so! According to the Laws of Physics and Electricity, this phenomenon is impossible, showing the Reality of some ever-present, energy-organizing principle permeating All That Is.

Kirlian photography clearly shows significant differences between commercial and organic foods. Organic to a chemist means a compound with the presence of carbon. To a slick businessperson looking for a fast buck, it means anything "natural" – another equally nebulous term. After all, cyanide is natural, so is strychnine. As peace is more than the absence of war... to an honest organic farmer, organic soil is more than the absence of synthetic herbicides and pesticides. Organic soil is cultivated and fed with compost rich in vital energy and is protected by flourishing worms, microbes and friendly insects; it is indeed, user friendly. We rarely hear reports about cancer epidemics among workers in organic fields, like we do among workers in commercial fields. Those who know are careful where they put their hands, and what food they put in their mouths. BioDynamics goes beyond organics... re-connecting the physical earth with the astral, etheric and spiritual forces – nurturing our strength of Will. From the humble soil we find the source of sickness or healing. We build healthy soil with nutrition, with compost.

"To bin, or not to bin?" that is the question
Compost – Latin: *compositus* – means: to put together. Mother Nature provides everything required... and we simply put it together:

> One-part green, two-parts brown...
> makes the compost turn to ground.
> Add some water, add some soil...
> turning is the only toil.

A tool called the Wing-Dinger largely diminishes the toil. Bio-Dynamic compost avoids turning, creating mounds. Compost is truly worth its weight in gold. Awareness increases efficiency, while avoiding nuisances and odors. The use, even the sight of a bin, can get neighbors riled; assure them with proper aeration it is odor free. Others compost without a bin, following the Great Teacher – Mother Nature: the richest compost is an old forest floor.

DIY: simply mow the lawn... along with leaves, spent flowers, young weeds and garden wastes; spread it around plants as mulch. Leave about an inch of breathing space around the stalks of plants. This moisture saver breaks down from below into rich soil. You can blend table scraps such as fruit / vegetable peelings with water and pour it around Your plants.

Sheet composting is simple. Spread out a thick layer of leaves after harvest; they decompose during the winter. In the spring, turn the leaves into the soil when You rototill – or use the Garden Weasel, a non-motorized alternative – adding other natural organic material such as rock dust. Leaves may also be used as mulch around ornamental plants, bushes and trees. Apply the mulch thick enough to inhibit weeds without depriving soil of oxygen.

Mulch maintains moisture, suppresses weeds, and adds tilth to the soil by reducing soil compaction; mulch also stabilizes soil temperature, cooling the soil in the summer and buffering the harshness of winter. If Your neighbors rake their leaves and bag them for disposal, bring this treasure home. If they are dry, they can store in the bags until Spring; if wet, spread them around as mulch. As for You, be wise; save Yourself the chore of raking. Simply let leaves lie, and mow them right into Your lawn. Shredded leaves nourish the soil in the same way that grass clippings left on the lawn provide natural fertilizer. Grass clippings are 85% water and short clips decompose quickly. With grass recycling, fertilizers can be reduced or eliminated; mulching grass clippings saves the time and trouble of raking, bagging and disposal. 3" or more left on the grass blade promotes root growth and shades out weeds... encouraging deep roots, resisting drought and disease. Grass clippings and leaves contribute organic matter to the soil with lasting effects on texture, aeration and moisture-holding capacity. Building the compost pile is simple.

Select Location Although some prefer a garbage-type can with holes for air... the optimal location is directly on the soil, so decomposer organisms can move up the pile. Most gardens are near the house for easy access to the kitchen. Likewise, the logical place for the compost pile is in or near the garden, where materials are collected and will be used. Partial shade and partial sun are ideal, avoiding tree roots; they are smart and are attracted to nutrients. Keep away from Your neighbor's entertainment area. The far corner of Your

property may seem ideal at first. Yet, after walking it a few times with table scraps...? Make it convenient to both kitchen and garden – it may be an organized bin made from chicken wire and untreated 2x4s, or simply a pile on the ground.

Collect Materials Shredded leaves can make up 50% of the total volume. Bag extra dry leaves for use in the spring and summer. Green grass clippings and other green, nitrogen-based materials such as spent flowers, young weeds and garden wastes mowed or shredded, can make up 25% of the volume; branches and woody stalks can be shredded. Soil from Your yard or starter compost from a previous batch can be 25% of the volume. Chopped fruit and vegetable peelings and table scraps blended with water to deter rodents also may be added. Save the expense of artificial activators as microorganisms are abundant on grass clippings and in the soil. Variety is the spice of compost. Grass clippings are high in nitrogen, water and organic matter; leaves, a great source of carbon, provide food for microorganisms, as well as nutrients such as potassium, phosphorus and organic matter. Shred and keep moist for optimal decomposition.

Hedge trimmings help aerate the pile; pine needles may be used in small amounts, and as mulch with acid loving plants. Straw and sawdust add carbon. Coffee grounds are a rich source of nitrogen: worms love them; while caffeine can be a central nervous system irritant, used judiciously by health lovers, the local coffee shop will gladly give a supply of used grounds.

While virtually all organic matter will compost down... meat, fish and dairy products are excluded from the compost – as they are from the health lovers' diet – because animal products have the vibration of death... and we are encouraging Life. These products as well as cooked food and bread attract rodents, who gladly set up a nest and cause odors. Avoid weeds with seeds; they may survive and sprout where You use the compost; some diseased plants can survive the compost process.

Black walnut leaves contain a toxin that inhibits friendly bacteria growth and can kill other plants. Although paper decomposes quickly, it is usually easiest to recycle paper. Rodale says newspapers and cardboard spread out around plants can preserve moisture gradually decomposing; while newsprint *ink* is OK for the soil, avoid color ads on shiny paper.

Build Layers Begin with a 6-inch layer of shredded leaves to hasten decomposition time... alternate 2" layers of green nitrogen materials, brown carbon materials, and soil or compost. Green materials support growth and reproduction of microorganisms. Brown materials provide energy. Soil and starter compost provide microorganisms for the process, as bacteria and fungi eat and digest once living matter: the organisms require only food, air and moisture. In this manner, You can create the ideal composting environment for decomposer organisms to produce finished compost in a short time... bringing Your garden nutrient-rich humus... all the while avoiding odors. Moisture is essential for Your decomposer microorganisms to thrive. Keep the pile as wet as a wrung-out sponge. Water as You go and... to hold in the heat of decomposition... build the compost pile with a minimum volume of 3'x3'x3' and a maximum volume of 4'x4'x4'... any larger bodes for a stinking mess, due to lack of air circulation.

Chopping materials provides more surface area for the decomposer microorganisms. To aerate, turn Your pile at least once a week, speeding the decomposition process by adding air and mixing to create a uniform texture. Some build a fixed bin with two 3x3 sections side by side; when it's time to turn, they go from one side to the other with a pitchfork. A moist, warm pile turns to compost in 3-9 months.

Solutions for Common Challenges If the pile gets too wet simply add more raw materials when turning it over. If it gets too dry, add water and shade the compost pile. Some may cover it with black plastic, especially in the winter, to keep it from drying and to intensify the heat. While compost thermometers are available, the pile is "cooking" when it is hot to the touch in the middle; this would be between 130-150° – keeping in mind anything over 160° kills beneficial bacteria. If the pile gets too cold: turn it, and add grass clippings and other high-nitrogen materials. If it gets too hot: turn it, and add soil; water if required. If there is an unpleasant odor, turn the pile and add soil or high-carbon materials, such as shredded leaves; add blended fruit and vegetable peelings. If necessary, reduce the quantity making two piles. If it is too slow, turn more, adding water and green materials.

Compost Builds Healthy Soil
Composting is a wonderful way to recycle and re-use what would otherwise end up in a landfill. Reclaiming valuable resources, we add to the vibrational quality of our gardens - and Our Garden Planet. Finished compost is loose and crumbly. Compost may look different from what we normally perceive as soil. Good or finished compost smells earthy and somewhat sweet, similar to the forest floor. Temperature of finished compost is the same as the outside air. Some tough fibers or pieces of leaves may remain, suitable for the vegetable garden. For use in flower gardens around the house, sift through ½" hardware wire. 1-3" may be added in the Spring, after turning the soil... in the fall, add before the soil freezes.

For container gardening... mix compost 50/50 with decent potting soil such as Jungle Mix, peat moss, leaf mold, compost, and paramagnetic forces of *vermiculite* – mica expanded by heat, and *perlite* – a natural volcanic glass similar to obsidian, as well as charcoal. Before buying anything of this nature read the label. Watch for something that says "All-Natural Compost **Plus**" and see what they classify as "plus." Whenever possible use 100% organic, pure compost and soil. Always begin with some stones for drainage. Add nitrogen sources frequently... this element is quickly lost in containers; grass clippings are a great source; added as mulch at the top they retain moisture.

Every garden can benefit from compost; it is an excellent mulch spread around plants, under bushes, around trees. For young plants, 2-3" are usually sufficient. Mulching holds moisture, checks weeds, and slowly releases organic food for the soil. Compost is especially useful as mulch during hot, dry periods. Remember to leave breathing space around the stem. Compost is a versatile soil conditioner... when mixed with sandy soils, compost can retain and hold water... when mixed with clay soils, compost loosens the soil particles for aeration and drainage. With every soil type, compost retains nutrients and minerals essential for healthy plants, bushes and trees... releasing nutrients year-round.

Controlling Pests Naturally
Compost delivers nutrients, building the immune function of the soil. Always choose resistant varieties of plants... organic when available. For heirloom quality seeds visit: https://www.seedsofchange.com. Natural techniques such as raised beds for proper drainage... rotating flower beds, vegetable beds and fallow land, all bring optimal results. Diversify. Mow the lawn high. Keep the garden free of pest harboring

debris. Utilize companion planting; plant with the phases of the moon charted in the annual publication, *Llewellyn's Moon Sign Book* along with the annual calendar: *Stella Natura* indicating BioDynamic subtle influences.

Urine in the garden has already been mentioned in the section on fasting. Some spray "on the leaf above and underneath" a dilution of 32:1 – an ounce of urine per quart... or collect urine in containers and pour it around the outer perimeter of the garden to deter raccoons and rabbits. If that is beyond Your comfort zone, use other natural means of pest control: a spray can be made from one ounce of fresh-squeezed, strained lemon juice per quart of water, for indoor plants. Or soak one pressed garlic clove and one teaspoon of cayenne per quart of water for 24 hours. Strain and spray the outdoor garden. Shake red / black pepper at the perimeter to deter pests.

Hand pick insects. Hoe and hand pull weeds. Prune diseased or damaged plant material. Introduce beneficial insects such as ladybugs, lacewing and praying mantis. In temperate climates, set out a hummingbird feeder while it is still wintry; the scout finds it, somehow "marks" the territory as friendly... and brings the family when it warms up. The scout is able to attain a state of stasis and endure bitter, cold nights; if the feeder freezes during the night, it thaws during the day and the scout will find it.

Certain plants deter pests. Pennyroyal and tansy are effective, yet toxic to humans. Scatter calendula, marigolds, onions and garlic throughout the garden.

Planting the Outdoor Garden
Restoring paramagnetic energy to the soil can be creative, such as raised beds... ridge planting... stone mulching... and stone circles around the drip line of fruit trees. *From the Soil Up* by Donald Schriefer and *Secrets of the Soil: New Solutions for Restoring our Planet* by Peter Tompkins and Christopher Bird are recommended.

https://www.acresusa.com has an abundance of valuable resource material. As Knowledge grows... so grows Communion with Mother Nature. Know Thyself!

Once the soil is of decent quality... it is ready for planting. The following bird's-eye view is for the amateur gardener. One of Life's greatest pleasures, for

kids of all ages, is planting and nurturing seeds, watching them mature, then reaping the harvest. This pleasure begins with the idea... planning, selection of seeds, soaking the seeds in warm water to increase their metabolism and shorten germination time. Carrots, parsley and other slow germinating seeds are soaked for 24 hrs. Hard-coated seeds, morning glories or New Zealand spinach, can be started in water that is hot to the touch. Grass seed also sprouts faster if soaked in water for a few hours. After draining, mix the fine seeds with sand, or used coffee grounds, to prevent clumping when sowing. Keep the seeds moist after soaking – they dry, they die. You can soak all but the tiniest before planting.

To prep the seeds for sprouting, spread the soaked seeds on a damp piece of paper towel. Fold it in half and place in a plastic bag on top of the refrigerator or a warm place. Doing more than one kind of a seed at a time, write the name on the top of the paper towel with a waterproof marker before You dampen it. Check the seeds daily for germination; Your routine of peeking in the bag creates a bond and provides the seeds with a dose of oxygen. When the seeds have sprouted, the length of the tail equal to the length of the seed, plant them directly into the ground or a container. Plant before the roots grow long and get tangled. If the root grows through the paper towel, simply tear the towel and plant it together, taking special care to protect the tiny root; it is a lifeline for the seed. Tweezers are a great planting tool for tiny seeds; be gentle, they crush easily. If the seeds germinate before the moon is right to plant them... simply place in the butter-keeper of the refrigerator.

When You are ready to plant, prepare the seed bed the same for seeds as for transplants. Rake out bumps or valleys; break up large clots of soil. Seeds grow readily in soil that has been cultivated to a fine tilth. If You have heavy soil, backfill the rows and planting holes with a planting medium made up of equal parts: compost, sphagnum moss and potting soil, such as Jungle Mix. Saturate with water the night before planting.

Be sure to plant the seed at the depth recommended on the seed packet – from 1-3X the diameter of the seed. Planting too deep is one of the major causes of failure. It's also important to firm the soil over the seed after planting; seeds require contact with moist earth. Lettuce seed requires light to germinate; planting from seed, keep somewhat exposed; water with a fine mist.

In the heat of summer, mulch the area to protect from drying winds or driving rains. Branches pruned from juniper are helpful to keep the squirrels from digging in planted beds. Keep moist until seedlings appear.

To avoid the fungus known as potato scab… sprinkle pine needles in the furrow before planting potato eyes – for all kinds, including sweet potatoes and yams. To keep the onion-fly away… encircle newly planted babies with a solid dose of used coffee grounds, available from local restaurants and coffeehouses.

Most seeds remain viable for 3-5 years. Keep them cool and dry, in a glass jar or plastic covered container in the refrigerator; then to avoid condensation and ruining the seeds, allow the container to come to room temperature before opening it. When planning for the outdoor garden: *Eat Your Yard! Edible Trees, Shrubs, Vines, Herbs and Flowers for Your Landscape*, by Nan Chase. Also enjoy: How To Grow Lots of Food in a Grid-Down Situation: Even without Experience… or if Older, and Out of Shape.
https://thegrownetwork.com/i-can-grow-food-webinar/?oid=117&affid=128

Planting the Indoor Garden
Those without a yard can plant containers on the patio or balcony; plants thrive year-round in the house, next to the light of a window. During the dark days of winter use a plant light; for non-flowering seedlings, research indicates a cool-white bulb and a cool-blue bulb provide sufficient color for successful growth.

Keep seedlings a few inches from the light for 18 hrs/day. A mini-herb garden thrives in the kitchen with a container of a single basil plant, and separate containers for a plant each of parsley, rosemary, thyme, cilantro, chives, garlic greens, whatever Your heart desires. When harvesting, leave 2/3 of the plant to avoid shock; to trim a third from the top is tolerated by most herbs, as well as trimming side shoots. Feed plants with food peelings, such as a banana skin blended in water; they enjoy soak water from beans, grains and nuts as well. Raise their vibrational energies with a sprinkle of kelp before watering.

Growing indoors may be done without fancy lights, even without soil. While hydroponics grows plants in water containing dissolved inorganic nutrients rather than the soil, papyro-ponics grows 7/10-day sprouts and baby greens on newspaper saturated with water containing organic nutrients. This avoids the mess of soil in the kitchen or other areas of the house. Simply use solid planting trays and line the bottom with ½" of newspaper. Cover that with a couple of layers of unbleached paper towel free from dyes or dioxin, and saturate with water energized with powdered kelp, then spread the germinated seeds.

Grow baby sunflower greens by planting unhulled, soaked / germinated seeds… and nutritious wheatgrass by planting sprouted seeds. To germinate and sprout seeds, soak them in warm water for 12-24 hours. Sunflower seeds germinate readily and can be planted immediately after soaking; wheat or unpearled barley berries can be sprouted for a couple of days after soaking, and then planted. In both cases, after planting on the saturated paper or trays of soil, cover the seeds with a sheet of plastic, perhaps the bottom of another tray. This retains the moisture and creates a mini-ecosystem: as moisture evaporates, it collects on the plastic covering, holding moisture in the air.

Keep trays covered until the plastic is pushed up; as the plants are growing strong, the cover may be removed. Spray with energized water, keeping the babies moist as they grow. After 7-10 days it is time to harvest. Trim the sunflower greens close to the bottom; they may be eaten as they are or juiced, added to salads or juiced with other greens or vegetables for a nutritious, enzyme-rich drink.

Trim the wheat or barley grass close to the yellow part on the bottom where the lecithin and other powerful nutrients reside. If mold is apparent, cut above the mold; for future reference, some varieties of spelt seem to be mold-resistant. If You have a grass juicer, it makes a potent, strong tasting, chlorophyll-rich drink, that You may dilute with water. Otherwise, chew the grass sucking it dry; throw away the pulp. Doing this saturates the mucosal tissues and gums with potent, healing chlorophyll. It absorbs into Your bloodstream, purifies the liver and strengthens the immune response. Experiment growing other greens, soaking unhulled buckwheat… or whole raw peas – marrow fat peas, *Pisum sativum medullare* are exceptional.

Tower Garden - Juice Plus+ Insights When You run out of the mix that comes with it, replace with 2 Tbs of Sea salt per gallon of water; see: Dr Maynard Murray's *Sea Energy Agriculture: Nature's Ideal Trace Element Blend* to optimize genetic seed potential and to increase nutrient-density, overcoming genetic diseases & being able to handle high levels of environmental stress. Also:

HeartLand AutoSprout - Why Is This Happening To Me... AGAIN?! (whyagain.org)

Creating Enzyme-rich Foods

Theories of diet and nutrition can tend to be somewhat technical or complicated. Working with the criteria: is it ancient? is it simple? and following the easy guidelines of food combining to facilitate digestion, will simplify the matter providing a delicious diet to support our alkaline reserve, buffering our pH for health and happiness.

Preparing enzyme-rich meals is easy and enjoyable. Simply create new habits, such as soaking and germinating seeds. Actually, this is simple... it takes 15 seconds. Soak things when You think of it. Sprouts keep for days. After rinsing 3X put any grains, beans, nuts or seeds in a bowl, adding 3X as much distilled or r/o water with 1 Tbs whole sea salt. Warmth increases metabolism of all life, and cuts soaking time in half.

Over-soaking can waterlog and lead to rotting rather than germinating – especially chickpeas which can waterlog when soaked more than 12 hours in the same water; change the water. If things taste even a little off, make it part of the compost pile. Some seeds are hardier and take longer to soak – as much as 24 hours – such as almonds, hazelnuts Brazil nuts and beans.

Most things are ready after just a few hours – small seeds like sesame or millet: 1-2 hrs; medium seeds like sunflower or pumpkin: 5-6 hrs. Give soak water to the plants, and expose the germinated seeds to the air – in a colander covered with a plate maintaining an eco-system of moist warmth for a day. Rather than rinsing sprouts, give them a short bath with sea salt to nourish their growth... then well-drained, use or refrigerate.

Always begin any venture, especially in the kitchen, with an attitude of Gratitude. Preparing living foods is easy when we rid ourselves of the old concept of exact measurements and recipes. There are rarely any mistakes when working with living foods... except for improper combinations such as protein and starch – as in tree nuts made into a loaf served with a grain... or fruit with starch. Each dish comes out according to taste... adjusting with spices, herbs, agar-agar or chia for texture. Be creative: living foods are synonymous

with Freedom – both the freedom of a healthy body... and the freedom to create Your own masterful meals.

Kitchen equipment Begin with a sharp knife and a cutting board. While plastic or polyurethane cutting boards may appear clean, and wooden cutting boards may look like they could harbor bacteria, research shows the opposite. The optimal wooden cutting board is from hard wood such as oak or maple; slathered with bacteria then wiped with a damp cloth, the bacteria count was almost negligible; the synthetic boards show a high bacteria count – natural ways are healthy ways.

While the ancients may have mashed their sprouts and germinated seeds with a mortar and pestle... and while *suribachi* (Japanese: grinding bowls) are available and useful especially for dry items... a blender is a handy tool for the kitchen, with one admonition. When the spin is clockwise in nature, we observe sunny days. Storms such as tornados and hurricanes move counterclockwise on their destructive path. Salvaging an old blender, I cleaned it up and much to my delight there was a clockwise spin – a Hamilton Beach. So, I now use my old blender with its counterclockwise spin for fruit and veggie scraps to add to the compost pile and the garden. The energy here is to break down and destroy – a catabolic nature; whereas the blender used in food prep has an anabolic nature, building up the energies. Whatever brand You choose... You may wish to check and see which way the energy moves. Movement also applies to stirring a pot or a bowl. Many cultures teach their children clockwise movements.

Another handy tool is a vegetable grinder / grater / slicer. For fancy cuts on cukes and other veggies, there is a stainless grater called a mandolin. While manual graters are handy – the *Salad Shooter* is easy to use and clean; the *Vitamix* or other large blender used on Pulse is a blessing when dealing with large quantities. If Your kitchen is commercial-grade, the *Good Nature Juicer X-1* would be suitable for starters. The optimal home juicer is a Norwalk – it both triturates, and has a hydraulic press. Next is a *Solostar* – low-speed, or an *Omega* juicer and homogenizer; finally, a *Champion* can juice, homogenize and perform as a grinder... great for frozen bananas or other fruit for ice-cream. For a quality wheatgrass juicer, find a low-speed twin-gear with bio-ceramic magnets; it can also juice leafy greens and hard vegetables. With a dehydrator, set the thermostat <120° to preserve the enzymes.

Essenes understood about enzymes and living foods saying the Fire of the Sun is healing, life-enhancing. Fire we create destroys the life-giving qualities of food, interferes with health... and upsets inner balance. Ancient wisdom promotes eating fresh and living foods, especially avoiding cooked flesh. While yogurt or cheese made from unpasteurized goat's milk is tolerable for most on occasion, the ancients understood those who ate cooked foods and animal flesh displayed all manner of illness. In keeping with this notion, making bread they sprouted and mashed their grains, formed it into a flat loaf and placed it on a dish in the morning sun; at mid-day they would turn it over, and bring it in at sunset, creating enzyme-rich, chewy, tasty food. We can emulate their wisdom by using a dehydrator – keeping the thermostat at 120° retaining enzymes and vitality. Blending – better yet, mashing – sprouts to batter thickness, adding spices, perhaps diced onion, creates enzyme-rich crackers in the dehydrator. Get the kids involved, or let the kid in You come out and play. Add slivered onions or other vegetables, ground cumin and/or coriander seed. With a blender and a dehydrator, this new way of living and eating is a treat. As a bonus, the house is filled with appealing, soothing fragrances. This cracker or flat bread makes an enzyme-rich pizza... and much more!

You can also make fruit strips, such as dried bananas – whole, halved, sliced on the round, or poke Your little finger through the hole on the bottom of a peeled banana and it splits into 3 spears; dehydrated they each have their own consistency and texture. You can make nut burgers by sprouting sunflower seeds, or germinating sesame. Sesame can get bitter if soaked much more than one hour, which is enough to germinate such a tiny seed. You can also germinate almonds and hazelnuts, soaking for 24 hrs. Chop them all together in a food processor or mash in a suribachi bowl. Add some chopped onion, garlic, ginger or herbs; shape into burgers or logs and dehydrate until a crust forms, usually all day or overnight. Retaining enzymes, it provides a warmish taste for a chilly day. Any fruit or vegetable may be sliced thin and dehydrated; stored in sealed glass containers; they keep if thoroughly dry.

Another enzyme-rich food is nut and seed porridge... as a dressing for salad or steamed veggies. The difference is in the amount of water added. With digestive challenges, tree-nuts and ground-seeds are to be kept apart. If You choose to combine them, watch for signs of digestive disturbance. Tree nuts are more concentrated and digest easier by themselves. Tree-nuts (almonds, hazelnuts and Brazil nuts) and ground-seeds (sesame, sunflower and pumpkin) both come from Mother Earth and produce a healthy option to dairy known as Nut Milk or Seed Milk. To prepare this delicious, enzyme-rich treat, soak the seeds... soaking changes the fats into fatty acids, increasing absorption of nutrients from 75% to 100%; for those underweight and looking to build, use the unsoaked seeds for the whole fat. If You see broken, discolored seeds or powder in the bag, they are going rancid. If chewing burns Your throat, or with a bitter taste, they are rancid. Rancidity destroys Vitamin C; rancid fats are carcinogenic.

Soaking seeds raises their vibrational energies. Consider how You feel on a cloudy, cold day walking in the woods; the damp wind seems to go right through You. You sit down on a dry log near the sounds of a bubbling brook, protected somewhat from the wind. You zip Your jacket tight, pull down Your cap, fold Your arms, perhaps cross Your legs to retain Your body heat – sheltering Your life energy; You find Yourself rocking a bit; gradually You stop shivering; You are conserving Your energies concentrating them in Your core.

And then the sun breaks through the clouds, bathing You with its light and welcome warmth. You turn to greet the sun and see blue skies where before there was only gray. It makes You feel delightful. You uncross Your legs and arms; You may even unzip Your jacket a bit or take off Your cap to feel the warmth of the sun. Rather than focus on survival, You welcome the sun, the energy of Life.

Such an energetic shift takes place soaking seeds. For the preservation of the species, Mother Nature places enzyme inhibitors in each and every seed to keep it from sprouting at an inappropriate time. All the energies of the seed are concentrated within. In nature, for instance, the almond is encased in a hard, yet somewhat porous, shell. It falls from the tree, landing in a pile of leaves and gets buried; it lies dormant. Then with the arrival of Spring rains, the leaves and the soil get saturated. Water penetrates the almond shell and surrounds the nut within. The moisture leaches out enzyme inhibitors, phytates which block phosphorus and oxalates, which pull calcium out of circulation. The seed expands to twice its original size. It is fully energized, ready to grow to be a huge tree as programmed by its DNA. The seed begins to produce plant hormones and vitamins as well as the radicle to grow the root and the sprout to grow the cotyledon – the first 2 leaves – and finally the tree itself emerges. Energized, ready to grow.

Almonds are an excellent source of nutrition. In making the switch to a plant-based diet, some purchase almonds being concerned about the protein issue, clearly a red herring. They buy some roasted and salted nuts and munch on them as they watch TV. They end up with tightness in their stomach and say, "This vegetarian eating is not for me." Actually, it's the vibration of the food that challenges the digestive tract. After all, what would happen if You planted roasted and salted almonds? Would they grow? They would rot, decompose, and feed the earth. Nourishing when we soak raw nuts germinating them; plant these, and they would grow into trees.

When nuts and seeds are soaked, the enzyme inhibitors have leached into the water; Your houseplants love this energy and consider it a real treat. Rinse them and pour through a strainer or colander, let them air out somewhat before storing; they are ready to make Earth Milk, or a dressing for steamed veggies or salad.

King of the Nuts, Queen of the Grains and Their Court Jesters Making an Alkaline Ash of Themselves
Earth Milk There are many variations on the basic theme; blend 2/3C of nuts and / or seeds with 2C water; more or less water to taste. In the case of almonds and hazelnuts, blend for 4-5 minutes – until pouring through a strainer You are left with the brown skin, only a few flecks of white. If You have a lot of white with some brown flecks, simply blend more. Brown skins are high in oxalic acid; excess can interfere with calcium balance. To have a little on occasion is tolerable. Once blended and strained, the milk may be taken as is.

Some prefer to avoid the high fat content of unsoaked almonds and hazelnuts; soaking converts much of the fat into fatty acids. When soaking, change the water every 12 hours; after soaking for 24-36 hours, the skins come off rather easily. Blending time is reduced with soaked nuts, making a creamy, delicious drink.

You can also add a sprinkle of cinnamon or nutmeg or a sprinkle of dehydrated vanilla powder or a few drops of vanilla extract; toasted carob powder is a healthy,

tasty substitute for chocolate. For an alternative sweetener... consider liquid stevia: 1 drop / 8 oz liquid... or simply use dehydrated sugar cane juice available as Sucanat™. Earth Milks can have many flavors: almond, hazelnut, pecan, pumpkin, sesame, sunflower, walnut... individually or blended, interesting "kitchen chemistry" leading to new discoveries. These milks provide a source of enzyme-rich nutrition to be enjoyed any time of day, leaving You satisfied.

Seed Porridge may be eaten as is, or used as a dressing for salads or steamed veggies. When You feel like chewing porridge – perhaps warmed in the dehydrator – follow the procedure for Earth Milk using pumpkin, sesame or sunflower – add less water. Blend ingredients to attain desired consistency. For optimal digestion, chew Your liquids to add salivary enzymes... and drink Your solids, chewing until liquid. This also enhances the flavor to savor; having Seed Porridge, always chew it well. Why gobble food? If time is a factor, have a drink of water and wait until later; it will digest easier, and You will be happy.

Another option for Seed Porridge is found with wheat and rye. These take a couple of days to sprout. Once rinsed and thoroughly drained, they may be stored in the refrigerator. These may be used in place of the above nuts or seeds. You can create a tasty treat by using: 1C along with some germinated sunflower seeds or germinated pumpkin seeds, and a couple of spoons of soaked chia. These ingredients provide a whole, plant food source of Omega 3-6-9 essential fatty acids.

Flax Seed is "the exception that proves the rule." The theory is enzyme inhibitors from seeds leach into the soak water and is best given as nutrient energy for plants. European spas, however, have long used flax **water** to soothe an inflamed digestive tract, and assist cleansing. Mix ½ C flax with 2 quarts of water; let sit in the refrigerator for 24 hrs. The mucogenic water soothes and strengthens an irritated colon. Have a glass on an empty stomach in the morning. For serious issues, pour water off and refrigerate, drinking throughout the day; refill the pitcher with water and soak another 24 hrs. The same seeds may be used for a few days before losing their slippery, energetic qualities.

Flax seeds may also be soaked using less water. Half fill a container with flax seeds and top it off with water.

It becomes a gelatinous mass in a few hours and may be stirred, usually once is sufficient. This may simply be stored in the refrigerator and used as above in Seed Milk or Porridge, or used alone. Even though germinated, avoid excess flax due to its high estrogen levels. While 1 Tbs of flax per day is safe for most, it is wise to use caution. Agar-agar, Chia and Psyllium husk powder are alternatives for thickening.

Oil Dressings Soy and canola have a counter-clockwise spin and are energetically debilitating... wise to avoid. Besides canola, flaxseed oil, is considered the highest vegetable source of omega-3 essential fatty acid and has long been touted as healthy. Unfortunately, it can upset the hormonal balance. Hemp seed oil has the full-spectrum family of omegas. All oils are best avoided when cooking. Heating distorts the fatty acid turning it into an unnatural trans-form that raises total cholesterol levels and lowers HDL (good) cholesterol. Also avoid corn, peanut, safflower and sunflower oils. Extra Virgin Olive Oil means the first pressing, excluding use of heat and chemicals; safe to use for cooking... as well as Extra Virgin Coconut Oil. An excellent flavor for salads is Hempseed oil; it is the single most nutritious oil internally and externally. Hempseed oil is fragile and kept in the freezer it does not solidify; watch the expiration date. Sesame is tolerated by most, on occasion. **All oils require much *oxygen* to metabolize; use _sparingly_.** These oils with the juice of a fresh lemon... along with a sprinkling of herbs... make simple and flavorful dressings. Although avoid lemon with starchy meals; the sour taste inhibits ptyalin production, required to digest starch. Here are some healthier options to refined oils – tasty treats.

Seed Dressings are a delicious, nutritious option to processed oils, even to EVOO. Germinated seeds provide enzyme-rich vital nutrition. Follow directions for Seed Milk or Seed Porridge... a liquid dressing for salads or a thicker sauce for steamed veggies. Remember: fruits and vegetables digest well when kept apart – for veggie dressings, avoid the use of bananas, figs, etc., with Your germinated / sprouted seeds. Substitute a peeled cucumber, zucchini, some onion, garlic or ginger. Color? blend in a small piece of peeled beet for pink, or add ½ avocado at the very end for creamy green.

Whoever gives away their secret recipe? The real secret ingredient is the Love put into it, as well as the Love the gardener put into it, another good reason to

Go Organic! For proportions, here are a few dressing suggestions:

Beets All Peel and cube ½ blender of beets, add the juice of two lemons along with dulse or kelp powder to taste. Add water to cover and blend thoroughly. Then add 2-3C pre-soaked sunflower seeds, depending on taste and consistency. Once blended, add one diced avocado and pulse blend; over blending avocado can make the dish taste "off"; the same applies to dehydrating avos.

Creamy Nut Blend ½C each of soaked pine nuts, sunflower seeds and/or almonds with 2C water; add dulse or kelp powder to taste, 2 cloves of garlic... basil, cilantro, dill, oregano, rosemary or thyme. Play with combinations and make some pleasant discoveries.

Cuvocado Blend 3-4 peeled cucumbers with dulse or kelp powder to taste, one clove of garlic, 1Tsp fresh grated ginger root, and 1 bunch of fresh basil or cilantro. Once blended add avocado; pulse blend.

Greek Delight Combine 1oz fresh lemon juice, 3oz apple cider vinegar, 1tsp each of _dried_ oregano, basil and tarragon – 1Tbs each if _fresh_; a clove of peeled garlic, 2Tsp Dijon-style mustard; blend for 15 seconds, then while running slowly, add 1C extra virgin olive oil in a steady stream; process another 30 seconds. In a large salad bowl, place mixed, exotic leafy greens and add the dressing, tossing gently to coat evenly. Add thinly sliced beet, cucumber and red onion, and oil-cured Greek olives. Avoid starch at this meal; lemon taste delays amylase production for 15 minutes.

Vegetable Marinade 1C water and juice of one lemon; add ½C dulse powder, 1tsp dill and 1tsp turmeric powder, or 1 Tbs of fresh minced dill and fresh grated turmeric. Slice veggies and marinate for 15-30 minutes. Drain.

Pine Cream Blend 2C of soaked pine nuts with dulse or kelp powder to taste, 2 cloves of garlic, ½C fresh basil, ½C fresh cilantro (1C fresh herbs altogether) then only enough water to make a cream.

Triple Nutty Blend ½C each of soaked pumpkin, sesame and sunflower with 2C of water, 3Tbs dulse / kelp powder, 2Tsp fresh grated ginger and 1C parsley or herb blend.

Cole Slaw is antioxidant rich... select a medium head of cabbage with a freshly cut stem and dark outer leaves. Peel or scrape one pound of carrots and one *small* onion. Push the carrots and onion through the salad shooter with the grater attachment twice. This assures that the onion is distributed as well as sweetness of the carrots. Then push through the cabbage, minus the stem, including the dark green leaves. Sprinkle Brittany or Celtic (gray) sea salt and fresh-ground black pepper to taste. Replace the traditional mayonnaise with one of the above recipes, or a variation. Or use ½C apple cider vinegar and ½C water, to make *Twelve Day Cole Slaw* – so named because it keeps that long, although it seldom does... it soon disappears.

Rooty Mineral Salad is delicious and nutritious. Presoak arame or hijiki seaweed in plenty of water. Shred 4 carrots, 2 parsnips, 2 peeled beets and 6 sunchokes – also known as Jerusalem artichokes. Mix together, making sure there are at least 2C of soak-water from the seaweed; add 1Tsp fresh squeezed lemon juice and 1C pre-soaked and crushed walnuts. Add whatever available sprouts and enjoy.

Sprout Salad is a blend of whatever sprouts can be created with the seeds available. Lentils, especially Puy lentils... rye and wheat sprout in two days together or separately – soak in a bowl for at least 8 hours. Pour through a colander collecting the soak water to feed Your plants. A plate on top of the colander maintains a warm, moist eco-system. Since every living thing gives off wastes, these growing sprouts require a rinse then pour back in the colander to air dry. Do this for two days; twice a day in hot, humid climates. After thorough draining, store in a covered container. These create or embellish side dishes or a nutritious snack, as do sprouted garbanzos / chickpeas – which generally take 3 days of twice a day rinsing; mung in 18-24 hrs!

Enzyme Soup is a variable blend – 3C of green veggie juice... 1C of soaked almonds... or 1½C of soaked pine nuts... along with basil, cilantro, coriander, cumin, dill, garlic, ginger, oregano, rosemary, sage or thyme with dulse or kelp powder. Once blended... add a handful of lentil or mung sprouts... sprinkle granulated dulse or powdered kelp for color and flavor. At the end... add one diced avocado, stir in then pulse quickly. As a variation, instead of veggie juice... blend 1C water and 2C fresh asparagus or spinach; strain.

Vegan Borscht with Crème Topping is great for the blood and the liver. In 2C water, blend 4 medium, peeled diced beets, ½ onion, a stalk of celery, a Tbs of dulse or kelp powder; pour into bowls. Rinse out the blender; then in ¼C water with 1tsp lemon juice blend ½C pine nuts until thick and creamy. Top each bowl with 1Tsp of the crème; sprinkle with minced scallions.

Seed Loaf is enzyme-rich nutrition, a suitable entree. Simply germinate the seeds to activate dormant energy. With almonds and hazelnuts, remove the skins after soaking because of the oxalic acid factor. This keeps little fingers busy and is a great way for kids to help in the kitchen. To facilitate matters, scald the nuts by dipping a strainer full in boiling water – a few seconds. With the skins removed, homogenize 1C almonds and hazelnuts, ½C each of soaked sunflower and sesame, using the juicer, with the special solid plate on the bottom of the attachment. If You have time to chill the almonds and seeds before this process, it cuts down on the amount of heat generated and saves some enzymes... otherwise alternate ½C seeds with other ingredients chilled from the refrigerator – broccoli, carrots, celery, and beets. Add flavors of onion, garlic and/or ginger to taste... plus herbs such as basil, oregano, rosemary and thyme; mix by hand; at another time experiment with curry spices or the spices once added to meat loaf. This Seed Loaf may be shaped on a platter with garnishes of fresh parsley, basil and cilantro, and served with steamed veggies and/or a salad... keeping grains and starches for another meal. Left out for a few hours or overnight, it takes on a slightly fermented flavor the next day. Like natural Sauerkraut and Kimchee, this is pre-digested food, beneficial for our friendly bacteria – our biome.

Natural Sauerkraut is easy to make with red or green cabbage – or ½ and ½. Soak 3 strands of wakame seaweed in water. Carefully remove the large outer leaves from the cabbage; rinse and save for covering at the end. Grate, chop or homogenize the cabbage as You did for the Seed Loaf or, using whatever juicer You have, juice the cabbage and then mix juice and pulp together. Cut a sweet apple into eight pieces, removing seeds and core. Layer 1" cabbage, apple pieces and seaweed in a one-gallon ceramic crock or glass container. There should be plenty of juice, or add some seaweed soak water. Cover with the large outer leaves. Seal this mixture from the outside air by securing a heavy-duty plastic bag with water, placing it on top. Cover with a clean towel and let sit for 3 days at room temperature. Take off the coverings, remove apple pieces and any discolored cabbage, and store in glass jars in the refrigerator.

Kimchee is a variation on the theme using Napa cabbage, any hard roots, or combinations – beets, carrots, jicama, parsnip – with one small onion, 3 cloves of garlic, and as much cayenne as possible. Kimchee is delicious. In season, slice fresh-picked corn from the cob, mixing it all together.

Sprouted Hummus makes an enzyme-rich side dish or topping. Soak chickpeas 12 hrs – change the water and soak another 12. Rinse daily for 2-3 days, depending on warmth and humidity, until the tail is as long as the seed. In very humid climates, sprout them in the refrigerator. Blend 2C of the sprouts with ½C water, ¼C dulse or kelp powder, ¼C fresh lemon juice; add at least 4 Tbs raw sesame tahini, and 2-4 cloves of garlic. Marinate for 30 minutes, then refrigerate until using. Since chickpeas are a challenge to digest for some, substitute red beans and be surprised.

Guacamole is another enzyme-rich side dish or topping. Mash 4-6 avocados, and add 1Tbs lemon or lime juice per avocado; mix in 2C finely diced scallions, 2-4 cloves of garlic, and ¾C each of finely diced fresh basil, cilantro and/or dill. A diced tomato and finely diced red jalapeno pepper may be added for spice and color, or a finely diced red bell pepper. Avocados are a great source of lutein – an anti-oxidant for the eyes – and helps absorb other nutrient factors, especially eaten with greens.

Vegan Pate for stuffed celery, mushrooms, peppers, or to spread on Essene bread or dehydrated crackers. Blend 1C each of soaked almonds and pumpkin seeds, ½C of soaked walnuts, ¼C each of soaked brown sesame and sunflower, ¾C lentil sprouts, until smooth. Add 1½C mushrooms, 2-3 cloves of garlic, 1tsp kelp powder to taste. Blend until creamy smooth. Refrigerate before using.

Nori Open Face Sandwiches may be made by following the above recipe, and cutting the nori sheets in ¼s before spreading the paste, then place in the dehydrator at 120º until crispy. Imagine. Explore.

Enzyme-rich Seed Cheese Any single nut or seed may be used or any combination: almond, cashew, hazelnut, pine, pumpkin, sesame, sunflower, or walnut.

Blend 2C soaked seeds with 2C water, dulse or kelp powder to taste and leave it out 6-9 hrs, then pour into a fine-meshed bag. Let it hang above a bowl to collect the seed whey for dressing or soup for 3-6 hours, depending on sharpness of flavor. Experiment. Refrigerate or use as stuffing for celery, mushroom caps, pepper quarters, etc. Also use as a paste for nori rolls, or mixed in diced fruit.

Enzyme-rich Pizza Sprout a mix of wheat and rye, or other grains such as kamut and blend to a thick, batter consistency. Oil the tray lightly. Pour the batter and place the tray in the dehydrator overnight or all day. You may turn it when it looks almost done, to speed the process. Once finished, blend some red peppers, adding basil, oregano, or other herbs, and spread over the crust. Add slivered onion, olives, mushrooms or other toppings; dehydrate until warm & crispy.

For an alternative crust, soak 1 part each of chia and 2 parts sunflower seeds for five hours. Spread out on dehydrator trays... overnight or until crispy. Add toppings as desired; perhaps sunflower seed cheese, topped with veggies and tomatoes... which are allowed because this crust, rather than starch, is pure protein.

Nori Rolls {Caution: While nori sheets and seaweed are economically purchased at Oriental shops, they are probably contaminated. Most are dried on rocks sprayed with herbicides to control weeds growing between. Maine Coast Sea Veg has truly organic seaweed. Muscle test.} A bamboo roller facilitates rolling, although it can be done without. Put a clove of garlic, a small carrot, ½ onion, and ½ red or yellow pepper in a food processor. Mix with 1C of Seed Cheese and add 2Tbs kombu powder, 1Tbs kelp powder, ½C of dulse or nori flakes (or a little of both), ½C minced parsley, 1Tbs wasabe (Japanese hot green) mustard and 1Tbs ground ginger. Mix well, and spread over four nori sheets – adding fresh sprouts as available, and slivers of fresh cut avocado. Roll tightly. At the end, seal as You would an envelope by moistening with water. With a wet knife... slice into bite sized pieces.

Seaweed Variations Nori, as dulse, has a delicate flavor. Both may be eaten as a snack without soaking. Some find whole dulse a little salty so they soak it for a minute (that's all it takes) and squeeze off excess liquid. This liquid or any water from soaking seaweed may be used in cooking grains, making soups, or feeding Your plants. Seaweed are macroalgae – superfoods – optimally eaten raw.

Regarding seaweed, as with any food, the individual is the judge of taste. The way to know is to stretch out of the comfort zone... and experience something different. With something less than enjoyable, simply divide the rest in small baggies and give as samples to friends so they can determine whether they enjoy that flavor. Or cook them with beans or soups to minimize their strong flavor. These superfoods may taste strong; they also make You strong – and smart – worth incorporating in everyone's diet, especially with mental or emotional challenges.

The tough seaweeds are kelp and kombu. Purchased dry, broken in small pieces or cut with scissors... add water and let sit for 3-6 hrs. These expand considerably; have small pieces with of plenty water. The pieces may then be strained from the water, which can be refrigerated and used as broth or for cooking grains. Soaked it can be added to a salad, blended in a dressing or served with steamed veggies. Soak larger pieces and, once expanded, blend with the liquid and serve as a side dish; it keeps in the refrigerator in a covered dish for a few days. Eating the seaweed fresh and soaked gives the full complement of nutrition; cooking always alters protein structure as well as major minerals, such as calcium and magnesium.

Wakame is easily broken in pieces, and once soaked is a tasty addition to almost any dish. Some seaweed looks like spaghetti: hijiki is thicker, arame slender. Both may be soaked for a few hours until tender. All 3 make a lovely side dish, or even a filling salad. Simply soak the seaweed... saving the soak water for another time. Grate some beets, carrots, and daikon radish, dice some red bell peppers, mince some scallions and add some sprouts. Dice an avocado and mix all ingredients well.

Enzyme-Rich Desserts are to be eaten alone, perhaps with other enzyme-rich desserts as a meal in itself. Enzymes are at the core of our health care crisis, along with the lack of nutrition in commercial foods. Some people sit down and have their fill of animal protein and starches, with a glass of ice water and wine, then a cup of coffee and cake or pie for dessert, with a scoop of ice cream, followed by a liqueur. All this combines to guarantee digestive distress and ill health.

At a party and times for celebration, eat – then have other activities for 3 hours – then have dessert.

Dried Fruit Logs Mash dried figs, dates and raisins, formed into small logs or round balls and coat with shredded coconut, or crushed walnuts. Dehydrate.

Raw Fruit Pie begins with crust. Process 1C of soaked, skinned then dehydrated almonds in a food processor to create a fine texture. Add 1C raisins and continue to process until this mix forms a ball in the processor. You may have to add a splash of water. It may move, so make sure Your processor stays put. Press this ball into a 9" glass pie plate as Your crust. Then take 1C presoaked pecans, or ½ pecans ½ walnuts and mix in the food processor with a banana, 1C figs (dried or fresh), 1tsp almond extract, 1tsp vanilla extract, ¼tsp cinnamon, and ¼tsp nutmeg. Process until smooth; pour this filling into the pie crust shell. Chill for two hours.

Use the basic crust and make a filling according to what fruits are in season, such as a blend of fresh blueberries and a spotted banana. If You feel creative, peel and de-seed a ripe papaya or several mangoes; slice in half, then make thin slices that You can fan out as the first layer on the crust; pour on a blend of banana and strawberries. (Caution: Always use organic strawberries, even if they are only available frozen. Commercial strawberries are among the most highly sprayed produce.) Add another layer of thinly sliced papaya, more sauce, etc. topping with a layer of sauce; strawberry halves may encircle the finished product, or peel a kiwi, cut in half, then make thin slices on the ½ round and encircle the pie. Some may wonder about banana, a sweet fruit, and strawberry, a sour fruit being eaten at the same time. These fruits are, indeed, a poor combination because they have inherently dichotomous tastes... true if one were to have a banana in one hand and a strawberry in the other, taking alternating bites. Confusing messages would be sent to the brain via the taste buds. When we blend them together, we create a new sub-acid fruit and the taste buds experience them as one. During the season, load Your freezer with blended, nutritious desserts.

Candy Bars Combine 1C soaked hazelnuts, 1C soaked walnuts, 2C organic and unsulfured dried fruit. Mix these ingredients well in a food processor, shape into bars and dehydrate overnight or all day. As an alternate, make logs then roll in toasted carob powder and/or shredded coconut.

Mock Egg Nog is a treat for special times. Combine 1/3C cashews, 1Tsp flax, 1tsp lecithin, 1tsp grated lemon rind, 2Tsp maple syrup, 1½tsp vanilla extract, 3C hot water, a pinch of cinnamon, barley malt sweetener and Sucanat™. Blend well and serve with a sprinkle of nutmeg.

Optimal Fuel for HeartMindBodySpirit These recipes are based on the fact that animals in nature – of which we are primates of the human variety – remain healthy when they are eating whole, raw foods rich in fiber. Primates are healthy and socially amenable as herbivores. When primates such as baboons kill and eat meat, they become nervous and ill-tempered, with nasty, vicious ways. Facts are clear. The vibrations of our food choices determine the vibrations of our personalities... and our lives.

Alkaline Reserve... pH measures the potential of Hydrogen: Hydrogen (H+) acid ion concentration *or* Hydroxide (OH-) alkaline ion concentration. Values range between 1 (most acidic) and 6.9 (slightly acidic); 7 being neutral; 7.1 (slightly alkaline) and 14 (most alkaline.) Alkaline foods leave behind a negative ion charge surplus having a beneficial effect on one's body. The charge is the sum of negative and positive charges in amino acids, chelated minerals, electrolytes, organic compounds, vitamins and metabolic waste. Healthy individuals have slightly alkaline saliva and urine; since the pH of urine varies throughout the day, an assessment is made collecting urine for a 24-hour period. Use a container with a secure lid and keep it in the refrigerator. The optimal pH is 7.2 for both saliva and urine, buffering acidic metabolic wastes.

The nucleus of cells and protein-related digestive secretions are normally acid. Essentially the human body is electrical in nature. Organs and muscle systems require electrical voltage to function. Each cell is a battery with an acid nucleus and an alkaline cytoplasm surrounding the nucleus, bound by the cell wall... the membrane which we now recognize **is** the mem-brain.

Except for the stomach and most of the digestive tract, all the major organs – liver, pancreas, spleen, kidneys – as well as the muscles, can *survive* in a slightly acid state. For *optimal* function the body likes to be slightly alkaline. Arthur C. Guyton, in his *Medical Physiology*, wrote of maintaining the "alkaline reserve" and left us wondering what that meant... and how to do it.

The recommendations found here for optimal diet leads to that goal. Low fat, low protein, high fiber diet means eating more fruits, vegetables and whole grains. As fire leaves ashes... the fire of digestion also leaves a residue and affects our pH balance. The focus, in the past, has been on a high fat, high protein and low fiber diet found in animal foods and refined carbohydrates such as white flour, sugar and white rice; these leave an acidic residue in the body. The blood maintains pH between 7.35 - 7.45 and with 7 being neutral, that means the blood is slightly more attracted to alkalinity. Excess alkalinity, even though a real challenge given today's eating habits, can lead to diarrhea, dehydration and death. Acid forming foods are congesting and their chronic use forces an emergency response to survive; excess acidity leads to congestion, constipation and coma. Keep balanced and, like the blood, lean slightly toward alkalinity.

We already have acids forming in our system: day-to-day functioning and movement. When our diet has an abundance of acid forming elements, the body responds. One choice is to retain water as things move through the colon to dilute the acidity; even if we have edema... or feel bloated... even if we are overweight. It's better than the other option – too much acidity leads to death. Another mechanism responding to acid forming elements is to neutralize the acids with alkaline elements. Unless found in the diet, the body has a ready store... with calcium in the bones, and sodium in the gallbladder. Even if we develop osteoporosis, or if little concretions called gallstones are left behind, it's better than death! It is optimal to eat foods that build our alkaline reserve, those rich in calcium, iron, magnesium, potassium and sodium; with less emphasis on foods that leave an acidic residue such as chlorine, phosphorus and sulfur – alcohol, animal foods and refined grains and sugars.

The optimal fuel for the human HeartMindBodySpirit is 80% raw. We have already considered the fundamentals of raw foods. There are hundreds of fruits and vegetables, although most Americans recognize a dozen and maybe eat a handful. There is really a large variety awaiting exploration. Alkaline foods include virtually all vegetables and fruits except blueberries, cranberries, plums / prunes, and commercial citrus. The latter are picked while still unripe, for shipping – they are acid forming; although if allowed to tree ripen, the citric acid digests and leaves an alkaline residue. Canned, bottled or frozen, it is pasteurized and, therefore, acid forming. If You have a citrus tree in the yard, gently shake a branch and what falls to the ground is usually fairly ripe.

The nuts that are alkaline forming include almonds, hazelnuts and pine nuts – as well as small seeds such as flax, pumpkin, sesame and sunflower – alkaline when germinated (soaked) acidic when roasted.

Fresh beans are alkaline; the one alkaline dried bean is soy, and its products such as miso, tempeh, sprouts, as well as germinated / soaked raw soymilk or even cooked soybeans. Be especially aware of soy protein isolates. Fractionated food, such as tofu or okara, is less than optimal. Some have a challenge digesting any soy... so be aware. Muscle test. Like animal foods, the grains commonly consumed in our society are acid forming – wheat, rye, barley, oats, and white, brown or red rice. The following alkaline grains are ancient, tiny, quick to prepare and delicious:

Amaranth The Latin name *Amaranthaceae* means: does not fade, does not wither; it is the ancient grain of the Aztecs. Each plant requires 3-4 square feet and moisture, for the first 3 weeks of growth; it can then withstand drought and produce nutritious leaves. In a good year one mature plant can produce a half million tiny seeds. These may be sprouted, popped like corn or cooked like other grains. Typically, cereal grains contain little lysine to make complete protein in the body, so when cooking other grains, add a little amaranth. In fact, amaranth is in a family by itself; rather than a cereal grain, it is a seed high in protein.

Millet – *Panicum miliaceum* means: a thousand little loaves of bread; it is the ancient grain of Africa and China where it is known as "Queen of the Grains" – a balanced food, offering complete protein, a nutty taste.

Quinoa (KEENwa) means: mother grain; it is the ancient grain of the Incas, and a member of the goosefoot family, *Chenopodium*, with beets, chard, lamb's quarters and spinach. Each grain is covered with saponin, a natural insect repellent, that can be removed by soaking. Unlike cereals, in which the germ is usually located at the tip of each grain, the germ covers the entire quinoa kernel. As the quinoa soaks or cooks, the germ separates from the kernel making white, sprout-like rings. Plentiful lysine like amaranth, rather than a cereal grain, it is a seed high in protein.

Teff means: lost, because that is the consequence dropping any of this tiny grain; it is the ancient grain of Ethiopia. Five times richer than any other grain, it is high in calcium, iron and potassium... available in ivory and brown. Cooked together with amaranth, it has an interesting porridge texture.

Grain Medley These cook together nicely, and offer alkaline enhancing, whole grain nutrition. They may be used in a ratio of roughly equal parts: 2 parts each of millet and quinoa, and 1 part each of amaranth and teff. Once purchased – to save the measuring – simply combine everything in a large container, mix thoroughly and store in tightly sealed containers. As with any seed, if stored for longer periods, place a whole bay leaf at the bottom and top preventing bugs.

To prepare this grain medley, measure out one-part grain to 4-parts water and let it soak for 2 hours to germinate. Even though cooking this grain destroys enzymes, by soaking the vibrational frequencies change bringing them from a concentrated state, to a germinated, enlivened, energetic state of youth changing the energy of the food. After soaking, give it a stir to circulate the enzyme inhibitors leached out into the water; they may settle to the bottom becoming trapped in the grain while pouring off the soak water. Pour through a fine strainer into a large measuring cup. This water is nutritious for plants especially any that are less than vibrant. Note how many ounces are taken away, and replace that exact amount of water maintaining the 4:1 ratio of water to grain. Bring it to a slow simmer for 15 minutes and turn off the heat, keeping the lid on and keeping it on the burner. It is ready when the water absorbs. Meanwhile create Your side dishes of seaweed and salad. When cooking, perhaps add kelp for a touch of salty flavor or slices of ginger root for a savory flavor. When finished cooking, the ginger root may be taken out and, if desired, stir in some diced onion – giving a crunchy consistency, and a pleasant flavor. Once it is a bit cooler, add some hardy sprouts such as mung or kamut. A sprinkle of dulse powder on the finished product looks inviting.

Grain Burgers If You have leftovers, You may enjoy shaping them into burgers and placing them in the dehydrator... or warming them under the broiler.

Buckwheat is an ancient plant of Asia, a neutral grain; unrelated to wheat, it is part of the rhubarb / dock family. Raw buckwheat may be cooked as grains; it also cooks quickly. Toasted buckwheat – kasha – is beyond germination because of the toasting process. It is easily cooked by boiling 2 parts water, then add 1-part kasha, a diced onion, kelp or any flavors; stir, cover, and take off the burner until the water absorbs. Buckwheat also can be soaked for only 30 minutes, then dehydrated – simply spread out and left to dry – a crunchy topping on blended Cosmic Soup and salads.

Kamut is an ancient grain like spelt; it leaves a slight acid residue. Because it is new to most, it is usually well tolerated by those with allergic challenges. Mixing this, and any of the above grains, with cooked squash or sweet potatoes. Kamut sprouts are somewhat chewy, yet delicious... adding texture to many dishes.

Spelt is an ancient grain; higher in gluten than wheat, well tolerated because of its solubility. Nutrients go into solution rapidly, bio-available; minimal digestive effort. The mystic Hildegard von Bingen healed incurables with fruit for breakfast and spelt with vegetables later in the day. Spelt sprouts... like wheat and rye sprouts... may be added to salads or used similarly.

Grain Pilaf In addition to the earlier alkaline Grain Medley, some or all of the following acid-forming grains may be enjoyed on occasion: barley, brown basmati rice, kamut, rye, spelt and wheat. While it is always optimal to soak 5-6 hours, it helps to sprout them for at least one day; lessening their acid-forming nature.

Hokkaido Pumpkin originally from Japan, now grown in New England, these are the sweetest and most nutritious of the winter squashes. Green skinned ones are a little sweeter, cook drier, and may require steaming to keep them moist. Pumpkins keep well if undamaged and still have some stalk. Store them without touching each other on an airy shelf in a warm, dry living room or bedroom; there is generally too much moisture in the kitchen. For delicious pumpkin soup: lightly sauté a diced, medium onion in a soup pan. Add a Tbs dulse powder and stir. Add ½ medium pumpkin cut into small chunks, strips of kombu or other seaweed, and cover with water, cooking until soft (30 minutes); purée, add a pinch of pink salt, and 2Tsp of fresh grated ginger juice or 4Tsp fresh grated ginger to taste; simmer 2 minutes. Serve with a garnish of parsley or chopped scallions. For stuffed pumpkin, cut in half and steam until tender, making Your stuffing from cooking onions, mushrooms, celery, spices; mixing with Your grain of choice and a sprinkle of kelp.

Jerusalem Artichokes knobby tubers unrelated to globe artichokes: members of the thistle family, these tubers are a species of sunflower – healing for the pancreas and digestive system. The vegetable was brought from France to England in the 17th century as girasol artichoke; *girasol* is archaic French for sunflower. The name artichoke was attributed to the similarity in flavor to the globe artichoke; gradually there was a transition from girasol to the more phonetically similar and Anglicized word Jerusalem. After cleaning, they may be grated and added to salads, a side dish with some seaweed and light herbs, or cooked and mashed like potatoes; sliced on the round, they are used in soups and stews.

Millet Mashed Potato Over medium heat... 1tsp unrefined Sesame Oil in a pan; when warmed, add a diced onion and stir for 2-3 minutes. Add a splash of Nama Shoyu™ – unpasteurized soy sauce – stir again. Combine ½ medium cauliflower, or an equal amount of pumpkin or sweet potato, cut into small pieces, 3C water, 1C millet and a pinch of whole salt. Bring to a simmer... cover and cook until the water is absorbed – 20 minutes; then mash for a smooth, creamy texture. Serve with a garnish of chopped scallions and sprouts... enjoy Nightshade-free mashed potatoes.

Vegan Chili (cooked) Soak ¾C millet in warm water. While germinating, dice two stalks of celery, 1½C onion, 1 green pepper, 2 cloves of garlic... sauté in 1Tsp olive oil – or simply steam in a little water. Then add 1lb each of light red kidney beans, dark red kidney beans and garbanzos, all of which have been soaked for 10 hours – sprouted, if possible. Combine with 3-4 peeled, diced red peppers and cover with water. Add whole salt, black pepper or paprika to taste, roughly 1tsp each. Boil... then simmer for 1 hour covered. Give the millet soak water to Your plants, and add the millet to the chili. Cook for ½ hour, adding more water if required. Once it has finished cooking and once the pot has stopped steaming... add cayenne pepper to taste. {Avoid cooking with cayenne, as it irritates sensitive tissues.}

Vegan Chili (enzyme-rich) Place ½ gallon of lentil sprouts in a large bowl; grate a medium, peeled beet and 3 large, peeled carrots; add a bunch of scallions and 2 stalks of celery, diced. Blend 2 red peppers, 1 large onion, 3-4 cloves of garlic, 1 zucchini, 1Tsp kelp and 1Tsp miso until smooth... slowly add 4oz chili powder and jalapenos to taste; once blended, dice an avocado, and pulse blend. Marinate for 15 minutes before serving. Pour over sprouts and veggies; mix.

Other Factors to Build Our Alkaline Reserve

Have a large salad with any cooked meal to maintain the balance of 80% raw, 20% cooked; and, with any cooked food, take digestive enzymes to relieve Your pancreas and liver of additional burdens. So-called enzymes based on HCL, or pancreatin, are less than optimal; they are pancreas tissue from a cow or pig – or worse, synthetic. Although only effective within a narrow range of pH, papain from papaya, and bromelain from pineapple are suitable – the latter are superior when dealing with inflammation. Optimal enzymes are plant-based; these tolerate the wide range of pH of the digestive tract. One or two before a meal; more with digestive challenges, or if going to a banquet or a celebration. Enjoy!

In the interest of easy digestion and food combining, it is wise to eat cooked grains with whole grain bread; if something else is chosen to add to the meal, keep them apart from seed dressing or seed cheese. Germinated or sprouted grains usually combine well with germinated or sprouted seeds, and vegetables.

The Duc de la Rochefoucauld, 17th century French sage, said: "to preserve one's health by too strict a regime is in itself a tedious malady." What You do on occasion is of little consequence; what You do every day is important. A diet based on germinated and raw foods – fruits, fresh juices, sprouts and salads – as well as whole grains and lightly steamed vegetables, is what we are anatomically and physiologically designed to eat. Consider that 100g of spinach in 1948 contained over 150 mg of iron; today that same 100g is lucky to have 2 or 3 mg of iron. Why? Chemicals have depleted our soils of nutrients. That is why wild grown seaweed, macroalgae, as well as microalgae are so highly recommended. Raising the vibrations of the foods we eat is similar to changing regular gasoline for high-octane gasoline in a high-performance racing car. Using the proper fuel brings the desired results! We are living in conditions that require high-performance foods. Your health is in Your hands... and what Your hands... bring to Your mouth... and how You *feel* about it!

Certain things decrease our alkaline reserve by bringing acid-forming elements into our lives. Besides alcohol, animal foods, refined and processed foods, eating foods indiscriminately or improperly combined, along with overeating... shallow breathing... lack of rest... noise or other forms of stress... excess or lack of exercise... and insufficient water, all create acids for the physical body. At the emotional level, negative feelings like anger, resentment, helplessness or hopelessness, fear or grief inordinate in length or intensity... all keep us removed from True Self. At the mental level, apathy, confusion, denial, or dullness from drugs... lead to levels of acidity affecting our state of conscious awareness and attitude toward Life.

In addition to the enzyme-rich foods listed above, it's the simple, pleasant things in life that can influence the alkaline reserve... moderate sunshine: a minimum of 30 minutes outdoors every day; even if it's cloudy or cold, the healing rays come through. Summer months, avoid sun between 10 - 2, when possible.

Proper combinations along with frugal / reasonable eating, deep breathing, proper rest, pleasant music and nature sounds, relaxation and meditation, moderate exercise, adequate water and occasional fasting all contribute to the alkaline reserve.

At the emotional level: laughing, and even more so... a simple smile... positive feelings re-enforced by positive affirmations... build self-esteem and courage. At the mental level: create thoughts and feelings of joy and enthusiasm; learn from old issues, releasing the past. All these processes contribute to build our alkaline reserve – and facilitate a human being experiencing being human... with optimal efficiency.

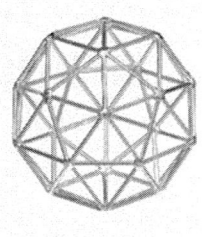

9 - ENERGY MEDICINE AS FOUND IN HOMEOPATHY

Homeopathy, perhaps the quintessential ancient Vibrational Medicine, was **re-discovered** around 1796; German physician Samuel Hahnemann popularized a therapeutic system of medicine – with roots in Ayurveda and is now used throughout the East and the West. Hippocrates studied Ayurveda and worked with the principles of ancient wisdom. There are ancient remedies in the Indian pharmacopoeia missing from the standard *Materia Medica* compiled by William Boericke, MD. An example is *Centella asiatica*, known as Gotu kola, commonly used as a blood purifier and diuretic... in India, it is useful in its homeopathic form to counter depression. The remedy *Kurchi* is useful with diarrhea and amoebic dysentery. These remedies are from Ayurveda – Life Knowledge.

While most people can grasp the ancient concept that colors and sounds can have a direct impact on our subtle energy fields, our emotions, our feelings... some have a challenge understanding how "inert" stones can impart vibrational energies... or how fragrances can influence the HeartMindBodySpirit. With these energetics of subtle energy fields, we flirt with the concept of quantum physics and informational medicine. With homeopathy... we go to the *heart* of quantum physics with the ultimate challenge for the Western Mind. Western scientists are now ready to grapple with this New Reality... their experience with acupuncture flexed their scientific imaginations.

Western science long denied the existence of chi (energy) and the meridian (distribution) system of acupuncture. Having performed millions of autopsies and operations, they never "saw" any evidence, nor any indicators of such a system. Then in preparation for a presidential trip to China in the 70's, noted journalist and later the editor of *The New York Times*, Jim Reston, had acute appendicitis requiring immediate surgery. It was out of the question for him to fly back to New York for the operation, which he had in China, and acupuncture was used to block his pain afterwards. Mr Reston wrote extensively of its merits, from his own experiences and observations. A veil was lifted, and Western scientists were forced to take another look. Acupuncture is now readily available in every large city, even small towns. Other scientists are studying various forms of Vibrational Energy Medicine, among them – homeopathy. There are two health systems to consider.

While some may see a source of contention in these diametrically opposed responses to a disease process, they each have their proper role to play at the proper time. If someone is stung by a bee and goes into anaphylactic shock – swollen neck, impaired breathing – this is hardly the time to consider herbs for a liver cleanse! *Arnica* and *Apis* may be given on the way to the ER... although the focus is on a shot of nor-epinephrine. Once the emergency is over, breathing is restored, then we can think about the liver cleanse.

On the other hand, if someone has angina or even a myocardial infarction, rather than a lifetime prescription of synthetic drugs... another prescription can be found in nutrition and Holistic Lifestyle Medicine – particularly aerobics. The nutritional program may include enzymes with and between meals, a saturation dose of Co-enzyme Q-10, and Hawthorn berries as tea, &/or homeopathic potencies of that herb: *Crataegus*.

For health and balance, utilize both: the conventional approach for the immediate emergency and short-term stabilization... the complementary approach for long-term. The blend of both worlds – Modern Technology and Ancient Wisdom – allows us to consider Integrated Healing of HeartMindBodySpirit.

The Conventional Approach

Allopathic uses remedies such as drugs or surgery based on what produces results **opposite** to the symptoms.

The process is complex.

The prescription is simple.

Diagnostic tools include sophisticated blood analysis, hi-tech machinery such as x-rays, ultrasound, MRI, EEG, EKG, etc.

Reductionist Model: the field is narrowed and targeted.

Deterministic, Analytical and Retrogressive.

Quick fix; best for emergency; danger of side-effects.

Aggressive and suppressive; treatment is for symptoms; when they subside or disappear, we are at the end of our quest.

The Complimentary Approach

Homeopathic uses remedies from the animal, plant and mineral kingdoms based on what produces results **similar** to the symptoms.

The process is simple.

The prescription is complex.

Diagnostic tools include consciousness on the part of the client *and* the therapist looking at the individual interactions regarding the set of symptoms, primary of which are mental symptoms: their aggravation and amelioration.

Holistic Model: the field includes physical, emotional, mental and spiritual "wholeness".

Probabilistic, Empirical and Progressive.

Gradual recovery, best in chronic cases; totally safe.

Gentle and cleansing; the cure of the symptoms leads to another level of holistic healing, where we are ready for the next aspect of our quest.

Homeopathy and Quantum Physics

The more we know, the more we know there is to explore and integrate. In 1906, J.J. Thompson was awarded the Nobel Prize for showing that the electron is a *particle*. Then in 1937 his son, G.P. Thompson won the Nobel Prize for showing that the electron is a *wave*. The truth is both... and neither. Sometimes an electron behaves as a particle in a deterministic manner... and sometimes it acts like a wave in a probabilistic manner... known as a corpuscular packet of energy... nicknamed a ***wavicle***!

In normal everyday living we are aware of the substantial aspects of matter. It is only in our labs, some stretching out for miles, that we empirically gather and quantify the more ethereal aspects of matter. We now know that quantum mechanical effects are present in the behavior of gases. Our choice to ignore them is merely a matter of convenience in getting workable or practical results. Potential vibrations at any point in a field are capable of producing quanta that move about in space and interact. Increasingly higher and higher energies are present in a smaller region of space. The exchange of these quanta, the carriers of the field interactions... evolves in time.   In quantum field theory, particles are not acted upon by force as classical physics had supposed; they interact with each other through exchange of other particles.

We live in a quantum mechanical universe; as fractal geometry shows, there is an intimate relationship between microcosm and the macrocosm. Our health challenges first appear on the quantum level of the microcosm, and progress to the level of the macrocosm where we develop signs and symptoms. Homeopathy, Energy Medicine, works at the energetic quantum level – where challenges first appear.

Holistic v/s Individualistic

The individualistic approach considers the universe as the sum of its parts. The holistic approach considers the whole universe as one unit. As an example: in a deuteron atom, we can measure:

0.000548 = The mass of the electron

1.007597 = proton

<u>1.008986 = neutron</u>

2.017131 = Total atomic mass unit

2.014740 = The **mass** of a deuteron atom

0.002391= The mass difference (**energy difference**)

Clearly, basic atomic elements prove the universe is more than the sum of the individual parts. The whole universe is interconnected, and the difference of mass is the energy spent to interconnect the particles. Seeking answers, scientists explore plasma physics – delving into our Electric Universe.

Rather than having specialties as MDs generally do... homeopaths see the whole person, analyzing signs and symptoms... with priority given to the mental aspects, which influence our feeling body. Homeopathy as Vibrational Medicine, Energy Medicine and Informational Medicine working with subtle energies, must consider intricate inter-relationships of HeartMindBodySpirit.

What is Homeopathy?

In nearly every country, Homeopathy relieves suffering. The Greek word *homos* = same, and *homoios* = similar. The homeopathic principle treats with **similars** – treating like with like – taking a substance that, in a healthy person, produces symptoms similar to those experienced by the sick. This substance is then diluted to varying degrees. The remedy may be so dilute the only thing left is the "imprint" – the fingerprint of its vibrational energy.

In conventional medicine, symptoms are caused by illness. Homeopathy sees symptoms as a natural reaction warding off illness and seeks to temporarily stimulate the symptoms rather than suppress them... allowing balance as the natural order of things.

Great-grandma kept Syrup of Ipecac in the medicine cabinet. If a child swallows a toxin, the doctor may recommend eating bread to absorb it, or... giving ipecac to bring it up – depending on what is ingested. Mysteriously, 1Tbs ipecac normally causes nausea and produces vomiting, yet in homeopathic doses, ipecac relieves symptoms of nausea and vomiting!

How Remedies Are Made

In Brazil, *Ipecacuanha* is widely known as vomit root. Homeopathic *Ipecacuanha* – Ipecac, derives from the Mother Tincture. Combine 100g of the powdered dried root with 150cc of distilled water and 750cc strong alcohol – pure grain alcohol: 190-proof. Store in a cool, dark place for 1 week and shake with Love, 2x day. Strain through an unbleached coffee filter into a sterilized jar: dishwasher cleaned, steamed & heat-dried is sufficient. To 1-part Mother Tincture, add 3-parts distilled water and 6-parts strong alcohol. This mixture is then succussed: shaken or pounded in the palm of one's hand **100x** imprinting the vibrational frequencies, the subtle energy field – into the remedy.

This consists of a 10-part solution, known as Ipecac 1X. (Roman letter X = 10) Take 1-part 1X + 9 parts water, succuss 100 times, for a solution 2X, and so forth. Take 1-part 1X + 99 parts water, and succuss for 1C. (Roman letter C = 100) Take 1-part of 1C + 99 parts water, succuss 100 times and You have 2C, and so forth. The process is repeated sequentially up to 30C, 200C, 1000C known as 1M, 100,000C known as 1CM, and 1,000,000C known as 1MM. While this is labor intensive, homeopathy remains an alternative that effectively, efficiently and economically deals with health care crises – bringing holistic balance.

According to Avogadro's Principle there is not a single molecule – not even an atom – of the original remedy left by 12C. So how can homeopathy work, especially at the higher, more dilute doses**?** Is it the placebo effect? If so, how can we explain success with babies... or dogs and chickens? The secret is succussion... which generates quantum waves... vibrations... trapped in the structure of the vehicle: alcohol and water. When we have sensitive enough instruments, we will be able to measure these waves. Until then... we marvel at their wondrous effects.

The Nature of a Wave

We can calculate the wave generated by a large mass. Earth moves 27,000km/hour which generates a wave of 10^{-64}m; a 1000kg truck moving 100 kph generates a wave of 10^{-33}m; a ball 500g moving at 100 kph generates a wave of 10^{-29}m; a cell 10^{-9}g moving at 1m/sec generates a wave of 10^{-17}m; an atom generates a wave of 10^{-2}m; radio waves vary from 1m>km.

Conclusion: as mass is reduced the wave factor increases. As the frequency of a wave increases, so does its energy. Waves behave as particles when they interact with other objects – other waves, even particles! Dual properties of matter are more significant at a small scale.

How Homeopathy Works

Using a wave-charged remedy... we introduce subtle energy fields into our bodies. For every action there is a reaction... and our body responds on subtle levels. The homeopathic approach is mild, gentle, curative, permanent and timely. Homeopathic remedies used to cure minor ailments can save an individual from major challenges. This is achieved by constantly evolving the body's natural immune defense system.

Our understanding of the immune response system has grown immensely. In the past, our understanding of the immune response system was limited to the spleen, the lymph nodes and the *beta* and *theta* cells – named because they are produced in the *blood* and *bones*, and in the *thymus*. Then someone discovered the limbic system of the brain was involved. Today we understand that <u>all</u> organs, glands, and in fact, every part of the body is involved in our immune response. Immune response systems are compromised with the overuse of antibiotics, synthetic drugs, chlorine in our drinking water, which also destroys the friendly intestinal bacteria, and fluorine, historically used by despots to control the masses. All of these over-acidify and upset our delicate ecosystem.

Candida Albicans: Life out of Balance

Homeopathy, in conjunction with a wholistic lifestyle, builds the *immune response*. One remedy is the Mother Tincture of *Echinacea angustifolia*: 10 drops in 1oz water 3x/day; followed 15 minutes later with the Mother Tincture of *Hydrastis* (Goldenseal): 10 drops in 1oz water; wait 15 minutes before any other taste.

Exemplifying the homeopathic approach for a common immune response system challenge... consider the prevalent, yet barely understood condition of *Candida Albicans*. Normally present in small amounts, it is a mold, a fungus, found on the skin and mucous membranes along with many other microorganisms... they all help maintain balance. When growth increases drastically, it is devastating. In a healthy body, Candida is kept in check by friendly bacteria. Unfortunately, our modern lifestyle destroys large amounts of friendly bacteria, upsetting the delicate balance of Mother Nature, allowing Candida to flourish. Candida thrives on sugars and refined carbohydrates such as white flour and white rice; Candida also has a penchant for moldy foods such as bleu cheese... and fermented foods such as beer, wine, pickles and vinegar. In a word, Candida relishes an acid environment created by refined, processed foods, and all animal foods. Over-acidity can have mental and emotional contributing factors in addition to dietary, so identify and root out frustration, anger, resentment, at home and work.

Besides muscle testing or the pendulum, we can easily observe Candida out of balance with the Spit Test. Awakening in the morning, before getting up, gather whatever is in the mouth and spit into a glass of water, that has been waiting at the bedside. If it floats, all is well. If it sinks a bit and then floats... or if some bits dangle much like a jellyfish... watch Your diet and frequently monitor morning mucus. If all or any portion sinks it is time to take action. Check the glass every 15 minutes. Usually after an hour floating spit dissolves.

As Candida fungus multiplies, so do their waste products... and they enter the bloodstream... wreaking havoc with the immune and nervous systems... with cravings for foods Candida thrives on: sugars, chocolate, alcohol, etc. The wide variety of symptoms includes: allergies, bloating, constipation, diaper rash, diarrhea, earaches, excess weight, fatigue, food sensitivity, gas, headaches, irritability, numbness, obesity, PMS, vaginal infections, as well as mental and emotional situations: memory challenges, irrational or unclear thinking, inordinate crying, depression, being easily upset, even suicidal tendencies.

Living out of balance with sweets and alcohol... living in the fast lane... consuming drugs habitually – to get us going and help us sleep – is it any wonder we are in such a sad state of affairs... spending >3 billion annually on the over-consumption of OTC drugs alone! Over 75m Americans take one or more prescription drugs every day! Through the media, we are programmed and led to believe depression is a Prozac deficiency, headache a Darvon deficiency, and osteoporosis a Tums deficiency. Most drugs and all antibiotics result in the wild growth of competitive yeast organisms. Antibiotics actually prepare a feast for the yeast – the dead and attenuated toxic bacteria, as well as the friendly bacteria killed by the antibiotics – providing a smorgasbord for them to enjoy.

Progesterone in birth control pills nourishes yeast, as do: laxatives – causing Vit D and calcium deficiency; mineral oil – reducing absorption of fat-soluble vitamins, ADEK; and antacids – which also depletes calcium levels and reduces B12 absorption.

Some people keep Candida in check by dietary habits. Guidelines include avoiding all refined, processed foods. Refined carbohydrates convert to sugar, and excess sugar is stored as fat. Avoid canned and dried foods, sugars, processed cereals, and all animal foods... especially pasteurized dairy products. Avoid all fruits... high sugar vegetables such as corn, lima beans, okra, peas and potatoes... as well as beets and carrots. Avoid all fermented foods except raw, enzyme-rich Sauerkraut or Kimchee; 1 tsp/meal is allowed.

Balance can be restored with full-spectrum pro-biotics, coconut oil, fermented foods – rich in friendly bacteria, green vegetable juices – leafy greens, broccoli stems, celery, cucumber, parsley, string beans and zucchini, eating sprouts and vegetables as well as germinated nuts and seeds. Making these dietary / lifestyle adjustments, and as the spit test shows improvement, eat sparingly of germinated alkaline grains high in protein: quinoa and amaranth. If conditions persist or if from deeply-rooted emotions... homeopathy can help.

The Homeopathic Treatment for Yeast

The process is simple... the prescription is complex. The first thing to ascertain is the set of symptoms, primarily mental symptoms. If mental symptoms are abundant and forceful, we could base our remedy on those factors alone – anxieties, aversions, cravings, desires, dreams, fears, neurotic, and psychotic behavior patterns. Thus, we see the complete picture.

In the absence of mental symptoms, we must look at the physical. Some symptoms are generic and can apply to various conditions; some contradictory such as bouts of constipation and diarrhea... look at all symptoms before drawing conclusions.

As with all homeopathic remedies, keep the mouth free from other tastes 15 min before and after taking them. With more than one remedy – keep them 15 minutes apart. If symptoms recur, the person didn't take the remedy for the whole 4 weeks; repeat for 1 week.

Prevent contamination: tip the globules or tablets into the cap or a plastic spoon which is inert – having neither a negative nor positive charge; if using the cap, keep it away from Your lips when placing them under the tongue, where they can dissolve. When taking liquid remedies, add the drops to 1oz distilled or r/o water; savor a moment before swallowing.

Kept in a cool, dark place away from strong smelling substances and chemicals... the remedies remain effective for years – much like the seeds from the pyramids that sprouted... and grew.

Classical homeopathy considers mental and emotional challenges as the primary, most profound clues. Otherwise, we play detective. What are the symptoms? If the yeast is in the G-I tract, look at specifics.

If in the mouth with a white, fungal, thrush-like growth... the mouth being hot and tender... if the mouth tastes like cellar mold or has a bitter taste – also if a child cries during nursing, or an animal has problems eating – *Borax* 6X, 3x/day for 4 weeks.

If in the throat with tonsillitis, especially when it changes from side to side quickly, or diphtheria-like symptoms, tonsils appearing glazed and shiny, or the appearance of a deposit, pearly white like porcelain – *Lac caninum* 30C, 3x/day for 4 weeks.

If in the stomach with a burning sensation from mouth to stomach, accompanied by a thirst for small amounts of water taken frequently, food allergies that result in diarrhea – *Arsenicum album* 30C, 3x/day for 4 weeks.

If in the stomach where only a little food – especially starch and sugar – creates a bloated feeling... or fullness with burning and belching – *Lycopodium* 200C, take only once, or only as required, a characteristic unique to this particular remedy. Or *Lycopodium* 30C or 1M, 3x/day for 4 weeks.

If in the stomach where digestion is slow and food putrefies before it digests, where even the simplest food distresses; if there is a weak pulse and the person hates heat and wants a fan, even on a cool day; if the person feels relief by passing gas or belching – *Carbo vegitabilis* 30C, 3x/day for 4 weeks.

If in the stomach with flatulence, belching with a bitter taste... or no relief from passing gas or belching – *China officinalis* aka *Cinchona* 30C, 3x/day 4 weeks.

If in the intestines where there may be pain or burning... a slimy stool that may be whitish or gray... where the person likes cold water... where bad breath fills the room (the GI tract still may be stressed from antibiotics) – *Mercurius sol* aka *Mercurius vivus* 30C liquid, 10 drops in an ounce of water, 3x/day 4 weeks.

If in the intestines where constipation and diarrhea alternate... where there is frequent ineffectual urging... where there is bad breath, especially after a meal... where the person gets up in the morning feeling unrested with a headache or constipation... or gets up in the morning and feels fatigued all day with diarrhea – *Nux vomica* 30C, 3x/day for 4 weeks.

If in the intestines where chronic constipation leads to hemorrhoids – *Nux vomica*, 30C at bedtime and *Sulphur* 30C when getting up... for 3 months.

In the ears for the first time – *Hepar sulphuris* 30C, 3x/day for four weeks; if it persists, *Hepar sulph* 200C, 3x/day for four weeks; if it still persists – *Tuberculinum* 200C, 3x/day for 2 weeks.

In the ears recurrently – use *Tuberculinum* 200C, 3x/day for two weeks; if it still persists – *Graphites* 30C, 3x/day for 4 weeks.

So here we have one condition... Candida albicans... and a dozen remedies depending on symptoms. There are 1000s of homeopathic remedies; completely safe, free from side effects, non-addicting, safe for babies, children, when pregnant, the elderly, and all types of animals. As always, proper diet... probiotics, enzymes and whole superfoods... regular exercise... adequate re-mineralized and re-energized distilled or r/o water... and sleep... enhance the immune response.

Immune response system Booster – *Hydrastis* ... Mother Tincture, 10 drops in ½ glass of re-mineralized, re-energized or r/o water, 3x/day. This may be taken alone or alternated with any of the above, keeping them apart by 15 minutes. While an effective use of homeopathic Goldenseal... it is usually recommended to use the *herbal* form as well as herbal echinacea for a couple of weeks... and then take a couple of weeks off, to strengthen Your immune response system.

Many homeopathic remedies are combinations dealing with general symptoms: *cold extremities* or *runny nose*. They contain 4 or 5 remedies... hoping, with this shotgun approach, one will hit the target. Classical homeopathy takes an extensive case history, including emotional and mental trauma, and physical symptoms.

In lieu of a classical homeopath... if time is a factor... until You put together the case history... this palliative has been used successfully over the years:

Arising: *Sulphur* 30C

Mid-day: *Calcarea Carbonica* 30C

Bedtime: *Nux Vomica* 30C

Following the admonition of Hippocrates: *primum non nocere* – first do no harm – homeopathy is free from allergies, complications and side effects. With normal usage, it is impossible to hurt anyone; it either works... or another remedy is appropriate. Symptoms may intensify during the first few days – a wonderful, positive sign – merely a cleansing reaction; keep up the remedy, watch symptoms disappear. Cleansing may then go to a deeper level: the feeling body, the thinking body, or the spirit body. Use the appropriate homeopathic remedy.

There are homeopathic crèmes for specific purposes. Any injury, especially with bruises, will benefit using Arnica crème, along with Arnica pellets 10X or 30C, whatever is available. However, if the skin is *broken*, use Calendula crème with the Arnica pellets.

Proper diet and Holistic Lifestyles: Probiotics, Algae, Enzymes, Living Foods discussed elsewhere are guaranteed to enhance the cleansing at all levels of HeartMindBodySpirit.

To facilitate Your explorations:
Homeopathic Materia Medica, W. Boericke, MD
Repertory of Homeopathic Materia Medica, J.T. Kent, MD
The Complete Book of Homeopathy, Dr Michael Weiner
A Dictionary of Homeopathic Terminology, Jay Yasgur, R.Ph., M.Sc.
Dogs: Homeopathic Remedies, George McLeod, MRCVS
Homeopathic Medicine at Home, M.B. Panos, MD and Jane Heimlich
Homeopathy Medicine of the New Man, George Vithoulkas
The Prescriber, John H. Clarke, MD
J A Satti, PhD: http://www.nanopathy.com/

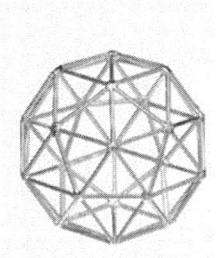

10 – ENERGY MEDICINE FOR DAILY LIVING

Rather than tell me
what kind of disease a person has,
tell me what kind of person has a disease.
-Hippocrates

There are no incurable diseases...
only incurable people.
-Dr Bernie Siegel

Abundance Affirmations

I *Am* & You *Are* Pure Awareness in this world of polarity exploring human consciousness. The Divine explores through us regardless of what we think, or others say. If we allow ourselves... if we *feel* we truly deserve it... we are A-Bun-Dance personified. Many are wealthy, yet unhappy; others happy, yet financially challenged.

You Possess Free Will, You really *can* have it all. If You choose to win at the Money Game... be sure to clear Your money motivation. When driven by Ego, Your money is based on separation from the Divine – so, the richer You get, the lonelier and more spiritually impoverished You feel. Being spiritually bankrupt and materially wealthy is true Shakespearean tragedy. Panic-driven, survival-consciousness catches many in a vicious circle. Some people tally how much they give and how much they get, figure the difference and arrive at the balance of their emotional savings account. This choice promises anxiety and frustration.

Rather than relying on Ego... feeling separate from the Divine... Trust in the Infinite – the Divine Presence Sustaining All, that *is* all. Go within and feel Oneness. Be confident and Know that Success is Your birthright. The Book of Enoch says: Be still and know... I Am God! I Am the Source of Prosperity beyond mere money. In our own Divinity... we experience Peace and Love. We are able to give and receive freely, while experiencing complete harmony. As the Divine, we have eternal internal safety. While this may sometimes lack the superficial appearance of external security, it is ultimately wholesome and satisfying and brings Harmonious Healing for HeartMindBodySpirit as One. Internal safety is the optimal launching pad for external security. Placing trust in the Divine Self, we can explore consciousness and experience the Kingdom of Heaven within. You can have worldly goods *and* riches of the Spirit. Open Your mind to Infinite Possibilities. Open Your heart to Universal Love.

These affirmations are optimal with **Mirror Therapy**: looking deeply in Your eyes. Relax; focus with 3 deep, caressing breaths before and after doing affirmations. These may be recorded over a background of Nature Sounds, listened to while working, playing or sleeping. Affirmations produce major miracles in Life *only* when *felt* in Your heart. Whether speaking or recording affirmations, say them – with *feelings* – in the first, second and third person: using Your Name or Nick-name (N) – as though making an announcement!

~~~~~~

I Am so Blessed – fit & trim!

My glands and my organs are happy…
doing an excellent job keeping me healthy!

My Life continues to be One Blessing after anOther!

~~~~~~

You Are so Blessed – fit & trim!

Your glands and Your organs are happy…
doing an excellent job keeping You healthy!

Your Life continues to be One Blessing after anOther!

~~~~~~

(N) is so Blessed – fit & trim!

(N)'s glands and organs are happy…
doing an excellent job keeping (N) healthy!

(N)'s Life continues to be One Blessing after anOther!

~~~~~~

Perhaps this is the Ultimate Affirmation. It can apply to every situation affecting our intimate experience of HeartMindBodySpirit – as One. Affirmations *affirm* and *confirm* we *are* the Source of All – the Word made flesh. I Create as I Speak! I Create My Wish Fulfilled! Indeed, as pure Spirit having a physical experience, **each in our own way**… a radiant expression of Infinite Being – Pure Energy expressing and experiencing all shades of human consciousness. ABRACADABRA**!**

Doing affirmations in this manner engages Your thinking body as well as Your feeling body… stimulating Your subconscious to first accept… and then to create… Your New Reality. Affirmations are especially useful before bed and upon arising; these are the optimal times to approach Your subconscious. Use affirmations that truly excite You, resonating with Your HeartMindBodySpirit. Other examples follow:

{With Gratitude to The Light Center: Black Mountain, NC https://urlight.org/} The first seven affirmations are offered as a precursor for whatever final affirmation You may choose – as You set the stage for Your new Playbook… creating Your New Reality!

I release all of my past… negativities, fears, judging, human relationships, inner self, and future human desires… to the Light.
{Our highest potential can only be limited by ourselves. The first step in being abundant is to release all things that hold us back. With each challenge, we can repeat the above affirmation.}

I Am a Light Being.
{We have, in the past, thought and spoken negatively about ourselves. The time has come to boldly affirm the Truth: I *Am* a Being of Light and Love.}

I radiate the Light from my Light Center throughout my being.
{By radiating the Light from Your solar plexus throughout Your being… You begin to consciously raise the vibrational rate of every part of Your being – HeartMindBodySpirit.}

I radiate the Light from my Light Center to Everyone.
{The first 3 affirmations concentrate on self. In this affirmation, You begin to support others. Radiating the Light from Your Light Center to Everyone influences everyone's Light Center, bringing about an important evolution in Your life by supporting others, who are Other aspects of Divine Self.}

I radiate the Light from my Light Center to Everything.
{By radiating the Light from Your Light Center to the mineral, plant, animal and angelic kingdoms… You support these kingdoms in fulfilling their work – and they graciously and gratefully support You in return.}

178

I Am in a bubble of Light, and only Light can come to me, only Light can be here.
{With billions of us on Planet Earth, some are thinking negative thoughts and experiencing negative emotions which can influence *Your* thoughts and emotions; thus, the bubble of Light.}

Thank You Divine Self for everything.
Thank You Divine Self for everyone.
Thank You Divine Self for me.
{Being thankful for *all* that exists is essential to spiritual growth... which requires Gratitude for everything and for everyone – especially ourselves. Together we all comprise the full-spectrum of God's creation – which is, Infinite Being exploring Free Will along with Infinite Possibilities on the finite plane of human consciousness – with every possible choice from Brilliant Light to Dazzling Darkness.}

The ancients speak of creation as a glorious illusion known as Maya – One huge Leela – a Divine Play... a Divine Dance. It is up to each One to choose the part that is **exciting**. We Voice our Choice and with Free Will, we can change... we *can* choose differently... in a heartbeat. We are all *so* Blessed!

Having set the stage by affirming Your connection to All, with *feelings* of Love and Compassion... it is now time to proceed with an affirmation that gives "flesh and bones" to Your Wish Fulfilled – an affirmation that *can* create Your New Reality.

I recognize my negative programming, and I now choose... to <u>change</u> my Playbook. I Am Love and Compassion to all... including mySelf!

You recognize Your negative programming, and You now choose... to <u>change</u> Your Playbook. You Are Love and Compassion to all... including YourSelf!

(N) recognizes the negative programming, and now chooses to <u>change</u> the Playbook. (N) is Love and Compassion to all... including the Divine Self!

Smile at Yourself in the mirror... and know You are being Showered with Blessings on Your Sacred Journey – in Perfect Divine Order!

{For the Best Affirmation eVer, as well as using tools of technology, see below: **Relationships.**}

Acne
Anyone suffering from acne, take courage. The answer is simple. Microbes are normally present in our gut, in our biome... and on the skin as part of our defense system. *Corynebacterium acne* is one of many... and this particular microbe thrives **only** when oleic acid levels are unnaturally high. Frequent use of soap (an alkali) wipes out the colonies of acid-loving microbes and weakens our defense against unfriendly air-borne bacteria. The body immediately responds by secreting oil and oleic *acid* to feed the surviving microbial flora. Soap, in fact, compromises our immune response and **aggravates** acne. Rather than soap, use a loofa sponge, splash on apple cider vinegar, and use clay.

Witch Hazel water is one of the very best remedies. This natural astringent can help control acne by reducing inflammation, decreasing oil and redness. It can lessen bacteria growth on the skin while speeding up the healing of scars, scabs, and infection. After using Witch Hazel, apply a few drops of Coconut oil, which may be taken internally as well as externally to normalize *C. acne*, preventing and reducing redness or blemishes... and can soothe flare-ups with eczema and psoriasis as well. In time, acne will be history. (See Chapter 5: **Soap: Dirtier than Dirt**. See also below: **Diatomaceous Earth**)

Acquired Immune Defense Strategies (AIDS)
Stress suppresses the immune response system. Concentrating sympathetic nervous system energy on the "Freeze! Fight? or Flight?" mode leads to muscle tension, tightness, constriction and consequent aching. Repressed, suppressed and prolonged negative emotions inhibit our immune response system... as do anger, apathy, bitterness, depression, intense or prolonged loneliness, or grieving, and various levels of unconsciousness... which result in negative lifestyles.

Strategies to support our immune response can be as **simple as a *smile***. Living with tensions of a stressed immune response system, we tend to frown, wrinkling our eyebrows. Activating these muscles sends a message to the brain: **Trouble** – so the hypothalamus directs the pituitary and adrenals to produce hormones to respond to this negative state of affairs, and our body is saturated with negative, tension-filled juices geared for survival. A simple smile activates other muscle groups, sending another message to the brain: Life is wonderful – so the hypothalamus directs the pituitary and adrenals to produce hormones of happiness, and we are filled with positive, loving juices to rest, digest and rejuvenate.

A smile in slow moving traffic – can completely change Your perspective. It can lead to laughter – realizing how silly it is to be upset about external "reality" when the only true *Reality* is what we experience inside. This nourishes the immune response system. For someone, perhaps elderly, who seriously lacks the *strength* to smile, hold a pencil between the teeth at the back of the mouth – smiling is effortless, muscles activated, and hormones of happiness are released.

Norm Cousins, renowned editor of *Saturday Review*, says: Laughter is the best Medicine! In 1964 diagnosed with ankylosing spondylitis, destroying connective tissue and leading to spinal degeneration, doctors gave him a 1 in 500 chance of surviving, so he *fired them* and took charge of his own treatment. Replacing his painkillers with large doses of Vitamin C, he watched Candid Camera, the Marx Brothers and other "belly bouncers" as he calls them. He found that a few minutes of genuine laughter acted as an effective anesthetic, and provided a few hours of pain-free sleep; he said: "Laughter activates the fighting spirit!"

His book, *Anatomy of an Illness* – as perceived by the patient – turned heads in the medical community when parts were published in *The New England Journal of Medicine* in 1976. He went on to be an influential faculty member at UCLA School of Medicine before he passed in 1990. Laughter is the best medicine... along with a positive outlook, supported by a life-enhancing, empowering, Verbal Diet. Visualizations and affirmations offer positive re-enforcement.

Meditation is a powerful force maintaining positive energy within... keeping You centered through the rush of life. Maintain a meditative attitude of Gratitude in Your heart. Exercise and diet can do much to facilitate an improved immune response. In addition, important nutrition comes from enzymes and probiotics, Co-enzyme Q10 and AFA: Klamath Lake blue-green algae. {See below: **AFA**.}

Addictions

Drug use is epidemic in the West. Men addicts drink and use drugs to rebel; they feel caught; indeed, they are caught in the trap of drugs! Women addicts drink and use drugs to relieve depression; they also feel caught, indeed, they are caught in a vicious circle. Men and women alike drink and use drugs to forget their problems only to wake up with the same problems... and feeling even more rebellious and more depressed. Progress on the Road to Recovery is made with an understanding how our body, mind, and spirit function.

In *The Addictive Brain*, Gabriel Cousens, MD, explains that current research verifies what many have long suspected. There is a biologically altered brain from both genetic and environmental stress that predisposes a person to drug abuse. The biological effects of long-term drug abuse of alcohol also tend to mirror the biochemical effects of the gene defects that led to the predisposition. Irresistible craving is associated with a problem in the reward centers of the brain involving neurotransmitters and enzymes that control them. Hundreds of experiments suggest that the craving for alcohol, drugs and food are, to a major extent, the result of defects in the neuronal transmission systems in the mesolimbic area of the brain, the reward-pleasure centers in the brain. These abnormalities play a primary role in compulsive behavior disorders and addictions involving drugs, alcohol, and food... possibly sex and gambling addictions as well.

Poor nutrition – actually malnutrition – people get today with fast-foods, junk foods, high sugar diets, synthetic foods, foods with pesticides and herbicides... all serve to create the preconditions of a non-genetically, but altered brain neurochemistry of the addictive brain. There is a significant increase in hyperactivity today that can often be treated with proper nutritional supplements and organic whole-food, plant-based diets. The modern diet creates the environmental conditions that predispose children to developing the addictive brain neurochemistry and makes them susceptible to the plague of alcohol, psychoactive drugs, and other compulsive disorders. Through proper live-food nutrition and holistic lifestyles, we *can* repair most of these disrupted neurotransmitter pathways and repair the addictive brain... *if* the person is committed to rebuilding his or her life.

Optimal results are obtained if those involved in the healing process avoid nicotine, sugar and caffeine, avoiding the symptoms that act as a buildup to drinking or drug usage and at least a portion of the dry-drunk syndrome. Part of the cycle of repair is being aware of the overall nutritional deficiencies that develop from all sorts of drug use. One of the most obvious is the nutrient destruction caused by alcohol abuse. This loss of nutrients includes critical minerals: zinc, chromium, manganese, magnesium, calcium, copper, iron, and Vit B-complex. Deficiencies in these can alter the brain biochemistry and cause cravings and symptoms. The four key neurotransmitters disrupted are the serotonin system, GABA, glutamine and dopaminergic systems.

To restore neurotransmitters, avoid the addictive substances that destroy them and eat whole foods, as well as seaweed and microalgae from Klamath Lake... especially rich in neuropeptides – building blocks of neurotransmitters.

Addictions are usually associated with alcohol, caffeine (coffee, tea, cola and sugary commercial chocolate), OTC, prescription and street drugs, food, nicotine, sugar, or another substance, such as money. There are intangibles to consider as well: co-dependent relationships, gambling, media, shopping and sex being the major players... yet, 1st on the list is screen-time, with the device of Your choice discreetly at Your side! Addiction blocks our ability to experience Life's Joys and to achieve our potential as conscious individuals. Put devices "away" whenever possible.

We are meant to function as energetic, happy, healthy, independent, joyous spiritual beings resonating with the Source of All. Anything less than this glorious experience of Life throws us into a state of disharmony marked by confusion and conflict leading to anger, boredom, depression, failure, fear, guilt, poor self-esteem, sadness and self-destructive lifestyle. These experiences wear down the immune response system... opening doors for dys-function, dis-ease, degeneration and death – first the spirit, then the mind, the emotions, and then the body.

We have Choice. We can play "poor me" looking for sympathy. We can sigh, "This is the hand Life dealt me... what can I do, but play it?" We can even throw our hand in and get, hopefully, better cards. Wilson W. Wilson once quipped: "If You place a small value on Yourself, the rest of the world will not raise the price!" Stand up for Your limitations, and You shall own them.

Ask questions... create other choices. What is it about this situation that I have yet to understand? How can this situation benefit all concerned? What else is possible? With the support of others in healthy inter-dependent relationships, we can stand up and choose Life with confidence and enthusiasm.

To deal with cravings and mood swings as we shift from varying degrees of unconsciousness to a conscious, loving experience of Who we are and what Life is about: Go Within. Jung says, "Who looks without, dreams; who looks within, awakens." To permanently heal, releasing addictions and co-dependent behavior, requires openness and honesty to recognize the factors that created our current situation. Once identified, we can accept, understand and release them knowing they are experiences for our growth and spiritual development.

First change our thoughts as well as our food and drink. Creating our Verbal Diet is as crucial, as sound nutrition. Energy work is supportive. Life is a process of learning and we are given growth opportunities assisting evolution to higher states of consciousness. Addictions are growth opportunities presenting us with choices. We can choose to be disempowered... either a martyr or a victim. We can also choose the Path of Healing and function with optimum energy as we connect with High Self... True Self, recognizing we are One with the Universe, One with Love. With Free Will and Choice... we explore.

To recognize our addictions is to recognize our choices. We can stay in the darkness of unconsciousness or turn toward the Light and Love that beckons us to Awareness of Who We Are. Our immune response system, our whole Being yearns for the experience of... and the expression of pure Universal Love. The only way for any of us to create Love is to give it away... to be open channels of Light. *Healing and Recovery* by David Hawkins, MD, PhD is a wise choice to facilitate transmutation of addictions.

AFA: Aphanizomenon flos-aquae

May 18, 1980; Mount St. Helen's erupted with a force that was calculated to equal 1,500 Hiroshima-size bombs. Over one and a half cubic miles of rock were blown across the Washington countryside, lowering the peak by 1300 feet! The blast was heard 200 miles away and volcanic ash, rich in minerals, was blown over an area, from Canada to the Mississippi River. Newspaper reports expressed concern about the loss of cropland and forests buried in ash. Then, a few years later, articles appeared detailing how fast the forests were returning, plants popping up, streams revitalized, and nearby farmers delighted with crop output from the power of paramagnetic (volcanic) ash.

17,000 years ago... Mount Mazama erupted and rocked the northern hemisphere sending volcanic ash over an even wider area. A 150 lb rock was found 450 miles away in Idaho. This eruption left Crater Lake, tremendously rich in minerals and trace elements. 17 volcanic streams and rivers feed Upper Klamath Lake, rich in *Aphanizomenon flos-aquae* which means: invisible-flower-of-the-water – known as AFA or Aphan; arguably the world's most perfect food, it is manna from the heart of the earth with an amino acid ratio virtually identical to human milk with all the essential fatty acids. The algae grow according to Mother Nature's specifications; to address concerns: we cannot over-harvest these algae causing extinction. As more algae are harvested, the remaining algae rejoice and reproduce vigorously. A win-win for the algae... and for algae eaters who know minerals are essential for optimal health.

We can consider net protein utilization (NPU) as an index of how well amino acids can be assimilated by humans. Red meat is approximately 19% protein and has an NPU of approximately 60%. Since it is only 67% digestible, this means 100g of sirloin nets about 13g of usable protein. In the algae family, chlorella has 20% NPU, spirulina has 37%, and AFA or Klamath Lake blue-green algae, has 75% with virtually 100% digestibility. These vital amino acids are used during times of stress and disease.

One interesting difference between Spirulina and AFA can be traced to one fact: Spirulina is tropical algae... AFA is a heartier cold-climate species. In the warmer climates of the tropics, the membrane of a Spirulina cell can easily maintain its flexibility by producing a rather high percent of saturated fatty acids. AFA algae, on the other hand, are far from tropical luxury. The colder climate of Upper Klamath Lake forces AFA's cell membrane enzymes to compensate by ingeniously manufacturing poly-*unsaturated* fatty acids (PUFAs) that enhance their life-sustaining membrane flexibility. To be sure both forms of algae are blessed with a rich array of phytochemical antioxidants such as carotenes. Although Spirulina contains slightly more beta-carotene than AFA algae, one must be careful to take a more educated look. The presence of more PUFAs allows for wider variety of other carotenoids – such as alpha and gamma carotene – to be spread out within the cell membrane itself. The true healing power of beta-carotene can be fully realized along with a variety of other structurally related carotenoid compounds.

Carotenoid compounds in all forms of blue green algae are also particularly sensitive to the type of harvesting techniques employed. The sun-drying and spray-drying techniques often used in processing Spirulina invariably cause a marked decrease in beta-carotene as well as the concentration of methionine, which is a sulfur-containing essential amino acid. Prof. Karl J. Abrams has a more complete scientific explanation for those interested: *Algae to the Rescue: Everything You Need to Know about Nutritional Blue-Green Algae.*

In a double-blind, cross-over study performed at the Royal Victoria Hospital in Montreal (Manoukian, 1998) it was discovered that, unlike anything else *ever* tested... Klamath Lake blue green algae triggered the migration of 40% (nearly 1 billion) of the circulating Natural Killer (NK) cells from blood to tissue within 2 hours of consumption; obviously playing an important role in the immune response system. They are mainly responsible for the detection and removal of sick cells altered either due to malignant transformation or viral infection. When infected by a virus, or when a cell becomes cancerous, it produces a chemical message on the external surface of its membrane recognized by the immune response system. In effect it says, "Hey, I'm infected; either kill me or I will damage other cells around me." When NK cells detect these messages on infected cells, they move forward and eliminate them.

Eating these algae also triggered a 2- to 4-fold increase in the expression of adhesion molecules on the surface of the circulating NK cells. Adhesion molecules allow NK cells to adhere to the capillary wall and migrate out of blood circulation to wherever the sick cells are. To be successful, the immune response system requires killer cells that are active and can travel. To prevent the development of cancer or the spreading of viral infections like colds and flu, NK cells must migrate from the blood so they can provide effective immune patrolling of all tissues. Many substances are known to improve the *activity* of NK cells, such as green tea and Gingko biloba. Until this study using Klamath Lake blue green algae, no substance... not even pharmaceutical ones... were known to stimulate NK cells to *migrate* into the tissues to search and destroy sick cells.

This recent research, therefore, suggests that eating *Aphanizomenon flos-aquae* daily may stimulate the immune response system to help prevent cancer and illness associated with viral infections. In fact, much evidence already exists suggesting that blue green algae contain high concentrations of chlorophyll, phycocyanin and beta-carotene, and may play a valuable role in any cancer prevention program. Other recent research indicates AFA helps stimulate the increased production of red blood cells, an effect that may be due to its high content of B12; it may also help in reducing cholesterol, eliminating abnormal intestinal permeability as measured with the lactulose / mannitol test; and another study suggests AFA stimulates specific areas of the brain, supporting prolific reports of increased mental alertness. Enjoy: *Primordial Food: Aphanizomenon flos-aquae* by Christian Drapeau.

While commercial foods are rich in a handful of vitamins and minerals; organic foods are rich in only a few dozen; algae provide the 60+ nutrients our bodies require. Optimal nutrition is in seaweed, which are *macro*algae, growing in a pH of 8+ and the *micro*algae found in Klamath Lake, AFA, which grow in a pH of 9-10. Most AFA available is freeze-dried. 21st century technology with refractance window drying (RWD) takes place in the middle of the lake; in the sunlight, the dried algae look like sparkling sapphires and emeralds! RWD Klamath Lake algae is available by the pound for economy: www.algaeworld.com

Aloha! = alo Ha!
While Aloha is filled with various shades of meaning… the literal translation **alo** means being in the presence of **Ha**, the Breath of Life. The very word beckons one to follow the advice found in The Book of Enoch: "Be still… and know… I Am God!" Get out in the peace and quiet of Nature, in *meditation*… come to reconciliation first with true Self, then family, then with society.

Hawaiians recognize and honor Nature. Reflecting this in their culture when giving directions, they often say, go mauka… or go makai. Go mauka simply means – turn toward the mountain. Go makai – turn toward the sea. Hawaiians honor both of these special places in Nature where You can experience Your true Self and… possibly Ho'oponopono… to make things right once again… to *reconcile*, particularly after wrong-doing, or after neglecting one's obligations.

Ho'oponopono recognizes the powerful energies of Repentance, Forgiveness, Gratitude and Love. To make things right once again, with deep feelings in Your Heart… say those four words and meditate on their vibrations… one at a time… either out loud, or simply in Your head. The power is in the *feeling* and in the willingness to forgive and love. God *is* Love! https://www.laughteronlineuniversity.com/hooponopono-4-simple-steps/

Alzheimer's, Aluminum, Mercury & Other Heavy Metals
Several independent, international studies show that aluminum, rather than being a cause of Alzheimer's accumulates in the brain *because* of the disease. Aluminum is also present in Down's Syndrome. Aluminum is found in antacids, anti-perspirants, cooking utensils, cosmetics, deodorants and pharmaceuticals. When foods are highly acidic, as tomato-based or dairy-based sauces and soups or highly acidic liquids, whether soda, beer, wine or fruit juice… aluminum migrates *into* the food and drink – a process known as adsorption!

Studies also show mercury, rather than being the cause, accumulates on degenerating brain cells. The principal sources are amalgam fillings: mostly mercury and silver, contaminated waters and fish. British scientists have (ab)used sheep, drilling their perfectly good teeth and placing a few amalgam fillings; two years later, the sheep were found to have mercury in their brains and kidneys!

Conscious eating assists the liver in the detox process, especially Vitamin C, garlic, and seaweed, as well as microalgae from Klamath Lake. Prevent Alzheimer's with a pure diet avoiding aluminum and mercury; if these are found in hair tissue analysis, use homeopathic *Alumina* or *Mercurius*. Use 30C 3x/day for 2 weeks; then 200C once every morning for 2 weeks; then 1M every third day for 2 weeks. For arsenic detox use *Arsenicum album*; for cadmium: *Cadmium*; and for lead: *Plumbum* – with the same protocol. Consult *Materia Medica with Repertory*, by William Boericke, MD; look up the individual remedy… and read: Relationships to fine-tune the approach.

Alzheimer's studies incriminate estrogen. In addition to avoiding animal foods, especially dairy, it is wise to wear natural fibers, organic when possible, avoiding polyester like the plague – it contributes to many diseases. (See below: **Estrogenic Pesticides**.)

Angel Interventions

Often our Healing Journey involves people who are out of touch – physically, emotionally, mentally or spiritually. As an example, someone may have old issues yet to be resolved with a person who has passed on... moved to an unknown location, is belligerent, or incommunicado. With such a situation, write a letter to Your Guardian Angel and the other person's Guardian Angel. In the letter, relate the circumstances explaining why You seem to be at an impasse. Thank the Angels for working together, resolving things at another level. Sleep on it for a couple of days... read it again... having made any changes... re-write the letter with Your finest handwriting on quality paper. Keep the paper close to bed. Read it for 30 days before going to bed, and when You wake. At the end of 30 days, surround Yourself with Love and Light; standing at the sink, hold the bottom corner of the paper diagonally and light the top edges, letting the flame consume the sheet from above. When the ashes fall in the sink... wash them down the drain, along with the negativity. Thank Your Angels. It is amazing how things can change as You focus with Intention on Your Healing Journey.

The four Archangels have a specific Service: Gabriel – strength, Michael – compassion, Raphael – healing, Uriel – light. To explore Angels: *The Physics of Angels: Exploring the Realm Where Science and Spirit Meet*, by Matthew Fox and Rupert Sheldrake, 1996.

Animalia

To facilitate our understanding of who we are in the Grand Scheme of Things, possibly to help determine the optimal diet, human beings are classified as *Animalia* – animals; *Chordata* – having a notochord and a nervous system; *Vertebrata* – hard, bony vertebrae; *Mammalia* – nursing their young. The classifications of Mammals are as follows: *Artiodactyla* having an even number of toes – camels, cattle, deer, goats, hippopotami, pigs; *Carnivora* flesh eaters – bears, cats, dogs; *Cetacea* water mammals – dolphins, porpoises, whales; *Chiroptera* literally: hand-wings – bats; *Insectivora* insect eaters – hedgehogs, moles, shrews; *Marsupialia* nursing their young in a pouch – bandicoots, kangaroos, koala, opossums, wombats; *Perissodactyla* having an odd number of toes – horses, rhinoceroses, tapirs; *Primata* the first, the highest in the order of things – apes, humans, lemurs, monkeys, tarsiers; *Proboscidea* literally: to feed in front, having a long flexible snout – elephants, mammoths, mastodons; *Rodentia* those who gnaw – beavers, mice, rats, squirrels.

Among these classifications of mammals – those who nurse their young – only *one* thrives as flesh-eaters: Carnivora; one primate, tarsiers eat insects, as do the Insectivora and Chiroptera, although some bats are strict fruitarians. Some Rodentia, such as rats, are omnivores yet most eat nuts, grains and roots when plentiful – all the rest are herbivores, vegetarians.

Anthroposophy

In the meetings of the Anthroposophical Society
a great truth can be experienced.
When human beings meet together
seeking the Spirit with unity of purpose,
then they also find their way to each other –
they find the path from soul to soul.
—Rudolph Steiner

Since Steiner re-founded the Anthroposophical Society, many people mistakenly think he had coined the word. Actually, Thomas Vaughan first used the word in 1650. He allied himself with the Rosicrucian movement and translated its primary documents into English. Vaughan, under the pen name Eugenius Philalethes, wrote a short work: *Anthroposophia Theomagica: A Discourse on the Nature of Man and His State after Death* that considered "human nature in the light of divine wisdom." This 17th century source, with alchemical and Neo-platonic overtones, allows us to conjecture. *Anthroposophy* is a reference to Hermetic cosmology – the science of subtle states mediating between the divine and earthly realms. The 19th century idealist philosophers Schelling and Fichte, Swiss holistic physician Ignaz Troxler, and Viennese philosopher Robert Zimmermann, all wrote about Anthroposophy. As a young man, Rudolph Steiner was influenced by lectures of Robert Zimmermann at the University of Vienna, and was inspired to investigate Goethe, which transformed his life and teachings.

Theosophy means the wisdom of God. Anthroposophy means the wisdom of the human being. Anthroposophy is a form of human self-knowledge that unites science, art and religion – or as expressed in the motto of Waldorf schools: it unites "Head, Hands and Heart." As we develop cognitive feeling, a thinking heart – we connect the spiritual in humans with the spiritual in the universe.

For the serious student of anthroposophy, four basic works of Rudolph Steiner are recommended: *Theosophy, The Philosophy of Freedom, Knowledge of the Higher Worlds and its Attainment* and *An Outline of Esoteric Science*. As an introduction: *What is Anthroposophy: 3 Perspectives on Self-Knowledge*, also by RS. https://www.rsarchive.org/ You may also like to explore https://neoanthroposophy.com

Antioxidants: Anti-aging

Vitamins A, C, E, and minerals like selenium and zinc are well-known antioxidants. Beta-carotene is also famous. Research showing beta-carotene causes breast cancer used ***synthetic*** beta-carotene. Found in whole-foods like the algae, it is present with the other dozen or so carotenoids; they synergistically clean up free radicals. We learn from such studies that isolated and synthetic extracts are a burden on the body. Use wild, whole superfoods: seaweed and microalgae.

All herbs have antioxidant qualities. Special mention may be made of echinacea, gingko biloba and milk thistle. Culinary herbs: dried alfalfa leaves, allspice, anise, basil, black pepper, capsicum, caraway, celery seed, chili peppers, cloves, cumin, garlic, ginger, lemon balm, lemon grass, licorice, mace, marjoram, nutmeg, oregano, rosemary, sage, thyme are all beneficial – especially the last four, members of the mint family. These are easy to grow, even indoors in front of a sunny window.

Whether as a preventive or a response to a situation, it is crucial to build our natural defense system with probiotics, acidophilus and bifidus for the intestines… with Co-Q10 for the heart and liver. Especially with cooked food, plant-based enzymes that tolerate a broad spectrum of pH are equally important, as are adequate re-mineralized and re-energized distilled or r/o water, exercise, and rest. With any great recipe… the real secret is the Love put into it. Let love flow in a special, intimate relationship as well. Express Your love, appreciation and gratitude verbally, and by massaging each other's feet, holding, caressing, hugging and kissing… a wonderful preparation for sacred sexual union – the ultimate experience to build the immune response system and keep us forever young.

Arthritis: Causes and Relief from Pain

The root causes of chronic pain and inflammation are lack of enzymes and lack of free electrons. The Earth has an abundant source of the latter. All we have to do is make contact. Originally, humans walked with bare feet; then once our ancestors learned to cure animal skins and make leather, their crude moccasins segued into various forms of footwear that always allowed continued contact with Earth's energies. While leather is not a conductive material, the moisture from our feet makes it so. Although free electrons are plentiful, modern shoes insulate us from Earth's energies. There is an answer. Get Your bare feet on the ground… simply sit with feet on the ground and be one with the sounds of Nature, a glorious time and space to meditate; or lie down on a natural fiber sheet – polyester blocks the flow of Earth's energy, as well as modern footwear with synthetic soles. For inclement weather, see below: **Grounding**.

Diet also aggravates various forms of inflammation. The nightshade family is notorious, especially cooked. This includes eggplant, tomatoes, all peppers, all potatoes, except yams and sweet potatoes, as well as *tobacco*. The way to know for sure is to avoid them for a month and then start using them again, paying attention to what You feel. All nightshades contain a certain amount of *nicotine* which is why they are so addictive. Explore: https://www.westonaprice.org/

Citrus as well as dairy aggravate certain forms of arthritis. Some can tolerate orange juice if it is picked ripe and freshly squeezed, rather than picked green for shipping and/or pasteurized for bottling, canning or freezing. Ripe, fresh squeezed provides citric acid, and when digested properly it has a positive, cleansing effect on our body – actually adding *alkaline* minerals to our reserve. Proper digestion of fresh squeezed orange juice means it is taken alone, or at a fruit meal with sour fruits – like kiwi.

The real benefit of juice is enzymes… active in *freshly* juiced fruits and vegetables. If bottled, assume it's been cooked with all vitality and enzymes destroyed, unless it is in the refrigerated section and is stocked daily by a local company.

If juice can sit on the shelf, it makes sense to leave it there. Juices high in natural sodium are beneficial for someone with arthritis: celery, cucumber, green beans, parsley, spinach, zucchini… with a piece of ginger root.

Without the convenience of a juicer, blend well and strain out the pulp; squeeze out the vital nutrients in a mesh bag held over a bowl. Some of the juice absorbs through the skin. You can soak aching hands in this juice for a few minutes, or Epsom salts or baking soda.

The pains of arthritis originate from inorganic minerals and acidic build-up in the body, the primary source being animal foods, especially dairy, refined foods such as white flour, white rice, sugary processed and fried foods. Eliminate these for 30 days; feel the difference. Since achy tissues are saturated with acids, the natural solution – add 2 lbs Epsom salts and 2 lbs baking soda to a tub of warm water and soak for a while. Chemical solutions seek equilibrium. The skin acts as an osmotic membrane and the alkaline solution draws acids from the body… relieving aches and pain.

For over-acid conditions, indicated by pain, some find relief by taking 1Tsp unpasteurized, organic apple cider vinegar in a glass of warm water on an empty stomach am & pm. Avoid apple cider vinegar or lemon juice with starchy foods: sour tastes interfere with production of ptyalin and amylase.

For painful joints, dissolve as much Epsom salts as You can in a few ounces of warm water. Add and stir, until it no longer dissolves and just sits in the bottom of the bowl: a super-saturated solution. Dip a tea towel or kitchen towel in the solution to absorb it. Then fold the towel lengthwise in thirds, using the residual salt; wrap around the knee, or aching joint. Pin it in place. To protect the bed from wetness, cover with plastic cling wrap. Keep it on all night. Do this for a few nights and see the difference. In the morning, unwrapping the towel, splash vinegar on the aching joint; this vinegar splash also works well with varicose veins, providing relief. 1Tbs apple cider vinegar in a glass of water upon arising, before meals and before bed is often helpful. Always use good quality acv, indicated by a brownish ring at the bottom of the bottle – called the "mother".

Ayurveda

The ancient medical system of India is their philosophy of life, or Life Knowledge – Ayurveda – offering keys for harmony and balance. The ayurvedic physician studies 5 years and is supervised 1 in the hospital. Although some spas in the US are designed as ayurvedic medical centers, most spas neglect the treatment of disease. Instead, they adopt elements of Ayurveda that focus on positive lifestyle choices, general detoxification, relaxation, enhanced spiritual awareness, and gentle exercise. Ayurvedic massage called panchakarma is one part of the traditional detoxification and rejuvenation program of India, in which the entire body is vigorously massaged with large amounts of warm oil and herbs removing toxins from the system. With permission, oil is also poured into the ears, between the eyebrows and at specific energy points, to maximize benefits.

The *Vedas*, meaning: Knowledge, are several ancient scriptures. There is an ancient Hindu medical treatise – sometimes called the Fifth Veda – that is known as *Ayurveda*: Life Knowledge, or the Science of Life. Early physicians, such as Hippocrates studied Ayurveda.

Ayurveda also has herbal extracts in a non-alcohol base, in powder, tablets or vegetarian capsules, both individually, and formulations from antiquity. An example is Vit C: the common type is from ascorbic acid, or ascorbates added directly to a natural base of acerola or other materials. Another type is called "food grown" where the ascorbic acid or ascorbates are added to a medium such as yeast, allowing a label claim of "food grown" or "natural source" – reality, the Vit C is added indirectly; the label is misleading. Naturally occurring Vit C comes from the whole natural nutrient concentrate material itself, free from synthetic ascorbic acid or any other ascorbate.

The Ayurvedic Amla-C is made from fresh, organic whole fruit – Himalayan Amla (*Emblica officinalis*) reputably the highest known naturally occurring Vit C of any edible fruit in the world. Camu-camu (*Myrciaria dubia*) found in the Amazon rainforest, runs a close second. Since both are from a whole food source, they contain the complete family of bioflavonoids – as do the white insides of juiced citrus, best eaten rather than discarded, by scraping the insides of the rind with a spoon for an extra bioflavonoid boost.

B-12

B12, rather than a vitamin is a bacterium, a group of cobalt-containing compounds called cobalamins: 5-deoxyadenosylcobalamin (also known as adenosyl cobalamin) and methylcobalamin – coenzyme forms of B12 found in human metabolism. Vit B12 plays a role in DNA synthesis, red blood cell formation, and in both the nervous system and immune response system.

Some feel meat is necessary for iron as well as B12. (See below: **Iron Efficiency**) Meat-eaters, however, are the **majority** of people with pernicious anemia, or B12 deficiency!

Since B12 is a bacterium – rather than a true member of the Vit B family – it is tricky. Once believed sea vegetables and certain cultured or fermented foods, such as tempeh and miso, were sources of B12... some of these contain what are called B12 analogs. These are B12-like compounds that have no vitamin activity and could actually compete with real B12 for absorption. Therefore, relying on these foods for B12 might increase a vegan's risk for deficiency. Indeed, humans may produce B12 from bacteria found in the large intestine, the first 1/3 of which reabsorbs water and, hopefully, some B12. Unfortunately, B12 is absorbed in the small intestine much higher up, rendering the B12 from the colon mostly unusable. B12 gets into the organs and muscles of ruminants because B12 is created from bacteria fermenting in their stomachs, and absorbed in their small intestines.

The easy way to add B12 to the diet is with a supplement. Vegans enjoy soil-based micro-organisms and can also use fortified foods. Cereals, meat analogs, and plant milk alternatives enriched with B12 are popular sources, as are certain brands of nutritional yeast, such as Red Star Vegetarian Support Formula. B12 used to fortify these foods is obtained from bacterial cultures, rather than animal products, and is vegan. Sub-lingual B12 is best.

Some nutrients come from sunlight (photosynthesis = chlorophyll) and some nutrients comes from the air. Traces of B12 may be found on *unwashed* greens, including wheatgrass and barleygrass. Going out to Your Garden of Eatin' pick salad greens and simply brush off any organic soil with Your fingers; when buying at the store simply inspect for critters. Rinsing greens washes away the B12 that may be present – such as "pre-washed" spinach! Enjoy Your meal!

Interestingly enough, human feces has significant B12. A study showed a group of Iranian vegans obtained adequate B12 from unwashed vegetables fertilized with human manure! Such fertilization of vegetables and other plant foods make a significant contribution to dietary needs, particularly in areas where hygiene standards are different from ours. This may be responsible for the lack of anemia from B12 deficiency in vegan communities found in developing countries as well as in China. (See below: **Vegetarian Power**.)

Babies on a Conscious Diet
The optimal food for any baby is Mother's milk, presuming the mother had nutritional consciousness during gestation. The first few days are crucial for bonding and to impart important immune factors in the colostrum. Nurse as long as possible. For the first few days, nurse the baby uncovered... out in the sun. This efficiently deals with the normal jaundice that comes after the first few days of life – while the liver learns how to re-cycle hemoglobin. Alfalfa sprouts make the milk sweet... fennel juice or fennel tea makes milk abundant. Nettle tea promotes easy flow.

When we look at mammals, we see two types of mothering and their species-specific milk is designed for them. We have **nest & cache** mammals... who can nurse their babies and leave them in a nest or safe place from 4-15 hours before the babies must be fed again. They are able to space out feeds throughout the day because their milk is high in fat and protein, and low in water. Then we have **carry & hibernate** mammals... who keep their babies close to them at all times, feeding them continuously through the day. These mammals nurse their babies often because their milk is low in fat and protein, and high in water.

Human milk is among the lowest in fat and protein, and highest in water. Humans by design are carriers. That's why our babies constantly nurse and love to be close. Many new mothers nurse their baby and since the baby craves to nurse again so soon, they worry about making enough milk or worry their baby has a sleeping issue because they wake so often to be fed and held close. Human babies and human milk are genetically designed to be breastfed and kept close, continuously.

We are carrying mammals living in a nesting mammals world with only a short time allowed for maternity leave! Society sets us up and supports us to be nesters: from spreading the message that baby should be sleeping rather than feeding throughout the night... and that baby should only eat in designated intervals... so, they sell expensive gadgets with the promise of long stretches in between. However, our babies are programmed differently and so are we. This is one reason why parents are so exhausted – we have little support from our society and our health care system to be the carrying mammals we are meant to be!

One might think babies require large amounts of protein since they grow by leaps and bounds... yet Mother's Milk has only 2% protein, similar to watermelon! In a word, we are over-proteinized to $ell food products and then OTC$ for the resulting acid-indigestion! Interestingly enough, studies show the peoples of Vilcabamba, Ecuador... the Hunza Valley... and Georgia... consume only 35g protein and 1500 cal/day... with 1/10th the fat in the Standard American Diet {SAD!} and 10X more fiber. These countries show high rates of Health, Happiness and Longevity. Be a Wise Wom(b)an Warrior with Your baby... Our future!

Regarding nursing, if circumstances are otherwise, the most nutritious food for the baby is seaweed known as Sea Moss: commercially-grown is usually a creamy color; wild-grown is darker. Soak it in hot water; when the water is then warm enough to handle, work the seaweed with fingers searching for small crustaceans or other bits of extraneous matter. Give a little of that soak water to each houseplant; then add fresh warm water to the seaweed, and let it gel. Scoop some out, blend with water and a touch of cinnamon. When feeding from the bottle, cut a larger hole in the nipple allowing easy passage of this thicker liquid. Some children have been raised on this *alone* their first year and turned-out smart and healthy because Sea Moss is nutritious marine algae.

Soy protein isolate is the main ingredient of soy-based infant formulas... a toxin with trypsin inhibitors, high phytate content and high aluminum content – it is best avoided These formulas lack healthy cholesterol, lactose and galactose, required for a developing nervous system. Soy allergies are as common as cow's milk allergies... especially among children.

Children with autism especially deserve optimal nutrition, with a deficient detoxification pathway that uses sulfate to excrete toxins... and the pathway gets clogged when low on sulfate. Epsom salt baths are the answer: simply put sufficient warm water in the baby's basin and add salt until it no longer dissolves, creating a slight build-up on the bottom; super-saturated water raises the sulfate levels, to get the detoxification pathway flowing again.

Several teeth indicate it is time to introduce solid foods. While most have mashed bananas as their introduction to solids, this creates a memory of, and a craving for, sweets. Salad materials: carrots, spinach and deseeded cucumber may be fresh grated and strained or merely finely grated... a couple of minutes, well worth the effort; cooked, prepared foods are devitalized and compromise baby's delicate system. Enzyme-rich foods are always preferred. If on occasion the young one has something cooked take an enzyme capsule and sprinkle 1/2 the contents, mixing it in.

Avoid grains until all 20 baby teeth come in. It is only then that the salivary glands begin to produce amylase, the starch-digesting enzyme. This means avoid cream of rice, cream of wheat, oatmeal and other forms of baby gruel... and even whole, alkaline-forming grains such as millet, quinoa and amaranth. You can begin feeding alkaline grains after 2 years, with all 20 teeth.

When we feed babies pasteurized dairy and starches, they let us know something is amiss by their runny noses, croup, rashes, and other symptoms of discomfort. Earache is a common symptom. Sometimes babies fed dairy eliminate mucus through the Eustachian tube and out the ear, causing much pain. The old-world remedy of a thimbleful of urine in the ear, with a small cotton ball to hold it in place, brings quick relief. If You can, catch the baby's urine while changing a diaper; otherwise use mother's urine – the middle catch, as described in Chapter 7, in the section **Urine Used in Healing**. As an alternative, mince a clove of garlic and marinate in a few ounces of warm olive oil for several hours. Strain and use a few drops, holding in place with a small cotton ball.

A diaper wet with fresh urine wiped over baby's face and body is healing. If there is a diaper rash, check out the cause: acids in the baby's food or, if nursing, Mother's diet. Change diapers more frequently; older urine forms ammonia and is irritating. Air and sunshine in moderation work wonders. Rather than talcum powder that blocks the pores, sprinkle diatomaceous earth or clay powder from the health food store. Use corn starch if organic to avoid GMOs. Water-based homeopathic crèmes are preferred. Oil blocks air!

After the 1st year, germinated seed milks add another dimension of nutrition and allow for additional blended factors such as sprouts, dulse and algae. Be strong enough to graciously refuse candy and other unconscious offerings from people. When something does slip by, get rid of it subtly – by substituting something healthy. If it's a done deal... give extra breast milk, water, fresh juice and/or enzymes.

Even after solid foods are introduced, many mothers choose to continue nursing, especially at bedtime, many times until the child is four or older. This deepens the feelings of confidence for the children, and compassion for the mothers – creating a Bond for Life.

Baking Powder
Most baking powder is undesirable. Aluminum salts accumulate in the brain affecting memory loss and brain deterioration. Baking powder free from aluminum salts is available, or make Your own with 1Tsp baking soda, 2Tsp cream of tartar, and 2Tsp of arrowroot.

Barefoot is Best
Studies show children going barefoot have healthier feet, fewer deformities, greater flexibility, and greater mobility than those who wear shoes. Walking, running and playing while barefoot releases toxins and strengthens the feet. Most orthopedic physicians agree the more closely a child's shoe resembles the barefoot state, the better – lightweight, flexible, shaped like the foot, room for toes, free from arch inserts or stiff sides. Most orthopedists are particularly opposed to shoes labeled "corrective" or "orthopedic" which some doctors still advocate to strengthen foot and leg deformities, flat feet, pigeon toes, knock-knees or bow-legs. Most experts agree: there is complete lack of evidence showing benefits of corrective shoes; for the vast majority... the supposed deformities correct themselves. Simple cloth tennis shoes may be the optimal choice after all.

Walking barefoot on wet grass or sand draws out toxins through the soles of the feet, bringing in negative ions – free electrons – and is healing for HeartMindBodySpirit. Encourage children to play outdoors in bare feet. When children climb trees, rather than saying, "Get down from there! You could fall and hurt Yourself!" create an empowering Verbal Diet and encourage them: "Take off Your shoes and socks; that way You can hold on with Your legs and feet as well as Your arms and hands!" Even indoors, encourage the children to be barefoot and to use their toes to pick things from the floor. It's amazing how agile they can become. John D Rockefeller used his toes to turn the pages of the daily newspaper!

Beans and Gas
To de-gas beans, soak and sprout for a couple of days, rinsing every day. If time is a factor, soak in hot water until the water becomes cool. Soak a second time in hot water for eight hours – overnight or all day. Give all soak water to houseplants. Cook in fresh water until skins begin to peel or until a cooled bean is easily mashed between tongue and the roof of the mouth. To lessen the gas effect, beans may be cooked with seaweed and / or other carminatives such as coriander, dill, fennel and garlic.

Being Human
Everyone is given a physical body. It is Yours for the entire time... like it or not... that is Your choice. Everything / everyOne are reflections of Divine Presence here with a purpose. Why judge or coerce anyone? Live Your own Truth, and allow others to experience their own Journey, their own Path to Truth.

You are enrolled in a full-time, informal, School of Life. Every day has opportunities and experiences that You may enjoy, think irrelevant, painful or boring.

Everything is in Perfect Divine Order. Why think there are mistakes? There are only opportunities for growth – a process of trial and error. Failed experiments are as much part of the process as the ones that work.

Every aspect of Life contains its opportunities. The same opportunity will be presented to You in various forms, until You have grown from it. Then You can go on to the next opportunity for growth.

"There" sometimes appears better than "here." When "there" has become "here," You simply obtain another "there" that may, again, appear better than "here."

Others are mirrors of You. If You love or are uneasy about another person, it reflects something You love or are uneasy about in terms of Your Self. You are merely experiencing a reflection of Your own energy vibration.

What You make of Yourself is up to You. You have the tools and resources required. What You do with them is Your choice.
All answers to Life's questions are found within. Simply look... listen... and trust. Meditation allows awareness in the present moment. Now is forever.

You will forget all this. All previous experiences are a preparation for Your Journey as the Pure Experience of Infinite Being. God is Light and Love. God is in the Kingdom of Heaven – which is within. Take a deep, caressing breath... and experience the Light and Love within. Explore inner dimensions. Let that Light and Love fill the day with Peace and Joy!

Better than Butter

Changing recommendations about foods is evidence of fluctuating "science" compared to the steadiness of Mother Nature's Ways. Take the issue of butter and margarine. Butter is a food. Margarine is **1** molecule away from being plastic... and shares two dozen ingredients with paint! It was thought to be a cheap way to fatten turkeys; when it killed the turkeys, they wondered what to do with their "invention".

After the Depression, butter became quite expensive and margarine was used as a substitute – sold much more economically as "white butter." For years the dairy interests fought using yellow dye to color "fake butter." In fact, at their insistence, restaurants had to cut margarine into triangles... so customers would know the difference! Free trade prevailed and packets of yellow liquid dye then were sold with the "white butter" to mix at home. Finally, it came pre-mixed, touted as "better than butter" because of the fat and cholesterol issues. Now we realize with hydrogenation in margarine, "butter is better" although not by much. Actually, margarine is deadly – saturated fatty acids congest our delicate mechanisms. Commercial butter is close behind, with added dangers – cows are inoculated with synthetic antibiotics, growth hormones and other chemical toxins, which to a large extent are stored in fats. Beware of butter... at least get organic butter from pasture-raised, contented cows.

For the health conscious, avocado or nut butter is the optimal choice. Avocado has a high monounsaturated fat content and benefits the arteries; it is wonderful for the HDL / LDL ratio, and suppresses blood changes that lead to clogged arteries, as well as clots that can trigger heart attack. Avos decrease blood insulin levels that directly damage the arteries; and for diabetes, heart disease, or high blood pressure they are excellent balancing foods.

Choose avocado somewhat firm to the touch with stem intact; when slightly soft near the stem, it is ready. Put hard avos in a paper bag and place in a warm spot such as on top of the refrigerator. This traps ethylene gas normally given off as every fruit ripens, hastening the process... a green banana in the bag speeds the process even more. Mashing them, 1Tbs lemon or lime juice per avocado slows the natural change of color.

BioDynamic Gardening

Rudolf Joseph Laurence Steiner, born 27 February 1861 to Austrian parents in Kraljevic (meaning King's Village) on a remote Hungarian plain, that is now Yugoslavia, gave 6,000 lectures and wrote hundreds of books on topics ranging from agriculture, architecture, economics, education, eurhythmy dance, medicine and knowledge of the higher worlds; perhaps best known for his system of education: Waldorf Schools, used world-wide, educating Head, Hands and Heart. His BioDynamic system of agriculture is used around the world – AU, CA, EU, IN, JP, MX, NZ & US.

In his younger years he was a member of the esoteric Theosophical Society. The leaders, Annie Besant and the Rev Charles Leadbetter, had asked Krishnamurti to take over – thinking he was the Star in the East. He knew otherwise... declining due to philosophical differences. Asking Steiner to take over, he also declined for the same reasons... and founded the Anthroposophical Society. The Theosophical Society was covert with arcane overtones; the Anthroposophical Society, under Steiner's guidance, freely and clearly brought Knowledge to the masses, evidenced by his classics: *Christianity as Mystical Fact and the Mysteries of Antiquity,* and *Knowledge of the Higher Worlds and its Attainment.*

Asked about diet, he spoke about nutrition and the soil. Actually, shortly after cataloguing the works of Goethe... Steiner – like Goethe – became a vegetarian. While he recommended vegetarianism... he felt it was personal, and declined proselytizing. Some strict vegans – who eat no animal flesh or animal produce, including dairy and honey, and avoid wearing leather or bone jewelry – wonder how to reconcile their views with Steiner's BioDynamic methods, with their absolutely clear results. While personal preference is sacrosanct... there are certain things to consider.

Really strict vegans avoid animals as food and clothing, as well as things like photographic film because of the gelatin involved – so they take no pictures, although digital photos put this issue to rest; some avoid the movies (although discerning people do that for other ethical reasons); they even avoid cars because the tires and interiors have some animal-derived components. Other more moderate vegans, while avoiding animal foods, do wear leather shoes for either comfort, warmth or durability. Free from judging choices of others, they reason that the animals are being killed as a food source by the undiscerning, and the leather is a by-product. While some may avoid cars because of their polluting effects, they realize animal parts go into bicycle tires **as** well as car tires – yet they ride their bikes and do what they can to respect Mother Earth. Indeed, if a committed vegan investigated the common products used… to completely avoid animal by-products, one would almost have to be a hermit.

Different cultures have different standards. Westerners love dogs and eat cows. Many oriental cultures consider dog meat a delicacy, and cook them alive for the additional flavoring from adrenalized blood! In India cows are held sacred and given the right of way in the streets. Steiner based his homeopathic soil preparations on the cow. In his view, the cow is a ruminant calm and peaceful; having its four feet firmly planted on the *earth*… with horns pointed to the *heavens*… the cow digests the grass… as well as the earthly and astral forces; by virtue of this etheric digestion, the cow passes a veritable treasure trove used in the preparation known as BD 500. All preparations are available from the Josephine Porter Institute of Applied BioDynamics. It is possible to DIY. https://jpibiodynamics.org/

With bucket and shovel in hand, walk through a pasture of organically raised cows looking for fresh cow pies, noting if they have a smooth or rippled surface. The smooth ones are from an aged or sickly cow; rippled ones are more energetic. When You have enough, take some cow's horns that have been cleaned out, and pack them with the fresh manure. Use a tablespoon; tap the tip of the horn on a rock, reaching to the tip with a wire hanger to release any air pockets – otherwise the bacteria and oxygen begin to ferment. When the horns are full, bury them at least 18" under the surface. Mark the spot well.

Steiner instructs to do this at the Autumnal Equinox… preferably on the Feast of Michael the Archangel, September 29th. {See Steiner's: *The Four Seasons and the Archangels* and *The Archangel Michael.*} Steiner says the Earth inhales and exhales on one level every day with nightfall and daylight – and on a subtle level once a year… inhaling in the Autumn / Winter and exhaling in the Spring / Summer. These horns remain buried all winter… as Mother Earth *breathes in* the Cosmic Astral forces. They are to be dug up near Summer Solstice… preferably on the Feast of John the Baptist, June 24th, under the guidance of Archangel

Uriel. During Winter, we are under the guidance of Archangel Gabriel; in Spring, Archangel Raphael. When dug up and tapped out from the horns, the cow pies were transformed into sweet-smelling humus known as BD 500, which is then homeopathically potentized to enrich the soil with Earth Energy.

In a 5-gallon ceramic or clay crock, or even a plastic bucket, place 3 gallons of water and stir in a handful of the BD 500; stir vigorously either by hand or with a wooden paddle. Create a vortex of swirling energy… and when the vortex is nicely formed {order}, immediately reverse – stirring in the opposite direction {chaos}. Order soon is restored and when it is, reverse again – alternating between order and chaos for one hour… obviously it is helpful to take turns with friends. This is a wonderful time for chanting, meditation, blessings, or reading from Steiner's *Agriculture: Spiritual Foundations for the Renewal of Agriculture* {The American English translation is superior, by Catherine Creeger and Malcolm Gardner.}

Once this is complete… take the end of a branch from a pine tree and, dipping it in the potentized water, sprinkle the soil. This amount is sufficient for 1 acre. Rather than being concerned about covering every square inch, focus on Intention. Sprinkle even the other side of the fence, blessing the neighbor's land as well.

The following day… bless the land with BD 501, homeopathically potentized to enrich the soil with Light Energy. Other horns are buried, packed with quartz crystal ground between sheets of glass to a fine powder. These are buried from the Feast of John the Baptist, June 24th, until the Feast of Michael the Archangel, September 29th, as Mother Earth *breathes out* – capturing the forces of magma from the core of the Earth in the quartz powder. Use the same directions and procedures as with BD 500.

Using this energetic treatment of the soil – one day BD 500… the next day BD 501 has transformed cracked, arid soil into fertile cropland. See *BioDynamic Agriculture* (2 vol) by Alex Podolinsky. If serious, as was his situation Down Under in AU, do these procedures at the Spring and Autumnal Equinox for a couple of years, and watch Mother Nature self-heal. The process is enhanced using BD preparations (preps) for the compost pile and lightly coating the land with this composted energy as well. Alex's neighbors were shocked as he produced bountiful harvests, while they still had arid, cracked soil! As with the BD 500 and BD 501, Steiner gives specific instructions in *Agriculture* for the 6 BD compost preps.

BD 502: fresh yarrow flowers packed in a stag's bladder are hung up to dry in the sun, away from the reach of animals. Left there all summer, it is buried in the Autumn {Archangel Michael} and dug up in the Spring {John the Baptist}. This pulls in the energy of Venus and potentizes the minerals sulfur and potash.

BD 503: fresh chamomile flowers packed in a section of cow intestines, are wrapped in a fine plastic screen, and buried from Autumn to Spring. This pulls in the energy of Mercury and potentizes the minerals calcium, sulfur and potash.

BD 504: fresh stinging nettle – end leaves, stems, blossoms – are wrapped in a fine plastic screen and buried for a whole year when the blossoms present themselves, usually near the Feast of John the Baptist. This pulls in the energy of the Sun and potentizes the minerals sulfur, potassium, calcium and iron.

BD 505: chopped oak bark packed in the skull of a cow is covered with peat moss, and buried from Autumn to Spring. This pulls in the energy of the Moon and potentizes the mineral calcium.

BD 506: fresh dandelion flowers folded in the mesentery of a cow, wrapped in a fine plastic screen... is buried from Autumn to Spring. This pulls in the energy of Jupiter and potentizes the mineral silica.

BD 507: fresh valerian flowers are juiced and, rather than bury, allowed to ferment. This pulls in the energy of Mars and potentizes the mineral phosphorus.

These 6 preparations are placed in a specific order buried in the compost pile in glass jars... and remain untouched for 3-6 months before using. As indicated by dowsing and the pendulum, this greatly enhances the energy of the compost.

Over the years, experiments using other animal parts – goat, for instance – or using these herbs free from animal involvement – show there is absolutely **no** comparison regarding the potentizing energies that accrue, when following the specific instructions of Steiner. Other experiments used a cow that died naturally; this cow, being older, lacked vitality as well

as potentizing results! In BioDynamics, the cow to be sacrificed is raised with kindness and gratitude... surrounded with Love and Light – only a few years old, this vibrant energy imparts vitality to the preps.

Another prep **BD 508:** fresh horsetail herb, *Equisetum*, as a tea, is sprayed to control fungus and mildew. This pulls in the energy of Saturn and potentizes the mineral silica. Fermented horsetail tea is also used in another BioDynamic protocol to attract rain.

Harvey Lisle, student of Steiner for over 50 years – personal chemist for Dr Ann Wigmore and Hippocrates Health Institute – gives a formula for paramagnetic tree paste in *The Enlivened Rock Powders* protecting from insects and animals... and protecting cracks in the bark, and at trunk-limb junctions... acting as anti-bacterial and anti-fungal... while providing a paramagnetic force field. Blend 2C BioDynamic compost, 1C fine-ground basalt or silica rock powder – both impart paramagnetic qualities – and 3Tbs raw linseed {flaxseed} oil, which acts as the drying agent imparting resistance to the weather; add sufficient water to blend into a good brushable consistency. Brush this on the tree trunk to a height of several feet... every Spring, Summer and Autumn.

Consciously connecting with the other Planets... we raise the vibrations of our beloved Mother Earth. Enhancing the vibrations of our foods... we raise the consciousness of humankind. Advanced students will enjoy homeopathic BioDynamics, connecting the science and medical lectures of Rudolph Steiner from Garuda BioDynamic Institute: www.garudabd.org The Steiner e-Library: https://www.rsarchive.org/ Scientific studies of water verify the theories. What is water? Coherent? Intelligent? Source of Bio-photons? Explore. Conversations with Dr. Cowan & Friends| Ep16: Dolf Zantinge (bitchute.com)
Home - ANALEMMA (analemma-water.com)

Biological Transmutation
"If You are working with rock powders, You should know a little something about the transmutation of elements. This is a subject science avoids since its practitioners know so little about it... and yet it happens continuously in the mineral, plant, animal and human kingdoms. Transmutation is easy to understand if You consider the elements not so much material as spiritual – with strong enzymatic forces. Rather than chemical reaction... Transmutation is spiritual digestion.

"The name Louis Kervran is synonymous with the subject of his book, *Biological Transmutation*, (1962, translated 1980). As a youngster he noted the chickens his folks kept, picked up pieces of mica grit found in the yard. When they were butchered and the gizzards inspected, the mica grit was not to be found. Presumably it had been digested. Although no lime grit was given to the chickens, their eggs had strong calcareous shells. It wasn't until later in life that he determined the silica in the mica grit had transmuted to the calcium found in the shells.

"How many of us have wondered where dairy cows get the calcium they require? Many dairy cows give at least 20,000 pounds of milk a year. They give birth to a calf weighing from 75-90 lbs and at the same time keep up their own calcium metabolism – those cows are putting out more calcium than they are taking in. Where is that extra calcium coming from? At the same time, they are eating pasture grasses, hay, corn silage and grains, all rich in silica. Extra calcium they require comes from the silica they take in: silica is transmuting to calcium.

"Silica has an atomic weight of 28, carbon an atomic weight of 12. Add the two together and You get 40, the atomic weight of calcium. Sounds simple, yet more complex than we can fully understand.

"A similar phenomenon takes place in my compost pile. While I am building up the pile, I work in some basalt… a gray powder. After several months in the compost pile, I see the basalt powder has turned white, and is now lime. No one can tell me I may be mistaken because I am a chemist, and I have tested that white material carefully. It is lime. It is more than lime; it is nascent lime. The word *nascent* comes from the Latin: 'in the act of being born.' This nascent lime is much more active than regular lime. It combines with humic acid to form humate, a highly desirable end product. Other silica rock powders should act in a similar fashion, although I have not made the confirming observation as I have with basalt. Of course, the sure-fire way of producing a humate in the compost pile is to add a little lime during the site's construction. By adding a rock powder to the compost pile adds another dimension, enhancing the properties of the compost as You add it to Your gardens or fields or fruit trees."

{*The Enlivened Rock Powders*: Harvey Lisle worked with Dr Ann Wigmore for years as her personal bio-chemist. She usually called early in the morning, and (before the days of caller ID) if the phone rang before 6 am – he'd simply pick up & say, Good Morning, Ann how are You? He loved her spunk! Seeing the first edition of *Harmonious Healing*… he gave permission to quote his writings. Dr Ann and Viktoras Kulvinskas co-founded The Hippocrates Health Institute in Boston in the '60s. Both have books worthy of consideration… *Be Your Own Doctor* by Dr Ann Wigmore. *Survival in the 21st Century – A Planetary Healers Manual* and *Love Your Body* by Viktoras Kulvinskas.}

Bones

In addition to dietary recommendations of dark leafy greens and any other sources of chlorophyll… air and sun baths are healing for the bones, perhaps while doing aerobic exercises or lifting light weights. Play or listen to cello / drum music, let it vibrate the bones. When performing Tai Chi practice of Shake the Earth bouncing and landing on Your heels also strengthens the bones – as does tapping wrists together… also, briskly rubbing fingernails together. Nurture Your inner life with visualization and meditation. Diatomaceous Earth is a tremendous source of silica. Stinging nettle has 6,500 ppm! Horsetail has 386 ppm. Homeopathy: silica tissue salts; *Symphytum* 30C or 200C – 3x/day.

Braggs™ Liquid Aminos

Soy sauce is from *chemically* fermented soybeans, with *commercial* salt. Tamari is *naturally* fermented soybeans, with *sea* salt. Braggs is made from heating hydrochloric acid breaking down the soy protein into amino acids… then using baking soda to temper the acidity. Unfortunately, heat denatures protein; while it may increase the bio-availability of amino acids – it also increases the bio-availability of MSG which gets degraded during the fermentation process.

Oriental Wisdom understands through centuries of experimentation, soy must be sprouted or fermented. Purists may love the taste, yet avoid Braggs™ preferring Nama Shoyu™ organic, unpasteurized soy sauce – even safe with Candida or sensitivities to fermented foods. Use mellow low-salt miso or use kelp for salty flavoring. {See below: **Soy**.}

Breath: Physical – Sacred (3X3)

HA! Laughter Affirms Life: HaHaHa! Interestingly enough, alo–Ha means: Be-ing in the Presence of – the Breath of Life – aHa… Breath IS Life: exchanging what is useful for what is useless. Breath is the sOurce of our physical Life; also the vehicle to engage Sacred Space – experiencing HeartMindBodySpirit as One.

Anatomy studies structure. Physiology studies function. We know even *thinking* You have exhaled completely – such as, blowing out the BreathDay candles, or blowing up a balloon – You *still* retain 1/3 lung capacity and plenty of oxygen reserve. Studies of Wim Hof verify this. https://www.wimhofmethod.com

Exploring Breath at the personal level leads to fascinating discoveries both physically, emotionally and spiritually. For instance, the brain of a cigarette smoker knows from habit... when inhaling, smoke comes in... *along with* extra air. Ironically, when the brain requires oxygen, the smoker reaches for the nearest pack to inhale! Instead, take deep breaths and breathe out forcefully, through *pursed* lips. This creates *backpressure* driving oxygen from the lungs into the bloodstream. After 2-3 breaths of this nature, cravings for a cigarette diminish. Lungs are the bellows of Life.

In acupuncture, the lung and large intestine meridians are referred to as The Essential Rhythms of Life. The real Question: What IS this "Life"? Are we physical accidents, who may seem to experience the *ethereal* on occasion? Or are we spiritual beings having a physical experience – The Word Made Flesh? To answer that, we explore the Vibration that sustains All.

Guardian Angels and Others who hold the Frequencies of Love, Truth and Beauty, Trust, Harmony and Peace on this planet are Force Fields: Beings experiencing truth, awareness and bliss on a level *between* Pure Consciousness and Human Consciousness. We humans, men and wom(b)en – unlike the angels – can experience minor things like taste, and major things like the vibrations of our hearts... our feelings and emotions. Opening our Heart of Hearts, we go beyond our human inhibitions... and experience Pure Love, taking us to Conscious Awareness: Self-Realization – Enlightenment – Being Aware of *being aware* as the One... All That Is... knOwing All–Ways: OM... as the *vibration* within... is Home Sweet hOMe!

Sacred Breath is the Key that opens the door. Practicing Sacred Breath in meditation builds Inner Strength – supporting our spiritual immune system. Practicing meditation, we becOMe stronger. Eventually... when we leave the meditation place... we bring with us... the meditation space: Breath by Sacred Breath. At first, we find it easy being with Sacred Breath: making juice... preparing food... Love energizes HeartMindBodySpirit – as One. With practice... we extend awareness of Sacred Breath with family and friends... being *with* them in the mOMent... the Here and Now. Practicing Sacred Breath through the day, strengthens our spiritual immune system so when someone purposely pushes our buttons or caught in traffic... we easily slide into Sacred Breath with anOther hOMe-run. Peace being our goal we are Victorious with the Main Lesson of Life!

Beginners Note: Rather than attempt to *still* Monkey-mind, it is easier to give it *focus*. Many focus on the inner *sounds* as an internal mantra: sooo... on the inhale, hummm... on the exhale. This technique of meditation is found in the *Vedas* along with the mantra So-Hum, which in Sanskrit literally means: I Am That! Others focus Monkey-mind on the *temperature* at their nostrils: coool... inhaling – and waaarm... exhaling. Some focus on counting. Enlightenment... which is really Self-Realization... can be as esoteric as **3X3**, or as simple as **1,2,3** – inhale slowly stretching out the word aaand... then exhale completely thinking of the number: and... 1... and... 2... and... 3... and... 1... and so on, repeat in 3s.

Enlightenment! Exoteric meets Esoteric. Simple as 1,2,3 – 3X3. Experiment. Eventually, losing track, being in the Meditation *space*... and experiencing Peace within. The Kingdom of Heaven is within. Practice. Practice. Practice. Breath by Sacred Breath.

Great Spirit... Father Sun... Mother Earth... every Sacred Breath is my re-birth... every day a chance to be... Love and Compassion with all I see... including Me!

Love YourSelf All–ways. Blessing Your Sacred Journey!

Burns, Bites and Boo-boos
While sunshine is healing – moderation is key. Tanning rays are more abundant before and after peak time. Rays promoting Vit D production are present only *during* peak time... prudence is in order. Avoid prolonged exposure during the peak hours 11-3... 20-30 minutes is sufficient for Vit D. Use Caution around reflective surfaces – water, sand, snow, and metal. Cloudy days have almost the same ultraviolet rays.

Repeated abuse of the sun leads to wrinkling, aging and possible melanoma.

Sunscreens actually *prevent* Vit D production, which interferes with melanoma growth and other cancers. There is a direct link between the introduction and sales of sunscreens and the rise in melanoma rates... wisely avoided. Keep covered or in the shade, especially mid-day. Sunscreens have PABA (para-aminobenzoic acid) as a key ingredient; the most effective and natural source of PABA is found in fresh fruits and vegetables. Unless spending time outdoors in warmer climates... it's prudent to supplement with D3. 5000 IU with every meal.

A healing miracle for burns is being taught beginner firefighters. First Aid consists of spraying cold water on the affected area until heat is reduced, which stops the continued burning of all layers of the skin... then spread egg whites onto the affected area. One woman burned a large part of her hand with boiling water. In spite of the pain, she ran cold faucet water on her hand, separated 2 egg whites from the yolks, beat them slightly and dipped her hand in the solution. The whites dried forming a protective layer. She learned the egg white is natural collagen and continued for one hour to apply layer upon layer of beaten egg white. By afternoon she no longer felt pain and the next day there was hardly a trace of burn. 10 days later, her skin regained normal color. The burned area totally regenerated thanks to the collagen in the egg whites – a placenta full of vitamins.

For casual sunburn and insect bites use cold compresses; splash apple cider vinegar for relief. Still irritation? Use 2-parts apple cider vinegar and 1-part olive oil. Blisters? *Aloe vera* jelly may be used. In both situations, freshly voided urine – most effective if applied immediately. Homeopathic protocol for stinging or burning: *Urtica urens*. Bee-stings: *Apis mellifica*. Ticks: *Ledum palustre*. Poison ivy, impetigo other watery, blistery irritations, and for itching: *Rhus tox*.
For injuries: if the skin is intact and black or blue... Mother Tincture or *Arnica* crème. If the skin is broken... *Calendula* crème. For serious wounds: *Calendula* Mother Tincture: 1-part – 9-parts coconut or olive oil. Take a few doses of *Arnica* before and after surgery.

For injuries to ligaments from exertion, lifting, using weights or stretching: *Rhus tox* 30C, 3x/day... still without relief: *Ruta graveolens* 30C.

For lacerations of muscles... damage to nerves, deep cuts at the fingers or toes: *Hypericum* 30C, 3x/day.

For a puncture wound literally involving a rusty nail near a source of fecal matter in the barnyard: *Ledum* 3X to ward off tetanus... or taken as prophylactic.

For old sprains... for bruised-like pain in the bones, joints and cartilage... for sprains of the ankles and wrists and for carpal tunnel: *Ruta graveolens* 30C... still without relief: 3C or 3X, and directly apply the Mother Tincture mixed in oil.

For injuries to bones or fracture: *Symphytum* 3X-12X. Old injuries in the head: *Natrum sulph* 6X.

For sharp cutting pain, as with a knife... or clean-cut wounds and symptoms traceable to surgery: *Staphysagria* 30C, 3x/day. J A Satti, PhD, homeopath: http://www.nanopathy.com/ Serious **Pain**, see below.

Caffeine
Caffeine from coffee and black tea leads to symptoms similar to anxiety neurosis: recurrent headaches, mental irritability, cardiac arrhythmia and gastrointestinal disturbances. According to *The British Medical Journal* it is the most utilized and most abused drug. The most potent form of caffeine is found in coffee that is boiled or percolated: 120 mg/cup; drip: 90; instant: 70; decaf: 3. Energy drinks vary from 69 to 200. Coke: 65; Pepsi: 43; Excedrin: 65; No-Doze: 100; Vivarin: 200; Cocoa: 10; 1 oz of bittersweet chocolate: 20; dark chocolate: 12; milk chocolate: 10 mg and 70 mg theobromine – not as powerful as caffeine, still a stimulant. If a child has 3 oz of chocolate, intake is roughly 30 mg caffeine and 200 mg theobromine. Multiply the above numbers by 3 for a young child, by 2 for a young teen. This can precipitate mild delirium or hyperactivity. Added sugar intensifies the results. We know how school kids behave after snack and lunch. Pregnancy prolongs the effects of caffeine 3X. The normal ½ life of caffeine for adult is 6 hrs; for a smoker: 3 hrs; in pregnancy: 18 hrs; a newborn: 4 days! Decaf has a bit of caffeine as well as methylene chloride, a carcinogenic solvent used to extract caffeine.

The Journal of the American Medical Association reports that women who had 1½-3 cups of coffee a day doubled their chance of miscarriage. Duke University Medical Center suggests caffeine intensifies stress. There was an average 37% increase in adrenaline among subjects who consumed 2-3 cups of caffeinated beverage in 4 hours. When adrenaline rises – a natural occurrence with threatening situations – blood pressure, heart rate, muscle tension and perspiration increase. Caffeine heightens the length of the adrenaline rush. Under this influence, employees can stay with a simple clerical task longer – although it does have a negative impact on performing complex tasks. James Lane, professor of behavioral medicine, warns: "Coffee has hundreds of chemicals; most have yet to be studied." Many of these chemicals are absent with organic coffee, as well as organic black and green tea.

Rudolf Steiner speaks of different qualities of caffeine. A coffee house is a place for discussion... philosophy... and poetry, all requiring intellectual concentration – focus – attention to detail. Embassies and other diplomatic venues serve tea – promoting a superficial, lighthearted exchange: "How do You do. Lovely to see You again." Perhaps if our diplomatic negotiators would replace their tea with a cup of coffee, we might see thoughtful and dramatic results. The caffeine in guarana offers no crash along with focused concentration – an entirely different physiological effect from caffeine in coffee and black tea. Perhaps the high fat content of the guarana seed – even in powdered form – leads to slower release of caffeine.

As with Life, moderation is a virtue – excess is dangerous. To have an occasional cup is probably okay; muscle test: ask Your body. Caffeine, however, is a calcium robber promoting osteoporosis. It has been shown to exacerbate psychotic symptoms in those with mental challenges. Those with fibrocystic breast disease, palpitations, heartburn or infertility are told by the medical establishment to avoid caffeine.

According to *The American Academy of Pediatrics*, caffeine and other stimulants contained in beverages are best excluded from the diets of children and adolescents as it inhibits the neurological, immune and cardiovascular systems. Parkinson's has also been linked to caffeine, which also negatively affects stroke patients; those who consume caffeine had far *less* blood flow to the brain than non-coffee drinkers. Even the NYT bought into the myth, saying it raises the IQ. Clearly, if caffeine reduces blood flow with its contingent oxygen and nutrients – as well as waste removal – caffeine reduces intellectual function!

Some feel caffeine keeps them "regular" with morning bowel movements. When too much enters the system at once, red flags go up: get rid of this poison! The body empties the colon, stimulating the eliminative process. Caffeine is a central nervous system irritant: sciatica and low back pain is reduced by 50% in just a few days when avoiding caffeine.

As with any true addiction, caffeine – especially in coffee and black tea – brings severe withdrawal symptoms such as crashing headaches. To avoid this, simply withdraw more slowly. Cut Your regular dose in half for a few days; then cut that in half for a few days; drink more re-mineralized and re-energized distilled or r/o water. The rare cup is usually problem-free.

Cannabis and Bamboo
Two plants can save the planet if put to proper use: cannabis and bamboo. Books are being written about the benefits of Cannabis as a sacred herb, and society's understanding is going through a paradigm shift. Originally: *Tell Your Children*, sometimes titled: *The Burning Question, Dope Addict, Doped Youth*, and *Love Madness* – the 1936 American propaganda film *Reefer Madness* revolves around melodramatic events that ensue when high-school students are lured by pushers to try marijuana aka Mary Jane or weed. Depicted as Evil and the Gateway Drug to heroin leading to certain destruction... cannabis is now vindicated as the Heroine bringing healing for HeartMindBodySpirit! Surprisingly, cannabis is the **Exit Drug** from alcohol addiction for *many* people! Laws vary. Research. Relief comes in a variety of ways, including CBD suppositories.

Bamboo – the resource of the future bids Caution, *and* can be delicious. Some types are known to contain varying levels of cyanide, unsafe to eat! Thinking of growing bamboo to eat? 35' clumping *Nastus elatus* is the best for eating bamboo shoots raw. Snap them off, peel them and eat the big shoot right where it grows! Raw is Best! 80% Raw and *maximum* 20% Cooked – preferably steamed – has been shown to strengthen the immune system. *Phyllostachys Nigra* 'Henon' is a beautiful, hardy giant bamboo... cold and drought tolerant, low maintenance... that emerges green and turns ghostly gray with sunlight exposure. Tasty, edible shoots emerging from the ground are safe to eat. Younger shoots are optimal... 6-9 inches. Quality wood is perfect for crafts and building construction.

Bamboo is stronger than maple... with more compressive strength than concrete... and the same strength-to-weight ratio as steel! There are many varieties. Some bamboo grows 3-4' in a single day; a green living resource, bamboo alleviates environmental concerns with traditional materials... the lumber of the future. Bamboo re-grows when it is harvested and grows for decades. Replenished from an intricate network of roots, some bamboo grows to its maximum height of around 80' in two months. As it thickens, the walls of each hollow stalk grow hard and dense, and soft internodes convert into fibrous cellulose. Bobby Grimes, Black Belt Steiner student living on the Big Island, has multiple resources for all matters agricultural... aware that Discipline and Sacred Breath is Key to Success! On the mainland, involved in bamboo research since 1991 in Appalachia http://earthadvocatesresearchfarm.com/ https://www.bobbygrimes.com

2020 as our collective **Year of 20/20 Vision** was an open invitation to All: Grow Your Own Garden of Eatin' – Take Charge of Your Life with Appreciation. Care. Compassion. Gratitude. Minimalism. Permaculture. Return to Mother Nature's Ways and explore the Essene Tradition which nurtures HeartMindBodySpirit as One and promotes holistic, Harmonious Healing. Engaging Ancient Wisdom in Modern Times helps One find the Way back to Source, Home Sweet hOMe! Sacred Breath is the Key.

Cancer

"The most thrilling experience I can recall
was to see cancer cells taken from a human body
and thriving on cooked food...
yet unable to survive on the *same* food
when it was uncooked."
Be Your Own Doctor, Dr Ann Wigmore

Every degenerative disease... especially cancer... thrives where the environment is highly acidic, lacking in oxygen and rich in sugars. Symptoms of oxygen deficiency are fatigue... slow healing of wounds... and infections. Chronic manifestations are found in altered brain function, arthritis, cancer, diabetes, heart challenges and other chronic degenerative diseases. While our external environment suffers from oxygen depletion... we can change our internal environment.

What are dietary sources of oxygen? Oxygen in fats is less than 15%; depending on amino acid profile,

proteins range from 20-40%. Combined, fats and proteins in animal foods require large amounts of oxygen to metabolize – also true of refined carbohydrates such as white flour and white rice, alcohol, caffeine, nicotine, sugars and sodas. Cooked food and all forms of junk food are low in oxygen and high in toxins. Junk food uses available oxygen to oxidize synthetic chemicals and preservatives, and to metabolize pitifully few nutrients.

Foods high in oxygen: fresh juices, fresh vegetables, whole grains, nuts and seeds – especially germinated and/or sprouted. Oxygen comprises over 50% of the weight of these foods. Greens are a wonderful source of oxygen and nutrition. While commercial produce is used in studies and shows healing results with members of the cabbage and onion families, even more profound results are obtained using organic produce, sprouts, seaweed, as well as microalgae from Klamath Lake. In addition to including oxygen-rich foods, avoid sugars. Cancer thrives on fruits, carrots and beets, especially juices, with high sugar content.

These simple dietary changes along with re-mineralized and re-energized distilled or r/o water, reasonable exercise, proper rest and positive thought-forms empower us – healing HeartMindBodySpirit. Negative thought-forms and stress – whether physical, emotional or mental – also deplete oxygen. These acid-forming factors suck up oxygen like a sponge to neutralize acidic toxins; the body does what it must for survival. In times of stress – it is crucial to breathe deeply, consciously. Even the NIH has said for years: Why medicate? Meditate! The recommendations and their benefits are documented by decades of research at Hippocrates Health Institute, Tree of Life Rejuvenation Center, and Optimum Health Institutes. (See below: **Curing and Healing**)

The Goal: strengthen the immune response system, and restore balance. Cancerous cells replicate wildly; these suggested protocols promote healthy cellular replication. Dr Linus Pauling (twice Nobel Laureate) noted every unhealthy condition can be traced to a mineral deficiency. Minerals in seaweed are full-spectrum; dulse has a tendency to absorb mercury, perhaps because it has less iodine; kelp has outstanding integrity and purity. The microalgae – chlorella and blue-green algae – are exceptional: micronutrients and minerals are absorbed through the upper portion of the stomach. Our DNA resonates with

Earth's First Food: algae – especially *wild-grown* seaweed and Klamath Lake's **AFA**. (See above.)

Carob

Carob is known in other cultures as locust bean. Is this because it's the only thing that would survive a swarm of locusts... or because the locusts would feed on them? Carob is known as St. John's bread. Scriptures say John the Baptist fasted in the desert, eating only locusts and wild honey. Rather than John being an insectivore... we can understand that he ate the locust bean, carob. He likely was a vegan, as other Essenes who lived near Mt Carmel near the Sea of Galilee... and others on the spiritual path. (See below: **Vegan Life and Religions**)

Carob has a naturally sweet taste, unlike the bitterness of cocoa, usually masked with sugar to make chocolate. Carob, high in fiber and low in fat (1/10 that of chocolate), has 4X the calcium of chocolate. Chocolate has oxalic acid interfering with the utilization of calcium... caffeine, an addictive substance... and theobromine, a related stimulant. Unlike chocolate... carob, being a legume, has few allergic reactions.

Carob pods, growing on tall trees, have been used for thousands of years. This tasty, nutritious, large brown bean-like fruit can be eaten whole or ground into powder. The pods can be chewed: swallow the juice, discard pulp. Carob, 6% protein and 60% complex carbohydrate... contains calcium, phosphorus and iron, facilitating digestion; a mild laxative. Carob is safely given to babies: ½ tsp in 4 oz water... even to dogs. Raw carob has a mild flavor; toasted carob is more flavorful... a delicious addition to nut, seed, grain milks... dehydrated treats... and banana ice cream.

Cashews

Like soybeans and garbanzos, cashews can be a challenge to digest. Cashews are heat-treated in the harvesting process; specifically, they are roasted to get rid of the sap which burns – badly – and to open the husk, partially destroying enzymes. Labels saying raw are false. They are soft and ship poorly, so beyond the enzyme issue, cashews are complicated by rancidity as all soft nuts, especially when broken. Some buy pieces to save money – at the expense of health. Use whole cashews, and give the broken bits to the birds.

When making cream of vegetable soup... such as asparagus, broccoli, or spinach, use ½C blended whole cashews per quart of soup. For a delicious milkshake: blend 2/3C cashews and 2C water – flavorings: vanilla, carob, or stevia – for a sweet treat leaving blood sugar levels stable; perhaps make it thicker, freezing for an occasional ice cream treat. Alternative to cashews: blend macadamia and pine nuts.

Chocolate: Organic and Healthy

Commercial chocolate is decaying the world we live in: physically, morally. Huge areas of tropical rainforest are being cleared to grow cacao in Brazil, Ecuador, Indonesia and Malaysia. Cacao is heavily cultivated in Africa, the Caribbean, SE Asia, South Pacific Islands. Pesticides used poison women and children sprayers, who are beaten and kept as slaves, especially on the Ivory Coast of Africa. Chemical residues are found in commercial chocolate, as well as milk and sugar.

Studies say a little dark chocolate is beneficial for the heart and endocrine energy system... women especially resonate with chocolate. Chocolate benefits the brain – enhancing memory – although it must be >60% cocoa for therapeutic value. If You choose an occasional healthy chocolate treat, avoid the varieties with dairy and sugar, choosing organic.

When chocolate was discovered, health and nutrition were common sense; a chocolate drink would produce a sense of euphoria, a "warm-all-over" sensation. Aztec, Incan and Mayan peoples wondered whether to call it food? or medicine? Montezuma and the Royal Court drank it for energy and vitality. Eventually, they called it Theobroma Cacao – Food of the Gods.

Clay

While potter's clay has possible contaminants such as lead... clay from the health food store is suitable for internal and external use; there are several types. Aluminum always assumes the center position in the formula of clay compounds: CaO Al2O3 SiO2. The first group in any clay formula is always a member of the lime group, and the last group is always a silicate. Because of the rhythmical element aluminum, clay becomes a *rhythmical* rock powder, both *diamagnetic* and *paramagnetic* forces, bringing balance. Internally, clay has been used to draw toxins from the intestinal tract. Bentonite clay, widely known, is a mixture of aluminum and magnesium silicate minerals, coming from weathered volcanic ash – both safe and healing.

When introducing Your system to the healing powers of clay, place 2Tsp of dry, pure clay in 12 oz water... stir and leave at the windowsill, taking in the sun, moon and astral forces for 24 hrs. Slowly... gently... tip the glass and drink until clay is about to be swallowed; then refill the glass leaving it until the next day. Repeat for up to 1 week, then rinse the glass and clay making a gift for Your plants; then refresh, and leave at the windowsill for 24 hrs. Stir and drink on an empty stomach in the morning for 3 - 30 days.

Externally, clay can draw out toxins – first "cure" the clay. A small wide-mouthed glass jar is suitable. Fill it ½ with clay then top off with distilled or r/o water. Leave it near a window at least 24 hrs – outdoors: cover with cheesecloth. Do this around the Full Moon. When the sun shines, the clay is charged with paramagnetic forces; when the moon shines, the clay is charged with diamagnetic forces. If it looks cracked, add more water; otherwise, cover this thick paste, and keep it as part of the First-Aid Kit... useful for insect stings, boils or rashes. Spread a ¼" layer on the area to be treated and allow to air dry. As it dries, it pulls out toxins rejuvenating the skin.

As toothpaste "a little dab'll do ya!" – any medium, even water will suffice, and a soft brush. After brushing, use a tongue scraper. Rather than rinsing, allow mucosal membranes and gums to absorb the healing energy of clay for 15 minutes: time for Sacred Breath.

As a skin rejuvenator, spread on clay and take an air bath until it cakes and dries; use for facials. Wash with a loofa and see how the skin looks and feels. Read: *Our Earth, Our Cure* by Michel Abehsera.

Cleansing Gently
Some traditional herbalists claim a "cleansing crisis" or discomfort is good – almost necessary – following the general philosophy: no pain, no gain. This approach can drain vital energy from the body and leave it cleaner and leaner, yet lacking energy to maintain future health. Cleansing crises occur when too much, too strong, or too strong a combination of herbs have been used – precipitating a variety of symptoms, such as diarrhea, headache or rash; discontinue and flush the system with water, fresh vegetable juices or broth, resuming the cleanse at lower doses. Generally, a week is adequate for most constitutions to cleanse the small and large intestines, kidneys and liver. Physical

exercise, deep breathing, herbal baths, salt baths, saunas, massage, and dry skin brushing facilitate.

Gentle diuretic herbal teas can cleanse the kidneys: corn silk for pain... cranberry for a rinse... hydrangea to dissolve stones... marshmallow for lungs and kidneys... nettle for kidneys and liver... parsley leaf or watermelon seeds for kidneys. To cleanse the liver: alfalfa, artichoke, dandelion, gentian, milk thistle and yellow dock. Chlorophyll-rich foods tone the liver, additionally cleansing the kidneys.

An herbal bitters formula can improve digestion, prevent mucus in the intestinal tract and encourage peristalsis... discouraging incompletely digested foods from accumulating as wastes. Bitters are liver tonics – artichoke, fumitory, gentian, goldenseal, milk thistle, Oregon grape root and wahoo bark. For balance, mix a few of these with a stomach-soothing herb such as cardamom, cinnamon, ginger, licorice or peppermint.

Eating high fiber whole foods with fresh herbs and spices maintains a healthy colon. Sometimes vigorous cleansing may deplete friendly bacteria, so supplement with acidophilus: predominant in the small intestine... bifidus: predominant in the large intestine... or use bioactive Sauerkraut or Kimchee; build Your biOMe.

Chlorophyll implants after colonics and enemas restore friendly energies known as prebiotics and... through the portal vein, the liver gets a boost.

9-days organic juice fast detoxifies and regenerates the organs. Drink only what is recommended each day; while quantity may vary, two quarts is average. With profound health challenges, avoid the high sugar of days 6 & 7, substituting day 8 for those days.

Day 1: Drink plenty of re-mineralized and re-energized distilled or r/o water to rinse the body... and to alert the system – something serious is happening.

Day 2: Cranberry juice – free from sugar or corn syrup, from the health food store – either straight, one ounce diluted in 8 oz water, or with apple or pear as a sweetener; or a ½ dozen frozen cranberries blended in 8 oz water to adjust pH of the urinary tract as a preparation for cleansing.

Day 3: Comfrey root tea detoxifies the stomach by stimulating pepsin production.

Day 4: Pineapple juice – rich in bromelain – cleanses the small intestine – juice at least 5 pineapples.

Day 5: Lemon and water... ½C fresh squeezed lemon per quart of water to detoxify and cleanse the liver.

Day 6: Carrot juice – made fresh, with the possible addition of ginger root for flavor – coats and lubricates the liver, kidneys, lungs and brain.

Day 7: Beet juice – make 12 oz fresh in the morning from leaves and peeled root to pull toxins from the liver into the blood stream. Add a capsule of probiotics – through the day it will slightly ferment. Russians call it kvass. Always dilute: 3 oz 4x/day with a pint of water.

Day 8: Green juices freshly made from kale, collards, cucumber, celery, green beans, parsley, and wheatgrass juice if You have a slow-gear juicer, causes an exchange of toxins across cellular membranes: a systemic flush.

Day 9: Drink plenty of re-mineralized and re-energized distilled or r/o water to rinse and cleanse the system.

Congratulate Yourself for this wonderful accomplishment! Guaranteed, it was different from what was imagined. Empower Yourself. Experiment. Explore. What would it be like to be *free* from cooked foods? to have raw and living foods, and germinated nuts and seeds for 30 days? Many have gotten off insulin by doing so! What might happen? Explore.

Co-enzyme Q10: A Miracle Enzyme

Everything in creation has a purpose... mosquitoes provide larvae, making fish food... and fish keep our waters clean. Tobacco, arsenic, opium and other poisons can be made into helpful homeopathic remedies for a wide variety of ailments. Another beneficial use of tobacco is Co-enzyme Q10. This anti-oxidant serves as a foundation stone for the production of energy at the cellular level – adenosine tri-phosphate – ATP. Who benefits? Anyone under 35 who is challenged with any degenerative disease can benefit from ubiquinone. Anyone over 35 can benefit from the ubiquinol form for maximum absorption.

Co-Q-10, isolated in 1957 by Dr Fred Crane of the University of Wisconsin, was expensive, costing $1,000/g to produce. Then a Japanese company discovered it grows from a mold on tobacco leaves!

They have worldwide rights as the only producer, so all other companies buy from them: some add lecithin or other nutrient factors, and put on their own labels. Research indicates soft-gel capsules are more easily absorbed because Q10 is fat-soluble. Take powdered capsules with something oily such as avocados, nuts or seeds. In addition to energy... Q10 provides a co-enzyme factor assisting other enzymes to function.

More Q10 is in the heart than *any* other tissue... and research indicates those with heart challenges have greatly reduced levels. This wonder nutrient is useful for treating heart disease and high blood pressure, and can protect the heart from further damage... improve the effects of heart surgery... and defends the heart from potential toxic drugs as a preventive.

Besides effectiveness with the heart, Q10 can correct periodontal disease, increase the competence of the immune cells, serve as a factor in weight regulation, and act as a factor in rejuvenation. Repeated tests with old mice saw the shiny coats and bright eyes of youth return... some had a life span equal to about 150 human years. Research shows beneficial effects with diabetes, muscular dystrophy, MS, lupus, allergies, and various respiratory and brain challenges. Natural sources are found in whole grains, nuts, and dark green vegetables.

Experiment. First have a *saturation dose* and then a maintenance dose. This is calculated by weight... 1mg per pound. Divide the dose and take with meals. Do this for 6 weeks. Then cut the dose in half for two weeks. Then take 50-100 mg per day thereafter, depending on body size – double that with *any* statin drug. You may choose to prepare for this saturation dose by taking 30mg a day for a week to introduce the system. Those aware of serious heart challenges may choose to take 2-3X the recommended saturation dose for 6 weeks; then taper down to a maintenance dose.

European natural physicians recommend as much as 1000-1500mg per day for people with Parkinson's disease... and use that amount for the saturation dose, then reduce the amount as above. While this may lead to expensive urine – there are zero adverse effects, and it's only for a short period of time.

Medical science calls Q10 *ubiquinone* meaning, it's everywhere: some doctors see this as a waste of money. Obviously, they have yet to do serious research. Generally, they say... when in doubt – don't! Generally, natural physicians say... when in doubt – dare! Simply muscle test. If You always do what You've always done, You'll always get what You've always gotten. With little to lose and much to gain, experiment Being Well. It's Your Body. It's Your Choice!

Cotton Growers Go Organic

Cotton has been cultivated for >4000 years. In the last several decades, however, the cultivation of cotton has changed dramatically; it is a toxic undertaking. Cotton's public image – natural, healthy and pure – has little connection to its production, involving the ever-escalating use of synthetic pesticides, fertilizers and defoliants. In recent years, however, the cotton industry has begun to roll back the inroads technology has made in farming, in favor of sustainable and environmentally friendly methods.

Recognizing the changes some farmers were making in cotton farming, the clothing manufacturer Patagonia announced in January 1996 it would begin using only organically grown cotton in its products. In addition to switching to organic cotton, Patagonia demonstrated its commitment to reducing environmental harm by *publicizing* the *problems* inherent in conventional methods of cotton cultivation, and encouraging support of *sustainable* agricultural practices. Drawing attention to the environmental cost of conventional cotton cultivation, Patagonia encourages other clothing companies to go organic... as well as aid organic farmers to increase production, and prompt consumers to choose items made of organically grown cotton.

Modern cotton cultivation and the devastation wreaked upon the environment, began after WWII when chemical manufacturers created powerful pesticides, herbicides and fungicides, now used in worldwide agriculture on a massive scale: >6b lbs/ year, much of it on cotton. Although cotton production accounts for only .05 percent of the total worldwide agricultural acreage, **10%** of *all* pesticides used worldwide are used in cotton cultivation. *Cotton uses 20X more pesticides than average farming!*

In conventional cultivation, a cotton seed begins with fumigation to prevent the growth of fungi, then planted in soil *sterilized* to kill organisms that could attack the seed or the roots. The seed and resulting plant are fed synthetic nutrients to promote growth: sprayed with fungicides, herbicides and pesticides to control insects and weeds. Finally, after growth regulators have forced all plants to mature at the same time, they are treated with a defoliant, killing the plants in preparation for harvesting the cotton.

Chemicals in cotton cultivation affect human health in a variety of ways. Unintentional pesticide poisoning is believed to be responsible for innumerable deaths worldwide each year. Pesticides contaminate wells upon which people rely for their drinking water, and have been linked to cancers and other health problems among those who use them, as well as those who live in the areas where they are applied. Pesticides may harm even those who are far removed from cotton farming – through cottonseed oil in foods they eat.

Conventional cotton's impact on the environment is appalling. The sterilization and chemical treatment of soil decreases the ability to hold water or support life. Easily eroded... often highly toxic... pesticides also kill harmless, beneficial species: threatening wildlife coming in contact. Pesticides find their way into groundwater, air and surrounding soils, interfering with reproductive cycles of birds and mammals. Perhaps most disturbing of all... they are ultimately ineffective.

Over a long period of use the insect and plant pests that do not fall prey to the application of chemicals designed to eradicate them, develop resistance to those chemicals. Increased doses may be effective for a time, and natural selection guarantees some always survive, and create new generations of chemically immune pests. As pesticides eliminated predators, superbugs are free to reproduce and damage crops.

To maximize profit, crop rotation is ignored; soil becomes functionally dead, capable of supporting the cotton crop *only* in a mechanical way. Soil degradation, toxification and monocultivation ultimately result in destruction of entire ecosystems. Plants and animals cease to inhabit areas of intensive cotton cultivation, leaving behind an empty, brown landscape.

Environmental awareness led some farmers to adopt organic cultivation, promising to halt devastating effects of conventional cotton farming. Many methods used are not new in the sense of recently discovered. The primary difference in organic methods is, rather than relying on synthetic compounds to aid production, they utilize natural processes and interaction among species to create a cotton ecosystem. A variety of techniques, skills and knowledge is required.

In place of synthetic fertilizers, organic farmers plow under special crops and use off-site composting and crop rotation to add nutrients to the soil. Cover crops are grown around the cotton; they combine hand and machine weeding; they release beneficial insects to replace pesticides. Near organic cotton fields, farmers plant "trap crops" attracting pests away from the crop. To avoid mixing leaves with the cotton during harvesting, organic farmers hand pick, stop applying irrigation water or rely on frost to kill the plants.

Organic cotton cultivation is more labor intensive than conventional cultivation; hence, it costs more. At each step, more human skill and knowledge is required to replace the more efficient, yet detrimental, chemical applications. The organic farmer and a trained workforce *must constantly attend to the crop to ward off hazards, to* maintain soil fertility and to eliminate weeds. Although organic methods make an enormous difference in environmental impacts, the countries that currently cultivate organic cotton see little change in the amount or quality of the harvests.

To lend validity to organic labeling, groups have formed to certify organic cotton production. There are currently hundreds of organizations to certify organic cultivation. Groups range from private, non-profit organizations like the California Certified Organic Farmers, to government agencies like the Texas Department of Agriculture. Recently, the International Federation of Organic Agricultural Movements developed a program to assure groups use the same standards and procedures.

The majority of certifying groups require soil free from synthetic chemical use for 3 years before the cotton produced can be called organic. Cotton grown with natural methods in the interim is termed transitional. Certification also requires the gin and spinning equipment be cleaned to remove chemical traces before organically grown cotton is processed. Consequently, clothing companies and consumers who purchase organic cotton can be sure production assisted the environment; fibers are free from toxins.

Organic cotton cultivation, and sustainable agriculture in general, highlights the gap we get to bridge between economically viable and environmentally viable. Chemical-intensive cultivation maximizes monetary profits, but carries hidden costs: pesticide regulation and testing, hazardous waste disposal and cleanup, and incalculable environmental losses.

Although organic farming methods appear new and innovative, in some ways they resemble the traditional methods employed a century ago – labor intensive... reliant on natural materials. Perhaps it was then agriculture reached sustainability. The environmental damage evident today is the result of humans' attempt to go beyond sustainability. If that is the case, then we must now look back in order to move ahead.

Patagonia, Inc. partnered with The Nature Conservancy and Ovis XXI – a group of sheep ranchers in Argentina and southern Chile – to protect and restore Patagonia's multi-million-acre grasslands. The Patagonia Grassland Regeneration and Sustainability Standard (GRASS), is a voluntary system; ranches reaching specific rangeland conservation goals earn certification. Patagonia, Inc. has committed to buying the certified wool to be used in its clothing. Restored grasslands mean more grazers like rodents and rabbits, which means healthier populations of predators like red foxes and pumas, as well as large birds and wildlife in general. As conscious consumers, it behooves us to support holistic management of Our Beloved Mother Earth. Explore: The Pesticide Action Network of North America www.panna.org

Diabetes

Diabetes is the leading cause of blindness, and accounts for 50% of leg and foot amputations. Diabetes can cause impotence, gangrene and hearing impairments. Our first known description of the disease is from an Egyptian papyrus from 1500 BCE. The Greek physician Aretaeus of Cappadocia named it diabetes around 100 CE meaning, going through... increased urination being the first sign. Ancient physicians, noticing ants were attracted to the urine of diabetics, and that the urine left a white deposit, assumed that salt was being lost. Then in the 17th century a physician named Thomas Willis tasted diabetic urine and proclaimed it "wondrous sweet." Then another physician named it diabetes mellitus – sweet urine. Usually seen as a disease of affluence, affecting the overweight... particularly those who carry their weight at the waistline, rather than the thighs.

While a few doctors still recommend a high protein diet, as they did in the late 18th century, actuality a low protein, low fat, and high complex-carbohydrate diet brings optimal results. Fat, specifically animal foods, directly impairs the function of insulin, and causes obesity. Dr James Anderson, of the University of Kentucky, has produced diabetes in healthy, lean men by feeding a very high fat diet for two weeks! Now with widespread use of fast-foods and hydrogenated fats, the disease of affluence is imposed upon the indigent – a consequence of so-called civilization. *Super-Size Me!* is an eye-opening documentary.

Avoiding animal foods and refined, processed foods is essential to support normal functioning of the body. Taking plenty of extra plant-based enzymes along with probiotics and Co-Q10 supports pancreas, liver and kidneys – bringing dramatic benefits.

Dr Anderson found that with appropriate diet, "95% of adult-onset diabetics on oral drugs could be off such drugs in less than eight weeks, and 50-75% could normalize blood sugar and get off all insulin within weeks." People achieved the same results after 30 days on a raw diet... some Type 1 Diabetes can be insulin free! This has proven by Gabriel Cousens, MD.

In the respected magazine *Diabetes Care,* November, 1997, "Diabetic Peripheral Neuropathy" praises advanced technology that can restore circulation... and actually has avoided many amputations. Overcoming lymphatic and circulatory stasis, the instrument is available for both doctor's office and home use. https://www.h-wave.com/

Diarrhea

The body knows what it is doing... getting rid of toxins and waste. Avoid animal-based foods; eat high-fiber, plant-based foods. Drink plenty of fluids to replace those lost. Green banana is constipating and garlic is normalizing. In chronic cases, drink whole watermelon juice rich in electrolytes; use Homeopathic *Kurchi*, in recurrent cases.

Diatomaceous Earth

DE is a whitish powder rich in silica, composed of the shells of diatoms – various minute unicellular, colonial algae of the class Bacillariophyceae... having siliceous cell walls consisting of two overlapping symmetrical parts. Used on field crops, as food for livestock or household pets, there is a version for human consumption, that is easy to use. 10 Amazing Uses for Diatomaceous Earth in the Home | Wellness Mama

Most deposits of DE are useless... some are dangerous. Optimal DE is food grade... known as fossil shell flour that is suitable for animals; the formula for human consumption is *grain storage* or *D-10* from Biocontrol: www.biconet.com 1Tsp in a glass of water on an empty stomach once a day, cleanses the intestinal tract, providing abundant silica the body can transmute, perhaps into calcium... enriching hair, skin and nails. It may be applied to any rash or slow-healing wound, perhaps with coconut oil. Silica also helps fight free radical damage in a way similar to antioxidants as it remains stable and carries a negative electrical charge, attracting positively charged free radicals. As the precession of the equinoxes in the zodiac brings us into the Age of Aquarius... the Age of the Crystal... DE, along with the ancient, edible forms of Blue-green algae, provides elite, superior nutrition; highly recommended.

DO-IN: The Art of Self-Massage

Do-In (DOE-in) the Ancient Art, also called Tao Yinn or Dao Yinn meaning: The Way of the Voice of Nature... opens energy channels and keeps them flowing, by rubbing and generating heat. For a grounding, centering experience to *relax* and *release*: rub counter-clockwise; to *tonify* and *strengthen*: rub clockwise.

Rub fingernails against each other briskly, generating heat and energizing the acupuncture meridians.

Rub hands until warm, as though giving a good washing.

Rub the crown and temples for mental clarity.

Rub the ears to heat the body, vitalizing the kidneys.

Rub the eyes to vitalize the liver, refreshing the spirit.

Rub the nose to vitalize the heart, feeling One.

Rub the mouth to vitalize digestive processes.

Rub nostrils and cheeks to eliminate mucus, cleansing the lungs.

Rub the neck for emotional balance and poise.

Rub the arms to ease nervousness and resolve emotional challenges.

Rub the chest and upper back to release depression, fear and grief.

Rub the heart to enhance circulation and increase Love for All of Life.

Rub the liver to sustain energy, strengthening the eyes.

Rub kidneys to clear ear challenges, improving hearing.

Rub the feet for physical strength and mental grounding.

Rub the legs to release past challenges... being here and now.

Rub the buttocks to relax the sciatic nerves, tension and stress.

Rub the sacrum to relax lower back, hemorrhoidal and menstrual challenges.

Rub the belly for abundant health and centering, enhancing intuition and wisdom.

Doctor and Physician

The Latin word *doctor* means teacher... perhaps, referring to someone who has a doctoral degree such as DC, DDS, DO, MD, ND or PhD, or someone with a degree from the School of Life – Scola Dura Saxa. Whatever the schooling, the holistic approach incorporates an understanding of the relationships between the physical, emotional, mental and spiritual aspects of Life. The Greek word *physis* means *nature* the title physician implies: one who brings about the natural order of things by returning to Nature's Ways. Doctor and physician both imply spending time... listening... honoring queries and comments.

The true doctor teaches what has been overlooked or ignored... restoring natural order internally and externally. The true doctor / physician understands the caduceus: known in ancient times as the Staff of Hermes. The vertical line represents the spinal column, the central nervous system, the Path of Kundalini or coiled energy... rising from the base of the spine as Pure Consciousness with the origin being the *sacrum*, the Latin word meaning, sacred. The ancients recognized the sacred bone as such, and named it so:

os sacrum – THE sacred bone. Two serpents twined around the central staff represent female and male energies... symbolizing the feeling body and the thinking body wrapped around the acting body. Kundalini {coiled energy} rises from the sacrum in a double helix spiral... similar to DNA... culminating in the right and left hemispheres of the brain, coordinated by the corpus callosum. The wings represent lift off of coiled energy rising from the Root to the Crown energy centers, where the experience is conscious communion with High Self as One. Nirvana.

Dowsing

Everyone has intuitive capacities... called by science: Innate Intelligence, tuning-in or tapping into Infinite Mind, Divine Intelligence! Perhaps this is why L-rods are often called divining rods. As with all skills, using L-rods or dowsing rods requires balance, determination, trust and persistent practice. Every object, animate and inanimate, has energetic radiations, and our expanded senses perceives them intuitively – and even measure them. The subconscious or super-conscious mind is the recipient of this information. L-rods facilitate communication between conscious and subconscious establishing the required communication between the two aspects of Self. With practice, the subconscious will become acclimated and respond accurately. Be in a meditative space and approach dowsing with Thanksgiving... Enthusiasm... Optimism... and Confidence... Knowing You *can* do it.

American pioneers found water using L-rods or other means of dowsing, bringing this knowledge from the Old World. A tree branch that forked into a Y was most often used – usually from Witch hazel, *Hamamelis virginiana* or even the common willow, *Salix alba*. Some people call it dowsing for water... others say "witching for water". Interestingly, Witch Hazel has nothing to do with witches – *wiche* in olde English literally means: pliant. Branches from this tree were favored, also used for archery. *Hamamelis* is the primary ingredient in the ointment Preparation H and because of its astringent qualities it is commonly used on hemorrhoids; many think the H refers to the condition... rather than associating the H with the tree from which it was derived!

You can easily make L-rods from a hanger and a straw. Cut the hanger in two with 4" handles that bends at 90°, extending 10". Cut the straw in two 4" pieces to cover the handles; holding the straws allows for free movement. Walking, hold the rods steady. At first, they may move to the center crossing each other, or move sideways. Meditate. Practice.

Once comfortable, walk to one side of a room, then walk toward someone. Depending on the power of their auric field, when You are 4-8' away, the rods spread apart at their secondary aura, and You have just done Your first reading. Congratulations! Practice.

Having used a *pendulum* for years, and quite comfortable with this means of accessing information, I received a set of L-rods as a gift; it was quite the conversation piece. Then one night someone came for a treatment. Borrowing a car, the owner gave her a single key for both door and ignition. She took a short cut from her car to the door and, being emotionally distraught, inadvertently dropped the key in the grass! After the treatment she made the discovery. Being without a flashlight, the L-rods came to mind. It was the first time I used them, so I practiced walking slowly from my office to the front door, holding my hands steady. Honestly, there was little hope – only trust. Imagining a line from her car across the grass to the front door, I slowly moved in that direction. Surprisingly, the rods converged toward the center and crossed. At first – chiding myself for being distracted, vowing to hold them with more attention to steadiness – I thought: Wait a minute! Squatting to the ground... between my feet... was the single key among the blades of grass! You can do it too!

Several years later... with Harvey Lisle (*The Enlivened Rock Powders*), we walked to the center of a property and clearly stated our specific intention: "I am looking for a water source that will give 10 gallons per minute!" Harvey slowly began turning in a circle... eventually, the L-rods crossed and he declared: "It's in this direction." He walked until they crossed again. "Here... here's the spot." They dug their well... built their house... and are still enjoying plentiful water.

There are professional water dowsers who have a success rate of 95%+ – never quite 100%... still it is phenomenal! On page 173 of his book, Harvey declares there is "a rational reason why this can be done, and succeeds most of the time. Water travels through the ground in veins of gravel or sand because there is less resistance to flow. As the water travels through the veins, there is a certain amount of friction generated – and friction generates an electrical force field. Nearly everyone has had the experience of walking across a thick carpet on a dry day, touching some metallic object and a spark flies; the person jumps. As the dowser walks along dowsing for water, he enters the electrical field created by the water flowing through the gravel vein, and L-rods or pendulum respond to this force.

"Picking up the forces emanating from paramagnetic rock powders is the key to determining whether they are paramagnetic and not inert. Certainly, dowsing a rock powder is easier and simpler than dowsing for water. Either rock powder has a force field or it doesn't. If the force field spirals upward, counter-clockwise, it indicates paramagnetism; if it spirals downward, clockwise, it indicates diamagnetism. Healthy soil balances the two forces."

Harvey says to make such a determination: use one L-rod and ask, "Does this soil have more paramagnetic or diamagnetic forces?" If it points to the left, it indicates counterclockwise paramagnetic forces, as it would over a bucket of basalt; if it points to the right, it indicates clockwise diamagnetic forces, as it would over a bag of lime. Plants by their nature pull in more lime (calcium) forces, so they are a little more diamagnetic, or slightly alkaline; good soil pulls in more silica and basalt forces, so it has more of a paramagnetic, or slightly acid force. Dowsing opens many doors. Explore! See also below: **Muscle Testing, Pendulums and Switched Energies**.

Ear Candles
The function of the ear is to change sound waves to mechanical vibrations that can stimulate nerve cells and facilitate communication. The key to the system lies with the 3 small bones of the ear, hinged together inside the middle ear cavity. Incoming sound waves are funneled along the ear canal where they strike the eardrum and make it vibrate. Hard wax or other debris can interfere with those vibrations. Those using a hearing aid may secrete more wax than others, clogging their hearing; also true for swimmers, transcribers, telephone operators and others with ears plugged or covered for extended periods... wax and fungus may become a challenge.

Ear candles made & used properly create an energetic vacuum drawing debris from the ear canal... restoring free flow of sound vibrations: painless, effective, convenient and economical. Avoid flying for one week.

To rinse the ear: mix equal parts rubbing alcohol and hydrogen peroxide, letting it sit until the bubbling sound disappears; without bubbling, the H2O2 is >90 days from opening the bottle; ineffective. For earache: use fresh, middle catch urine – or warm, garlic-infused olive oil... held in place with a ball of cotton.

Earth's Energies

North: Wisdom and Knowledge – White.
Northeast: Communication and Wisdom.
East: Illumination and Communication – Yellow.
Southeast: Loving Communications.
South: Place of the Heart – Green.
Southwest: Self Love and Understanding.
West: Introspection – Brown.
Northwest: Wisdom of Self.

"Earth, rather than a planet with life on it, is a living planet. The physical structure – core, mantle, mountain ranges – acts as the skeleton or frame of its existential body.

"Soil covering its grasslands and forests is a mammoth digestive system where all things break down, absorb, and recycle into new growth.

"Oceans, waterways, and rain, function as a circulatory system that moves life-giving "blood" – purifying and revitalizing the body.

"Algae, bacteria, plants and trees provide the planet's lungs, constantly regenerating the entire atmosphere.

"The animal kingdom provides the functions of a nervous system, a finely tuned and diversified series of organisms sensitized to environmental change. Each species is a unique expression of life, with its own consciousness... and its own gifts to the whole body.

"Humankind allows the planet to exercise self-conscious awareness – reflexive thought – the human enables Earth to reflect on itself... and on the Infinite Mystery out of which it has come... in which it exists. We are a means by which nature can appreciate its own beauty, feel its own splendor... or destroy itself.

"Shifting from seeing ourselves as separate beings placed on Earth – the world was made for us – to seeing ourselves as a self-reflexive expression of Earth – we were made for the world – is a major shift in our understanding of who and what we are... a shift at the deepest possible level: our **identity**... our sense of self." (Michael Dowd, *The Big Picture*, quoted in *The Enlivened Rock Powders*, by Harvey Lisle.) Perhaps more accurately put, "our identity: our sense of **Self**."

From time immemorial, we have been invited to Know Thyself! ...a paradigm shift equivalent to the chick leaving the egg. Having looked outside at the world around us – the macrocosm – here's a fascinating look at the physical world within – the microcosm. Stretched out... the DNA in a *single cell* would measure 1 meter long. All DNA in a human body stretched out in a single line would reach from Earth to the Sun and back 50X! Since the Sun is 93m miles away... this means we are comprised of approximately 4.65 trillion miles of DNA!

EMFs – Protection from Electromagnetic Frequencies

Some 21st century frequencies throw our immune response system out of balance, wreaking havoc with our health and well-being; electromagnetic frequencies: EMFs, and electromagnetic radiations: EMRs, emanate from everything that runs on AC: cell phones and cell towers – cameras and Wi-Fi on the roadways, cars, computers, cordless phones, vacuum cleaners, blenders, power tools, hair dryers, etc.

The situation came to light when people sued carriers, claiming brain tumors were in the shape of cell phones – some tumors, even including the shape of the antenna! Industry spent several millions to conduct a study, hiring Dr George Carlo to disprove such claims. In fact, his study substantiated the claims: Dr George Carlo's: *Cell phones: invisible hazards in the wireless age; an insider's alarming discoveries about cancer and genetic damage,* 2001, as well as *Wireless phones and health: scientific progress,* 1998, and *Wireless phones and health II: state of the science,* 2001.

Obviously, we've known about this danger for a long time. Many countries are reasonably cautious with children. In Sweden, it is illegal for kids under 17 to use a cell phone; other countries in Europe and the UK strongly discourage use until 16. Studies show when a child uses a cell phone for two *minutes* it takes two *hours* for brainwaves to return to normal. Why so long? The human skull gradually thickens – and is fully-wired – only at age 26. Sweden also warns that the antenna on the base of a cordless phone is like having a cell phone tower in Your home or office. EMFs are constant, even when the phone is sitting idle. Sweden and Canada warn about Wi-Fi: disrupting the immune system and the brain.

The fine print in current cell phone contracts states that the person will not sue the company or phone manufacturers – either individually or in a class action suit; most people fail to pay attention to that clause signing the contract, and... it's impossible to get a phone without a signed contract! In addition, instruction booklets state that the user should hold the phone *at least* an inch from the head and limit calls to *5 minutes*. Who does that? Think of our teens; think of our future. It is wise to be aware – to use protection, especially with items we hold in our hands so close to our heads – such as a cell phone or hair dryer, and those items we practically hug – computers, laptops and other electronic gadgets.

Technology developed in the Russian space program was bought by a German company; they tweaked the technology and verified its effectiveness with European as well as American university studies. This technology was bought by an American company and is now widely available. There is a specific Cell Guard that does not *block* EMFs, otherwise the cell phone would not work; rather, they *modulate* and *harmonize* the frequencies making them compatible with the frequencies of the body. All other applications use the Universal Guard – one on the base unit of the cordless phone and one on the handset; use 2 two inches apart on the router; 2 on a desktop: both monitor and tower; 1 on a laptop; 2 on machines: the motor & the switch.

Thermography pictures without the Guard after 15 minutes of cell phone use – show intense red, orange and yellow – indicating heat in the brain; the next day, same person using the same phone with a Guard, after 15 minutes – show cool blues and greens... normal.

Some people see remarkable improvement in a week. Headaches, neck and shoulder pain, mental confusion, and tiredness – can disappear. One mother reported her son recently complained about knee pain and she thought it was simply "growing pains" all kids experience. When her Guards arrived, she called to her son to bring his cell phone. He always wore cargo pants, slung low around his hips, with deep pockets. As he reached for his phone, she realized it was at the level of his aching knee. She knew cell phones give off the biggest burst of radiation when ringing and when dialing; his knee pain disappeared within a week.

Also available is a state-of-the-art pendant – Bio*life* – developed by Robert Richards of *Clarus* fame, made of surgical steel and copper. We live in a Sea of Radiation; this is wonderful protection – especially when in a store or working someplace likes a hospital... or an office where there may be multiple computers and other electronic paraphernalia... or on a plane and Your neighbor pulls out a laptop for the duration of the flight. Using protection is a necessity of Life. Dr Robert Becker says: "The greatest danger we face is not global warming, or even chemical pollution. It is clearly electromagnetic pollution!"
https://www.giawellness.com/23215/products/energy/

Energy and Vibration
Energy derives from the Greek *en ergon*, at work, referring to vigor or power in *action*. Vibration refers to rapid linear *motion* of a particle or elastic solid, about an equilibrium position; (slang) a distinctive e-*motion*-al aura, or atmosphere, capable of being sensed, or experienced as "vibes".

Energy Boost – DIY
Do It Yourself energy boost is free and costs only concentration, intention, and time. Focus. Meditate. Be One with Self and feel Energy within.

Jin Shin Juytsu means: Divine-Human-coming-together. Using Your hands as jumper cables to boost energies throughout Your body, there are 6 basic contact points. Breathe slowly and deeply, exhaling completely... with Your tongue gently caressing the bump at the roof of the mouth – connecting Your heart and pineal centers. "Be Still, And Know: I Am God."

As You breathe in, visualize... Love filling You. As You breathe out, visualize... well, traditionally it would be said: negativity leaving; that, however, honors duality; others say: blockages leaving – and that gives credence to the blockages. Besides... what You resist persists; what You allow changes. Simply visualize... Love coming in, dancing around Your heart... healing everything... and let Love move through as You exhale, healing everyone... healing all Life everywhere. Words help the flow initially, then it becomes automatic. Tongue caressing the roof of the mouth, slowly breathe in: I bring Love into my life. Exhale completely: I express Love to the world. After some practice, there may be a build-up and release of energy compared to pleasurable waves after orgasm.

The 1st contact of Jin Shin Juytsu – **Total Harmonizer** – energizes the Central and Governing Vessels in charge of all the meridians, and influencing... through the navel and diaphragm... Your feeling body, Your thinking body and Your acting body – Your Whole Being – balancing the hypothalamus, the Motherboard of Your brain, which controls the endocrine glands producing hormones orchestrated by Your Heart.

Bring Your thumb webs together at the navel, hands resting comfortably on the skin of the lower belly – Your hara – Your power center. Probably, Your dominant hand is on top. Switch hands now and feel the difference. One is more comfortable than the other – lightly hold *that* contact with the thumb underneath and the fingers on top of the other hand. As You do 9 breaths described above, visualize Love doing a delightful dance all around Your diaphragm and umbilicus. Continue caressing, gently moving Your tongue; breathe in rounds of 9 until You feel pulsing of energy in Your hands. {Doing this the first time, and then seasonally... traditionally to do four rounds of 9, regardless of when the pulsing may occur.}

The 2nd contact – **Sustenance** – energizes the spleen / stomach meridian. With Your dominant hand, gently grasp and hold the opposite thumb, with thumb-webs touching... hands on hara. Caressing during the 9 breaths, visualize Love doing a delightful dance around Your spleen and Your stomach.

The 3rd contact – **Essential Rhythms of Life** – energizes the lung / large intestine meridian. Insert Your ring finger into Your gently closed dominant hand. Caressing during the 9 breaths, visualize Love doing a delightful dance through the intricate pockets of Your lungs and Your large intestine.

The 4th contact – **Harmonizer of All the Elements** – energizes the liver / gall bladder meridian. Insert Your middle finger into Your gently closed dominant hand. Caressing during the 9 breaths, visualize Love doing a delightful dance throughout Your liver.

The 5th contact – **Flow** – energizes the kidney / bladder meridian. Insert Your index finger into Your gently closed dominant hand. Caressing during the 9 breaths, visualize Love doing a delightful dance through the fine tubules of Your kidneys... and through Your bladder.

The 6th contact – **Inner Knowing** – energizes the heart and small intestine meridian. Insert Your little finger into Your gently closed dominant hand. Caressing during the 9 breaths, visualize Love doing a delightful dance through every chamber of Your heart and around the villi of Your small intestine.

Further enhancing Harmonious Healing for the meridian systems, bring the fingertips of both hands pressed together, with fingers spaced apart and do the 9 breaths; then, while briskly tapping the fingertips together, conclude with 9 final breaths.

After 3 months of daily practice, **Advanced Jin Shin Jyutsu** may proceed: with energies flowing harmoniously through Your body, You can use Your hands to harmonize with the Source of all Life everywhere: the Divine Presence that sustains all. Take a deep, caressing breath; exhaling, visualize energy moving down the center front of Your body; inhaling, visualize energy moving up the center of Your back. Picture this unbroken circle... caressing... breathing in and out 9 times.

Place Your right hand on the top of Your head and hold it there until instructed otherwise. Bring the thumb and fingertips of the left hand together, placing between the eyebrows. This revitalizes energy deep within... improving memory, dissipating mental stress, senility. 9 caressing breaths until pulsations are felt.

Then open Your left hand and let the palm gently rest at the tip of Your nose. This revitalizes both the reproductive and circulatory systems. 9 caressing breaths until pulsations are felt.

Bring the thumb and fingertips of the left hand together, placing them on Your mid-sternum. This revitalizes both the lungs and the pelvis. 9 caressing breaths until pulsations are felt.

Move Your fingertips to the tip of the sternum. This revitalizes the Source of Life energy – both descending and ascending forces. 9 caressing breaths until pulsations are felt.

Move Your fingertips to the pubic bone. This revitalizes the descending Source of Life energy, strengthening the spine. 9 caressing breaths until pulsations are felt.

Leaving Your fingertips at the top of the pubic bone, now move Your right hand from the top of Your head; place Your palm at Your sacrum with the tip of Your middle finger at the coccyx, the tip of the spine. This revitalizes the ascending Source of Life energy... aiding circulation to the legs and feet. 9 caressing breaths until pulsations are felt.

To explore beyond these basics – *The Touch of Healing: Energizing Body... Mind... Spirit with the Art of Jin Shin Jyutsu*, by Alice Burmeister with Tom Monte.

Other ancient mudras or hand gestures improve concentration, memory and overall mood... as well as increase neural activity. With Your right hand: join the tips of the ring and little fingers with the thumb – keeping the other two fingers straight; with Your left hand: join the tips of the middle and ring fingers with the thumb – again keep the other fingers straight. 5 minutes, 4x/day. Affirm: I have clear goals... clear priorities... and a loving sense of satisfaction.

For another energy boost to recharge Your batteries day or night, simply go outdoors, away from electrical interference of motors – air conditioners and refrigerators – as well as the router, Wi-Fi, computers and TV, and... stay away from overhead wires. Hold hands stretched above Your head, much like antennae; turn slowly until You feel tingling in the palms of Your hands. The first time, it took a few minutes to feel; and only a few seconds for Monkey-mind to appear.

"Wait a minute... of course, You feel tingling in Your hands; they've been over Your head for a few minutes and the blood has drained down Your arms, silly!" So, keeping my arms stretched to the heavens, I turned away and the tingling immediately disappeared. Returning to that direction, it started again. To be sure, turning in the other direction... again it disappeared; returning to the original position, so did the tingling!

My kahuna-mentor Mr Ting laughed. "Such skepticism is normal" he said. "That is the direction of Your birthplace." Fortunately, it was a clear night and I quickly checked the North Star – I was facing east-northeast, an accurate direction from Maui to Detroit. "What about in Detroit?" "You will find the tingling in the direction of the hospital or home where You were born; and, except for electrical interference in a hospital, You could find the room where You first saw the light of day.

If You were born at home, You could find the room!" Find Your direction... surround Yourself with Love... breathe deeply with tongue caressing: 3X3 Sacred Breaths as energies recharge. Feel the power. Feel empowered. Be the Power!

If You are doing "all the right things" and still feel somewhat out-of-sorts, here's a simple, time-honored remedy for what ails You... wild-grown kelp and / or Klamath Lake blue-green algae taken with water... adequately provide Mother Nature's powerhouse of minerals and trace elements to get the electricity flowing. First, prepare Your body: take 1 cap or 1/8 tsp morning, and mid-day before 4 pm for 3 days; double that for 3 days; continue doubling to 8 caps or 1 tsp taken 3x/day. Even if 3 meals are not eaten, take the dose with a glass of water. Maintain until symptoms subside. Gradually reduce, should one wish to do so, until symptoms reappear... then bump it up a notch; maintain that dose. Some situations require a high amount. Your body has the answer – muscle test. Cleansing? Simply have those nutrients with 2-3 quarts of re-mineralized and re-energized distilled or r/o water, depending on body size, mostly in the morning – for 1-3 days. It is such a powerful experience You may be inspired to do another 3 days, or longer. Experiment. You Are the Power!

Given the wide and balanced nutrient content, be open to miracles as the body returns to homeostasis. In fact, as the commercials say: "Ask Your doctor if this is good for You!" Rather than asking... You are informing so any medications can be monitored and possibly discontinued.

Will Tuttle, PhD, author of *The World Peace Diet: Eating for Spiritual Health and Social Harmony*, clarifies: "We have cast our culture out of the garden and into the rat race of competition and consumerism. As we repress the shame of our routine violence toward nature and animals, our resulting hidden low self-esteem drives the profits of corporations that enrich themselves through our craving for gadgets, drugs and entertainment to help distract us from what we know in our Hearts, and to gloss over the violence of our meals. As we question this mentality of domination and choose compassion, healing and peace by eating plant-based meals, we find our joy rising, our spirit deepening, our mind quickening, our feelings softening, energy increasing and creativity flourishing." Follow Your Inner Voice Intuition. Or, simply ask Your High Self. See below: **Muscle Testing, Pendulums and Switched Energies**.

Enlightenment

Rather than attaining, developing or *having* something, enlightenment is recognition of Be–ing the I Am that I Am expressing Infinite Being in this finite temporary form, exploring human consciousness. Enlightenment is truly liberating. Recognizing there are infinite expressions of Infinite Being frees us from judgment or coercion. Our consciousness becomes transparent to its own Intrinsic Nature, as being the One... in action.

Echu, the Zen poet, says "It is a rare privilege to be born a human being, as we happen to be... if we do not experience enlightenment in this life, when do we expect that we will?"

Fritz Perls says: "When we lose our minds... we come to our senses." Go beyond Your mind, go beyond Your senses in meditation; turn Your mind and Your senses within, You can *feel* You Are the One... *I Am that I Am*. I Am the Vibration that sustains All – I Am the Source of All. I Am the delightful expression of the I Am!

We have glimmers of this feeling, a moment here or there... and when that feeling becomes habitual, it is Enlightenment – when we truly feel there is nowhere to go, nothing to do – or attain, and nobody You have to be, except exactly who You are right now. You *Are* the One, the epitome of Free Will, exploring human experience through the unique circumstances of Your precious Life.

There are many forms of meditation that claim to facilitate the process of Realization resulting in Your Enlightenment – from basic Raja Yoga, turning one's senses within... to highly complicated techniques discussed below in the section on **Supernatural Breathing**. There are many excellent books as well, such as *A Course in Miracles*; also, *The Power of Now: A Guide to Spiritual Enlightenment*, by Eckhart Tolle. Especially consider: *The Impersonal Life* and *The Way Out*, by Joseph Benner. These and other books and videos are inspiring – highly recommended to explore.

An articulate prosaic expression of Enlightenment can be found in Erwin Laszlo's *Science and the Akashic Field: An Integral Theory of Everything*:

Come, sail with me on a quiet pond.
The shores are shrouded, the surface smooth.
We are vessels on the pond
and we are one with the pond.
A fine wake spreads out behind us,
traveling throughout the misty waters.
Its subtle waves register our passage.
Your wake and mine coalesce,
they form a pattern that mirrors
Your movement as well as mine.
As other vessels who are also us
sail the pond that is us as well,
their waves intersect with both of ours.
The pond's surface comes alive
with wave upon wave, ripple upon ripple.
They are the memory of our movement;
the traces of our being.
The waters *whisper* from You to me...
and from me to You,
and from both of us to all the others
who sail the pond:
Our separateness is an illusion;
we are inter-connected parts of the whole –
we are a pond with movement and memory.
Our Reality is greater than You and Me,
and All the vessels that sail the waters,
and All the waters on which they sail**!**

When all is said and done... perhaps the simplest and easiest way to achieve and experience Enlightenment is to find a pond... or somewhere else in Nature... and consider the advice found in seven words from the *Book of Enoch*: Be Still... And Know... I Am God!

Essene Benediction Celebrating Life

Essene tradition encourages empowerment through Consciousness and Awareness. There is a difference between the two. Think of a snowstorm. Each flake is a unique expression swirling and dancing – enjoying the Experience of Being a radiant, 6-sided crystal of *singular* beauty and importance, supporting the action of the mighty blizzard! Stroking the ego with thrilling experiences forms the basis of Awareness. Consciousness happens as the snowflake meets the ocean, enjoying Harmony, Singularity & Peace. That *feeling* of Awareness is possible here & now.

Essene tradition cherishes Communing with Nature as a Way of realizing the intercourse between Awareness – the blizzard... and Consciousness – the ocean. Divine play between Father Sun and Mother Earth beckons! Communing with Nature is a Way of realizing the connection between the feeling body, the thinking body and the acting body, and a Way of realizing the relationship of All Creation Everywhere. There is only Oneness... captured, perhaps, as Divine Presence providing an ocean of sustenance for all Creation that we know... and the oceans we have yet to discover.

Planet Earth, for our particular experiment, or experience, requires both Polarity and Free Will. In our polarity reality, the Divine Presence – OM, All That Is – first expressed creation as Mother Goddess and Father God... from which Creation flows. Everything we experience is an aspect of blended female and male energies. We have estrogen and testosterone floating in our systems via our gonads and adrenals.

The Divine Presence explores Infinite Imagination. Each One of Us is a multi-faceted manifestation somewhere along the infinite continuum stretching from Brilliant Light, such as Mary Magdalen, to Dazzling Darkness, such as Mao. Each person chooses their own comfortable shade of gray – everyOne manifests Divine Presence exploring. OM in a phrase, All That Is... in a word, OM is hOMe. Welcome hOMe! The Kingdom of Heaven truly is within. We choose our Reality to experience our Own Lessons. We explore Infinite Possibilities as One Infinite Be–ing. In the Essene Tradition, rather than prayer or petitioning... let it be a Celebration of Life. Rather than begging *for* something to be received, or a change of heart *from* someone, Essenes fill their Hearts with Joy... as they *stand in* their Wish Fulfilled!

When Gregg Braden left IBM, he traveled for years to remote cultures, staying in various monasteries on his quest to discover what is behind their power of "prayer". When he returned to drought-stricken Taos, NM, he was excited when a Native American friend asked, "Would You like to come along to a Rain Dance." Like to? Gregg was ecstatic! Arriving at a nondescript, albeit dry, circle of stones it was just the two of them... his friend removed boots and sox and started moving around the stones – for about 15 minutes. He then abruptly sat down and said, OK, we can go now. Astounded, Gregg said: That's it?! Yes, his friend said... he danced until he heard the rumbling of thunder and sharp cracks of lightning... until he heard the rain moving through the corn fields... and the children dancing exuberantly, splashing in the streets... he danced and danced and when he felt mud

oozing between his toes... he knew his service was complete. He had entered his Heart of Hearts... feeling Joy... being *in* his Wish Fulfilled!

In fact, an unexplained pocket of air moved in bringing some minor relief. You may enjoy Gregg's books, especially *Walking Between the Worlds: The Essene Science of Compassion* and *The Isaiah Effect: Decoding the Lost Science of Prayer and Prophecy*, and his recent writings; and the video: *The 3 Amigos* with Drs Bruce Lipton, Joe Dispenza and Gregg Braden. The 3 Amigos are more than 3 Friends, or 3 Kindred Spirits – 3 Wise Men with a knack for explaining, each from their own particular scientific background, the process of standing in... feeling... and thus creating... Your Wish Fulfilled!
https://www.youtube.com/watch?v=P_FlYwg2oU4

The following may help find Your Heart of Hearts, and *feel* the Joy which is the Essence of the Divine Presence. *Feel* the power... Feel *empowered*... *Be* the Power! The roots of the Essene Tradition go back to Chaldean times, long before the Jewish sect of the 2nd century. While there is much speculation – the Essene community is far from being a static group of celibate monks. Many chose to change the **i** to **e**, add the **r** and... cel**e**b**r**ate Life! We know Essenes are from the Yogic tradition – the primal *holistic* healers: honoring the intimate connection between feeling body... thinking body... and acting body. Contemporary understanding of the word yoga is reduced to exercises, stretches and holding postures... Yogic tradition teaches Inner Communion – inner yoking – connecting the flesh and blood of the acting body with the thinking body... it is then, the feeling body begins to make a connection with the spiritual body.

Ancient tradition also teaches there is a physical, embryological connection between the tissue at the root of the tongue and the tissue forming the pericardial sac that holds the heart. With the tip of Your tongue find and caress the little bump at the roof of Your mouth. Since the g-spot is spoken for, we can call it the G-spot, connecting with the God and Goddess within. Since the Kingdom of Heaven *is* within You, some may call it the H-spot – connecting Heaven with Your Heart. Caressing the little bump, {a small percentage of people have a tiny hole} it expands slightly; the palatine nerve being stimulated increases blood flow to the area making it expand... much like caressing Your lover's nipple. With tongue stimulating this area, a message goes by way of the palatine nerve to the Pineal Center; connecting with the Heart Center... and Love gushes forth! Eventually, connecting the Third Eye center with the Heart center, we begin to *see energetically* with our Heart of Hearts. See below: **Tongue Awareness**.

Being aware of, being Mindful of this connection – caressing with the tongue... breathing slowly & deeply... tells Your entire system that all is well. Being in a safe place, the sympathetic nervous system – freeze! fight? flight? – goes on stand-by; the para-sympathetic system is activated... resumes normal functioning – digest, rest and rejuvenate. Keep Your Focus on Appreciation, Care, Compassion and Gratitude for 3 minutes... creating a signal of .1 Hz – Harmonizing HeartBrain as One.

The optimal experience is in Nature... soaking up free electrons and negative ions barefoot at the seashore, riverbank, lakeside, a bed of grass – or, indoors using a grounding pad. If possible, cross Your ankles, whichever way feels comfortable activating subconscious access; with thumb webs touching at the navel, hands resting comfortably on the skin of the lower belly – Your hara, Your power center – moving Your tongue... loving YourSelf... HeartMindBodySpirit *in* Your Wish Fulfilled!

Estrogenic Pesticides

Hormones occur naturally in small concentrations maintaining delicate balance – regulating growth, development, and sexual traits, among other functions. Naturally present in women, regulating menses, pregnancy, lactation and menopause... estrogen is naturally present also, to a lesser extent, in men – created by their adrenals.

Certain synthetics that kill weeds, insects and pests, and certain chemicals incorporated into plastic, both mimic *and* be mistaken for estrogen. These chemicals contain chlorine, and are stored in fat; they accumulate – interfering with the menstrual cycle, increasing the risk of breast cancer, decreasing certain male characteristics in boys, decreasing sperm counts and interfering with the immune response. Over 50 years, breast cancer rates went from 1 in 20, to 1 in 8; sperm counts dropped 50%.

Unfortunately, estrogen mimics are found everywhere: lawn care chemicals such as 2,4-D, with the offspring Dicamba; atrazine, an herbicide commonly found in domestic water supplies; styrene and phthalates, BPA and elements of plastic that can *ad*sorb into foods... and the ubiquitous environmental toxins dioxin and DDT... now found in the body fat of everyone on Earth.

Avoid lawn care chemicals. What is so important about a lawn free from dandelions? Is it worth getting cancer? Lawn care services and products use broad leaf weed killers containing 2,4-D, called by various names... and the dioxin found in it mimics estrogen. If toxins are on the lawn... You breathe it... Your skin absorbs it... and You track it into Your house.

Avoid chemicals in the home. Instead use an all-purpose cleaner for virtually everything: 2 quarts of water, 1/2C vinegar and 1/4C baking soda; double that for the toilet – after a few minutes, scrub and flush. Sluggish or clogged drains: 1/2C baking soda, then 1C vinegar; wait 20 minutes then flush with hot water for 3 minutes.

Buy food wisely. The safest food is grown organically – free from synthetic chemicals. Because our government subsidizes chemical-intensive agriculture and generally ignores organic agriculture, organic foods are somewhat more expensive than conventionally produced foods. Many organic distributors sell food wholesale to co-ops or clubs... even so, be aware: certain foods contribute a larger share of estrogenic residues... the largest share of atrazine in our diet is from milk, corn, sugar and meat. Fish swimming in contaminated waters concentrate fat-soluble chemicals, including most estrogen mimics. Consider avoiding animal foods, and replacing sugar, honey, and maple syrup with Stevia: 1 drop /8 oz.

Use paper products that are chlorine bleach free. Chlorine bleaching of paper products produces dioxin, some of which remain in the product and some of which are released into our water by paper mills. Use recycled, napkins, towels, toilet paper and filters.

Avoid plastic food packaging. Plasticizers, making plastic flexible, easily migrate into foods, especially those containing fats or alcohol. This migration is intensified with microwaves. With frozen foods of this nature, it is safest to warm them in a Corning Ware dish on low heat. Simplify the process: take from the freezer, and store in the refrigerator before use.

DDT is found in the bark of trees all over the world: low concentrations were found in remote parts of Venezuela and New Zealand; high concentrations of DDT and other organo-chlorine compounds used in insecticides and fungicides were measured in bark from the US, Europe, India, Middle East, Japan, Brazil, Australia, Taiwan, South Korea and Russia. In the US, farming areas in the midwestern and eastern states, California and the South show high contamination. DDT was banned in 1973, yet high concentrations are still found in parts of the Midwest and the Southeast.

A report by the Danish EPA, *Male Reproductive Health and Environmental Chemicals with Estrogenic Effects*, reports dramatic changes in the last 50 years brought about by dioxin and other estrogenic mimics. Besides the decline in sperm counts, a rise in testicular cancer, undescended testicles and hypospadias: malformation of external genitalia. Dioxin has also been linked to endometriosis in women – a painful disease where cells of the tissue lining the uterus, the endometrium, escape and become attached to other pelvic organs, as well as other parts of the body.

The Danish Report identifies many consumer products as possible sources of estrogenic chemicals; in addition to these, watch for any of the 100+ types of PCBs, dioxins and furans, and alkylphenols – breakdown products of alkylphenol polyethoxylates widely used in cosmetics, detergents and paints. Phthalates are the most abundant man-made environmental pollutants, and human intake per day is measured in tens of milligrams. Some plastics contain 40% phthalate esters by weight, leaching out over time. Most plastic packing in the US contains phthalates. Amazingly, blood for transfusions is many times packaged in such plastics. BeAware!

Facial Care

Gently wash with a loofa sponge, then enjoy a facial sauna: bring a pint of water to a boil... add herbs, cover, steep for 5 minutes; bring the pot to the table... tie hair or cover with a scarf... bend over the pot, draping Your head and the pot with a thick towel. Let the steam bathe Your face... keeping eyes closed for ten minutes. Opening the pores, toxins and impurities are released. Lightly scrub again with the loofa, then cold rinse... and a splash of apple cider vinegar.

For oily skin... mix 3Tsp licorice root, 2Tsp lavender, 1Tsp each: comfrey leaf, lemon peel, pansy, parsley, peppermint and strawberry leaves. Boil the roots for ten minutes, then steep the rest for ten minutes. For dry skin... mix 3Tsp licorice root, 2Tsp chamomile, 2Tsp comfrey leaf, 1Tsp each of comfrey root, dulse, sea moss and red clover. Boil roots 10 minutes, then steep the rest 10 minutes.

After the facial sauna, use a mask to rejuvenate: For oily skin... a chlorophyll mask consisting of clay mixed with parsley or other green juice. Mix minced parsley with a small amount of water and add to some dry clay. For dry or chapped skin... oat flour mixed with applesauce. For acne... 1tsp comfrey root powder / 1tsp wheat germ oil. Flabby skin... mashed cucumber.

Follow a mask with a natural astringent to close the pores: apple cider vinegar, aloe-vera water or gel, rose or orange water. Follow with a few drops of moisturizing oil. For the ultimate luxury: use microalgae, such as Aphanizomenon; the same organic nutrients that we take internally can be applied externally nourishing the skin.

Fever

When fever occurs, we can take a deep breath, relax and be grateful: the immune response system is functioning properly. Clearly designed as intelligent beings we innately know what to do for survival.

Childhood diseases exercise the immune response system... and present an opportunity to look at diet and lifestyle. When feverish and eliminating large amounts of mucus, consider the mucus-forming foods: all dairy products, refined flour, white rice, potatoes and sugar. Eliminating these supports smooth functioning, and brings relief for acne, allergies, asthma and other breathing challenges; and that's only the ABCs, the list goes on: diabetes, eczema, fibromyalgia, gangrene, headache, influenza, jaundice, kidney stones, liver challenges... and on and on. Eliminate the congestive factors and dissolve the health challenges.

Beginning the elimination process, there may be a slight to moderate cleansing reaction for a few days, such as headache or body aches. Simply understand what it is, and assist the cleanse by rinsing out, drinking plenty of re-mineralized and re-energized distilled or r/o water.

For a dry fever free from mucus discharge, the body's Innate Wisdom knows turning up the thermostat can eliminate certain intruders. Keep warm… drink warm water or peppermint tea to encourage sweating. Let the body work things out… trust… the body knows what it is doing, knows what is optimal and heals itself.

Small children can peak at 106° free from brain damage – 102-104° is common. An adult with sustained 106° risks brain damage… 104° is tolerable, though uncomfortable. A cool cloth on the head, hands and wrists moderates a high fever. With any fever, take an enema to assist. Fever cleanses… eliminating toxins and congestive factors. Rather than feeling "sick" – be grateful. Your body is responding… and getting well. Fever is Your friend.

After the cleansing, restore balance to Your system by taking prebiotics, probiotics and other friendly bacteria found in raw Sauerkraut or Kimchee. Turmeric, ginger, garlic and onions act as Mother Nature's antibiotics – add to veggiekraut, neutralizing harmful bacteria.

Fleas

Fleas avoid pets regularly fed nutritional yeast and garlic, mixed in their favorite foods. To get rid of fleas, shampoo with undiluted Dr Bronner's peppermint oil soap. To remove fleas from carpeting, before going to bed place a casserole dish with an inch of water on the floor, with a desk lamp shining on the water. Attracted to the light, the fleas fall into the water… moving on to the next dimension of consciousness.

Food Combining

Improper combinations stress the digestive system because larger than normal molecules get absorbed into the bloodstream bringing biochemical impurities to joints, muscles, organs, causing swelling and inflammation such as arthritis, bursitis or fibromyalgia. There are basic principles for easy food combining: Fruit is best eaten as a meal by itself… preferably the first meal of the day. After a night of digesting, fasting and resting, it is the optimal break-fast with cleansing action. Most fruits combine except: Melons: eat them alone or with other melons.

Sub-acid fruits: apples, apricot, grapes, mango, nectarine, papaya, peach, pear, and plum.

Sour fruits: berries, citrus, kiwi, pineapple, pomegranate, sour apples, strawberries.

Sweet fruits: bananas, persimmons and all dried fruits.

Like melons… all fruits combine within their own category. Sub-acid fruits also combine well with *either* sour or sweet.

Sour fruits and sweet fruits… are best kept apart.

Improperly combining may produce digestive stress or gas; an example is a fruit salad made with apples, grapes, citrus pieces and… banana slices. The exception that proves the rule is when You blend sweet and sour fruits creating – for the taste buds – a new sub-acid fruit: a blend of bananas and strawberries, as a sauce for papaya pie – add thin slices of kiwi halves around the rim and You have an example of Chef Aris' Sunfired Paradise Pie! https://www.sunfired.com/

Fruits combine with protein, such as a handful of nuts – germinated, changes most fats to fatty acids; raw nuts will help put on weight, especially germinated, blended and slightly fermented into sunflower (or other) seed cheese. For those on a transition diet… organic, raw goat cheese combines with fruit.

Fruits with starches invite digestive distress and gas, such as cinnamon raisin bread… or basmati rice pilaf with peas, cashews and raisins. The simple reason: starches and sweets when combined create alcohol; while minimal alcohol is normally present in the digestive process, this combination is too intense. Always avoid fruit with starch for superior digestion.
Another combination best avoided is starch and protein; their digestive juices have different pH values. Rice pilaf with cashew or brown rice with nut loaf and salad, sounds nutritious… yet invites digestive stress and gas. While Mother Nature combines protein and carbohydrate – as in beans and grains. The exception that proves the rule is when starch and protein are raw and sprouted, with enzymes intact. An example is salad greens, seaweed, and grated vegetables, with sprouted wheat and rye berries… topped with a dressing of germinated sunflower seeds blended with cucumber and avocado. See Chapter 8: **Enzyme-rich Recipes**.

Full-Spectrum Lighting

A two-year Canadian study found full-spectrum lights in classrooms improves academic achievement, attendance, growth rates, and even lessens tooth decay! Dr Warren Hathaway, the psychologist who conducted the experiment and subsequently presented it to the American Psychological Society –

comments: "Lighting systems are designed more for electrical efficiency than their physiological or psychological effect. This is a huge mistake!"

They collected health and school records of 327 children from five similar suburban schools near Edmonton, Alberta. Students in schools that used yellow-orange high vapor sodium lamps (like street lights) had the worst academic, attendance and health records; students in schools that used the daylight-like fluorescent bulbs that have a low ultraviolet frequency had superior results. Hathaway adds caution to the effect of the lights: since the lights provided a dose of UVB radiation, "You have to be careful about the sun exposure they get outside school in mid-day."

Gall Bladder and Liver Cleanse

The liver creates bile daily... storing it in the gall bladder. Normally when we eat oily or fatty foods, the gall bladder releases bile to emulsify fats and facilitate digestion. When we avoid fats in our diet... bile collects. After 3 or 4 days, the body being efficient, stops production of bile; the gall bladder is full and ready. With a large amount of fat intake, the gall bladder opens... and bile gushes out, carrying any residual build-up, including small gallstones. This procedure empties the gall bladder and stimulates the liver; it has been used with great success by young and old, even while pregnant.

Avoid all fats for 4-5 days; this includes all animal products, oils, nuts, seeds, and avocados. Watch for hidden oils, such as cheese and ice cream made from oil. Drink fresh apple juice, high in pectin and if sweets are tolerated... some beet, carrot and ginger root: dilute ½ and ½ with water. Have salads with lemon juice and Nama Shoyu™ dressing.

Many eat whole apples chewed with as much fresh diced or pressed garlic as possible. Alternative: eat a whole apple – or more, then a heaping tablespoon of pressed garlic – or more, washed down with a minimal amount of water. Simply avoid all oils & fats.

After 4-5 days: upon arising have 2 Tbs of Epsom salts in a glass of warm water as a purge. After an hour, have apples for breakfast. Have a large salad for lunch and skip dinner or have a glass of fresh vegetable juice. When ready for bed, squeeze 4oz of fresh lemon juice and mix with 4oz of organic extra-virgin olive oil. Drink it. Shivering or feeling nauseous is normal. Go to bed and lie on the right side; right knee drawn to chest will open energy pathways for the liver... stay for at least ½ hour... or until falling asleep. Surround Yourself with a cocoon of rose-purple light; surround that with a cocoon of white light. Affirm: I perfectly reflect the rhythm and flow of life. I Am so blessed!

Your bowels may move immediately upon arising; if not, have a large glass of warm water; otherwise, 2Tbs of Epsom salts in warm water. Eliminating many green globules is normal; to explore they could be retrieved, cut in half and analyzed. Once a year is sufficient to increase energy and improve digestion; twice, if there are liver challenges.

Gelatin

Whether found in Jell-O™ or gelatin capsules or powder, the source is animal connective tissue. Some say it comes from horse or cow hooves; actually, a large percentage of gelatin is derived by scraping the inside of the hides of these animals after slaughter. The vibration of death, along with chemical residues, provides adequate reason to avoid these. Better food stores carry vegetarian capsules made from rice starch. Agar-Agar and sea moss – whole rather than powdered – makes a vegan gelatin dessert.

Glandular Support

Pituitary: Alfalfa, *Medicago sativa* – 30C or 200C. Connecting Spirit with Earth, it controls growth, puberty, pregnancy and vitality.

Pineal: Passionflower, *Passiflora incarnata* – 30C or 200C. Known as the seat of the soul, it relates to the Spirit side of Your Nature.

Thyroid: (hyper) 4-6 kelp caps 3/day; (hypo) kelp or dulse liquid, 20-70 drops 3/day. Ancients link thyroid with creative expression.

Thymus: Echinacea, *Echinacea angustifolia*; Goldenseal, *Hydrastis*, both as Mother Tincture, 10 drops, 15 minutes apart, 3x/day, 3 weeks on, one week off. There is a close relationship with the heart. Compassionate, generous, loving, peaceful thoughts and feelings... energize both Your thymus and immune response system.

Pancreas: (in general) Juniper berries, *Juniperus communis*; (diabetes milletus) 1-part Licorice, *Glycyrrhiza glabra*, 2-parts Goldenseal;

215

(hypoglycemia) Licorice. (See below: **Liver Lore**.) The pancreas relates to Your feelings, or cravings for sweetness and joy in life. This is the organ of balance. (See below: **Stevia**.)

Adrenals: Licorice, *Glycyrrhiza glabra*. These small glands, triggered by the "freeze... fight... or flight" response, regulate the blood pressure and blood sugar... maintaining a close relationship with kidneys in filtering blood.

Gonads: (female) Blue cohosh, *Caulophyllum thalictroides*, for easing pains of childbirth, and menstrual flow; Black cohosh or black snakeroot, *Cimicifuga racemosa* for most other female challenges; Stargrass, *Aletris farinosa*, to tonify a uterus stressed from having multiple childbirths, miscarriages, or abortions; (male) Sarsaparilla, *Smilax ornata*. These glands represent sharing with others, ultimately... expressing sacred sexual intimacy with a special someOne.

As a general *Endocrine Tonic*: combine 1tsp each: chicory root, dandelion root and willow bark... boil in a quart of water 10 minutes; steep for 10 minutes... drink ½ cup throughout the day.

God: An Evolving Energy

While this notion may seem shocking – starkly heretical to some – it is worthy of consideration. Scriptures proclaim we are "made in the image and likeness of God" and since *we* are evolving – in our consciousness – why not God?

We all have our notions of God: Hindu, Jewish, Christian, Muslim, atheist, agnostic... and, whether we admit it or not, God is far beyond our conceptions... we can only experience amazement at what we may term Infinite Being – the genderless Godhead, Infinite Mind. Rupert Sheldrake expands our awareness:

"If the fields and energy of nature are *aspects* of the Word, the Spirit of God... then God must have an evolutionary aspect, evolving with the cosmos, with biological life, and humankind. God is not remote and separate from nature, but immanent in it. Yet at the same time, God is the unity that transcends it. In other words, God is not just immanent in nature, as in pantheist philosophies, but both immanent and transcendent – a philosophy known as panentheism. 15th century mystic Nicholas of Cusa says: 'Divinity is the enfolding and unfolding of everything that is. Divinity is in all things in such a way that all things are in divinity.'

"The creative polarity of Spirit and Word, like other creative polarities, can be modeled in terms of gender but in an ambiguous manner. If we think of the feminine principle as active – like Shakti – then the Spirit is feminine; the Word is masculine. The word for spirit in Hebrew, *ruah*, is feminine. {For an illuminating discussion on this matter, see *A New Vision of Reality*, by Bede Griffiths.} In Greek, the corresponding *pneuma*, is neuter; in Latin it is masculine, *spiritus*.

Alternately, taking the masculine principle as active, then the Spirit is masculine and the Word feminine. While this is an unfamiliar way of thinking, given the identification of the Word with the Son... there is no doubt that the biblical concept of the Word of God has much in common with the feminine divine Wisdom, Sophia. {See: *The Coming of the Cosmic Christ*, by Matthew Fox.} In the Book of Proverbs 8:22-3,27,29-31... Wisdom (Sophia) speaks of herself as follows:

'The Lord created me in the beginning of his works
before all else that he made, long ago.
Alone, I was fashioned in times long past, at the
beginning, long before earth itself.
When he set the heavens in their place I was there,
when he prescribed the limits of the sea
and knit together earth's foundations.
Then I was at his side each day,
his darling and delight,
playing in his presence continually,
playing on the earth, when he had finished it;
while *my* delight was in mankind.'

"The prologue to John's Gospel: the Word is like Wisdom. In a Christian context, (energy) fields can be thought of as an aspect of the Word, and (pure) energy as an aspect of the Spirit. If the Word and Spirit of God are immanent in the realm of nature and immanent in the creative process, then God must be evolving along with nature. At the same time, God somehow gives this process an overall purpose which the mystic Teilhard de Chardin conceived of as the Omega Point... the state of unity toward which everything is developing. Such conception is necessarily obscure since it goes beyond anything that has happened so far, beyond our powers of thought.

'By its structure, Omega – in its ultimate principle – can only be a distinct center radiating at the core of a system of centers; a grouping in which the personalization of the All and the personalizations of the elements reach their maximum – simultaneously and without merging, under the influence of a supremely autonomous focus of Union.' (*The Phenomenon of Man*, Pierre Teilhard de Chardin.)

"New forms of theology have recently been developing in an attempt to conceive of a God of a living, evolutionary cosmos. Evolutionary theology involves a radical break with traditional theological ideas of God… as timeless, uninfluenced by worldly events, acting on it but not really interacting *with* it. However, the God of the Bible was intimately involved with the history of the world and humankind. This remote, impassive image is *not* biblical but developed in the early church under Greek philosophers. In the spirit of Platonism, the mind of God was identified with the transcendent realm of eternal Forms; under the influence of Aristotle… God was conceived of as the unmoved mover.

"By contrast here's a new, evolutionary view of God: 'Like all living things, God not only acts on others, but also takes account of others in the divine self-constitution. God is not the world, and the world is not God. But God includes the world, and the world includes God. God perfects the world and the world perfects God. There is no world apart from God, and there is no God apart from some world. Yet, there are differences. Whereas no world can exist without God, God can exist without *this* world. Our planet as well as the whole universe may disappear and be superseded by something else, and God will continue. But since God, like all living things perfectly embodies the principle of internal relations, God's life depends on there being some world to include.' (*The Liberation of Life: From the Cell to the Community*, Birch and Cobb.)

"Each of us – faced with the mystery of our existence and experience – must make sense of it. It appears we have 3 choices of philosophies:
The mechanistic theory of nature and human life – in which God is an optional extra…

The theory of nature as alive but without God… or:

The theory of a living God together with living nature.

"Each view can be elaborated intellectually… each can be defended on rational grounds, and each is held with deep conviction by many people. In the end, we choose between them by intuition. Our choice is influenced by our acknowledgement of mystery… and in turn affects our tolerance of it.

"Those with the lowest mystery-tolerance thresholds are drawn to the mechanistic-atheistic worldview that as a matter of principle denies the existence of mysterious entities like souls and God, and portrays a disenchanted, unmagical reality proceeding entirely mechanically.

"Those who acknowledge the life of evolutionary nature admit the mystery of life and creativity. And…

"Those who acknowledge the life of God… are consciously open to the mystery of divine consciousness, grace and love.

"What difference does it make to think of <u>nature</u> as <u>alive</u> rather than inanimate?

First, it undermines humanistic assumptions upon which our civilization is based.
Second, it gives us a new sense of our relationship to the natural world and a new view of human nature.
Third, a grand re-sacralization of nature happens.

"When we allow ourselves to think of the world as alive, we recognize a part of us knew this all along. It is like emerging from winter into spring. We begin to reconnect our mental life with our own direct intuitive experiences of nature. We can participate in the spirits of sacred places and times. We can see that we have much to learn from traditional societies who have kept their sense of connection with the living world around them. We can acknowledge the animistic traditions of our ancestors. And we can begin to develop a richer understanding of human nature, shaped by tradition and collective memory, linked to the earth and the heavens, related to all forms of life… and consciously open to the creative power expressed in all evolution. We are reborn into a living world." (*The Rebirth of Nature: The Greening of Science and God*, Rupert Sheldrake.)

In biology… Charles Robert Darwin and Alfred Russel Wallace first proposed the idea of evolution in scientific papers *written jointly*, and read before the Linnaean

217

Society on 30 June 1858. Is everything a matter of blind chance, as the materialists believe? Or is a guiding intelligence at work in the evolutionary process?

Charles Robert Darwin, on the one hand, developed a gloomy materialism that now pervades the thinking of Neo-Darwinism – the orthodox doctrine of academic biology. They theorize: everything happens by chance – through unconscious laws of nature – and has no meaning or purpose. We see the Light began to dawn for Charles Darwin, as witnessed by his later writings. https://www.wakingtimes.com/2014/06/10/plant-intelligence/

Alfred Russel Wallace came to another conclusion: evolution involves far more than natural selection; evolution is guided by creative, intelligent forces he identified as angels. His conception is summarized in the title of his last book: *The World of Life: A Manifestation of Creative Power, Directive Mind and Ultimate Purpose*. Today we hear a great deal about Darwin. How many have heard of Wallace? Together they co-founded evolutionary theory. If You are a materialist... evolutionary creativity can only be a matter of blind chance. Wallace gives us the option to believe there are other forces... expressing evolutionary creativity: the Forces *or* Angels of Love, Truth and Beauty... Trust, Harmony and Peace. Perhaps Wallace was aware of Essene writings. Certainly, his theory of Intelligent Design is vindicated by knowledge of the Genetic Code, as well as computer programming. Perhaps this is the reason Richard Dawkins, the world's most famous atheist, abandoned evolution favoring the idea of Intelligent Design. Imagine! See *The Myth of Evolution:* https://www.youtube.com/watch?v=HxjFLzOThck&feature=youtu.be

Grounding
Earth experiences lightning 5-6000X / hour – averaging **100X / minute**! Each bolt carries up to a million volts... travels 100,000 miles per hour... reaching a temperature of 60,000 degrees. And yet it's usually an inch in diameter. Why the constant bombardment of lightning? Is Mother Nature lashing out causing fires & floods? Actually, Mother Nature is charging Earth with negative ions – free electrons – for our well-being; reducing inflammation, neutralizing wandering free radicals, to promote normal functions,

including hormone production – such as regulating the stress hormone cortisol.

Mother Earth blesses us with the gift of free electrons through skin contact. When our ancestors learned how to cure animal skins and make leather, people started wearing moccasins to protect their feet. While leather is not a conductive material – such as metal or water – the feet tend to sweat and the moisture allows conductivity through the porous leather. Animals are in direct contact with the earth. Domesticated animals, being as ungrounded as their owners, suffer similar symptoms of inflammation and stress.

There is serious Trouble... with a capital **T**... and that rhymes with **G** and that stands for Grounding. From time immemorial we have been grounded – until recently. Now we wear synthetic shoes with hard rubber, insulating us from free electrons Mother Nature offers as stress relief. How often do we get our feet on the ground? After a walk along the seashore or barefoot in nature... with negative ions in the air as well as underfoot... we feel wonderful... exhilarated. What about other times... and Winter?

You can reconnect with the free electrons emanating from Mother Earth by literally plugging into the ground. You can DIY! At a plumbing supply, get a piece of copper sheeting, 6-9", a 3' piece of electrical wiring and a grounding plug that You can disassemble. Take out the blades that plug into the electricity; attach the wiring to the ground – reassemble the plug. Then solder the other end of the wiring to the plate; rather than regular lead solder – which interferes with energetic flow – use *silver* solder. Plug it in and enjoy underfoot – barefoot is best, although natural fiber sox are OK... lie or sit on it. Contact and connect!

This technology may well be the most important health discovery of our time. A simple investment brings peaceful sleep promoting health. The New Earthing Starter Kit includes the book *Earthing*, which details double-blind studies, as well as an Outlet Checker – important because sometimes the green & white wires get crossed and, although there is power... the outlet is not truly grounded. Research and details are available. https://www.earthing.com/

Grounding with crystals and far infrared. In the 1970's, NASA developed the first infrared therapy devices to put into America's space shuttles. NASA was looking for something to ensure the astronauts' immune response systems were functioning at their best. Today there are many applications of far infrared. BioMat therapy is backed by 20 years of international, peer-reviewed studies using natural light wave technology, derived primarily from Far Infrared light generated by natural amethyst crystals and 21 other components. The Biomat converts electricity from Alternating Current to Direct Current, eliminating concerns of EMFs associated with AC products. You can safely enjoy infrared light energy, and heal HeartMindBodySpirit as One.

Negative Ions control balance in the Autonomic Nervous System regarding *insulin* and *adrenal* functions, resisting disease and sickness. Wearing or sleeping on synthetic fabrics, calcium in your blood exits through urine... blood becomes more acidic... and neurosis may occur causing an exhausted feeling. Synthetics decrease negative ions, and**... as our negative ions decrease, the amount of sugar in our blood increases.** Diseases like diabetes occur. Wearing or sleeping on synthetic fabrics also decreases the amount of Vitamin C, the resistance of our body to disease weakens, and this causes stress. Absence of the right amounts of negative ions can result in headaches, insomnia and fatigue.

Amethysts are known for producing very high vibrations and negative ions, as well as being sources of far infrared light waves. This combination can penetrate the body up to 6" and reaches areas more traditional heat sources cannot. This broader reach of the ions and light waves creates profound muscle relaxation, helping relieve pain faster and longer (especially when well-hydrated, and taking enzymes am/pm and with meals).

This natural, deep penetrating therapy is safe for people of all ages – even pets often try and share the Biomat. Why? These infrared and negative ion therapy delivery devices, help boost the immune response system, detoxify the body, and relieve pain... helping relax, helping sleep.

The Biomat is constructed of 17 layers, each with its own useful purpose. One layer produces infrared rays, one blocks EMF waves; the top layer is filled with the finest amethyst in the world; the controller is made by Texas Instruments, America's oldest electronics manufacturer. https://victorkulvinskas.thebiomat.co

You can design Your own **Med-Bed** with the Biomat and the Quantum Energy Scalar Wave Wand of Light: https://terahertzforwellness.com/joycec/ The Biomat creates infrared heat underneath, and the Wand of Light creates a Quantum Energy field of heat above... You can facilitate holistic healing on all levels: HeartMindBodySpirit.

Hippocrates said: "If there's a way to heat the bones, then all diseases can be treated!" And... Einstein wisely said: "Future Medicine will be the Medicine of Frequencies!"

Using these two tools of technology as a **Med-Bed**, the optimal affirmations are three-fold, as found below: **Relationships**. Only You can make the magic happen. This is the miracle ONLY You can perform!

Survival means taking Charge of Your Life. How do we do that? Create Your Garden of Eatin' indoors and out! Follow Mother Nature's Ways. Holistic Lifestyle Medicine, conscientious MDs and even psychiatrists suggest taking Your MEDS... every day! See the basic handbook: *ABRACADABRA – Your Wish IS Fulfilled!* https://store.bookbaby.com/book/abracadabra For $5 off shipping **in the US**, click Add Coupon Code: abracadabra – click Apply! **OUTSIDE USA...** support Your local bookstore – the ISBN# 9 781098 383145.

Hair and Skin Care
After footwear, people assess others by their hair and skin. Hair shows inner strength: wavy hair represents vitality. The skin indicates our level of hydration as well as our emotional state; a rash shows irritation at some level; a boil indicates unexpressed anger bursting.

The average head has 100,000 hair follicles, and goes through a 2-6-year cycle of growth and loss. Cells at the base of the follicle elongate to form a thin filament and then push upward, differentiating into a hard, outer cuticle and an inner cortex. Hair growth continues at a rate of ¼ -1½ inches per month for 1000 days or so... until the follicle enters a quiescent phase for 100 days before it falls out. On average, we shed 50-100 hairs per day**!** More than this, especially when coming out "by the handful" indicates metal toxicity, parasites, and / or hormonal imbalance and emotional stress.

After childbirth, high fever, use of certain drugs, or after profound emotional stress, the cycle is accelerated – leading to diffuse hair loss. This can explain the bizarre phenomenon of sudden whitening of the hair following emotional trauma... or where pigmented hairs all fall out together. In *alopecia areata* there is inflammation and sudden, catastrophic hair loss.

Emotional stress leads to accelerated hair loss. Long-term anger or stress is a burden carried by tightened shoulder and neck muscles, inhibiting blood flow to brain and scalp – leading to headaches, vision changes, hair loss... and contributing to baldness. Meditation restores integrity and resolves many of these issues. Visualizations and affirmations work wonders. "Even though I have my challenges... I totally love, accept and respect myself." Repeat while tapping energy points around the cranium and heart, as in the Emotional Freedom Technique.

Proper nutrition and circulation are essential for healthy hair and skin. Trace elements and minerals in both fresh-water and marine algae are fully utilized. Wheatgrass and barleygrass juice add luster, and may also be applied to the skin and rubbed into the hair and scalp. Silica is recommended: the most abundant being stinging nettle (*Urtica dioica*) with 6500 ppm; or a water extract of horsetail (*Equisetum arvense*) with 386 ppm as well as horsetail tea, taken internally and as a rinse; these and food grade diatomaceous earth also strengthen the nails. Brushing hair brings natural oils from the scalp to the tips... bend at the waist and brush with hair hanging down; much more than 20 strokes/day damages with excess friction; follow with a brisk fingertip massage, promoting circulation.

Commercial soaps and shampoos have synthetic chemicals that absorb through the skin. Use pure castile soap only when necessary – once a week is sufficient. Why? Soaps are alkaline, and our hair and skin thrive in a slightly acid environment. To clean hair more frequently, rinse with straight apple cider vinegar to restore acidity and add luster. After any shampoo, an apple cider vinegar rinse also helps the hair control dandruff. After an Epsom salt bath, spray or splash on some straight apple cider vinegar... let it air dry.

Henna powder may be mixed with water, worked into the hair and left for 20-30 minutes. For darker color... use coffee instead of water; for redder shade... use red wine; "set" with a rinse of apple cider vinegar, restoring color and luster. Strong chamomile tea is for blonds, and brings out highlights for others. {Chamomile comes from the Greek, meaning grated apple, because its fragrant aroma is thought to be reminiscent of ripe apples.} After the chamomile tea has been worked into the hair and left for 20-30 minutes, set with lemon juice rinse, renewing brilliance of blond hair.

It is also possible to nourish and nurture hair: after shampooing with vinegar or lemon juice rinse, allow hair to dry. Towel it well, then begin at the back and work fingers loosely through the hair several times, speeding the drying process. A dryer makes hair brittle leading to split ends... brushing wet hair stretches and weakens the shaft, diminishing natural waviness. Fingers are best.

After it is fairly dry... take 1Tbs oil (two with a lot of hair); work it in, massaging the scalp to stimulate circulation. The first day, use extra virgin olive oil... on the second day, use hemp seed oil and let it blend in with the olive oil. On the third day, use coconut oil and let it blend in with the other two oils. After that, massage Your scalp every day until the oils are all absorbed.

Skin likes to be slightly acidic; soaps are alkaline. With any skin condition such as acne, avoid soap. In general, use soaps appropriately: when there is grease or grit to deal with, before preparing food, after the toilet. Otherwise, a loofa sponge with an apple cider vinegar rinse suffices. (Ch 5: Soap: **Dirtier than Dirt**)

Hair Tissue Analysis
Blood tissue analysis can change from day to day depending on diet... and from moment to moment depending on emotions and thoughts. Doctors working in mental hospitals have noted people with multiple personalities have blood drawn several times during the *same* day... exhibiting different aspects of their personalities: each personality has an individual blood profile; one exhibited diabetes, another personality: cardiovascular challenges, another was normal – one gentleman's other personality showed he was pregnant! Clearly our mental and emotional frame of mind influence blood chemistry. A blood profile tells the average person about the presence of viruses, liver, kidney, and endocrine function. It gives an accurate assessment of what is going on in the present moment.

Hair tissue, on the other hand, gives an accurate long-term record of vitamin and mineral excess or deficiency, as well as levels of heavy metals. Hair contains a unique record of the fluctuating levels of trace elements and drugs in the body. A rich network of capillaries surrounds the base of the hair follicle and, as the hair grows, chemicals move out of the blood to be incorporated into the shaft. Hair, being non-degradable, provides chemical data with astonishing permanence. Dr Angela Springfield of the University of North Texas has shown hairs plucked from ancient Peruvian mummies contain high levels of cocaine, confirming the chewing of cocoa leaves was long established in South America. Similar drug residues are also seen in Egyptian mummies.

Healing Journey

Some feel the Golden Years have turned to bronze. Once that thought-form settles in... once that *feeling* takes hold... that's how they begin to act. Holistic health recognizes feelings, thoughts, and actions determine the life experience. Choose longevity and vitality. Watch the spoken words and see Yourself as active and energetic. Visualizations and positive thoughts create *feelings* producing juices that allow us to be... forever young!

Be daring... do things associated with children... play monopoly or put together a puzzle with friends. If fingers are less than nimble, finger paint. It's fun – filled with memories of childhood. Especially during cold months, put on energetic music and dance. When weather warms, get a bike or tricycle; go for a ride. Feel sun on Your face... let wind blow through Your hair.

Rather than looking for Dr Fixit... Jonathon Swift suggests we "arrange for personal and intimate contact with Dr Diet, Dr Exercise, and Dr Merriman." Attitude is the **1** thing over which we have total control. It's all choice... and, quite simply, every time You open Your mouth – You Voice Your Choice. Enjoy a brisk walk, swinging arms in every direction... go out on a date with Mother Nature... Breathe... Smile.

You choose every second of the day... with every breath. Shallow breathing acidifies the system, making You feel tense and nervous. Conscious breathing makes You feel relaxed and happy. Breathe deeply; exhale completely; smile! As You go through Life, everyone experiences a certain amount of stress that instantly is relieved with a smile. And since the AMA says 90% of illnesses are stress related... we can use this most economic prescription from Dr Merriman: Be active! Smile! Be well!

Herbal Teas

Green and black teas are touted for antioxidants. There are plenty of antioxidants, everywhere... caffeine in these teas may offset the benefits. If You are nervous, or develop a headache unless You have them on a daily basis... reconsider. Most decaf varieties still have some caffeine, as well as chemical residues such as nickel – a heavy metal – and methylene chloride, a carcinogen. Organic herb teas are abundant. Experiment with a double-bag of nettle for over-all health. Pick-me-up? Double-bag of organic peppermint. Books: *The Scientific Validation of Herbal Medicine* by Daniel B. Mowrey, PhD and, the classic: *Back to Eden* by Jethro Kloss.

When making tea: boil barks, roots and seeds for at least 10 minutes, then cover and steep for another 10 minutes. To preserve volatile oils in flowers and leaves, bring the water to a boil, remove from heat, add herbs and cover steeping for 20 minutes. Tea can be charged with photon energy from the Sun in a glass jar... cover loosely with a lid or use cheesecloth and a rubber band. Be patient.

Herbs in Cooking

When using dried herbs, pour the desired amount into the palm of one hand and then briskly rub both palms together over the food; this freshly releases their essence, further enhancing flavors. Fresh minced herbs contribute to culinary renown in both cooked and fresh foods. While normal use is a sprinkle here and there, some herbs are used as successful substitutes for pasta or rice: 1C finely diced cilantro + 1C lentil sprouts, perhaps diced onion and / or jalapeño, makes a lovely bed for the topping of Your choice. Experiment. Enjoy.

Holistic Health: Personal and Planetary Balance

The basis of Holistic Health is relationship... beginning with our physical, emotional, mental and spiritual bodies, which affect our social body. Quite often physical challenges or accidents reflect emotional stress. Emotional challenges reflect mental anguish; mental challenges reflect spiritual imbalance. Dr Constantine Hering, homeopath, cites Natural Law: Healing happens from above down, from the inside out... with symptoms reappearing in reverse order of their appearance. When dealing with core issues, healing is complete and we are whole: HeartMindBodySpirit as One.

Professionals have recognized psychosomatic *illness*: a hypochondriac can create a real disease, sometimes death, with the power of the mind. Today we recognize the Reality of psychosomatic *wellness*. Intriguing studies in psychoneuroimmunoendocrinology such as *Deep Feeling, Deep Healing: The Heart, Mind, and Soul of Getting Well* by Andy Bernay-Roman reveals Truth. Tuning into the spiritual powers of the mind... we can totally reverse the disease state creating balance, harmony, health and... Happiness.

As a spiritual person is different from a religious person, spiritual healing is different from faith healing. The fact is: corporate religions are divisive of society. My church is the one true church. Come with me to **my** church, temple or mosque. Accept **our** dogmas and moral codes... and pay Your dues before leaving. You can rest assured, eternal salvation is Yours. Every war, crusade and jihad has been in the name of religion, in the Name of God. Yet the Supreme Source of All That Is... is free from boundaries and limits, philosophies and beliefs.

Asked where she went to church... a Wise Woman said: "I go to the little round church where the devil can't corner You." That Little Round Church is in Your Heart of Hearts. The dogma: Universal Love and Compassion. The moral code: The Golden Rule. Dues paid are challenges we experience, turning them into opportunities for growth and healing. Salvation is *here* and *now* as Love, Truth, Beauty, Trust, Harmony and Peace permeate our emotional, mental, physical and spiritual Tapestry of Life. This is the **core** of Holistic Health, the groundwork for evolution of conscious Awareness, inviting You to become aware of Your relationship with Self, first of all... with each Other... and with All Life Everywhere.

"Truths" are often discarded. What Einstein's Unified Field Theory did to Newtonian Physics is still having repercussions... the Hubble Telescope continues to tumble theory after theory. We are confronted once again with the age-old question: What is Truth? Two other questions are appropriate: Is it ancient? Is it simple? We recognize that Truth is Truth – and always has been found to be so. Falsehood aspires to be perceived as Truth – and always has been found out. We know: Truth is simple. Falsehood is ever complex. Holistic Health is far from New Age; it is Ancient Wisdom rediscovered in modern times: aromatherapy, chromatherapy, sound therapy, as well as crystals and affirmations, massage, reflexology, herbology, and meridian work such as acupressure, acupuncture and polarity therapy... are from time immemorial recalling wholeness to our cellular memory, and refresh HeartMindBodySpirit as One.

Holistic Health goes back to Sumerian times. As Abraham was 2000 years before Jesus, the Sumerians were 2000 years before Abraham. The primal holistic healers are Essenes... from ancient Aramaic: '*yssyn – healer*. While most know of Essenes as authors of the Dead Sea Scrolls, written the century before and after the birth of Jesus, few realize other Essene scrolls exist in the Archives of the Vatican, the Library of the Hapsburgs and the British Museum – all 3 great storehouses of confiscated or stolen treasures. Many of these other scrolls predate the Dead Sea community and even predate Jewish times. Essene or holistic influence is clearly evident even in Sumerian culture.

Essenes recognize the intimate relationships between our feeling body, our thinking body and our acting body – as well as the relationships between humankind, the planets and the cosmos, with daily morning invocations to the Earthly Mother and Her Host of Angels – Angels of Earth, Life, Joy, Sun, Water, and Air – and daily evening invocations to the Heavenly Father and His Host of Angels – Angels of Eternal Life, Creative Work, Peace, Power, Love and Wisdom. {See: **Appendix A**}

Essenes have few dogmas and freely believe whatever they choose based on their *studies* and their individual *experiences*. Essenes recognize we are made in the image and likeness of God. As we are both women and men the Divine Presence – Infinite Mind, the genderless GODhead **G**enerator, **O**perator, **D**estroyer – initiated our world of polarity creating Mother-Goddess and Father-God as the primary Children of the OM... the Source of All... forming the Holy Trinity as understood by most Essenes. Made in that Divine Image, we find in this world of polarity we have Free Will... indeed, we have Choice.

We can explore, experience and express a life of "eat, drink and be merry for tomorrow You will die!" and live in Fear that there will not be enough – perhaps terrified others will steal what we have, or maybe kill us for it. That is one choice. Or we can explore, experience and express Universal Love as found in the Golden Rule and, with confidence... know we can create and share abundance and prosperity here and now.

Divine Unity exists among All Beings everywhere: having Free Will there are infinite choices available between Bright Light and Dazzling Darkness. On the lighter side of the spectrum, conscious beings are free from Fear... choosing to live in their Heart of Hearts, permeated by the Forces of Love, Truth and Beauty, Trust, Harmony and Peace, reflecting the Nature of OM – the Source of All – exploring infinite possibilities in the finite world of human consciousness... expanding exponentially throughout Infinity! With Free Will we can always change our choices – after all, we are God... seeking Self-realization in human terms... creation is a glorious experiment in conscious Awareness.

Essenes recognize we are spiritual energy exploring a physical experience, having utmost respect for Mother Earth from Whom we physically come, and to Whom our physical vehicle shall return. Essenes recognize our ultimate Return is to Awareness as Consciousness. Fasting and meditation facilitate contact with High Self. Scientific studies and socio-psychological data reaffirm the ancient and valuable recommendations of the Essenes: eating biogenic, life-enhancing, foods along with a lifestyle honoring and respecting Nature's Laws... and respecting Each Other as One-anOther... indeed, we are, each One... anOther Expression of Infinite Being, the One. Conscious beings realize OM is Our true hOMe where Peace prevails all–ways!

Essenes recognize care of the physical form, like everything, is a matter of choice... individual preferences are wide and varied. What works for One, may be quite different from anOther. It is paramount to *feel* comfortable in Your Heart of Hearts. The choice in this world of polarity is between the **conventional** and the **holistic** health paradigms.

The conventional health paradigm focuses on the treatment of symptoms; emphasis is on efficiency – what is timely and cost-effective. Emotional neutrality is paramount because elimination of the symptoms and disease is the ultimate goal. Body systems are seen as mechanistic; disease and disability are seen as an entity; pain and disease are wholly negative – to be eradicated. Prevention focuses on the external... the environment. Usually, the patient is entirely dependent on the Doctor as Authority Figure... running objective and quantitative tests, recommending primarily invasive treatments revolving around drugs and surgery. The mind is only of secondary importance in an organic illness.

For the conventional practitioner, the Physicians' Desk Reference (PDR) is the Bible, noting contra-indications and side-effects. Unfortunately, certain drugs, especially antibiotics, destroy harmful bacteria as well as friendly. To survive, the body learns to build defense systems. While antibiotics were almost 100% effective when they first appeared, they are now only 10% effective. New ones must constantly be devised. The Center for Disease Control in Atlanta admits antibiotics are close to their own demise. The *Staphylococcus aureus* strain in Japan was the first to thumb its nose at the all-powerful drug Vancomycin. Some drugs drive disease processes so deeply into the tissues that stronger drugs must be used to counteract life-threatening situations, unfortunately, leading to liver and kidney damage, and iatrogenic – which literally means: physician-generated – *illnesses* that account for an ever-growing number of hospital admissions. These factors invite people to investigate alternatives. NIH, the National Institutes of Health notes billions are spent on alternative and complementary medicine. For years now NIH has said: **"Why medicate? Meditate!"** At the suggestion of the NIH... insurance companies now include many holistic modalities.

The holistic health paradigm focuses on a search for patterns and causes between body systems that are seen as energetic and dynamic. Emphasis is on human values; caring is an integral component in healing. Pain and disease are seen as useful information about conflict and disharmony in the life of the individual. This fundamentally non-invasive complex, is a *process* in the achievement of wellness. Prevention involves wholeness emotionally, mentally, physically and spiritually, co-equal factors in all illness and wellness.

Doctor (Latin: teacher) is seen as therapeutic partner, while the individual is autonomous; both rely on subjective, intuitive and qualitative input. This is a challenge for those in the left-brained conventional paradigm... while comforting for those in the right-brained holistic paradigm. 21st century medicine blends them as Holistic Lifestyle Medicine, sometimes called Informational Medicine. Holistic health honors the relationships between emotional, mental, physical and spiritual realities reflected in our society. As humankind becomes whole... Consciousness expands and reaches out to Mother Earth – Gaia – creating planetary Balance, universal Harmony... Cosmic Joy.

Honey

Raw honey has been used from time immemorial. There are two cautions: spores in raw *or* cooked honey may cause infant botulism, so only use honey when a baby is over 1 year old; by then their intestinal flora can deal with the spores.

Bees are being weakened and vast numbers are being wiped out, only partially due to killer bees. Another reason is many beekeepers take honey from the hives, replacing it with sugar water. The nutritious food collected to raise their young and feed themselves during the long winter months, is taken and substituted with a non-food producing progressively weaker strains of bees, leading to Colony Collapse Disorder – which is, by and large, absent among organic beekeepers. Bees pollinate our flowers and our crops – 40% of our food supply.

Do Gaia a favor... leave the honey at the store and use something else, such as Sucanat™ – whole sugar cane juice dehydrated into crystals. With sugar sensitivity – such as candida, or where sugar is to be absolutely avoided – such as cancer, use stevia – 1 drop / 8 oz.   A few drops in some water as a general tonic, lessens cravings. See below: **Stevia**. Perhaps for Your medicine cabinet, rather than daily use: **buckwheat honey** for coughs, sore throats and even the common cold – 1tsp 3x/day. In these cases, buckwheat honey is found to be superior to OTCs and prescription drugs. Buckwheat is thicker with renowned healing qualities, found useful during winter. Alfalfa and clover are thinner, cooling for summer months.

Humming for Holistic Health

Simplicity profoundly impacts HeartMindBodySpirit. A simple smile, such as Mona Lisa, and humming, like a contented child – both send a message to the subconscious: All Is Well... producing hormones of happiness. Ancient Wisdom gives evidence to consider. 7,000 yrs ago, Megalithic Temples were built in Malta, exhibiting knowledge of architecture, while emanating vibrations of 111 Hz – bringing trance-like meditation, leading to higher states of consciousness, raising the IQ as well as the EQ... social intelligence, and Creativity.

Essenes taught Mother Nature's Ways, with a holistic lifestyle that is Life-affirming, earth- and nature-oriented. They recognize Great Spirit as Source of All: Creator of both polarities – the Divine masculine: God... and the Divine feminine: Goddess. Essenes honor the natural rhythms and cycles of Sun, Moon and Earth, and the change of seasons... they tuned-in to the Sacred Music of the Spheres. The Pythagorean musical scale actually had A = 111 Hz!

111 HZ Pure Tone - YouTube This link runs for 1:11:11 so hum along with binaural headphones. With Your lips closed... completing the microcosmic circuit with tongue caressing the roof of the mouth... breathe in as deeply as comfortable, then slowly and forcefully exhale humming this sacred tone for as long as possible. Continuous nasal breathing in this manner will generate nitric oxide, bringing its multiple benefits. Perhaps first prepare with a **warm-up**. Practice.

The cranial vault contains Your Motherboard, a complex neurovascular network directed by the hypothalamus, which takes cues from Your Heart. Speech 101 teaches through breath and vibration, how to project Your voice through the several facial sinuses to be heard in the back of a hall should the sound system fail. These vibrations stimulate Your entire cranial neurovascular network.

Exhale completely... being comfortable with the emptiness for a moment. Fill Your lungs and exhale the long vowel sounds, ending with a vibrating hum: Haaame... Heeeme... Haaahm... Hooome... Huuum... repeat again and again, until Your voice is *felt* coming from Your *face*, rather than from Your vocal cords. Opening the resonant sphenoid sinuses, vibrations eventually felt... at the top of Your head.

The **warm-up** to Reprogram Your Subconscious and Recreate Your Life continues, as does Your cranial awakening. Let Your tongue rest with teeth apart, lips lightly closed, unsmiling – think of the farmer and daughter in Grant Wood's painting: *American Gothic*. Breathe in deeply, as much as possible, and exhale humming with Your deepest, most resonant tone as long as possible. You will feel Yourself vibrating. Having exhaled completely, bring teeth together and swallow; then separate Your teeth and rest Your tongue for the next round. Do 3 rounds.

Then, do 3 rounds with the same protocol except: teeth touching, smiling throughout, with the tip of the tongue caressing the roof of the mouth. Finally, 3 rounds as above with eyes focused center and up, and thumbs firmly fixed in Your ears, thumbnails facing posterior, with fingertips spread out among the cranial bones. Swallow after every exhale. You may notice a fragrance or taste... engaging the olfactory nerve among the other cranial nerves being stimulated.

Through breath, vibration and energetic contacts, Your HeartMindBodySpirit is One, and now fully awake. Your subconscious is fully Alert. Attentive. Receptive.

Feel Gratitude, Joy, and Humility as You approach Your subconscious through Your Heart of Hearts. With eyes closed, touch Your heart center; feel the warmth. Breathing slowly, a clear signal is sent: I Am now safe! With the sympathetic nervous system disengaged, Your parasympathetic nervous system of rest and digest, repair and rejuvenation, is fully engaged; with facial muscles free from tension especially around the eyes, and with the corners or Your mouth in a slight smile, a look of contentment, Your immune response is relaxed... yet fully alert. Awareness engages Your entire being: HeartMindBodySpirit! You are ready.

Those who are Wise, warm-up before doing exercise. Having completed these warm-up procedures, You are now ready to fully engage with the link: **111HZ Pure Tone** referenced above. Blessings on Your Sacred Journey... Breath by Sacred Breath!

Ho'oponopono Reconciliation. See **Aloha! = alo Ha!**

Hyperactivity in Kids of All Ages

Besides the stimulating effects of artificial colors and flavors... caffeine, meats, sodas, and sugars... TV also accelerates the nervous system. The light on the screen flickers on and off 60X/second. Fleeting images mesmerize... reducing attention span. Fluorescent lights have the same flickering effect that can lead to eyestrain, headaches and multiple symptoms associated with imbalance in our subtle energy fields. Avoid them and You will feel focused and centered... happy and contented. Conscious food and drink, as well as conscious visuals and sounds enhance the quality of our lives exponentially.

Ice Cream and Chemicals
"I scream... You scream...
we all scream for ice cream!"

Ancient Wisdom says:
Craving salty things is craving our father's love.
Craving sweet things is craving our mother's love.

Human milk, a sweet, alkaline-forming food, is nutritious for our precious babies, with a ratio of casein-to-whey designed to primarily develop their sophisticated brain. Baby stands at 9-12 months, and doubles its birth weight in 6 *months*.

Raw cow's milk, also an alkaline-forming food, is nutritious for calves... with a ratio of casein-to-whey designed to build muscle and bones. Baby calf stands immediately, and doubles its birth weight in 6 *weeks*!

The difference between human and cow milk is notable.   Milk contains two major proteins; humans have a ratio of casein to whey **40:60** and cows have **80:20**! Humans have saturated fat at 1.8g/100g, monounsaturated at 1.6 and polyunsaturated at .5; cows have saturated at 2.5, monounsaturated at 1 and polyunsaturated at .1! DHA, absent in cow milk, is found in human milk at .9g!

Pasteurization changes milk from alkaline-forming to an acid-forming food, and is deadly even when fed to calves – they die from congestive heart failure in about 60 days! Certainly, it is toxic for us contributing to allergies, all respiratory challenges, congestion of tissues, and other complicating degenerative disorders. Manufacturers are not required to list additives, and being interested in the bottom line, most ice creams are loaded with petroleum-based synthetic chemicals. While a Banana Split may sound appealing... even healthy, because it has some fruit... it is worthy of investigation: Diethyl glucol, replacing eggs as an emulsifier, is the same chemical used in antifreeze and paint removers. Piperonal, replacing vanilla, is also used to kill lice. Aldehyde C-17, replacing cherries, is a flammable liquid used in aniline dyes, plastic and rubber. Ethyl acetate, replacing pineapple, is a cleaner for leather and textiles with vapors known to cause lung, liver and heart damage. Butyraldehyde, replacing nuts, is an ingredient in rubber cement. Acryl acetate, replacing bananas, is an oil paint solvent. Benzyl acetate, replacing strawberry, is a nitrate solvent. While we think of it as a tasty treat... the average Banana Split is antifreeze, lice killer, oil paint solvent, and nitrate solvent... in a base of frozen liquid that, out of date, is converted to glue!

We can easily avoid this cacophony of chemicals, creating our own enzyme-rich desserts. Many juicers have an attachment for a homogenizer, making delicious ice cream. Simply take spotted bananas – the more spotted, the sweeter – peel and freeze. {The peels may be blended as fertilizer or composted; they are especially healing for any ailing house plant.} When frozen, push the bananas through for a creamy, nutritious ice cream. A blender also works well. Break a frozen banana in pieces, cover with some water and blend. Add dry ingredients such as carob, cinnamon, etc; then add more frozen pieces, perhaps strawberries, mangos or black mission figs until it gets thick, and the motor sounds like it's beginning to strain... then enjoy a cold, creamy, delicious, natural treat.

The more creative You get in the kitchen, the more control You have over Your health... and Consciousness. Peace on Earth begins at home, especially in the kitchen. As You avoid blood on Your cutting board, You raise consciousness on the planet. We *can* avoid bloodshed in our society. Refusing frozen bovine mucosal secretions, we avoid cruelty to animals on battery farms. Conscious choices create a compassionate world. Invest in a dehydrator.

"We have cast our culture out of the garden and into the rat race of competition & consumerism. As we repress the shame of our routine violence toward nature and animals, our resulting hidden low self-esteem drives the profits of corporations that enrich themselves through our craving for gadgets, drugs and entertainment to help distract us from what we know in our hearts... and to gloss over the violence of our meals. But as we question this mentality of domination and choose compassion, healing, and peace by eating plant-based meals – we find our joy rising, our spirit deepening, our mind quickening, our feelings softening, our energy increasing and our creativity flourishing!" *The World Peace Diet: Eating for Spiritual Health and Social Harmony* by Will Tuttle, PhD.

Immune Response System: Physical and Metaphysical Applications
Recognizing and honoring relationships between the physical, emotional, mental and spiritual aspects of Life, we can decipher subtle messages. Your subconscious, both individual and collective, knows Your Life's Purpose: What You are here to Know... and to Remember. Your conscious mind is left mystified, searching Your memory banks to figure it out. The subconscious gives clues... assisting Your Quest in the form of physical symptoms.

For instance, someone may seek health care because of aching and tightness in the neck, arms and shoulders. There may be a physical reason. Did the person spend a weekend helping a friend complete a building project? Was there a lot of lifting and carrying involved, sawing and hammering? This calls for a therapeutic massage or a soak in a tub with Epsom salts... or both.

Without physical cause, however, look at metaphysical or symbolic possibilities. The neck relates to flexibility, seeing both sides of an issue. Arms and shoulders are used for carrying things, and if not something physical... what other burdens does the person carry – burdens relating to feminine issues have left-sided symptoms... masculine issues have right-sided symptoms. There can be some surprisingly clear metaphysical applications at the emotional level.

To understand the physical and metaphysical reasons for an impaired immune response is a daunting task; we know the immune response system is more than the thymus, tonsils, spleen and limbic system of the brain. Our immune response system is a complete composite of who we are: HeartMindBodySpirit.

Physical reasons for impaired immune response include: a workday spent in the midst of toxic fumes such as smoke... drinking tap water – a cocktail of anti-biotics, chlorine, fluoride, hormonal and pharmaceutical residues – destroying friendly bacteria in the colon... satisfying natural cravings for pure water with sodas, caffeine and alcohol... over-acid systems due to animal foods, fried foods, refined foods... all these factors, day after day, impair the immune response system – compromising health. Some play the victim... others take control of their lives creating changes. Find a job that supports healthy living... one that truly *excites* You. Begin to make **T**herapeutic **L**ifestyle **C**hanges. HeartMindBodySpirit thrives on **TLC** that supports Consciousness.

If someone still finds immune challenges, even with a healthy way of living and thinking... look at metaphysical applications. The immune response system represents strength, vitality and enthusiasm. Corresponding issues relate to self-esteem and vulnerability. Criticism... judgment... coercion... whether directed at Self or Others... boil down to self-esteem. Are there feelings of resistance to being open, being vulnerable... feeling disappointment with self or others... feeling attacked or beaten... defenseless, defeated... helpless, hopeless? This is time to take charge... and *do* something. Discipline begins with sound nutrition – leading to vitality and self-esteem. Increase biogenic – living – foods and power-foods such as diatomaceous earth. Aphan {see above: **AFA**} bentonite clay, charcoal, chlorella, spirulina and seaweed – especially bladderwrack, kelp and sea moss – pull heavy metals from the system, offering superior nutrition. Beets, blueberries, cilantro, garlic, ginger, lemon, onions, turmeric – raw as much as possible – with enzymes and probiotics from hOMe-made Kimchee and Sauerkraut will support Your Sacred Journey. Dietary Discretion builds strength in HeartMindBodySpirit. True strength merges total honesty with open vulnerability. All other defenses attempt to conceal fears... or mask hidden emotions. Metaphysical causes can be transmuted with holistic healing work, which begins with creating Your optimal Verbal Diet.

As for Current Events, to build Your Immune Response... in addition to Your Lifestyle **MEDS** – **M**editation, **E**xercise and **E**nzymes, **D**ietary **D**iscretion and **D**iscipline, **S**ensuality **S**acred **S**exuality and **S**leep... consider Suramin which has been available for >100 years. Although it is chemically derived, simply make pine needle tea (a hot water extract of pine, fir, cedar, and / or spruce needles). Evergreens are virtually everywhere – add the energetic outer tips to both Your morning and afternoon tea as a boost! 23MedicinalPlantstheNativeAmericansUsedonaDaily Basis.pdf (usda.gov)

Ultimately... Everything is Vibration – Frequency. With frequencies of AI – Artificial Intelligence – in the air: graphene oxide, GMO foods, water, everywhere... orchestrated by wi-fi, most intensely with 5G... explore antidotes: TERMINATE A.I NANO BOTS - YouTube. Get out in Nature. Experience the Ultimate Healing Frequency... within!

Simply be aware of Your breath. With deeper breathing – technically called diaphragmatic breathing – You contract the diaphragm, the muscle sheet separating thorax from abdomen. This allows Your lungs to totally fill and offers a rhythmic massage for the small and large intestines by creating an experience of the Buddha-belly: slowly fill completely, slowly empty completely. Be Still. Be Aware.

Awareness creates a shift through conscious breathing. Taking Your time... You realize You are free from time. Experiencing eternity... You are in the here & now... and nOw is forever. Gently caressing the bump at the roof of Your mouth, slowly fill Your lungs and upper chest; pause: comfortable with the fullness. Gently caressing, slowly exhale... completely, drawing navel to the spine; pause: comfortable with the emptiness.

Breathing has been studied at Harvard and the secret is a pattern. Different patterns bring different results: when someone experiences *profound pain* in the chest the recommended pattern is the Ha–Ku Breath – with open mouth make the sound Ha on the inhale, then forcefully exhale saying Ku – until the pain disappears. Patterns also found in Ancient Wisdom focus on Your center: Breathe in deeply – count to 9... hold – count to 3... exhale completely – count 9... hold – for 3. Develop Your own pattern with or without counting, remembering to pause with the fullness... as well as with the emptiness... often in this stillness Spirit speaks. Be open to Your Inner Voice Intuition.

With repetition of consciously breathing... You notice and experience the different sounds of Your breath inhaling... and exhaling; free from judgment or comment... simply, being aware of Be-ing Aware... being the experience of Awareness – Being – Breathing – Listening – Observing. So Be It. And so, It Is. And It Is Done. And I Am One with All, And All Is One. Ecstasy is found with Sacred Breath!

Insect Repellant
While DEET and PMD products are available, they are often synthetic or have contaminants. Rather than combine lemon and eucalyptus essential oils, purchase Lemon Eucalyptus Oil. The Lemon Eucalyptus tree is native to NE Australia; the oil works against mosquitoes because its main ingredient – p-menthane-3,8-diol, or PMD – blocks mosquitoes from

sensing human presence masking signals such as carbon dioxide and lactic acid.

Mix 25 drops Lemon Eucalyptus Essential Oil... 4 oz Rubbing Alcohol or Witch Hazel... 1 Tsp Real Vanilla Extract... 2 oz Coconut Oil (optional)... store in a small spray bottle. Shake well before use. Spray over exposed skin and clothes; oil can stain. Re-apply every 4-6 hours, as required. Neem is derived from an evergreen tree native to India, and has similar repellant qualities. Always dilute when applying to the skin: 1 oz neem oil to 4 oz coconut oil.

Living life on the wild side? Being in Nature, especially in the tropics, if insects on a Nature walk are problematic, find a termite nest: a large, black soft nest usually found in between branches and the trunk. Push Your hands inside and little critters will swarm all over exuding a defense enzyme that actually has a pleasant fragrance – wipe over exposed skin and You will be insect-free!

Iron Efficiency
Anemia, iron deficiency – reduced hemoglobin in the blood, makes people feel "run down" or "tired all the time." An easy way to check is to bend the fingers of Your hand backwards, and look at the lines in the palm of Your hand. Also look in a mirror under Your lower eyelid. Bright red is a healthy sign; mere pink indicates: pay attention. Some people think meat will build up their iron. Consider:

"Years ago, Dr Hans Fischer and associates won a Nobel Prize for their work on red blood cells. During their research, they noticed human blood... which carries oxygen to all our cells... is practically identical to chlorophyll on the molecular level. Red blood cells are characterized by the oxygen-carrier, hemoglobin, which has as its central nucleus the mineral element iron. Green plants, on the other hand, are characterized by chlorophyll, which has magnesium as its nucleus. Careful examination of the two molecules shows them to be strikingly similar. (*Biology: A Human Approach*, by Irwin and Vilia Sherman.)

"Scientists J.H. Hughes and A.L. Latner of the University of Liverpool reported in the *Journal of Physiology* in 1936, a number of animals were made anemic by daily bleeding. After their hemoglobin levels were reduced to less than half the norm, the animals were divided into ten groups. Five of the groups were fed various types of chlorophyll in their diet. The other five groups of control animals did not receive any chlorophyll. Those animals receiving 'crude' or raw, unrefined chlorophyll were able to increase the speed of hemoglobin regeneration by more than 50% above average, to approximate their previous blood values in about 2 weeks. The group receiving synthetic chlorophyll, however, showed no improvement in the speed of hemoglobin regeneration. Their report concludes: 'It seems that the animal body is capable of converting chlorophyll to hemoglobin.'

"Raw, unrefined chlorophyll is most suitable for this purpose because it preserves the enzymes. Chlorophyll is a green (sometimes purple) pigment found in growing plants, containing mineral and protein compounds; the blood of the plant – it is condensed solar energy. Wheatgrass juice, raw, fresh greens and vegetables: cucumber, celery, zucchini and sprouts 'concentrate' sun power firsthand." Iron deficiency is foreign to cultures who regularly include seaweed or black salt in their diet!

Kidney Cleanse
The Kidney Cleanse is similar to the Gall Bladder / Liver Cleanse. Preparation is key, with several days of watermelon juice... red or yellow... seeds, skin and rind. With only a blender, first put in the soft portions; when liquid, add bits of the rind and skin, then strain... use cranberry juice for sugar sensitivities. If You suspect kidney stones, fast for a few days drinking plenty of water and hydrangea tea, which facilitates dissolution; with associated kidney pain, add corn silk to the hydrangea.

If You know there are stones, drink this tea from the Full Moon to the New Moon. Then, for 3 days, drink ¼C fresh lemon juice every 2 hrs; brush Your teeth when You have lemon, protecting the enamel. In between... drink at least 12 oz re-mineralized and re-energized distilled or r/o water. At the end of the 3rd day just before bed... drink 2oz castor oil or sesame oil, mixed with 2oz of lemon juice. In bed, surround Yourself with a cocoon of orange light... and then surround that with a cocoon of white light. Affirm: "My glands and my organs are happy doing an excellent job keeping me healthy. I welcome what is useful in my life... and I now comfortably and easily release the rest."

Know Thyself

Ancient Wisdom from the Essene perspective understands Divine Presence manifests as a Trinity of Energies. OM – All That Is – the I Am that I Am, mentioned to Moses, is the genderless Godhead... the Infinite Mind... seeking to explore Infinite Possibilities. At least in the world *we* perceive and experience... Infinite Mind – the I Am Presence – manifested in terms of polarity, first creating Mother Goddess – the Principle of Vision and Imagination... and Father God – the Principle of Being and Action.

Ancient Wisdom of almost every persuasion, perhaps best captured in *The Kybalion*, teaches the Principle of Correspondence: As Above... So Below! We experience our Self as a trinity of One indivisible Being manifesting as Mind, Body and Spirit **modulated by our Heart**: we are HeartMindBodySpirit – as One.

While we recognize our right-brain governs our feeling, receptive, feminine side... and our left-brain governs our thinking, outgoing, masculine side... we consider the Self in charge of both aspects. Each person, each One – each Self – is a trinity of radiant energy: our Divine Self as Source of All, with aspects of Mother Goddess and Father God. As our microcosm reflects the Divine macrocosm, our trinity of radiant energy is a macrocosm reflecting an Inner microcosm – the trinity known as Self.

The *High* Self is our superconscious mind holding profound Universal Wisdom... connected to the Akasha – the Knowledge of All That Is – often experienced as our Inner Voice Intuition. The *Middle* Self is our conscious, rational mind that thinks it is in charge – although research shows feelings are the ultimate creative factor, rather than plans or decisions made from our rational, egoic mind. The *Low* Self is a powerful combination of our somewhat muted unconscious mind taking over while driving, or doing repetitive tasks, and our *very* muted subconscious mind... that operates the vast majority of the time based on programming received during the first several years of life... relates to self-esteem, and issues of empowerment or disempowerment.

As we mature on our Journey of Self Knowledge, High Self begins to develop – really, unfold – as we spend time out – in Nature... as well as time within – in meditation. We become aware of choice: known as Free Will. We can apply ourselves at every opportunity to cleanse and purify our physical body with pure water, healing foods and sufficient exercise, and... our emotional / mental body with pure, empowering feelings and thoughts; both of these engage our spirit body, our creative Self, to make choices leading to growth on our Sacred Journey.

Eventually the realization dawns: I *Am* an expression of the Source of All – fully Aware – with sovereign power over my feeling body and my thinking body. I both choose and create... the Reality that I experience. Simply put, we are *all* the Word made flesh. Science tells us we are photon energy... we are the Divine Presence in flesh and bones – as is *every* One. The Divine Presence *is* the Essence of All That Is!

Jesus over-turned the tables of the money-changers in the Temple as well as our understanding of God – encouraging us to go beyond the puerile notion of God as Yahweh, the Avenger, who *rages* at our misguided actions. Indeed, how can *we* push God's buttons? And what sense does it make that we can rectify our misguided actions by slitting the throat of an innocent animal upon the Temple altar? Didn't the incident of Abraham and Isaac make it clear that blood-letting... so called "sacrifice" – making holy, restoring holiness or wholeness – is a mistaken notion of our relationship with the Divine? Jesus over-turned their tables scattering their blood-money, liberated the animals, and created general chaos in the Temple – that practice was clearly more for the profit of the Temple priests, than the "benefit" of God. It is beyond comprehension **how** mere humans possibly could either upset *or* appease Divine Serenity – the Quintessence of Love, Truth and Beauty, Trust, Harmony and Peace!

When Jesus commands: Love Your neighbor as Yourself, the pre-requisite is – to Know Yourself. The sin Jesus addresses is the sin of ignorance. Knowledge is salvation. *Knowing oneself* is coming to salvation *through* one's Self... Self-Realization! Jesus saves us from ignorance – the real sin whereby we "miss the mark" – sharing Knowledge and an Experience of Self as Source. Jesus rejects the notion of separateness in favor of Unity Consciousness; although John the Baptist was the re-incarnation of Elijah (Mt 11: 13-15) his experience baptizing Jesus was Unity Consciousness; his beheading, symbolic of leaving the physical behind while embracing the Life of the Spirit, liberating him from future re-incarnations.

As a child, Jesus studied in Egypt. The proverb posted at the External Temple is: "The body is the house of God, And So, It Is said: 'Know Yourself'!" At the Internal Temple, the proverb is: "Know Yourself, and You are going to know the gods!" Experiencing the Source of All <u>within</u>, filled with Wisdom, he shared Knowledge:

**Rather than coming to Salvation
through Faith or through the Law…
Salvation comes from Within
through Insight and Creative Thought.**

Through his life and teachings, Jesus replaced the Old Testament with the New Testament, a New Way to look at, and relate to Life… really, it is returning to the Old Way: Mother Nature's Way… Dao Yinn… which is the Way of the Voice of Nature, and also happens to be: the Way to Create the New You.

In the current parlance of quantum physics – rather than *matter* being somehow used to change matter… **energy changes matter**! Rather than a pill, a potion or injection being used to change matter… it *can*, albeit most times it is only temporarily… the *energy* of our <u>thoughts</u> and *especially* our <u>feelings</u> can change matter, most often permanently and painlessly! As we increase time spent Standing in our Wish Fulfilled… we experience *that* Reality in our Heart of Hearts, and our current reality eventually gives way to our New Reality. With Free Will… if You so choose… You *can* do so!

Mystery School Matriculation in Egypt was simple. Those who would enroll, learning *how* to Know Thyself, were led to a large pool, with a wall going across the middle. There were crocodiles on the one side, and for them to matriculate – they must find a way to get to the other side of the pool; they were assured there was a safe passageway to get there. Many struggled to find a narrow window or door, and would keep coming up for another gulp of air before resuming their search, feeling up and down all along the wall. Most were discouraged and gave up. Those with true courage soon realized there was no passage *through* the wall… so they must face their fears and dive deep, where the crocodiles were, to slip *under* the wall. In like fashion, You may find the following bit of esoteric information useful on Your Sacred Journey.

As You matriculate into the Next Dimension of Reality, consider the words of Ezekiel: "They have eyes to see but do not see and ears to hear but do not hear, for they are a headstrong and rebellious people." Also, consider the words of the Master: "For those who have eyes to see, let them see, and for those who have ears to hear, let them hear!" Making the transition from this physical, material 3D world to 5D, many will go toward the "tunnel of light" when they see it, having heard from those with Near-Death Experiences. The question is: where will that tunnel lead?

Rather than finding the Next Dimension… You may find Yourself in queue to be born again, and perhaps with *this* rebirth You will learn to *really* pay attention, learning from the Masters. Perhaps You purposely *choose* re-incarnation to be of Service. We are Infinite Beings experiencing Free Will, with absolute freedom to choose our Heart's desire. After all, Jesus clearly indicated John the Baptist was Elijah, who was to come again. Jesus also clearly said, I and the Father are One and You are One with Me as I am One with You! And, quite clearly: The Kingdom of Heaven is *within* You!

Thinking God, the Kingdom of Heaven, as "out there" – perhaps at the end of the tunnel of light – is to **sin** which is an Arabic word meaning: "miss the mark" and some will even "sin" by missing the target altogether! The message, the Knowledge, of all Masters leads to Your true Goal – Your true Self. So, when You see the tunnel of light… if You would prefer to move on from the cycles of re-incarnation, have courage and face Your own fears. Dive deep within… where You will find the Kingdom of Heaven.

Another lesson from the Mystery School involves the Sacred Space of Your Heart & the Tiny Space within it. Channels of light energy flow through Your head and body. Each of us has a halo of light and the size of each tube of light varies from person to person; simply bring Your thumb and middle finger together to see Yours. {**Supernatural Breathing with the Human Halo** see below.} Another secret revealed at the Mystery School to experience the Kingdom of Heaven within, involves several 90° turns.

Focused in meditation, visualize and feel the Energy that enters Your physical form coming in through the tube of light at the 3rd Eye Energy Center… 1" above the space between Your eyebrows… the Energy then makes a 90° turn when meeting the tube of light traveling from the Crown Energy Center toward the Perineum. Moving down, arriving at the Heart Center… the Energy makes another 90° turn forward, to the

Heart itself. To arrive at the Tiny Space of the Heart, it makes another 90° turn *down*ward. This takes courage. Most assume to "ascend" into Heaven one would make a 90° turn *up*ward. This is only a test... fortunately, free from crocodiles! Turning downward, You arrive at the Tiny Space of the Heart, experiencing the blissful Kingdom of Heaven *within*. Some mystics have that direct experience simply closing their eyes!

We are spiritual beings having a physical experience; when the time comes to disrobe from this physical form – having Free Will – You have an opportunity to make informed choices, as situations present themselves. Take the Masters at their Word. Truly... the Kingdom of Heaven **is** *within* You! Know Thyself! Know the I Am that I Am, the I Am that You Truly Are: Pure Awareness exploring human consciousness: Your Own delightful, unique expression of Divine Presence on a Sacred Journey, explOring the Next Dimension of Awareness!

Know Thyself: Inside & Out – Resources for Lovers of Wisdom

Pyramids around the world and other megalithic relics show ancient wisdom far superior in all scientific fields. Engineers say they are literally impossible to replicate with the technology of today. The monuments declare to all that they **knew** more than we, even now in this "advanced civilization" – ruled by the Matrix who keep many ancient secrets to themselves. Ancient peoples left us Spiritual Wisdom. Worldwide... Love of Wisdom has been considered the highest virtue of humankind.

Philosophy derives from two Greek words: *philo* / friend, and *sophia* / knowledge or wisdom. Philosopher means a Friend or Lover of Wisdom. During the two centuries before the common era, to maintain control the ruling families created *counterfeit* philosophical organizations which became corporate religions with churches and temples; they prostituted the 3 branches of Philosophy: Logic, Ethics and Physics... replacing them with Dogma, Doctrine and Fear, each based on Superstition and Ignorance. Through their corporate religious, political, and monetary institutions, the Elite Oligarchies have continued to suppress true Science: *scientia*, Knowledge & Religion: *religio*, Bind-together! Since 1 BCE, continuing to this day, they demand strict adherence to dogmas and morals of the **official** *cult*. In classic antiquity, *religio* meant yoga: to *yoke* or bind *all* aspects of HeartMindBodySpirit – being Conscious, having a sense of right... of moral obligation or duty towards everyone and everything: both in personal and social contexts. Knowledge that bound things together included the study of numbers, the stars and the soul... bequeathed to us by the more advanced civilizations of Babylon, Persia, India, Egypt, Greece, and Türkiye. Is there any doubt the Ancients had advanced Knowledge? Consider the "simple" Dogon People of Niger who knew there was Sirius A *as well as* Sirius B, thousands of years before we did, inscribing such on their cave walls! All these mysteries of Ancient Wisdom deserve investigation freeing us from our shackles.

Ancient Knowledge has been obscured and hidden, because Knowledge is too empowering for the comfort of those who would control. Historically, the greatest enemy of Ancient Wisdom – the greatest enemy of Knowledge – is religion. Clergy of all denominations have been denouncing scientists, astronomers, alchemists, etc. and even killing them – Socrates, Seneca, Boethius, Hypatia, Giordano Bruno... and in our own living memory: Nicholas Gonzalez, MD and Andrew Moulden MD, PhD... among many others. Recently, Joseph Mercola, MD was forced to remove many documents from his website under severe threat, because they were incriminating evidence against the Matrix Medical Mafia. Things are now about to change. The age of Pisces has given way to the age of Aquarius: we just crossed over a galactic alignment that takes place **once** every 24,000 years! With a New World Awakening, Knowledge is Free and Open to All.

Leaving behind the *Frightened*... the truly Enlightened realize to "Know Thyself" has two vital components reflecting our brain and our heart. The heart is actually 100,000X stronger electrically, and up to 5000X stronger magnetically than the brain! Aptly named by the ancients, the corpus collosum: the *tough body* – is the largest connective pathway in the brain with >200 million nerves *orchestrating* right brain activity: Vision and Imagination... with left brain activity: Be-ing and Action... as billions of nerves fire away. HeartMath

Physics tells us: any moving electric charge (current) generates an electromagnetic force field **and** a *magnetic* field *perpendicular* to it. The Brain–Heart connection generates the toroidal field within which we live, breathe and have our being! Electron-microscopy shocks scientists: every Galactic discovery is found *reflected* within us. We are, indeed, a microcosm of the macrocosm. The Force Field is able to be experienced **"Inside & Out"** enabling us to realize Who we are – manifestations of Infinite Mind exploring human

231

consciousness – Infinite Mind seeing how it *feels* to explore our Sunny-side and how it *feels* to explore our Shadow-side. Both deserve our attention because both are found within each One of us, and both have lessons for us to learn. We are, in fact, learning from each Other.

We explore the Force Field **inside** – the *microcosm* – primarily through **M**editation, the 1ˢᵗ of our **MEDS**, which also include: **E**xercise and **E**nzymes, **D**ietary **D**iscretion and **D**iscipline, **S**ensuality, **S**acred **S**exuality and **S**leep – all of which hugely serve to influence our **M**editation experience! Various types of meditation are covered in this book. The basic treatise is found in the *Vedas* – Raja yoga: turn the senses within; experience: Celestial Light, Harmony, Nectar and Vibration.

In the 21ˢᵗ century, we continue to witness censorship in an effort to confuse and control; still, we can explore the Force Field **outside** – the *macrocosm* – and facilitate Our Sacred Journey. Infinite Mind created the Force Field of the macrocosm as the Cosmos, and the Force Field of the microcosm within You… and within each One of us. It behooves us to explore Great Spirit in Action. It is Wise to be aware of the Moon's sign which changes every 2.5 days, as well as Your energy flow cycles: physically (28 days), emotionally (30 days) and intellectually (33 days): Biorhythm Calculator (biorhythm-calculator.net). As an introduction to Quantum Physics, here's a free audio-book: Butterflies are Free to Fly – A New and Radical Approach to Spiritual Evolution (butterfliesfree.com).

In the 21ˢᵗ Century, Spiritual Scientists with their own specialty, weave together Philosophical Psychology (*psyche*: soul, *logia*: the study of) which studies the nature of Nature, including the nature of Human Nature – blending with various branches of science, exploring the nature of **first principles**, the problems of **ultimate reality** and ultimately… engaging Quantum Physics! Some names are familiar. All deserve investigation and consideration: *considera* – to sit with the stars, and contemplate. Look up the websites for Bruce Lipton, Caroline Myss, Gregg Braden, Joe Dispenza, Lynne McTaggart, Pam Gregory, Rupert Sheldrake… and: Viktoras Kulvinskas, to whom *ABRACADABRA – Your Wish IS Fulfilled!* is dedicated… and who, because of his "accidental" discovery of the taste and nutrition available in sunflower greens, thought to explore! Viktoras, born 23Feb1939 in war-ravaged Lithuania in Eastern Europe, was rescued by the Germans and

lived in a refugee camp from age 5-10. He wondered about buckwheat. What would *their* greens taste like – and pea greens! Viktoras is called "The GrandFather of Living Foods" – he sowed the seeds and nurtured the seedlings both literally and figuratively, as people began growing their Indoor Garden of Eatin' at hOMe! Viktoras, as the Sage of the Age, summarizes Singularity: "**You Are All God in Drag, all of You!**" (His translation of Psalm 82:6, quoted by the Essene Master Jesus in John 10:35.) Viktoras Kulvinskas

These resources to **Know Thyself** range from recent past to ancient times, beginning appropriately with the Ultimate Tools to distinguish Truth from Falsehood – Muscle Testing – as well as the Map of Consciousness. *Power vs. Force: The Hidden Determinants of Human Behavior*, published in 1995 helps discern whether a person, or link or the book You are now reading, is filled with Truth… worth Your time and effort, or Falsehood.

https://veritaspub.com David R Hawkins, MD, PhD gives the scientific explanation as the basis for discerning Truth from Falsehood by *dowsing*, using the *pendulum*, using *muscle testing* and/or the *sway test* – all of which are explained in the book You are now reading – in Ch 10. Dr Hawkins and his students at Veritas Publishing have tested every sentence in his 10 books; all are powerful resources for Your library. {As an example, a dog looking at You with a wagging tail calibrates at 500 – Pure Love.} His other tool known as the Map of Consciousness has 23 levels: beginning at 20 – Shame… going up the scale until 200 – Courage… then 400 – Inner Light and Inner Wisdom… 500 – Inner Love… 600 – Presence… 700 – Universal Consciousness… 1000 – Full Consciousness. ***Healing & Recovery*** and ***Letting Go: The Pathway of Surrender*** are basic tools for Success in Our 3D world.

https://iconnect2all.com Gail and Gregory Hoag founded Metaforms in the 80s to create tools based on Sacred Geometry helping humanity evolve an Awareness with Source – Heart consciousness. They are recognized, leading experts on Sacred Geometric technologies for improving health on the planet – so we can thrive and play in the New Earth Energy based on Ancient Wisdom – allowing the Joyful expression of unconditional Love and Service to flourish once again.

https://masterysystems.com Beloved Helena and Robert Tennyson Stevens created Mastery Systems in the 80s to facilitate their Sacred Journey, and to share that Knowledge with family, friends and co-workers. They began with the Mastery of Language – through conscious Choice of Words we create our Reality. Every challenge in Life can be corrected by simply upgrading one's thought, word and feeling patterns. Robert also takes the Science and Practice of Iridology to the Next Order of Magnitude: incorporating emotions – exploring HeartMindBodySpirit as One.

https://www.ourspirit.com Tyla and Douglas Gabriel, former Montessori and Waldorf teachers, invite You to Enter the Temple of Wisdom with a personal experience that will begin to awaken Your supersensible organs of perception and take You to a place beyond time and space. Their writings and teachings facilitate the understanding and experience of Rudolf Steiner's *Knowledge of the Higher Worlds and its Attainment* in the 21st Century. In human consciousness, faculties are sleeping that, if awakened, lead to life-giving Wisdom.

https://www.bobbygrimes.com Bobby Grimes, Steiner student on the Big Island, provides multiple resources for matters agricultural, currently applying Bio-Dynamics to bamboo, which grows 3-4' in a single day... is stronger than maple... with more compressive strength than concrete... and the same strength-to-weight ratio as steel! As a green living resource, bamboo alleviates environmental concerns of traditional materials. Bamboo re-grows when it is harvested and grows for decades. Replenished from an intricate network of roots, a stalk of bamboo can grow to its maximum height of around 80' in two months. As it thickens, the walls of each hollow stalk grow hard and dense, and soft internodes convert into fibrous cellulose. Bamboo research has been ongoing: http://earthadvocatesresearchfarm.com/ Explore both.

https://www.scienceandnonduality.com Science And Non-Duality is a community inspired by timeless Wisdom, informed by cutting-edge Science, and grounded in direct experience. The disconnect from Earth-based, indigenous Wisdom began in the early days of humankind, when male-dominated religions replaced fertility goddess worship as the prevalent cultural vehicle... and started pitting humankind against its natural environment. Separation was born: me vs you... us vs them... human vs nature. SAND brings people together to explore the Big Questions of Life while celebrating the Mystery of Be-ing... while exploring Quantum Physics.

https://universaltruthschool.com Astro-theology shows how all the Ancient Legendary Stories, Myths, Scriptures, Fairy Tales, etc. have a simple common origin. In all of these wonderful ancient classics, the Personae are always the same, using different names. Syncretism brings together all the fields of Knowledge and Wisdom and shows the interrelatedness of all things. Syncretism is the opposite of division and disunity and covers all major topics: Theology, Astrotheology, Natural Science, Astrology, Reclaiming Dominion, and Breaking the Fictions of Religion, Science and Law. Holy Science is ancient, based on the workings of the solar system and based on the science of 'as above – so below'.

https://www.summum.us *Summum: Sealed Except to the Open Mind* has 7 Ancient Hermetic Principles. **1** - The Principle of Psychokinesis: "The universe is a mental creation." **2** - The Principle of Correspondence: "As above, so below; as below, so above." **3** - The Principle of Vibration: "Everything moves; everything vibrates." **4** - The Principle of Opposition: "Everything is dual; everything has an opposing point; everything has its pair of opposites; like and unlike are the same; opposites are identical in nature, but different in degree; extremes bond; all truths are but partial truths; all paradoxes may be reconciled." **5** - The Principle of Rhythm: "Everything flows out and in; everything has its season; all things rise and fall; the pendulum swing expresses itself in everything; the measure of the swing to the right is the measure of the swing to the left; rhythm compensates." **6** - The Principle of Cause and Effect: "Every cause has its effect; every effect has its cause; everything happens according to Law. Chance is just a name for Law not recognized; there are many fields of causation, but nothing escapes the Law of Destiny." **7** - The Principle of Gender: "Gender is in everything; everything has its masculine and feminine principles. Gender manifests on all levels." These are foundation stones of Hermeticism, outlined by Hermes Trismegistus – thrice master – philosopher, priest and king, who is said to have written the Emerald Tablet and the Corpus Hermeticum – highly influential, ancient teachings.

www.hermeticfellowship.org/HFCollectHermRed.html Serves as a general resource for students and practitioners of the western Hermetic Tradition, and a specific resource for the Alexandrine Temple of the Hermetic Fellowship, located in Portland, Oregon. https://www.essene.com/Mysticism/Hermetic.html

Sir George, fondly is called: "Grandfather of the New Age Movement"! Rather than involving cult, fad and woolly notions, it involves a non-sectarian, holistic outlook – scientific and practical, as well as mystical – a compassionate, global-humanitarian Essene perspective – pertinent to today. Sir George inspired and encouraged emerging syntheses between science and spirituality. With faith in the transformative power of spiritual awakening with mindfulness and meditation… he inspired spiritual groups, communities, and universities worldwide.

Essenes, being the primal holistic healers, recognize the HeartMindBodySpirit as One. In ancient Aramaic, 'yssyn means *healer* and can also mean spade or trowel which, as farmers, they kept tied at their waist. From remote ages of antiquity, Classic Wisdom existed that is Universal in application. Fragments are found in Sumerian hieroglyphs and on tiles and stones dating back 8-10,000 BCE… even the Ice Age – 12,000 BCE. https://thenazareneway.com/essenes_and_their_teaching.htm

The esoteric part of their teaching is found in The Tree of Life, The Communions, and the Sevenfold Peace. The exoteric or outer teaching appears in *The Essene Gospel of Peace, Genesis, An Essene Interpretation, Moses, the Prophet of the Law*, and *The Sermon on the Mount*. Some believe Essenes derive from Enoch, and claim him to be their founder – their Communion with the Angelic world having first been given to him. Enoch is also thought to be Melchizedek. The teaching is also in the Zend Avesta of Zoroaster, who translated it into a Way of Life followed for thousands of years. It contains the fundamental concepts of Brahmanism, the Vedas and the Upanishads; the Yoga systems of India sprang from the same source. Buddha later gave essentially the same basic ideas and his sacred Bodhi Tree correlates to the Essene Tree of Life. In Tibet, the teaching was known as the Tibetan Wheel of Life.

Pythagoreans and Stoics in ancient Greece followed Essene principles and much of their way of life. The same teaching was an element of Adonic culture of the Phoenicians, of the Alexandrian School of Philosophy in Egypt, and contributed greatly to many branches of Western culture: Freemasonry, Gnosticism, Kabbalah and Christianity. Jesus interpreted it in its most sublime and beautiful form, in the seven Beatitudes – known as the Sermon on the Mount.

Essenes lived on the shores of lakes and rivers, away from cities and towns, and practiced a communal way of life, sharing equally in everything. They were mainly agriculturists and arboriculturists, having a vast knowledge of crops, soil and climatic conditions which enabled them to grow a great variety of fruits and vegetables in comparatively desert areas, with a minimum of labor. They had no servants or slaves and were said to have been the first people to condemn slavery both in theory and practice. There were no rich and no poor amongst them, both conditions considered deviations from the Natural Law. They established their own economic system, based wholly on Natural Law, and showed that all man's food and material needs can be attained without struggle – through this Knowledge.

They spent much time in study both of ancient writings and special branches of learning, such as education, healing and astronomy. They were said to be the heirs of Chaldean and Persian astronomy and Egyptian arts of healing. They were adept in prophecy – for which they prepared by prolonged fasting. They were likewise proficient in the use of plants and herbs for healing man and beast. They lived a simple regular life, rising each day before sunrise to study and commune with the Forces of Nature, bathing in cold water as a ritual and donning white garments. After their daily labor in the fields and vineyards they partook of their meals in silence – preceding and ending with benedictions. They were entirely vegetarian and never touched flesh foods nor fermented liquids. Their evenings were devoted to study and communion with Celestial Forces. Their simple way of life enabled them to live to 120 years or more and they were said to have marvelous strength and endurance. In all their activities they expressed Creative Love. They sent out healers and teachers, among whom were Elijah, John the Baptist, John the Beloved and the great Essene Master, Jesus.

https://thenazareneway.com is a gold-mine of Ancient writings, as well as the Esoteric Teachings of Jesus and the Nazarean Essenes, and is dedicated to recovering the original teachings of the historical "Iesous the Nassarean" and "Maria the Magdalene." This storehouse of information is best downloaded on a Thumb drive. Major sections are: The Sacred and Apocryphal Texts… Philo of Alexandria – who holds the keys to unlocking ancient Bible codes… The Forgotten Teachings… Origins of the Nazarenes… The Descendants and Bloodline of Christ… Pharisees,

Sadducees, Therapeutae, and Essenes... Essenian and Nazarite Theosophy... Mysticism and the Coming Kingdom of God... Of Women and Holy Order... Paul: Apostle or Adversary... Monks and Monasteries... The Essenic Scriptorium... Transcendental Wisdom... Crucifixion and Resurrection... "and then came 'The Church'" + more. From Enoch to the Dead Sea Scrolls (thenazareneway.com) The Essenes and Their Teaching... The One Law... The Essene Tree of Life... The Essene Communions – Their Purpose and Meaning... Their Actual Practice... The Sevenfold Peace... Essene Psychology... Individual Inventory.

Laws of Love

Always be True to Your Self... Always honor Your feelings... Always have a smile, at least in Your heart... All-ways live by the Golden Rule. Asking always increases Your chances of receiving. Cooperation is more effective than struggle. If something can go right, it will. As one door closes, a wider one opens. You are safe now. Danger seems real only in the future. Life is wonder-filled... it only improves. Death is merely a shadow. Life keeps finding new and more joyful ways to express Itself. Love is the Spiritual Law that always works... All–ways. Life conspires to support those who love. Breath supports Life. Remember:

Yesterday is history. Tomorrow is a mystery.
Each breath is a Gift...
that's why it's called the Present.
Make the most of each Sacred Breath... each Gift.

Lice

Schoolchildren know the feeling...and those close to carriers may find themselves also scratching. Mix ½ tsp pennyroyal, ½ tsp eucalyptus, ½ tsp peppermint and 2 Tsp olive oil. After a shampoo, apple cider vinegar conditioner, and a hot rinse – work it into the hair. Wear a bathing cap or wrap with cling wrap overnight or as long as You can. Repeat shampoo, apple cider vinegar conditioner, and hot rinse.

As an alternate, the same procedure with tea tree oil, or press 3 cloves garlic and mix with 1 Tsp cayenne in 2 Tsp olive oil. Mild cases may be managed using Dr Bronner's peppermint oil soap as a shampoo, along with an apple cider vinegar rinse. This castile soap may also be used as a shampoo with pets to control fleas – undiluted. For normal use as hand or body soap, follow directions on the bottle and Dilute. Enjoy the ancient wisdom about natural perspectives found on the label!

Liver Lore

Ancient Wisdom regarded the liver as the essential organ much as we consider the heart. Indeed, the liver has >700 known functions producing >13,000 chemicals and some 2,000 systems of enzymes along with thousands of synergists, to facilitate the body's everyday functions. This 4½ lb organ is given pre-eminence by the body – even over the brain and the extensions of the brain, the eyes. The liver requires Vitamin A and if necessary, it takes it from the eyes. Ancient Wisdom teaches the connection between liver and eyes. Oxygen deprivation as in drowning, the body sacrifices the brain before the liver is deprived.

One primary function of the liver is to remove poisons and metabolic waste. As may be suspected, food has a profound effect on liver function. Meat, fish, dairy products, processed foods, refined flour and sugar, all inhibit smooth digestion, eventually leading to a buildup of toxins in the colon... creating a perfect breeding ground for fungi such as Candida and multiple parasites such as liver flukes.

Another source of liver and colon toxicity is improper food combining. When proteins are eaten along with starches... putrefaction of protein and fermentation of starch leads to "acid indigestion" creating toxic gases and compounds that enter the bloodstream, such as cadaverine, guanidine, histamines, indoles, lactic acid, methane, phenols, putrescines and skatoles.

One of the buffer mechanisms the body has to neutralize acids is organic sodium found in bile. Eventually, the liver shuts down some functions to preserve its sodium (alkaline) reserve... so the body shifts gears using calcium to buffer the acids – leading to sclerotic formations in the muscles and osteoporosis. Synthetic calcium supplements are incapable of restoring the alkaline reserve or warding off osteoporosis, including all popular advertised vitamins – petroleum-based, rather than plant-based, they are a burden for the body to excrete. Fresh celery juice has bio-available sodium.

As the liver influences our physical, mental and emotional health, our feelings and thoughts influence liver function. With anger or resentment, feelings of discouragement or self-pity, hatred or fear... the liver shifts to the sympathetic function – freeze! fight? flight? – whichever is best for survival – and the parasympathetic functions – digest, rest, repair – are put on hold. Dealing with a negative mental state related to self-preservation, toxins can invade the cellular structure being low priority. This applies to dietary toxins such as alcohol, caffeine, nicotine and sugar, all of which further stimulates the adrenals into crisis mode. Conversely, a positive mental state radiates enthusiasm, joy and peace, so the liver shifts into parasympathetic function for repair, rest and rejuvenation... normalizing body functions. The power of positive thoughts – even a simple smile – creates a happy liver supporting a happy life.

A sluggish bowel indicates a sluggish liver. As movement of feces is slowed, toxins are released into the blood and enter the liver through the portal vein... creating additional sluggishness in this vital organ. If tap water or over-acid conditions predominate, friendly bacteria are decimated. A full complement of friendly bacteria will convert excess carbohydrate into lactic acid; otherwise, protein residues are putrefied by coliform bacteria E. coli, and converted into toxic elements. This overworks the liver and interferes with basic functions leading to discomfort, fatigue and pain.

Hypoglycemia indicates a sluggish liver, brought on by a lack of useable protein. There may be too much protein in the diet; excess protein interferes with proper digestion and proper handling by the liver. Enhanced assimilation of amino acids is found with whole, plant sources of proteins... taking enzymes with every cooked meal or snack... and probiotics occasionally, offers support.

Hypoglycemia, rather than a pancreas challenge, is a liver challenge: the liver sets the glucose level of the blood; the pancreas provides insulin to bring glucose to the cells. Lack of Bs can cause sugar cravings; ironically, high doses of Bs create those same cravings. Nutrition is found in whole foods such as germinated millet, if You are drawn to carbs; for protein: quinoa and amaranth; while these are usually cooked, they may be sprouted as well. Germinated sesame, sunflower and pumpkin are sources of the B complex, and complete proteins – most easily assimilated in their enzyme-rich, raw forms.

In addition to enemas and chlorophyll-rich foods such as algae, a liver tonic is also strengthening. Almost any root is strengthening. Four Roots Tea is ideal: burdock, dandelion, licorice and Oregon grape root, and if You enjoy ginger, it buffers the bitter taste of licorice. Boil 2

Tsp mixed roots in a quart of water for 10 minutes; cover, steep another 10 minutes; drink ½C every hour.

As part of a healthy, holistic lifestyle... Edgar Cayce recommends castor oil packs to rejuvenate the liver. Find hexane-free castor oil. Place a washcloth soaked in castor oil on the right lower rib cage; cover with plastic and then a hot water bottle; cover with towel and blanket. Rest in a cocoon of rose-purple. This is somewhat different from a wet clay pack. As the clay dries, it pulls toxins from the body... it is to be discarded or composted. Castor oil actually absorbs through the skin and is rejuvenating. More castor oil may be added... re-using the same cloth several times, if kept refrigerated. Cotton flannel cloth is traditional.

A simple mechanical means of rejuvenating the liver... treats it like a sponge, squeezing out stale blood and allowing a fresh blood supply to energize this vital organ. Many times, a dark or foul bowel movement the next day occurs indicating metals and toxins being excreted. For the specifics of this procedure... and to restore energetic balance to all vital organs... see below: **Rejuvenation of Organs**.

LGBTQIA+... QUESTioning?
Anyone seriously on a Quest about the most Sacred aspect of Self – Sexuality – is Wise to consider outside influences. In addition to Mainstream Matrix Media 24/7/365, the "elephant in the room" is Diet! Avoid All Dairy, Soy, and Flax products for **30** days... flush out!

Dairy is twice deadly**+**... pasteurized, it is an acidic toxin rather than alkaline nourishment directly from mother. When we lost our baby teeth, we also lost the ability to produce lactase – to digest the lactose: milk sugar. When did society become gender confused? About the *same time* farmers gave estrogen shots to dairy cows to produce gallons instead of quarts! Hormonal residues concentrate in mucus secretions! It actually takes 1 gallon of milk to make 1 lb of cheese. That extra "estrogen energy" multiple times a day would upset anyone's normal hormonal balance!

Soy is an estrogenic plant and was used originally in the Orient to fix nitrogen in the soil. Discovery of fermentation techniques led to creation of tempeh, miso and tamari. Originally, these products were served in small portions, unpasteurized, rich in living enzymes and microbes. Today's commercialized world is remarkably different. Phytoestrogens in soy may disrupt endocrine function and could lead to breast cancer and infertility. Cooked soy oil can be carcinogenic, especially in a weakened system... this includes soy meats and soy ice cream.

Flax reduces total testosterone levels in men, throwing the hormonal balance for a loop. Flax is best avoided – except by hirsute women (ladies with a mustache) who would like to manage their testosterone levels. Flax contains high levels of lignans, a group of phytoestrogens similar to the human body's estrogen, the key female hormone. Actually, flax has been shown to reduce androgen levels in men with prostate cancer. Flax is medicine... rather than a daily food.

Avoid these 30 days, and see the profound differences in Your HeartMindBodySpirit, and in the mirror as well. Experiment. Perhaps "reward" Yourself for Your discipline after those 30 days: enjoy a soyburger with a double-slice of cheese, some flax crackers for a treat, topped off with Your favorite soy ice cream. See how You feel the next day: physically, emotionally, mentally and spiritually. Your Quest will be over, one way or the other. Know Thy(true)self ~ Love Your(true)self! Follow Mother Nature's Ways. Honor Your Sacred Sexuality. The 'Two-Spirit' people of indigenous North Americans (firstpeople.us) Walter L Williams is the author of *The Spirit and the Flesh* (Boston: Beacon Press) Professor of Anthropology, History and Gender Studies at the University of Southern California.

Longevity

Excepting domesticated pets and humans, mammals live seven times what it takes to mature. Out of political expediency, some say humans mature at 18; scientists say we mature – at least our skulls are fully thickened, and our hardware completely wired – at age 26! Either way, the math is clear: we live far less than our potential. To nurture longevity, the most powerful thing is energize our flow of chi, normalizing our meridians.

In addition to Jin Shin Jyutsu discussed above – **Energy Boost – DIY** – certain plants from Mother Nature support optimal performance. Hawthorn berries provide balance for the heart, especially taken with cayenne. Although cayenne may feel like it is burning, it actually soothes and brings healing. Taking cayenne for health benefits – rather than flavoring – take it between meals, on a relatively empty stomach. Take ½ tsp or more in an ounce of water – only enough to swallow – and a glass of water on the side as a wash;

as an alternative, take a square of toilet tissue, placing cayenne in the middle, folding it, and swallowing with water. This gives sensations of burning the mouth and the stomach for a few moments... it will pass, and both heart and circulatory system will benefit. Cooking with cayenne irritates sensitive tissues, so add a little after the pot has stopped steaming to flavor Your creation. Too much cayenne in food acts as a stimulant pushing things through the digestive tract... interfering with proper absorption of nutrients.

Gingko biloba, Gotu kola and Fo-ti balance brain function, and may be taken regularly. As with everything, take a weekly day off. Goldenseal and Echinacea may be taken for 3 weeks on, and 1 week off to enhance the immune response. Continuous use of these latter two herbs dilutes efficacy; use wisely... only when necessary.

Even regarding food, 1 day/wk take only re-mineralized and re-energized distilled or r/o water, and give Your system a rest; rest for Longevity. As noted in Chapter 7 on Fasting: best results are obtained when fasting on water alone every 2 days. Rest as much as possible. You are on Mother Nature's operating table. With a 7-day week, fast and rest on Mondays and Thursdays... being horizontal is recommended as is meditation.

Siberian ginseng root, *Eleutherococcus senticosus*, is an adaptogen supporting the cardiovascular, immune and glandular systems; supporting the liver, it also enhances physical and mental stamina, and is especially beneficial for men, especially red – aged 5 yrs. Women who use ginseng on a regular basis, especially Siberian or Korean, may develop a fuzzy upper lip. Although American ginseng may be suitable for some women for a short time... overall the herb of choice is Dong quai, aka *Angelica sinensis* preferred over *Angelica archangelica*.

Garlic, *Allium sativum*, known as Russian penicillin is more than an antibiotic... it also has antifungal and antiviral properties. While value is lost in cooking... odor-free capsules of aged garlic have potency. A clove a day keeps troubles away. Mix in a salad or other food, or dice and wash down with warm water. Reishi mushroom, *Ganoderma lucidum*, known in China as Ling zhi, is the most revered herb of Oriental history. Along with tree grown fungi such as Maitake, they boost immune function and, as an adaptogen, are healing food.

To promote longevity, eat foods promoting a healthy life, and having the most longevity themselves. This brings us again to the treasures found in microbes, probiotics, and enzymes. For major minerals and trace elements, microalgae from Klamath Lake and macroalgae from the ocean aka seaweed.

Drink juice from the grasses, especially wheat and barley; wheat is somewhat sweet; sometimes large amounts cause nausea. Barley has a somewhat bitter taste – bitters strengthen the heart – yet large quantities can be taken free from nausea, even if You eat a meal fairly soon. Either grass juice can be used as a rectal implant... 2-6 oz after an enema or bowel movement. This nourishes and strengthens the colon... and through the portal vein energizes the liver. A pint of barleygrass juice daily brings glowing skin and feelings of euphoria – a natural high from chlorophyll – bringing Zest for Life.

In addition to these herbs and foods, exercise is vital for longevity, if only brisk walking in the fresh air... preferably near water or in a park, especially barefoot among the trees. (See below: **Lymphatic System**.)

Love

Wish others well – *bene volere* – benevolence: to stand in the spirit of pure love, to wish only good equally, sincerely, for the so-called "just" and the "unjust" alike! Pure Love – avoids judgment and sees all as manifestations of Free Will in this world of polarity. Infinite Mind, Pure Consciousness, is exploring Pure Awareness through the full-spectrum of human consciousness. Essene Masters all recognize how easy it is to love those who love You... to test Your love, extend it to those who persecute You. Realizing this 3-D Reality exists as a continuum, stretching between the Power of Good and the Power of Evil – each are powerful. The vast majority of us are in between as various shades of gray – somewhere between chalk and charcoal – we recognize All as unique expressions of Source... the Divine Presence sustaining Creation... as Infinity explores infinitely in finite fashion.

Be confident. Everything happens in Perfect Divine Order. When a calamity strikes – tragic accident, weather event, false-flag "terrorism" or riot, suicide bombing, even if staged to create FEAR to promote the Matrix UN Agenda2030, perhaps especially then, live with Love and Compassion. We can be vengeful... or compassionate. Who *are* We? As we mature in Spirit, we recall: "Whatsoever You do to the least of these, You do unto Me" – You do unto Infinite Being – anOther Expression of the Word made flesh... anOther whO is alsO One explOring their Own Options in this delightful Reality we call Mother Earth School.

The idea of gaining and getting... creates fear of losing – along with the guilt of knowing others may have been hurt along the way or left behind. The idea of serving and co-operating creates the Joy of Pure Love – along with confidence... knowing we are living in accordance with Natural Law. We can resolve to live and labor and love in our time, so that what came to us as seed may go to the next generation as blossom... and what came to us as blossom may go to them as fruit. This is what is meant by progress. Wise and Loving people plant shade trees, under which they know they may never sit... nurturing Mother Nature with unconditional Love.

Lover and Beloved

God is Love. And Love must love. And to love, there must be a Beloved. Now since God is Existence, Infinite and Eternal, there is no one for Him to love but Himself. And in order to love Himself, He must imagine Himself as the Beloved, whom He as the Lover imagines He loves. Beloved and Lover implies separation. And separation creates longing... and longing causes search. And the wider and the more intense the search... the greater the separation, and the more profound the longing.

When longing is most intense, separation is complete, and the purpose of separation – which was that Love might experience Itself as Lover and Beloved – is fulfilled, and union follows. And when union is attained, the Lover knows that He Himself was all along the Beloved whom He loved and desired union with and all the impossible situations He overcame, were obstacles He Himself had placed in the path to Himself.

To attain union is so impossibly difficult, because it is impossible to become what You already Are. Union is nothing other than Knowledge of Oneself as the Only One. -Meher Baba.

Lymphatic System

Each blood vessel has a lymphatic vessel going alongside, removing excess blood protein and water from spaces around cells. Excess protein in tissue spaces produces excess sodium and blocks circulation... reducing the amount of oxygen and nutrients for the cells. Cells get sick and die. In combination, excess protein and sodium produce swollen, unhealthy cells increasing pressure in tissue spaces... a major source of inflammation and pain.

Increased pressure causes increased lymphatic flow. Constant increase of flow decreases the quality of work the lymphatic system is able to do... becoming a real effort to neutralize or eliminate poisons and toxins. Result: excess toxins are continually being dumped into the bloodstream. First affected are the delicate capillaries... congestion short-circuits the electrical system of the body, draining energy, straining the liver and major organs, affecting the whole experience of HeartMindBodySpirit. Deep breathing and movement support lymphatic flow – along with plenty of re-mineralized and re-energized distilled or r/o water... 2 quarts is usually sufficient, fresh lemon when possible.

Dry skin brushing stimulates lymphatic movement. Find a vegetable bristle brush with a long handle. If it is also used in the bath, make sure it is dry for this purpose. Begin at Your toes... put the foot up... and ever so lightly... stroke the top of the foot, coming up the leg to the hip... ending the stroke at the navel. Then begin another aspect of the foot, coming up another aspect of the leg – each time ending at the navel. Repeat until You have brushed the entire foot and leg. Then do the other leg... one arm, and then the other. Reach over Your shoulder – gently brush down Your back as far as possible. Rather than canceling what You did by dragging it up Your back, lift the brush off Your back and bring it to Your shoulder again and repeat: pushing down, lifting off and repeating until covering Your entire back. Then reach around, one side at a time, and pull down from where You left off, bringing every stroke to Your navel. Compared to the rest of the body, there are only a few lymph nodes in the face; gently brush, moving down Your neck, then Your chest, ending every stroke at the navel.

C. Samuel West DN, ND, of the International Academy of Lymphology, recommends rebounding to stimulate the lymphatics and the cardiovascular system when continuous for >20 minutes. Lymphatics... like the venous system... operate through one-way valves. Put on music; be the conductor waving arms above Your head when rebounding. The longest average life of any profession is the conductor... bouncing up and down, moving from side to side, waving arms over their heads. This aids lymphatic drainage under the arms and along the torso, promoting longevity. A rebounder – any jumping action such as skipping rope – brings an instant of weightlessness: again, and again and again... in this instant the one-way valves open... and the lymph flows. This same mechanism applies to horseback riding, or any bouncing action. Toss a baby in the air. Baby is invigorated – that's why they giggle... happy for passive exercise, receiving a rush of energy.

A brisk walk can be modified to promote lymphatic drainage. Simply walk with a bounce to each step, and rather than swinging arms at Your side, reach to the heavens as though grabbing astral forces, pulling them down. Reach to the sides and behind... with a smile and deep, caressing breaths – Joy-fully Invigorated!

For the **Control Group**... those preferring passive lymphatic exercise... a Chi machine gently moves the legs back & forth allowing flow of lymph, creating miracles – especially incorporating strategic placement of the arms... 3X3 Breathing... visualization... and meditation. 15 minutes 3X/day is optimal.

Advanced lymphatic stasis: fibromyalgia, or any inflammatory process, circulatory complications, and diabetes may be reversed with technology that has saved many gangrenous amputations! Along with Systemic Enzymes. https://www.h-wave.com/

Men's Issues

Researchers at Harvard found men who ate 10 servings of tomato-based foods weekly, were half as likely to develop prostate cancer as men who only had four servings. They credit lycopene... a red pigment and a strong antioxidant that affords overall protection. Johns Hopkins research links pancreatic cancer to low blood levels of lycopene. University of Kentucky researchers found elderly nuns with the highest levels of lycopene were more physically and mentally active. Lycopene is unaffected by heat, so in addition to raw tomatoes canned tomatoes & sauces are acceptable. However, lycopene found in tomato *juice* is a challenge to absorb! Those who choose to avoid tomatoes along with other nightshades... will find a rich source in watermelon.

As *Dioscorea* easily converts to female hormones, *Sarsaparilla* easily converts to testosterone. In cowboy movies, they go to the bar and ask for sarsaparilla. Another restorative agent is Mother Tincture of common oats, *Avena sativa*, 5 drops in 1 oz cold water, 3x/day... 15 minutes later, Mother Tincture of damiana, *Turnera aphrodisiaca*, 3 drops in ½ oz cold water, 3x/day – for 3 months or more. <u>Caution</u>: excess damiana overstimulates & lead to nervousness.

Fenugreek sprouts, 5-600mg taken with AFA, have been found to increase total testosterone levels, and especially free testosterone. Pine pollen is another natural support, as is Qi gong and daily walking. Men of all ages can benefit from soybeans – either sprouted or made into tempeh. Asians who eat these products are less likely than Westerners to develop prostate cancer because of a plant hormone called genistein. This hormone is lacking in soy sauce, soy oil, and soy-based ice cream. For older men with frequent urination or dribbling, Saw palmetto and Pygeum africanum taken in large doses with and in between meals can bring relief; minerals and some Vit D3 can perform wonders. Get out in the sun daily with feet on the ground, or supplement with Vit D: 1-5000 IU, twice a day. Ask Your body – muscle test.

European studies indicate organic farmers who eat pesticide-free food produce a significantly higher number of sperm than others. The Danish study of how chemicals affect human fertility – published in *Lancet* – incriminates pesticides and food additives as being involved in the decline in male fertility. To their surprise, scientists found an unexpectedly high sperm density in semen from 30 men at an organic farming seminar.

Minerals: Colloidal or Chelated... or neither?
Of course, those on both sides of the issue scramble to prove their viewpoints, and the superiority of their *products*. Recently, doctors determined through radio-isotope tracing colloidal minerals are in a form the body cannot fully utilize; chelates, minerals attached to amino acids, are challenging to assimilate as well. Mother Nature knows best. Minerals found in macroalgae – seaweed or ocean vegetables – and microalgae from Klamath Lake are wild-grown, superior foods. Algae are the source of nutrition for most whales – the most intelligent mammal on the planet – we can learn from them and derive equal benefits from these primitive, whole-food sources of protein, vitamins and minerals. Muscle test.

Moon Signs and Surgery
The Moon's phase influences tides, as well as the flow of blood. *Time* reported on 1,000 tonsillectomy cases analyzed by Dr Edson J. Andrews – only 18% of associated hemorrhaging occurred in the 4th and 1st quarters. To reduce the hazard of hemorrhage following a surgical procedure, have the surgery within one week before or after the New Moon... on a date when the moon is in a sign far from the body part involved. The further removed the Moon sign from the sign ruling the afflicted part of the body, the more optimal the healing... having no lunar aspects to Mars, while favorable aspects to Venus and Jupiter are beneficial. Cosmetic surgery is to be done in the increase of the Moon (from new to full), when the Moon is not in square or opposition to Mars. Avoid days when the moon is square, or opposite Saturn or the Sun.

Moon Signs as They Relate to the Body
Aries... head, face (except nose), cerebral hemispheres.
Taurus... neck, throat, larynx, tonsils, carotid arteries, jugular vein.
Gemini... shoulders, arms, fingers, lungs, thymus, upper ribs.
Cancer... stomach, diaphragm, breasts, thoracic duct, lymph system.
Leo... heart, aorta, back, spinal cord.
Virgo... large and small intestines, pancreas.
Libra... kidneys, equilibrium and balance (inner ear and cerebellum), sometimes, skin by association.
Scorpio... nose, genitals, descending colon, rectum, blood, urethra, sometimes, the back by association.
Sagittarius... hips, thighs, liver, veins, femur bone, sacral region.
Capricorn... teeth, bones, kneecaps, skin.
Aquarius... lower legs and ankles, varicose veins, and circulation.
Pisces... feet and toes, sometimes lungs and intestines by association... the entire body system related to leaks (such as the gut) and the draining of fluids.

Llewellyn's Moon Sign Book, an annual publication with astrological calculations, gives accurate dates and times of the Moon's sign based on the zodiac, for almost every purpose. Other almanacs use astronomical calculations, unfortunately, based on the constellation. Be wise. Be aware. The Moon's sign changes every 2.5 days as it travels the zodiac through each Lunar Month which lasts 29.5 days.

Muscle Testing... Pendulums... Sway Test... and Switched Energies

What is Truth? Epistemology explores the philosophical theory, yet the question still remains: How do we determine Truth v/s Falsehood? From time immemorial this question has been answered with dowsing and/or the pendulum – through which we are able to ascertain truth and, access information – such as where to dig a well that flows at 10 gal/min. Where to dig for a gold vein... both literally and metaphysically. We really "strike gold" when we *realize* we are 70% water like Gaia! Therefore, when pursuing these and other modalities – stay hydrated with re-mineralized and re-energized r/o or distilled water.

Traditionally, dowsers used a branch from the Witchhazel tree – *wiche* in Olde English meant *pliant* or bendable... the first choice for bows as well. When used for dowsing, some call it "witching for water" in honor of the tree. Other dowsers use copper or brass L-rods. You can DIY: simply straighten a wire hanger and make a 5-inch handle, bending 90 degrees with 12 inches in length; cut a straw to fit the handles to avoid skin surface resistance. Voila! You now have L-rods. Practice. Check people's energy fields. Things unfold before Your eyes. Be prepared to be a-maze-d!

Using a pendulum is another ancient way of dowsing to access information. Almost anything can be used. Introduced to the pendulum in Japan, we used a piece of string with a 5-yen piece – the size of a nickel with a convenient hole in the middle! Practice holding it steady. Take a deep, caressing breath. Focus. Hold Your elbow at Your side to subdue movement, or rest on a table. Hold the string or chain between thumb and first two fingers, wrist bent, fingers pointing downward.

Simply gather Your focus and honor Your Spirit Guides. Protocol always begins with Four Statements. Say out loud, or to Yourself: **Please, give me a yes.** It generally moves front to back – like shaking Your head yes. Then: **Please, give me a no.** It moves sideways – like shaking Your head no. Then: **My guides are now with me.** These can be Guardian Angels, Spirit Guides, Nature Spirits or Ancestors. If it says no, invite to be with You. Say it again... until receiving a positive response. Finally: **I have permission to pursue this train of thought.** It is always polite to ask permission, especially when working with someone. Sometimes permission may be denied due to an unstable, emotional state; it is advisable to wait. Once You have gone through the protocol: a clear Yes... No... Guides... Permission... state anything to be verified. That statement will be recognized as Truth with yes, or False with no. Sometimes asking for yes, the pendulum moves clockwise and for no, it moves counterclockwise. This is a normal variant of front to back and sideways. Reading energy centers, an energetic clockwise spin is normal; a counterclockwise spin shows trauma, or feeling totally disconnected... standing still indicates blockage.

Your subconscious and Inner Voice Intuition tunes into and recognizes Truth, accessing the Information Grid surrounding Earth through dowsing and the pendulum... as well as through muscle testing. Dr George Goodheart, a chiropractor from Detroit, developed muscle testing to assist in the sophisticated form of Chiropractic: S.O.T. Sacral-Occipital Technique. Muscle testing is now widely known as Applied Kinesiology or AK, utilized in Touch for Health, Cranial Reflex Analysis, and many other healing systems such as The Body Code and The Emotion Code. Discovering the emotion code - Interview with Bradley Nelson - YouTube

With muscle testing... objectivity is crucial. Enough leverage, and enough pressure overcomes any muscle. Rather than being about *power*, it is about the muscle locking in with strength... or exhibiting sponginess... determined in 1 or 2 seconds – longer is an issue of strength and will... an invalid test. Any muscle or muscle group may be used. Perhaps the most well-known requires two people and involves the deltoid muscle, at the shoulder. The arm is held out, parallel to the shoulders, and slightly forward. Push down on the forearm, just above the wrist with 5 lbs of pressure. With a strong muscle, the arm locks in place. Ask the name of the person being tested. Say: Hold, and then immediately press down gently on the arm. It locks in place. Then, ask the person to claim to be someone else: Albert Einstein or Helen Keller. Say: Hold, and immediately press down gently on the arm. At the very least it is spongy... or simply weakens and falls to the side – showing the brain and muscles work in conjunction, and recognize Truth or Falsehood.

To show someone how subtle this can be, explore the realms of the telepathic free from spoken words, simply think: Give me a yes. Then say: Hold, and press down on the arm. It is strong. Then think: Give me a no. Say: Hold, and press down on the arm. It is weak. Amazing!

With positive and negative, yes and no, established... test anything. Have the person hold or think about a food, supplement or homeopathic remedy. Test for strength or weakness. Have the person touch any organ; test for strength or weakness. Have the person think about a personal or business relationship... moving... taking on a new career... test the possibilities. While this takes two, You can also DIY!

You can Do It Yourself with the **Sway Test,** having *feet somewhat* <u>*more*</u> *than shoulder-width apart*; this is critical. Challenges getting proper results means: dehydration, mineral deficiency, or the feet are too close together!

Relax with 3 deep, caressing breaths; gather Your focus. Have hands joined in front palms up, one on top of the other, with tips of the thumbs touching. Take a deep, caressing breath to focus. Honor Great Spirit and Your Spirit Guides with the basic protocol. State aloud or to self: **Please, give me a yes.** After a few seconds You will sway forward. Then say: **Please, give me a no.** You will sway backward. If answers seem uncertain – think of an inviting situation, being with Your Beloved; You will sway forward, or an unpleasant situation; You will sway backward. Then say: **My guides are now with me.** If no, take a deep breath inviting them to be with You all–ways. Say it until You have a positive response. Then finally: **I have permission to pursue this train of thought.** It is always polite to ask permission, even with Yourself. Once You feel sure of accuracy, hold whatever is being tested, or merely think about it. Swaying forward is being told: **Go for it**. Swaying backward is being told: **Back away**. This reflects Nature: cells move forward for growth... and backward for protection.

Once You establish something is beneficial... next is how much and how often. With a supplement, say: It is my highest choice to take more than one at a time. With no, the answer is clear; one is sufficient. If yes, say: to take more than two. If yes again, to take more than 3. Increase the number until swaying backward. As for frequency: Take this amount more than once a day. With no, the answer is clear; that is sufficient. If yes: More than twice a day. If yes: More than 3X. Increase until swaying back.

The Sway Test is useful for anything: whether to move... where to move... business opportunity... change of job or relationship... investing... anything imaginable. Simply be Love and Compassion in Service to Source and state: It is for the Highest Good of All concerned for me to (proceed with this plan... do whatever). Your Innate Wisdom answers: Yes or No. Your Inner Voice Intuition, having been recognized – as well as encouraged – is ever-ready. When proficient with practice... swaying during phone conversations and other times, is common.

Your Inner Voice Intuition awaits explOration!
The Universe conspires for Your success!

When looking for yes and the pendulum swings sideways or counterclockwise, and muscle testing shows sponginess... when looking for no and the pendulum swings front to back or clockwise, and muscle testing shows strength... or when the Sway Test is reversed... all indicate **switched energies**, perhaps due to dehydration, exhaustion, fatigue, toxins or trauma – physically, emotionally, mentally or spiritually. To restore proper energetic flow is easy. We know earth energy travels from south pole to north pole, and our energy travels from the base of the spine to the crown. This same procedure is performed with both hands; so, begin with either hand: Make a circle with fingertips and thumb, placing it with Your navel at the center. Keep it there during the following:

Reach down with the heel of the hand resting on the pubic bone, with the tip of the middle and ring fingers reaching toward the perineum, moving Your hand up and down... 3 Sacred Breaths.

Reach around the back to the Sacrum with middle fingertip at the tailbone, moving Your hand vigorously up and down... 3 Sacred Breaths.

At the Heart center, moving Your hand vigorously up and down... 3 Sacred Breaths.

Where collarbone, first rib and sternum meet on both sides – acupuncture: K-27 – with thumb on one side and fingertips of index and middle fingers on the other, moving vigorously up and down... 3 Sacred Breaths.

Place index finger above the upper lip and middle finger below the lower lip, moving fingers vigorously up and down... 3 Sacred Breaths.

Bring thumb, index and middle finger to the bridge of the nose, moving vigorously up and down... 3 Sacred Breaths.

242

With hand at the top of the head, moving from front to back... 3 Sacred Breaths.

When complete, switch hands and repeat. Then do the Protocol again: Yes, No, Guides, Permission. Everything is now recalibrated, and normal.

For a concise explanation of the physiology of muscle testing, see: David R. Hawkins, MD, PhD, who brilliantly presents the ultimate journey in muscle testing's various applications in his book: *Power v/s Force: Hidden Determinants of Human Behavior* {which also offers a Map of Consciousness} 1987, *The Eye of the I: From Which Nothing Is Hidden... I: Reality and Subjectivity... Truth and Falsehood... Healing and Recovery...* and appropriately, before his death in 2012... *Letting Go – The Pathway of Surrender*.

And that is what Your Sacred Journey is all about...
Letting Go...
Surrendering to Great Spirit Within...
Learning... and Experiencing Your Highest Choices!

As Pure Awareness exploring human consciousness, when You finally Let Go...
ABRACADABRA
Your Wish IS Fulfilled!

Natural Deodorant

A wonderful cleansing practice, supporting the liver – start each day with the juice of a lemon squeezed into a quart of warm water. In the interest of Permaculture, use the lemon halves turning them inside out, wiping a half on each underarm – an effective deodorant.

New Macro-biotics

George Oshawa coined the term Macrobiotics mid-20th century, based on ancient principles of Five Phase Energetics; under his System: avoid meat and dairy, avoid white rice and other refined grains and sugars, and eat fish sparingly. Eat seaweed (macroalgae), whole grains (principally, brown rice), whole beans, and roots: burdock (gobo), carrots, daikon radish, lotus root and parsnips. Since fruits cause indigestion when eaten with grains and beans, their use is discouraged. When eaten, he recommended cooked to lessen potency, and to inhibit their ability to cause indigestion. Everything is well cooked; brown rice is encouraged at every meal, with Gomasio as seasoning – ground sesame with sea salt. Unfortunately, this enzyme-deficient diet lacks Vitality and Enthusiasm.

Many people, however, reverse various forms of cancer and other dis-ease using these guidelines. Those who are successful have a strong constitution, and the dramatic shift from the standard western diet – heavy in meat, dairy, refined and processed foods – shocks the system and initiates the healing response.

If this appears to be far-fetched... consider the gentleman who lived on the straight and narrow, avoiding smoking, drinking and partying with friends; in his 40s, he was diagnosed with cancer. Extremely discouraged, chiding himself for living the austere life... and still facing this affliction... he figured, "I have nothing to lose." He began smoking, drinking and living life in the fast lane... after several months, the cancer was in remission! His previously complacent immune response system was shocked and fighting back dealt with the toxins, **and** the cancer.

Rather than traditional Macrobiotics... or life in the fast lane... follow the **New Macro-biotics**: new perspectives on the Big Picture of Life, avoiding all animal foods, including fish, following Essene principles regarding biogenic and bioactive foods. Consider their four classifications of foods:

Biogenic foods are capable of producing life, such as germinated or sprouted nuts, seeds, beans and grains. These grow if planted, full of vitality; filled with youthful, adolescent energy, they fill us with enthusiasm.

Bioactive foods grown and matured, are eaten with enzymes intact... including fresh fruits, and those dried at low temperatures <120°... salads and other fresh, raw vegetables, including dried ocean vegetables, and fresh-water microalgae. They have Vital Forces intact.

Biostatic foods have had their vital principle removed by cooking, destroying enzymes. Recommended in this category are small amounts of germinated, cooked grains, especially grains that leave alkaline residues – quinoa and amaranth – and germinated beans: mung and lentils; also, lightly steamed vegetables. Enjoy the flavors, and remember: supplemental enzymes replace those lost in cooking, and facilitate optimal digestion; take them – before, during, or after a meal.

Biocidic foods are refined or processed... white flour and white rice; pickled, smoked or cooked animal foods such as eggs, fish, meat; all pasteurized dairy; starches baked >220° as well as pressure-cooked, microwaved, and deep-fried foods... these destroy vitality and weaken our immune response. Be Wise... avoid them all, especially processes animal foods.

For longevity and vitality, the recommended diet consists of 80% biogenic and bioactive, and 20% biostatic foods. The former two categories are enzyme-rich... leaving alkaline mineral residue. A small amount of the latter category can be tolerated, especially steamed, with supplemental enzymes to facilitate digestion. Having something on rare occasion is tolerable. Celebrate... Enjoy Life! These celebrations can stimulate the immune response system.

If someone has a serious health challenge, stay with the biogenic and bioactive categories... avoid all sugars – fruits, as well as carrots and beets especially juiced; use Stevia {1 drop / 8 oz} as sweetener for teas... or even some in water. (See above: **Liver Lore** and below: **Rejuvenation of Organs**.)

Notable Words of Wisdom

Today...
As I began to love myself
I found that anguish and emotional suffering
are only warning signs that I was living
against my own truth.
Today, I know, this is Authenticity.

As I began to love myself
I understood how much it can offend somebody
if I try to force my desires on this person,
even though I knew the time was not right
and the person was not ready for it...
and even though this person was me.
Today I call this Respect.

As I began to love myself
I stopped craving for a different life,
and I could see that everything
that surrounded me
was inviting me to grow.
Today I call this Maturity.

As I began to love myself
I understood that at any circumstance,
I am in the right place at the right time,
and everything happens exactly at the right moment.
So, I could be calm.
Today I call this Self-Confidence.

As I began to love myself
I quit stealing my own time,
and I stopped designing huge projects
for the future.
Today, I only do what brings me joy and happiness,
things I love to do and that make my heart cheer,
and I do them in my own way
and in my own rhythm.
Today I call this Simplicity.

As I began to love myself
I freed myself of anything
that is no good for my health –
food, people, things, situations,
and everything that drew me down,
and away from my Self.
At first, I called this attitude a healthy egoism.
Today I know it is Love of Oneself.

As I began to love myself
I quit trying to always be right,
and ever since...
I was wrong less of the time.
Today I discovered that is Modesty.

As I began to love myself
I refused to go on living in the past
and worrying about the future.
Now, I only live for the moment,
where everything is happening.
Today I live each day,
day by day,
and I call it Fulfillment.

As I began to love myself
I recognized
that my mind can disturb me
and it can make me sick.
But as I connected it to my heart,
my mind became a valuable ally.
Today I call this connection Wisdom of the Heart.

We no longer have to fear arguments,
confrontations, or any kind of problems
with ourselves or others.
Even stars collide,
and out of their crashing... new worlds are born.
Today I know... This is Life!
Although there are other versions and translations, it is believed by many that Charlie Chaplin wrote this poem;

244

if anything, he may have tweaked the Inspired Wisdom of the Ancients; it is best attributed to -Anon.

Rather than filling a vessel,
education is kindling a flame.
-Socrates

Our deepest fear is not at all that we are inadequate. Our deepest fear is that we are powerful beyond measure. It is our light, not our darkness, that most frightens us. We ask ourselves, who am I to be brilliant, gorgeous, talented and fabulous? Actually, who are You not to be? You are a child of God. Your playing small doesn't serve this world. There's nothing enlightened about shrinking, so others won't feel insecure around You. We were born to make known the Glory of God that is within us. It is not just in some of us; it's in everyOne! And as we let our own light shine, we unconsciously give others permission to do the same. As we are liberated from our own fear... our presence automatically liberates others. (Attributed to Nelson Mandela in his inaugural address, he quoted Marianne Williamson.)

When we are at peace with ourselves,
we become the kind of person
who can be at peace with others.
-Peace Pilgrim
At her grave, a simple stone says:
Here lies Peace Pilgrim
under the only stone she left unturned.

Past and future are figments of memory and imagination. The only reality is the Eternal Present.
-Anon

The only person You are forced to live with... is the person You allow Yourself to become.
-Anon

We can easily understand a child afraid of the dark;
the real tragedy of life is adults afraid of the light!
-Plato

As I remember to smile and be Aware...
my happiness and contentment increase.
-Anon

Rather than filling a vessel,
education is kindling a flame.
-Socrates

It is my view that the vegetarian manner of living, by its purely physical effect on the human temperament, would most beneficially influence the lot of humankind.
-Albert Einstein

The doctor of the future will give no medicine but will interest patients in the care of the human frame, in diet, and the cause and prevention of disease.
-Thomas A. Edison

Life is like photography –
we develop from the negative.
-Anon

Absence is to Love as wind is to fire.
It extinguishes the small, and enkindles the great.
-Folk wisdom

Relationships generate conflict;
conflict generates choice;
choice generates movement;
and movement generates more conflict.
We can break free from this cycle
by making choices that transcend dualism
and the perceived divisions between ourselves
and others... and between ourselves and God.
-Caroline Myss

If I would live my life over again, I would devote it to proving germs seek their natural habitat, diseased tissue rather than being the cause of diseased tissue. For example, mosquitoes seek the stagnant water... rather than cause the pool to become stagnant.
-Rudolph Virchow

The person who will not read has the same
disadvantage as the person who cannot read!
To lengthen Your life, lessen Your meals.
Who is strong? The one who conquers bad habits.
Eat to live... rather than live to eat.
Many dishes, many diseases.
Many medicines, few cures.
Being ignorant is worse than being unwilling to learn.
Early to bed – early to rise...
makes someone healthy, wealthy and wise.
It is easier to prevent bad habits than break them.
Who complains, has too much.
The Golden Rule in Life is: Moderation in all things.
Contentment makes poor men rich.
Discontent makes rich men poor.
-Ben Franklin

Of the action of drugs, we know little... yet we put them into bodies about which we know less... to cure diseases of which we know nothing at all.
-Sir William Osler, MD

One who stops learning is older... whether this happens at 20 or 80. One who keeps on learning remains young - and becomes constantly more valuable - regardless of physical capacity.
-Henry Ford

You educate to some extent by what You say,
more by what You do, still more by who You are,
and most of all – by the things You love.
-Canon Drinkwater, English Theologian

Great minds talk about ideas.
Mediocre minds talk about things.
Small minds talk about other people.
-Anon

Once the door of appreciation is opened,
so is the door of healing.
There is always time to love, to appreciate,
and to be compassionate.
The energy of love creates the highest good.
Love is its own reward.
As long as there is room in Your heart
for one enemy...
Your heart is not a safe place for a friend.
-Sufi Sayings

Believe one who knows. You find more in the woods than in books. Trees and stones teach You things that You can never learn from masters.
-Bernard of Clairvaux

Feel like a boy (girl), act like a gentleman (lady), speak like a saint... work like a horse!
-J.W. Easton

Whatever I command is a perfect idea
registered in Divine Mind,
and must manifest under Grace in a perfect way!
-Florence Scovil Shinn

Mass transportation is doomed to failure in North America because a car is the only place a person can be alone and think.
-Marshall McLuhan

Gratitude is the Law of Increase.
Complaint is the Law of Decrease.

Some education You get in school,
some afterward. Both are important.
Put them together and You have wisdom.
Here are some things to know:
Don't sweat the small stuff,
and remember... most stuff is small.
The most boring word in any language is "I".
Everyone is dispensable.
Life is full of surprises,
just say *never* and You'll see.
People are more important than things.
Persistence gets You almost anything.
Most folks are about as happy
as they make up their minds to be.
There's so much bad in the best of us,
and so much good in the worst of us...
that it doesn't behoove any of us,
to talk about the rest of us.
Live by what You trust, rather than what You fear.
Character counts; family matters.
Eating out with small children isn't worth it...
even if someone else is buying.
Wait to have kids until You can afford help.
Baby kittens open their eyes 6 weeks after birth...
people take about 26 years.
The world would run a lot smoother...
if more men knew how to dance.
TV ruins more minds than drugs.
Life is so much simpler when You tell the truth.
Those who do the world's real work...
don't wear neckties.
A good joke beats a pill for a lot of ailments.
There are no substitutes for fresh air, sunshine and exercise.
A smile is the easiest way to improve Your looks...
even if Your teeth are crooked.
May You live life, so there is
standing room only at Your memorial.
Mothers always know...
and sometimes fathers know, too.
Understand that we're all human.
The most important thing in life is to love someone,
and let someone love You!
-Emery Styron: Graduation Address

The end of our exploring will be the place where we started, and we will know the place for the first time.
-T.S. Eliot

The Universe is a great, living, intelligent being we have yet to recognize – in the same way that one cell of Your body hardly suspects the intelligence or even the existence of the person reading this.
-Michael Schneider, *A Beginner's Guide to Constructing the Universe*

Just look at us.
Everything is backwards.
Everything is upside down.
Doctors destroy health.
Lawyers destroy justice.
Universities destroy knowledge.
Governments destroy freedom.
Major media destroy information.
Religions destroy spirituality.
-Michael Ellner

We have been programmed for sickness: clothing, food, even the sheets we sleep on are – *synthetic* – nurturing Big Pharma, making Big Buck$ for the Medical Mafia! Rather than a Health Care System, the Matrix offers a Disease Management System. Refuse the abuse! Reconsider Diet and Lifestyle. Reclaim Independence. Follow Mother Nature's Ways for 30 days and see how You feel... how You look in the mirror. Nurture Your biOMe to maintain homeostasis with friendly microbes both inside and out:

Outside: the body prefers slight acidity on the skin to nurture colonies of friendly microbes, protecting us from outside invaders. Hair & skin products and **all soaps** are alkaline and destroy the friendly microbes. The body then work to reestablish protective microbial colonies. Apple cider vinegar and freshly voided urine are slightly acidic and known to be helpful for rashes, and to promote smooth skin. Avoid soap. For toothpaste: cured clay "a dab'll do!" {See above: **Clay**}

Inside: the body prefers alkaline-forming foods – most plant foods. For optimal performance: 80% living and raw, 10% steamed, 10% cooked. Avoid all animal foods, refined, fried, and other processed foods, sodas, and especially distilled alcohol. Caffeine either in coffee or tea, &/or naturally fermented wine or dark beer may be tolerated by most on Festive occasions such as the New & Full Moon, BreathDays, anniversaries. Celebrate the day before, the day of, and the day after – then back to work... doing whatever Service for Self, for Family, and for All... until the next Moon Celebration**!**

Numerology

If humankind would only know the power of 3s... 6s... and 9s... it would be a completely different Universe.
-Nikola Tesla

3 / C L U	6 / F O X	9 / I R
2 / B K T	5 / E N W	8 / H Q Z
1 / A J S	4 / D M V	7 / G P Y

Top row = Mental Plane {Thinking body}
Middle row = Emotional Plane {Feeling body}
Bottom row = Physical Plane {Acting body}
~~~ ~~~ ~~~

3 6 9 = Line of Memory
2 5 8 = Line of Emotional Balance
1 4 7 = Line of Practicality
~~~ ~~~ ~~~

1 2 3 = Line of the Planner
4 5 6 = Line of the Will
7 8 9 = Line of Activity
~~~ ~~~ ~~~

Having 3 5 *and* 7 = the Line of Spirituality; without any of those numbers = the Line of the Skeptic, or the Line of the Inquirer – assuming the role of Devil's Advocate.

Having 2 5 *and* 8 = the Line of Emotional Balance; without any of those numbers = the Line of Hypersensitivity – easily hurt in their younger years, they may become shy; their natural sensitivity indicates a deeply loving and tender nature.

Having 4 5 *and* 6 = the Line of the Will with 4's organization, 5's freedom and 6's creativity; without any of these numbers = the Line of Frustration with a lack of connection between planning and action. Many have overcome this inherent frustration and turned it into the Line of Greatness, such as George Washington, Abraham Lincoln, Dr Ann Wigmore, Viktoras Kulvinskas, civil-rights activist/comedian Dick Gregory, Edgar Cayce, & popular figures like Gisele Bündchen and Tom Brady.

Pythagoras is called the Father of Number, living in the 6th century BCE. He laid the foundation upon which great philosophers and mathematicians have built their theories. He set in place the Theory of Sound, the Slant of the Zodiac Circle, the Sun as the center of the Universe, the 47th Problem of Euclid {$A^2 + B^2 = C^2$}, the diatonic scale, and the study of Number, which today we call Numerology.

Pythagoras spent 22 years {a Master Number} studying in the East. Records prove the Science of Number was in use >11,000 years ago. Writings still exist such as *The Book of the Master of the Secret House* aka *The Egyptian Book of the Dead*, the Chinese *Circle of the Heavens*, the Indian *Vedas* and the Hebrew *Kabbalah*. We know the Science of Number was taught to Moses as an Egyptian priest, which he shared with the Hebrews.

Pythagoras based his teachings on Mathematics, Music and Astronomy – calling these the Triangular Foundation of the arts and sciences. Mathematics could exist without the other two – yet, nothing could exist without Number and so... Pythagoras placed Mathematics at the top of the Triangular Foundation.

According to the Pythagorean System, zer**O**, rather than being emptiness or an expression of the void, is actually s**O**urce, the Source of All... Infinite Possibilities... **the** sacred number from which flows all of creation; the Fibonacci Sequence begins with the Sacred zer**O**: O,1,1,2,3,5,8,13,21,34,55,89,144, &etc to infinity. (See below: **Sacred Geometry** and **Who is Robert Anthony Kreucher** for practical application of these basic principles.)

The **Ruling Number** from one's birth date can give an indication of the energetics surrounding the person's particular incarnation similar to the astrological positions found in the zodiac – there are correlations with their subtle influences. Add DD/MM/YYYY to find Your **Life Path Tendency**. Reduce to a single digit, unless it is 10, 11 or 22 called Master Numbers by Pythagorean numerologists. If there is a zer**O** in the birth date, it indicates a special spiritual connection with Source of All. For Your **Personal Year,** add the numerical month, day and the year of Your *last* birthday, reduce to a single digit – Your Personal Year Tendency... until Your next birthday.

You can also add the letters of Your name to have a sense of *persona* or personal character; if someone always goes by a nickname or initials, that sends out a specific vibration as well.

All numbers indicate an aspect of Divine Energy.
1: Leader, Individual
2: Team, Partnership
3: Creativity, Witty
4: Steady Work, Loyalty
5: Freedom, Travel, Expression
6: Family, Duty, Responsibility
7: Inner Work, Spiritual Perfection
8: Money, Organization
9: Universal Love, Selfless Service

To find the numerical vibration of Your name, write Your name as it appears on Your birth certificate. Each name has a vibration, and all names together have another vibration, as well as the name You go by... giving a complete picture. Wonderful interpretations can be given to any name. From these vibrational energies, we can even derive a sense of Life Purpose.

You can also analyze Your name in terms of physical, emotional, mental and intuitional energetics. Create 9 squares # and see which predominates or is absent.
Physical: D E M W
Emotional: B I O R S T X Z
Mental: A G H J L N P
Intuitional: C F K Q U V Y

The Physical person is body-oriented and works with form and facts: I must touch it to believe.

The Emotional person is people-oriented and is led by the heart, feelings and imagination: If I feel it, it is real.

The Mental person is mind-oriented and logical, a leader or delegator: Seeing is believing.

The Intuitional person is spirit-oriented... and relies on hunches or intuition: I feel inspired.

{*Your Days Are Numbered,* by Florence Campbell, and *The Life You Were Born to Live*, by Dan Millman are popular; a scholarly interpretation based on Pythagorean teachings, which also details the cycles of life: *The Complete Book of Numerology: Discovering the Inner Self*, by David A. Phillips, PhD. See also: **Sacred Geometry** below.}

In selecting a phone number or house number, You may wish to consider the energetics involved. The phone company usually presents a choice, or You can request one. Your address may be adjusted easily, such as 1050 (6) may be changed to 1052 (8) unless the someone already has that number; or 1050½ (9).

1 as a house number, or multiple 1s creates intense individuality. Family members are opinionated and this can create conflict. The Chinese character 1 resembles a door latch, and an address with multiple 1s may deflect opportunity because residents are locked in their ways. Hang brass wind chimes near the back door or window to enhance clear thinking. Keep free from confrontation by encouraging cooperation and communication.

2 dwellings are unfavorable because it is the first number to break away from the wholesome unity of 1 creating a pair of opposites – polarity and antagonism. These are ideal dwellings for meditation and learning centers, places for writers and composers. Keeping plants and cut flowers in the living and sleeping areas encourage harmony and cooperation.

3 dwellings are busy with social activity and have little downtime. To keep centered and focused, place a statue, sculpture or a small rock garden at all doors. Get the top of the line answering service.

4 dwellings are preferred for bankers and investors and others planting roots for their security. Those who live in these dwellings must learn to finish what they start, and to be patient. Chinese gamblers say 4 brings bad luck. Keep the entrance, foyer, closets, bathrooms and kitchen tidy to attract wealth and blessings.

5 dwellings are prone to stubbornness and possible infidelity, yet because of the 5 Chinese Elements and the 5 senses, they are considered lucky. Curb any tendency to finish other's sentences. Open curtains and windows to let in light and healthy fresh air. Neatly store or recycle old papers and magazines.

6 dwellings promote love and peace, wealth and blessings – great for families, children, group homes and churches – 6 encourages a close-knit energy. Have the bed opposite the door to clearly view all that enter: ensuring peaceful sleep, relaxed lovemaking. Lots of live, fresh-cut or silk flowers enhance the energies of these homes.

7 dwellings bring good fortune with institutions, both governmental and legal. Did they reflect on this with 1600 {=7} Pennsylvania Avenue {=77}? Together the address is 84=12=3 creating the presidential residence for the Republic. As the number of perfection 7 promotes a sense of spiritual energy. These are great places to play music, sing and dance – and wonderful places to party. Always keep doorways, hallways and stairways free from clutter.

8 dwellings are characterized by happiness and abundance. Moving water, a waterfall or even water pictures, spread throughout enhances these energies. This fosters an ability to recognize opportunities, follow through with plans, and be able to handle success, power, and finances in a responsible way.

9 dwellings are characterized by a feeling of security and long life. These spaces tend to collect clutter – be wary. Clutter creates disturbance and restlessness, interfering with Longevity. Keep things clean and tidy.

Some people notice double numbers called Master numbers in numerology, denoting an intensification of the specific frequency. Many notice 11:11, symbolizing a Doorway recognizing Singularity Consciousness… and Our relationship with All Life Everywhere.

People notice triple numbers as well. 1 is the beginning after Unity – **O**… which e e cummings called: the "nO of all nOthing" of the sphere. **111** is Your Wake-Up call. Pay Attention! Energy Flow… a new beginning, cycle, or perhaps Initiation in the Mystery Schools. **222** something is about to happen – particularly in the area of partnerships and relationships – what… is determined by the next triple number You see. **333** known as the Holy Trinity has 3 meanings: it can indicate Balance is being achieved, or it can be a Warning of Imbalance in Your Life; either way it indicates choice is at hand – either 666 {out of harmony} or 999 {completion}. **444** indicates deep awareness: Your true hOMe is in Your Heart of Hearts and Your Family is Your dearest Treasure; this is time to read about spirituality and explore the Mystery Schools. **555** indicates highest completion of the Mystery Schools and change is in the air; as the number of Christ Consciousness – Unity – it honors the Singularity of All Life Everywhere. **666** traditionally the number of the Beast, refers to the material world being carbon-based: 6 electrons, 6 neutrons and 6 protons. Whatever You are thinking about, 666 is a warning on the spiritual level; with **repeated** 666… stop whatever You are doing – if You are driving, literally pull over to the side of the road – and take a breather. **777** as part of the Mystery Schools, indicates a move from study mode to practice. **888** is completion of the Mystery Schools. **999** is completion, many times related to a previously seen 222. 999 is a connection of Love with All Life Everywhere. When observing numbers, as the saying goes, govern Yourselves accordingly.

Rejoice in the sense of humor within the Universe!

Enjoy the Divine Dance,

the Divine Play,

the Divine Comedy!

Oils

Refined oils are excluded from the Health Lover's Diet. Organic coconut or hemp seed oil are OK externally. Commercial oils are hybridized and downright dangerous – such as cottonseed oil. You deserve quality. Go organic whenever possible. Cooking with oil coats the food and slows digestion. On the <u>rare</u> occasion cooking with oil, Extra Virgin Olive Oil has a stronger flavor and Extra Virgin Coconut Oil has a lighter flavor. A 3:1 ratio of Omega-6 to Omega-3 is a healthy balance, versus the SAD Standard American Diet with 15:1! Avoid canola, corn and soy with their trans-fats, oxidation and GMOs, and cottonseed oil with its burden of herbicide residues.

Hemp seed oil, with an abundance of all essential and non-essential amino and fatty acids, is comprised of 25% protein, including a rare protein known as globule edestins – similar to globulin found in human blood plasma. Hemp *seed* oil is the healthiest oil from the plant kingdom with >90% unsaturated fats; Nature's most balanced oil with the perfect 3:1 ratio. Since hemp seed oil is nearly identical to our own lipids, it is capable of penetrating our cells and lubricating the surfaces between them; externally, massaging with hemp seed oil nourishes and moisturizes the skin with fatty acids. Coconut oil has a lovely fragrance for massage, and somewhat rare medium-chain fatty acids as well as healthy Omegas.

The nutritional value of oils is destroyed by the extraction and refining process. Cheap and quick, most oils are produced by solvent extraction... beginning with seeds ground into a rough pulp and steamed until soft... mixed with petroleum solvents, to separate the oil... then heated to drive off the solvents; neutralized, usually by caustic soda, bleaching improves the color; heated again to remove any tainting smells and, finally, treated with chemical retardants – BHA or BHT – to prevent rancidity. This whole process is unfortunate.

Vitamin E is destroyed by heat. Some stages in this process are only necessary to correct situations created previously: for example: vitamin E, a natural antioxidant preventing rancidity, is lost by heat; chemical preservatives are added.

Oils turn rancid with heat or light. Extra Virgin Olive Oil processed w/o heat can be kept in a cool, dark cupboard. Sesame may also be processed without heat; expeller- or cold-pressed and unrefined are preferred, although some heat is used that alters the chemical structure of the oil. Organic is optimal. With serious health challenges avoid oil – too much oxygen is required to metabolize it. In these cases, get natural oil from avocados, nuts and seeds. If You are healthy – raw organic sesame tahini, organic hemp seed oil and extra virgin coconut oil. Nutiva products have a history of being 100% organic. The gallon of hemp oil keeps in the freezer without solidifying, easy to re-fill the smaller bottle in the refrigerator.

There is a drop of oil (tocopherol) in every grain and seed that is used in the sprouting and growing process – in the natural order of things. When exposed to light and heat, the oil can go rancid. Flour once milled can turn rancid if it sits around on a shelf, or in a warehouse. Rancid oils or flour have an "off" taste, burning the back of the throat.

Although fresh-made flour may seem optimal, germinating is preferable. Choice baked goods can be made from sprouted grains, ground and slowly "cooked" in a dehydrator at <120° to retain vital enzymes. Flour products, even whole grain, present a challenge to digest – avoid with allergies, respiratory, digestive or chronic challenges.

Hydrogenated oils, such as found in peanut butter and margarine, wreak havoc on the digestive system. Unless You are totally healthy, avoid even natural peanut butter. With a relatively high incidence of aflatoxin mold, peanuts are less than desirable, especially imported varieties.

Special occasions call for celebration, so make a delicious natural peanut butter: shell some fresh, raw peanuts; dehydrate overnight; put through a juicer with the homogenizer blank. Fermented peanut butter with sunflower seeds and tahini makes a delicious cheese... having a dehydrator brings many blessings!

Gold Medal Cream Cheese: 1C unsoaked sunflower seeds and 1C water blend to creamy consistency. Add 1/2C tahini, blend; add 1/2C peanut butter, blend on pulse; stir in 1/2C chia seeds rather than blending. Add 1Tsp sea salt and blend for a few seconds. Pour in glass baking dish or glass bowl. Dehydrate for at least 12 hrs, then refrigerate; it will keep 1 week.

Olives

Although there are 700 varieties of olive, the wide range of colors simply reflects the stage at which they have been picked. As they ripen, olives progress through the spectrum, from green to pink, becoming brown, mauve, deepening to purple, violet, and black.

Freshly picked olives are intensely bitter. Indeed, fresh green olives are inedible because of an acrid glucoside called oleuropein; they are treated to make them palatable. The barely formed "cracked green olives" are split with a mallet and soaked in water changed daily to leach out oleuropein. Fully formed green olives are immersed in lye, traditionally, an alkaline solution made by boiling wood ash in water, to remove the oleuropein. Today, caustic soda is the usual soaking solution; after 6 hours, olives are rinsed several times.

Black olives, being fully ripe, avoid the processing. These olives are washed repeatedly and then cured by steeping in brine at 10% salinity. Brine allows certain bacteria to grow as well as slight lactic fermentation helping to preserve the olives.

An alternate Greek method of curing is to pack the olives in baskets, with alternating layers of rock salt. Weighted on top, the baskets are left on slats in the cool and dark, while the bitter juices drain away. Using either method, olives are ready to eat in about a month. It takes about the same amount of time for oil-cured olives, which are superior in taste; when finished they look like little prunes; the advantage is they store well without brine. Whichever method, the ripe olives are softer, milder, oilier to the taste and darker. Olives, high in mono-unsaturated fat, lower blood cholesterol, acting as an anticoagulant and antioxidant.

OM... AUM... GOD

Most people have seen the OM symbol, or have heard an OM chant, the significance is often overlooked – as is the significance of the English word God – which it turns out, is actually an acronym for Divine Energies: G.O.D. = Generator... Operator... Destroyer! Some understand the Generator as being the Father, the Operator as being the Son, and the Destroyer as being the Holy Spirit. Others also accept we live in a world of polarity, and so we can also understand the Generator as being the Mother... the Operator as being the Daughter, and the Destroyer as being the Holy Sophia. Holy Spirit and Holy Sophia together will transform all things, creating the New Heaven and New Earth.

While the sound of OM is reminiscent of the primordial Vibration from which all creation flows – "the Spirit of God hovering over the waters" mentioned in *Genesis* – there is more to consider. Traditionally, chanting – AUM – the 3 sounds, relate to the Hindu Trinity. The sound of **A** invokes Brahma, the Creator, and relates to our Root energy center; the sound of **U** invokes Vishnu, the Preserver, and relates to our Heart energy center; the sound of **M** invokes Shiva, the Destroyer {from which the new creation begins} and relates to our Crown energy center – Universal Consciousness. Interestingly enough, Brahma, Vishnu and Shiva have as their energy consorts Divine Feminine: Saraswati, Lakshmi and Parvati. This is consistent with the **Essene Trinity**: OM is the **Source** of All, from which flows first: **Father** God and **Mother** Goddess, and thus **All** of Creation. Bless Us Every One!

Organics

The current trend toward organic and BioDynamic foods has roots in the late 1800s. Justus von Liebig (1803-1873) was a top chemist, giving us chemical agriculture. By the late 1800s... the soils were already sick from *abuse*; greed is the simple cause of mono-agriculture with its failure to rotate multiple crops, failure to nourish the fields with compost, and failure to rotate the fallow field... the immune response system of Earth has been compromised. Also driven by greed, industrialists chanted their meme: Better Living Through Chemistry. Julius Hensel in 1894, attempting to counter chemicals, wrote *Bread from Stones* {available from Acres, USA} saying more than N-P-K is required for healthy plants, suggesting rock dust, compost and organic methods. Early 1900s saw problems with the soil and bees. Count Keyserlingk of Koberwitz, Germany invited Rudolph Steiner to his estate in 1924. These 8 days of lectures are compiled in *Agriculture: Spiritual Foundations for the Renewal of Agriculture*. The American English translation is by Catherine Creeger and Malcolm Gardner. {See also above: **BioDynamic Gardening** and **Biological Transmutation**}

The chemical industry and the bankers saw more money to be made with von Liebig than with Steiner. After WWII, the war industry wondered what to do with warehouses of nitrates stockpiled for bomb making. They decided to market the nitrates as chemical fertilizers: N-P-K – Nitrogen-Phosphorus-Potassium in various formulations usually associated with numbers such as 10-15-10, or other ratios depending on soils and crops. Initially, bumper harvests were recorded, especially in the US – technology being plentiful with tractors, and cheap oil. Then pests began to multiply like never before, so other chemicals were used – pesticides, fungicides, herbicides. Scientists were ecstatic with the phenomenal harvests... hardly noticing disappearing microbes and earthworms – with their castings and aerating contributions. Studies verify that our crops are cosmetically beautiful, yet nutritionally empty. Shortly after eating, many soon find themselves in the refrigerator, looking for some snacks. We eat... We are full... We are *still* hungry. With plenty of calories, we are warm, yet hungry!

Commercial foods have only a handful of vitamins and minerals... while rich in herbicide and pesticide residues. Prepared foods, synthetically "enriched" with artificial and "natural" colors and flavors, are toxic. Organic means much more than free from chemical contamination... or free from GMOs. Organic means farmers have a deeply profound relationship with soil. The farmer loves and nurtures the soil as "one of the family" sparing no expense or effort to support the many factors required to maintain the soil, keeping it rich in nutrients and microbial factors; keeping the soil healthy means healthy produce, assuring health for all.

There are studies using Kirlian photography that *see* the energetic difference when comparing commercial v/s organic grown foods. It is more than worthwhile paying for vibrationally enhanced foods. The consumer saves more than on medical bills, saving misery and agony, pain and suffering. Support local farmers; support CSAs – Community Supported Agriculture. Love the living, breathing organism of Mother Earth... and All Her Children... to the 7th Generation.

JAMA: Journal of the American Medical Association – – recently released a preliminary 7-year study of 70,000 people in France which found a 25% overall decreased risk of cancer among people who ate the most organic foods as compared to those who ate the least. {jamainternmed.2018.4357}

Physicians Committee for Responsible Medicine (pcrm.org) says plant-based protein is the optimal choice for general health, especially athletes: Vimeo | The Game Changers (gamechangersmovie.com) Join the Elite! Eat Organic, Whole-food Vegan! Love YourSelf, Your Family and Love Your Mother Earth!

Pain

Pain results from a build-up of uric acid and other toxic elements, as well as from dehydration. Especially avoid central nervous system irritants found in alcohol, caffeine, sodas, sugars, pasteurized fruit juices, artificial sweeteners, refined and processed foods. Dilute acids; give Your lymph the vehicle to remove the toxins by drinking what You may normally consider an absurd amount of water 3-4 quarts daily to flush out acidic waste. Systemic Enzymes – 2 am/pm on an empty stomach – assist the process.

Exercise... balanced diet... and positive mental attitudes... beginning with an attitude of Gratitude facilitate this process. Massage increases vascular and lymphatic circulation. When heat is indicated, avoid electric current interfering with subtle energy fields – use a hot water bottle. A salt bath {2 lbs Epsom salts + 2 lbs baking soda} hot enough to last at least 20-30 minutes. Caution: too hot is debilitating. With intense pain, such as with sciatica, stay in the tub for a few hours – adding more hot water and salt as required... or go to the ocean and stay in the water as long as possible. After soaking... a refreshing, quick cool rinse... easy dry and a splash of apple cider vinegar restore an acid environment for the friendly microbes, refreshing tone to underlying blood vessels.

Sometimes simply avoiding caffeine and nightshades greatly alleviates pain. The nightshades are members of *Solanaceae*, and represent a huge family of plants common in our Western diet. *Excepting sweet potatoes and yams...* they include all potatoes – whatever color or variety, tomatoes, eggplant and peppers – including banana, cayenne, chili, habaneros and paprika peppers. Paprika sneaks into flavoring under "spices" on labels. Other nightshades are goji berries and ashwagandha – used in Ayurvedic medicine, ground cherries, garden huckleberries and Cape gooseberries. Nightshades include **tobacco** and in fact, traces of nicotine are found in all of them**!** This accounts for the addictive nature of mashed potatoes, baked potatoes, French fries, potato chips and sticks. Leaving them behind... 50% of the pain disappears!

Some people have nightshade allergy... and others nightshade sensitivity, both have a wide variety of symptoms. Nightshades can cause heartburn or GERD; knowing how they react to peppers or tomatoes, some people cautiously avoid them; others, many times are surprised. Many resist the experiment to see how they might feel without Nightshades. Research shows nicotine actually inhibits healing! https://www.westonaprice.org/

Acupuncture... colonics... enemas... all relieve pain. Alternate: 1st an enema with warm water and strained lemon juice... then an enema with room temperature, re-mineralized and re-energized distilled or r/o plain water. Repeat if necessary; eventually, it brings relief. Patience is a virtue. When doing multiple enemas, always end with cool water to tighten the musculature of the colon, which likes to be about 105°... the cool water sends a signal and blood, rich in oxygen, rushes to warm the colon, and the extra oxygen nurtures this vital organ. Someone with severe migraine began to notice relief after five rounds of warm and cool. Determined, after four more rounds she was headache free! Yes, that's a lot of enemas... severe pain is a real motivator! She implanted some probiotics mixed in a bit of green juice when complete, and has been free from migraines ever since.

For serious pain: use kosher or rock salt until the water is saturated... it collects at the bottom of the tub; have someone replenish the hot water and add salt as required; stay all day, overnight or both, while drinking water – one person took 20 hours... with the help of a friend maintaining a comfortable temperature and adding salt, eventually acids were neutralized. The skin acts as an osmotic membrane and the alkaline solution draws the acids out from the body. When pain appears with congestion in the extremities, especially when there is threat of amputation due to stasis &/or the beginnings of gangrene: https://www.h-wave.com/

Inflammation and pain can be relieved with Systemic Enzymes: 2 am/pm on an empty stomach with a full glass of water. If profound, also 20 minutes before each meal; take 1 Digestive enzyme with each meal. Symptoms subside quickly. Chronic inflammation due to digestive, heart and lung issues also benefit from enzymes and large amounts of water. Cordyceps, Curcumin, Green tea extract, and Japanese knotweed, 500 mg of each 3x/day, taken with the enzymes for **3 Moon cycles**. Rest and evaluate after 1 Moon cycle.

With *intense* **chronic** pain, the question arises whether to use ice or heat. The answer is both. When a flare-up occurs especially with *chronic* sciatica, usually due to emotional issues, and the pain is **intense**... protect the skin and use an ice-pack 20 minutes on and 20 minutes off until the pain is 50% improved; then 20 minutes on and an hour off – for 24 hrs. The second day use an ice-pack 20 minutes on and 20 minutes off, alternating ice and heat – 20 minutes off in between.

With *intense* **acute** pain, such as a twisted, swollen ankle... RICE is the acronym we have always heard: Rest, Ice, Compression, Elevation. **RICE... far from being nice... is simply poor advice!** First of all, ice is the *worst* thing one can do with **acute** circumstances. Ice stops the flow of communication, or at least severely masks messages between nerves, blood vessels and muscles. Ice also stops the flow of lymph which is critical for the first 48 hours for the body to deal with the natural reactions happening in the injured tissue: delivering "macro-phages" to the injured area – these "large-eaters" are the clean-up crew. Ice actually reverses the flow of lymph *back into* the injured tissue, contributing to further swelling! As for the Rest and Compression in the RICE equation that, too, is inappropriate. Easy motion is the answer assisting flow of blood and lymph to and from the injured area. Movement is desirable, including manual compression and release in the direction of the navel. *After* easy motion, You *can* Elevate the injured part in such a way to allow for easy flow, again in the direction of the navel, which assists the heart and lymph doing the necessary work to heal the injury; while elevated, continue the easy motion as much as possible. https://www.youtube.com/watch?time_continue=13&v=0UmJVgEWZu4

Parasites
Bring 3 thinly sliced red onions to a boil in 2 quarts of water... cool until warm, strain and use as an enema. With kids, also eat lots of grated carrots, possibly with some grated coconut the day before. Drink the juice of a lemon in 2 qts water... then 2 qts oak bark tea 3 days in a row. Drink throughout the day, eating only raw, unsoaked pumpkin seeds. Pharmaceutical grade hydrogen peroxide 5-10 drops in a glass of water, 4X/day, is another effective deterrent: on an empty stomach – at least ½ hr *before* meals.

When does the itching occur? Many parasites are active and reproduce 5 days before the Full Moon.

Begin Your program about a week before that; if severe enough, continue until a week after the next Full Moon, effectively taking care of adults, eggs and larvae. And, of course, Mother Nature has her Sunny-side and her Dark-side; other parasites celebrate the New Moon. Combining available herbs in liquid tincture form is an excellent way to take advantage of their many health benefits: Black walnut hulls, Holy basil, Clove, Sage, Tansy and Wormwood are traditional.

Peace is *only* possible Within!

Sacred Breath is the Key: opening the door to our true Home Sweet hOMe! Meditation is merely time set aside to *practice* following Sacred Breath… to knOw… Peace. Inner Peace comes from mastering the Lessons of HeartMindBodySpirit as One**:** revealing a healthy spiritual immune system! Dedication to Principles… Devotion to Purpose… Discipline with Practice… along with Divine Patience – brings *immediate* results. Please see above: **Breath: Physical – Sacred (3X3)** as a paradigm for Peace Within. Indeed, this is the miracle only **You** can perform. Practice. Practice. Practice.

Peace on Earth

To define our terms, rather than the absence of war or tension… Peace is the presence of Justice… opening the Way for Compassion and Love. As children of Divine Infinite Mind, we are Divine Children, equally endowed with… and charged to protect… the Gift of Life. When the command of every religion is to love one another… to fight in the name of the Divine is blasphemy. As rational beings, we can only demand of our religious leaders that they do their job – that they lead. **There will be Peace on Earth when there is Peace *among* the world's religions!**

Pelvic Balance

Standing on one leg or shifting from one leg to another, indicates pelvic instability. Stand consciously, both feet firmly planted shoulder width apart. If the low back registers discomfort, inclining You to shift weight… bend both knees, relieving pressure on the low back. As we begin to be conscious of our stance… as we begin to take charge of our well-being… we make an impression on the central nervous system – equally sharing the weight on both sacroiliac ligaments, maintaining balance.

Sometimes getting out of a chair in a hurry, we get up on one foot as we move with the other. When getting out of a chair, out of bed, off the couch, or a treatment table… get up on both feet, sharing the body weight on both sacroiliac ligaments. Getting in and out of the car, which some do many times a day, is a critical time to support pelvic balance. "Finishing school" teaches the optimal way… whether You are a woman or a man… the most conservative way is: open the door and sit down, then swing the legs in. To get out: open the door, swing the legs out, planting both feet on the ground. Now when standing, both sacroiliac ligaments are involved in carrying the body weight. Especially when carrying additional weight, getting in and out of the car the usual way is dangerous: torquing the pelvis and possibly straining one of the sacroiliac ligaments.

Hearing about this in chiropractic school, it made sense. Resolving to do so "from now on" the next time getting in the car, starting the engine, I realized what happened – and made another commitment, determining to get in consciously. The next time, the same thing happened… I *really* made a commitment to do it properly. The third time: "Strike 3, yer out!" Consciously getting out of the car… I walked around the vehicle and got in consciously. This happened only twice, before my brain reminded me. "It's second nature to me now… like breathing-out and breathing-in…" Some put a sticker of a heart, a flower, or whatever… inside the window, above the door handle. Reaching for the handle, it serves as a reminder to… Love Your body. It works**!**

Permaculture

Permaculture is principled Living in Harmony with Nature. Basic Teachings are common sense. Live simply that all may simply live. Recognize there is a connection between the affluence of some and the poverty of others. Resist the social and economic pressures to buy what is unnecessary. Avoid consumerism for its own sake. Whenever possible: repair, re-cycle, re-use. Challenge poor quality, over-packaging, and built-in obsolescence. Use non-renewable resources with care. Enjoy the natural world… show care for the environment, avoid wasteful use of resources. Avoid unnecessary travel especially by car… walk or cycle when possible. Avoid over-eating… find alternatives to foods whose production or distribution involves damage to the environment, or the exploitation of the oppressed.

Reduce water pollution: use less water; use less detergent in the washing machine; switch to phosphate-free liquids. Re-cycle rubbish and used oil. Re-cycle kitchen waste; if a compost pile is out of the question, blend the waste and pour it in the garden. Ban toxic garden chemicals and pesticides. Weed by hand... great exercise, and healing to be in the garden. Grow food organically; support organic food producers. Join Your County Organic Gardeners Association. "Just Say No!" to chemicals and pharmaceuticals. Find alternatives to animal foods: You will be healthier for it... and fewer animals suffer cruel incarceration. Save trees by recycling. Plant fruit or nut trees wherever possible. Wear natural fibers. Ban all aerosols... there are cheaper effective alternatives. Use less energy more efficiently – cook by gas. Use less power, reducing pollution from power stations.

Think before You buy. Is Your lifestyle costing the earth? Our consumerist lifestyle affects the environment, and destroys Earth's life support systems. Most goods require raw materials, energy and industrial processes – causing toxic waste... requiring transportation, documentation, and at the end of their life, they are a disposal problem. We are either part of the problem... or part of the solution, as Bobby Seale said long ago. Permaculture beckons. Live simply... so Mother Earth may simply live.

Enjoy things compatible with a commitment to care for the planet and her inhabitants. Be generous, free from ostentation... hospitable, free from extravagance. Develop personal skills... take pleasure in sharing them. Make time for reflection – as much as possible – out in Nature... deepening feelings for Mother Earth and all Her Children. Earth-friendly, friendliness begins at hOMe – with Family and Friends.

With talents, time and money – support organizations concerned with the environment... justice... peace. Meet Kindred Spirits and support each Other establishing commUnities of consciOusness. Ask what difference You can make... where You are. Why should food travel an average of 1300 miles, source to table? Why should our food system consume 10 cal fossil fuel energy to produce 1 cal food? What would it take for more stores to support local organic farmers and sell local foods? Why lose >3**b** tons of topsoil every year? Why put 2**b** pounds of pesticides into our environment and food chain... each and every year?

Effectively tell the food agencies to stay away from antibiotics, hormones, pesticides and radiation by simply leaving those items in the stores! Learn about Mother Nature's Ways. How can I create time to grow organic food in my **own** backyard and connect with Mother Earth? What are the alternatives to the present costly, inequitable and unsustainable system of production and distribution? Find Your local community supported agriculture {CSA}. Think globally and act locally... *free* from judgment and coercion – *with* compassion and love. Consider Principles of **Permaculture** to support a Simple Lifestyle. Why?

As an expression of personal integrity and personal commitment to a fair distribution of the Earth's resources...
As a way to reduce impact on the environment, halting the present slide toward ecological disaster, and eventually reversing course...
As a means of de-linking from global competition for scarce resources, increasing international tension and fueling the arms race...
As a move toward a person-oriented Way of Life rather than possession-oriented, work together and share resources with neighbors...
As a means of promoting physical, mental, spiritual and planetary health with wholesome foods to reduce tension and anxiety – allowing time for Creativity, Relaxation, Meditation and CommUnion...
As an act of anticipation of the era when self-confidence and assertiveness of the underprivileged, *force* us to acknowledge new power relationships and new patterns of resource allocation...
As an expression of Solidarity with 4/5ths of humankind who, at present, have *little* choice in lifestyle...

As an exercise of purchasing power... to redirect production from satisfaction of *artificially created desires*, toward the supply of goods and services meeting *genuine* social requirements – minimizing our destructive impact on the world's poor.

Some efforts to simplify one's lifestyle become a Catch 22: Do I wipe my hands on a paper towel and destroy trees, or use a cloth towel that must be washed, thus polluting with detergent? Paper or plastic? Save a tree or save petroleum? Perhaps use a box and re-cycle the cardboard in the garden. Some efforts to simplify one's lifestyle actually complicate it taking much longer. Guilt can lead to inactivity or over-activity. Leave the control mechanisms of guilt and fear behind, along with their corollaries of judgment and coercion. Base Your Life on Consciousness. Do what feels comfortable. By example, others take a conscientious look at *their* lives & *their* impact on Mother Earth. Gentle proselytizing is optional. Be–ing is essential!

Pharmaceuticals: Helpful? Harmful? Yes!!

Choose wisely. Pharmaceuticals – from *pharmakon*: magic charm, poison or drug, and *pharmakia*: sorcery, connecting with Source, creating alchemical and spagyric extracts. Today's pharmaceuticals are mostly synthetic substances created in a laboratory. Their underlying principles are patently false. Do each of us have some sort of synthetic deficiency? Hardly! Do synthetic substances such as GMO foods support health? Hardly! While western medicine and synthetic drugs **do** excel in times of **emergency...** with chronic situations, prolonged use of synthetic drugs *always* leads to side-effects – for which another synthetic drug is prescribed, with *further* side-effects! The answer for chronic situations is **T**herapeutic **L**ifestyle **C**hanges.

Emergencies, however, call for immediate action! Stop the bleeding with compression, clean the wound – cover it *only* if necessary, otherwise the sun and air are vital components for healing, making whOle once again. Soak the swollen ankle in warm Epsom salts for a while – then move it as much as possible to stimulate lymphatic flow. Most emergencies can be dealt with at home. True emergencies require ER. When a child is bitten by an insect and goes into anaphylactic shock – swelling at the neck, difficulty breathing – a blast of a synthetic substance can shock the system into action... the swelling will disappear, allowing the child to breathe normally.

If someone turns blue indicating hypoxia – lack of oxygen – go to ER and **insist on Your choice**. Rather than treating for symptoms of COVID19(84) with a ventilator, leading to almost certain death – ask to be treated for cyanide poisoning! Every ER has a kit: with a couple of injections, a couple of capsules, the person can breathe normally in about 20 minutes... then a day or two with capsules, things return to normal for $200.

Emergency situations may be treated with a course of synthetics a few days if required, then followed by a course of cleansing with herbs. Choose and use drugs wisely! Consider what caused the situation... *usually*, **TLC**... **T**herapeutic **L**ifestyle **C**hanges are the optimal answer – especially with chronic situations!

Plants: Toxic and Safe

Whether around children or animals, it is wise to know safe plants. While symptoms from eating or handling are unlikely, any plant may cause an unexpected reaction in sensitive individuals. Any plant in a young child's mouth may obstruct or get into the airway. In a very young child, any plant ingestion may cause mild gastrointestinal upset due to fiber content. Be safe with children, visit a local nursery; talk to the gardener.

Polio

Polio is a history lesson, suppressed – and the go-to disease to defend vaccines. Coincidently, it's also the greatest lie and medical con-job of all time. Toxins Causing "Polio" is well-documented. Polio is the Virus that *never* was! Consider history:

1824: Metal workers had suffered for centuries from a paralysis similar to polio caused by lead and arsenic in the metals. English scientist John Cooke: "The fumes from these metals, or the receptance of them in solution into the stomach, often causes paralysis."

1890: Lead arsenate pesticide was sprayed in the US 12X every summer to kill codling moth on apple crops.

1892: Polio outbreaks began to occur in Vermont, an apple growing region. In his report the Government Inspector Dr. Charles Caverly noted: parents reported some children fell ill after eating fruit. He stated that "infantile paralysis usually occurred in families with more than one child, and as no efforts were made at isolation it was very certain it was non-contagious." (Only one child in the family having been struck).

1907: Calcium arsenate is used on cotton crops.

1908: A Massachusetts town with 3 cotton mills and apple orchards suddenly had 69 children with infantile paralysis.

1909: The UK bans apple imports from the US because of heavy lead arsenate residues.

1921: Franklin D. Roosevelt develops polio after swimming in Bay of Fundy, New Brunswick. Toxicity of water may have been due to pollution run-off.

1943: DDT is introduced as a neurotoxic pesticide. Over the next several years it comes into widespread use in American households: wall paper impregnated with DDT was placed in children's bedrooms.

1943: A polio epidemic in the UK town of Broadstairs, Kent is linked to a local dairy where cows were washed down with DDT.

1944: Albert Sabin reports that a major cause of sickness and death of American troops based in the Philippines was poliomyelitis. US military camps there were sprayed daily with DDT to kill mosquitoes. Neighboring Philippine settlements were not affected.

1944: NIH reports: DDT damages the same anterior horn cells that are damaged in infantile paralysis.

1946: Gebhaedt shows polio seasonality correlates with fruit harvest.

1949: Endocrinologist Morton Biskind, practitioner and medical researcher, found "DDT causes lesions in the spinal cord similar to human polio."

1950: US Public Health Industrial Hygiene Medical Director, J.G. Townsend, notes the similarity between parathion poisoning and polio and believes that some polio might be caused by eating fruits or vegetables with parathion residues.

1951: Dr. Biskind treats his polio patients as poisoning victims, removing toxins from food and environment, especially DDT contaminated milk and butter. Dr. Biskind writes: "Although young animals are more susceptible to the effects of DDT than adults, so far as the available literature is concerned, it does not appear that the effects of such concentrations on infants and children have even been considered."

1949-1951: Other doctors report success treating polio with anti-toxins used to treat poisoning. "In the poliomyelitis epidemic in North Carolina in 1948, 60 cases of this disease came under our care. The treatment was massive doses of Vit C every 2-4 hours. Children up to four years received vitamin C injection intramuscularly. All patients were clinically well after 72 hours." Dr FR Klenner reported.

1950: Dr. Biskind presents evidence to the US Congress that pesticides were the major cause of polio epidemics. He is joined by Dr. Ralph Scobey who reported he found clear evidence of poisoning when analyzing chemical traces in the blood of polio victims.

{This was a no-no. The viral causation theory was above questioning. The careers of prominent virologists and health authorities were threatened. Biskind and Scobey's ideas were ridiculed.}

1953: Clothes are moth-proofed by washing them in EQ-53, a formula containing DDT.

1953: Dr. Biskind writes: 'It was known by 1945 that DDT was stored in the body fat of mammals and appears in their milk... yet far from admitting a causal relationship between DDT and polio that is so obvious – which in any other field of biology would be instantly accepted – virtually the entire apparatus of communication, lay and scientific alike, has been devoted to denying, concealing, suppressing, distorting and attempting to convert into its opposite, the overwhelming evidence. Libel, slander, and economic boycott were used in this campaign.

1954: Legislation recognizing the dangers of persistent pesticide use is enacted, and a phase out of DDT in the US accelerates along with a shift of sales of DDT to 3rd World countries. {Note: DDT is phased out *at the same time* as polio vaccinations begin. Understanding that... polio cases sky rocket only in communities that accept the polio vaccine, as the polio vaccine is laced with heavy metals and other toxins; the paralysis narrative starts all over again. As the polio vaccines cause huge spikes in polio – rather than DDT – the misinformed public demand more polio vaccine... and the cycle spirals skyward exponentially.}

1956: American Medical Association mandates: all licensed medical doctors could no longer classify polio as polio. All polio diagnosis would be rejected in favor of Guillian-Barre Syndrome, AFP (acute flaccid paralysis), Bell's Palsy, Cerebral Palsy, ALS, (Lou-Gehrig's Disease), Multiple Sclerosis, Muscular Dystrophy, etc. This sleight of hand was fabricated with the sole intent of giving the public the impression that the polio vaccine was successful at decreasing polio or eradicating polio. The public bought this hook, line and sinker and to this very day, many pro vaccine arguments are ignited by the manufactured lie regarding the polio vaccine eradicating polio.

It is interesting to note the greatest rise in polio (1952) was five years *after* the introduction of the pertussis vaccine. This rate declined greatly over the next 3 years *before* the introduction of the Salk vaccine

(1956). The Sabin vaccine was introduced in 1962. William F. Koch, scientist and physician, stated in his experience, individuals who had been vaccinated with other vaccines ran as much as 400% greater risk of contracting polio.

1962: Rachel Carson's *Silent Spring* is published.

1968: DDT registration cancelled for the US.

1970s: While people firmly believe vaccinations are responsible for eradication of disease, the British Association for the Advancement of Science (1971) and *Scientific American* (1973) presented records documenting facts: 90% of all contagious disease was eliminated by vastly improved *sanitation, water systems, refrigeration, nutrition,* as well as humane living and working conditions. Vaccinations and antibiotics were introduced a century *after* that enormous period of decline (1850-1940) and yet is given *full* credit! US Congress' Office of Technology Assessment's report entitled: **Assessing the Efficacy and Safety of Medical Technologies** states, "It has been estimated only 10-20% of all procedures currently used in medical practice have been shown to be efficacious by *controlled* trial." Meaning: 80-90% of all drugs, devices and surgeries in daily use are unproven. Almost every surgery subjected to controlled medical study has been abandoned!

One thing is clear; bacteria do not cause disease. Take a throat culture from healthy people and there will be multiple types of bacteria, such as diphtheria, staph, strep, etc. A healthy immune response system holds them in check; they are unable to flourish and cause disease, or dis-ease. Unfortunately, it is "normal" for vaccinated children to be plagued with rashes or fever, earaches and sore throats. Even with lowered vitality, their bodies seek the quickest route – skin, ears, and tonsils – to expel toxic vaccine material and waste from the vaccine's damage. Antibiotics suppress symptoms driving toxins deeper… complicating their elimination. Vaccines lower immune response and vitality.

2008: Acute Flaccid Paralysis (AFP) is still a raging in many parts of the world where pesticide use is high, and DDT is still used. AFP. MS, MD, Bell's Palsy, cerebral palsy, ALS (Lou Gehrig's Disease), Guillian-Barre are all catch basket diagnosis, all similar in symptoms, tied to heavy metal poisoning and high toxic load. With current COVID19(84) vaxxers pointing to polio as the poster-child, history proves otherwise. New guidelines of the CDC, quietly published in 2020, say unvaccinated people should be treated the same as vaccinated people, tacit admission that quarantines, vaccine passports, and mandates requiring people to take COVID **experimental** "vaccine" gene-therapy inoculations were totally unnecessary, because they have failed to block transmission.

Probiotics & Enzymes – DIY
Because of swift and shoddy inspection of carcasses, the meat industry frequently recalls products contaminated with harmful strains of organisms such as E. coli. We are warned of the ever-present dangers. Actually, a small amount of a certain form of these bacteria is normal in a healthy colon! Those with last names are dangerous: designated by letters and numbers – such as N236.

Actually, 90% of bacteria are friendly in a healthy colon – such as Lactobacillus acidophilus, Bifidus, Bulgaricus and other major bacteria... with which, >200 minor bacteria types are synthesized easily in a healthy colon. These friendly bacteria are known as probiotics: they encourage a healthy, happy neighborhood in the intestines – known as Your biome, Your inner hOMe!

Most people have reversed this ratio of intestinal flora with 90% unfriendly, and only 10% friendly bacteria – due to chlorinated drinking water, improper combinations of proteins and starches, and antibiotics that some seemingly take for every sniffle. Whenever there is any feeling of internal imbalance – an impending cold, or a feeling like flu may be coming – take large quantities of plant-based enzymes on the hour; probiotics on the half hour; drink extra water; enemas facilitate the process.

Research shows probiotics taken with algae or powdered green grasses increase reproduction rates in the small intestine by 2-600%! The logical reason… friendly bacteria are dormant when taken in capsules and when dissolved, the bacteria come alive. As with all life forms, the primary drives are: nutrition and reproduction. With algae, friendly bacteria feast on the finest food of all… and reproduce vigorously.

Reality: we have >10X more microbes in our bodies as we have cells with *our* DNA – these microbes are from inter-planetary dust often called plasma – we are more ET – extra-terrestrial – than we are earthly beings! Encourage Your microbial Friends with **Homemade Probiotics & Enzymes!** Why pay when You can simply Do It Yourself? So... **DIY!**

Sunflower Cream Cheese: 1C sunflower seeds, 2C water, 1/4C of ferment such as Sauerkraut (whole &/or juice) a pinch of sea salt. Blend on Hi to get a creamy consistency free from any granulation; it takes a few minutes; taste a teaspoon – blend more it You find "bits & pieces" – then pour into glass or stainless bowl, and put in a warm place – at least 80 degrees – or with a dehydrator set at 100; after 6-8 hrs it will smell lemonish with cheese floating above the whey. Pour through cheesecloth or fine strainer, or a sprouting bag (perhaps a paint-strainer bag from any paint supply house) and let drip for 4-6 hrs until it has a firm texture. Put the cheese in a glass container in the frig, and pour the whey into a glass jar: have 1 oz before meals, except starches. The cheese can be served on sunflower / chia (non-gluten) crackers – delicious with tomato & avocado, or papaya, or simply an apple... it will keep 1 week. For a slightly sharper taste: 2/3 sunflower and 1/3 sesame. Experiment. ExplOre!

Whey from the sunflower seed cheese may be used in various recipes. An ounce or so taken am or pm on empty stomach with blue-green algae, spirulina &/or chlorella, will enhance Your immune response. Taken right before bed, it can enhance Dream-time.

Lazarus Dressing: 1C each of tahini butter... lime or lemon juice... and whey. Add more tahini for a thicker dressing. Blend. Let it sit 2-6 hrs to slightly ferment, then serve and refrigerate the rest. Please Note: Even though the tahini may be pasteurized = cooked = dead, even a raw foodist will LOVE this recipe, appropriately named because fermentation brings the tahini back to Life. These microbial cultures feed Your biome... nourish Your biOMe – Home Sweet hOMe!

Red Bean Hummus: Organic red beans, cooked thoroughly in a slow cooker – the Low setting is generally <190° avoiding acrylamide formation and preserving hardier enzymes. In a Vitamix or other strong model, blend 3C with 1/2C lime juice & 1/2C whey; more for a slightly fermented taste. Sprinkle with Himalayan pink salt and dress with thin slices jalapeno, sweet red & yellow peppers.

Crackers: Whey could be used in making crackers. Since flax throws our hormonal balance for a loop, it is best avoided – except by hirsute women (with a mustache) who would like to manage testosterone levels. Chia and sunflower seeds make a delicious cracker. Blend some unsoaked sunflower and add to the chia for it to absorb; add some veggiekraut juice if desired as well. Sprinkle lightly with salt; let sit for a few hours to culture. It can be thick or thin. Dehydrated, the appetizers, also can be a surprise treat such as pizza!

Pizza: With a layer of Sunflower Cream Cheese on a larger cracker, add: **Pizza Sauce**: 3-4 fresh plum (Italian) tomatoes preferred, 1C dried tomatoes, 1/2C dried red pepper, 1 fresh red pepper, 1/2 peeled beet (for color), juice of 3 lemon or lime, 2 cloves garlic, sea salt, dash cayenne, at least 3 drops of Stevia {usually 1 drop for every 8 oz liquid}. A spoon of agar or psyllium may be used to thicken. Then chop or dice onion, tomato, and fresh herbs, such as cilantro; sprinkle on top of the Pizza Sauce and place in the dehydrator for 20-30 minutes to warm. Gluten-free.

Veggiekraut: Chop 2 peeled beets, 1 medium cabbage, green or red or ½ & ½, 1 small cauliflower, 2 carrots; fill Vitamix with ¾ solids and ½ water – avoid blending: PULSE ONLY until desired consistency – the smaller the piece, the quicker the ferment. Repeat as required. Scallions and onions may be diced and added, also 5-6 drops of Stevia and 1Tbs Himalayan pink salt. {Black salt if You'd like a gamey flavor for a change; or simply add seaweed of Your choice.} Add ½C whey or juice from a previous batch of kraut, or a capsule of Probiotics. This recipe gives many kinds of probiotic microbes as well as cellulase and amylase enzymes. You may embellish this basic recipe to create lipase and protease enzymes as well, simply stirring in ¼–½C caraway seeds. Fill a bowl to the brim and cover with a plate; keep another bowl under this one to catch the inevitable overflow as the microbes work their magic. Leave 6-8 hrs or until there's a slightly lemonish aroma and flavor... then refrigerate. Due to its acidic nature, 1 Tbs max per meal is optimal.

Green Energy Blend for smoothie, soup or salad dressing for two. Blend ½C water, 2C chopped cucumbers, juice of 2 limes, 2 cloves chopped garlic, 2 handfuls – solo or together – chopped baby greens, salad greens, spinach, kale, and favorite fresh spices to taste, such as arugula, basil, cilantro, dill, and ginger. Pulse for a few seconds, then blend to a creamy consistency. Add 2 medium diced Hass avocados, a pinch to ¼ teaspoon of Himalayan salt to taste, blend to a thick creamy consistency. As is, it's a smoothie. As a soup: chopped tomato, baby zucchini, green onions as garnish – sprinkled with dulse flakes or whatever seaweed granules available, and any other seasonings. Serve with Sunflower Cream Cheese and Crackers. As a dressing: pour over salad, sprouts, and / or non-starchy steamed vegetables.

Plant Protein Patties: For best results use an Omega-type juicer, or even a wheatgrass juicer, with a slow-rotating auger. To avoid long strings of fiber, cut the celery <1 inch. As for beets, carrots and cucumbers, cut as normal for juicing. Use approximately 1 large bunch of celery, 1 bunch of spinach, 1 lb of beets, 2 lb of carrots, and 2 cucumbers. Add other greens such as cilantro, kale, parsley. Juice each veggie separately, keeping the pulp from each in separate containers.

From the pulp, mix together: 3C carrot, 1C celery, 1C other greens, 1C beet, ½C cucumber. Peel and prepare 4 onions for the food processor; pulse only, to produce 3C well-chopped. With 3C unsoaked sunflower seeds in the Vitamix – making sure the inside & cover is dry – set the speed on High, then with one hand holding the pitcher, the other hand rapidly and continuously engaging all sides of the blender with the plunger... approximately 10 seconds produces a fine-ground flour. Almond, pecan, pumpkin or walnut also may be used. **Note well**: seeds & nuts leave a burning at the back of the mouth, if rancid.

Combine all the produce in a large salad bowl and mix well. Then sprinkle the sunflower meal over the mix, along with 1 Tbs Himalayan pink salt and 2 Tbs of ground spice mix such as curry, or whatever favorite flavor. Mix and knead thoroughly 2-3 min until it forms a sticky consistency. Then scoop a 1C measure and form it into patties – there will be 16. Place these on dehydrator trays... set at 150... for 5 hours. Flip them for another hour or two. Ready to serve, or perfect for the fridge – will keep for a week.

This recipe also may be shaped into Nutloaf, or served in Napa cabbage or Nori as a roll, a delightful stuffing for red pepper or purple cabbage leaf, spread on chia-sunflower crackers, or with ¼ C measure form into small balls & dehydrate; serve as croquettes in soups, with zucchini spaghetti, or as a treat in salads.

To nurture Your biOMe and maintain hOMeostasis with friendly microbes inside and out – 2 Rules apply:

Rules for Healthy Living:

Outside: the body prefers slight acidity on the skin to nurture colonies of microbes protecting from outside invaders. Commercial hair & skin products and virtually all soaps are alkaline, destroying those friendly microbes; the body must then work to re-establish microbial colonies. Apple cider vinegar and freshly voided urine are the best to put on rashes, and to promote smooth skin. Avoid soap. For toothpaste, use cured clay "a little dab'll do!" (See: **Clay** above)

Inside: the body prefers alkaline-forming foods, most plant foods. Avoid all animal foods, refined, fried, and other processed foods, sodas, and distilled alcohol.

Reflexology

Procedures in this section and the next are offered for couples, families and healers to nurture each other with the healing power of touch. It is interesting to note that pleasure receptors in the brain for the feet and the genitals are right *next to each other*. That explains why a foot massage is such a sensual experience!

Foot reflexology is simple. Holding each other's feet and massaging them is healing for both, healing HeartMindBodySpirit. Healing goes a step beyond the power of touch when we find and massage a tender spot, breaking down uric acid crystals. Traditionally, begin with the right foot. Always conclude by vigorously slapping the whole foot stimulating circulation... as blood arrives, it brings oxygen; leaving, it takes the fragmented acid crystals to the liver for elimination. Move on to the left foot. After massaging and slapping... hold both feet for 3 Sacred Breaths at the Achilles area... feeling the connection. Feel commUnion... let Love flow.

According to Oriental Wisdom, the feet have 150,000 nerve endings. Tenderness indicates blockage of energy, and releasing the tenderness brings healing... whether or not aware of the organ involved. Reflexology charts are available, with few discrepancies. The classic works are: *Stories the Feet Can Tell* and *Stories the Feet Have Told*, by Eunice Ingham. For some... reflexology opens awareness of healing abilities. Discovering a tender spot may inspire exploration. Consult the charts. Knowing the organ involved, what else can be done for support. Ask the organ: what would You like? Listen... there are many possibilities for herbs, &etc.

Rejuvenation of Organs

Healing energetics flow with intention and focus. Caressing the bump at the roof of the mouth with the tongue with focused breathing, connects Heart and Pineal Centers by completing the microcosmic circuit – allowing the subtle energy fields to flow through the Central and Governing Vessels, nurturing HeartMindBodySpirit as One.

On the physical level: of the 12 cranial nerves, the 10th – the Vagus nerve, in Latin: the wanderer – travels from the skull down the neck, going between the clavicle and the 1st rib into the thoracic and abdominal cavities innervating all the organs. **Using these procedures... begin and conclude by Directing the Vagal Energy:**

Place Your left hand on their right shoulder, with Your four fingers pointing around the top of the shoulder and down the back, and Your thumb running parallel to the collarbone. As a conscious instrument of healing, You energetically connect with the vagal flow. Your receptive left hand maintains this contact; the position of Your right hand varies, over the organ to be energized. The Vagal energy flows up Your left arm, Your feminine receptive side... through Your Heart center... down Your right arm, the masculine outgoing side... to the organ – refreshing the energetic and neurological connections of the Vagus and the organ. Gently move Your right hand up and down for 3 Sacred Breaths – head to feet – like shaking Your head Yes, as though waking a sleeping baby – You are really waking a sluggish, slumbering organ. Check reflex points; repeat if necessary. **{DIY** Recalibrate Your Own Vagal Energetic Flow: with the palm of Your left hand on Your right shoulder, fingers and thumb on the back... and the palm of Your right hand on the pubic bone, fingers toward the perineum, moving up and down – smile, caressing the roof of Your mouth for 3X3 Sacred Breaths: The 1st 3 Breaths – head straight, eyes open stretching to the left; the 2nd 3 Breaths – head straight, eyes open stretching to the right; the 3rd 3 Breaths – eyes closed, focused at the 3rd Eye. Engaging the parasympathetic system, this protocol recalibrates vagal energetics. With a slight smile, relaxing the muscles around the eyes, affirm aloud: My Life is One Blessing after anOther! My glands and my organs are happy, doing an excellent job keeping me healthy. I Am so Blessed! Repeat through the day.**}**

In addition to the Vagus nerve, spinal nerves also pass from the brain through vertebral motor units also innervating the organs. Each vertebra along the dorsal and lumbar spine relates to a specific organ. These procedures may be used when there is tenderness at the specific vertebral level, or with a known challenge.

D1 relates to the heart muscle. Tenderness at D1 or the *left* thenar pad calls for investigation. The thenar pad has two points: the area toward the wrist relates to the physical heart... toward the thumb relates to the emotional heart. With tenderness in the first area, check pulses bilaterally at the wrists, with the hands lying on the tummy. A lower and weaker left pulse is an indicator. Place Your thumbs over the bilateral pulse and extend the arms all the way over the head – parallel to the body; if the right pulse loses volume and the left pulse gains volume, it is a further indicator.

If the first thenar area is tender, and if symptoms are aggravated by exertion, place Your right hand on the left lower ribcage and gently manipulate under the ribs with Your right thumb; with Your left hand, massage the protuberance at the top of the left humerus until that point of tenderness clears.

If the second thenar area is tender, accompanied by emotional stress, the area under the left ribcage may be tight; place both hands on top of the left ribcage and work both thumbs under the ribs until the area softens.

Conclude either procedure by Directing the Vagal Energy with Your right hand directly below the sternum, having fingers parallel to the left lower ribs, gently moving head to feet, while both of You visualize medium lemon, with 3X3 Sacred Breaths.

D2 relates to the heart valves. Tenderness at D2 says look elsewhere... short, stubby fingers with short nails, pitting edema at the ankles, blue veins on the chest or bluish lips, swollen eyelids, all serve as indicators. Primary concern is the diaphragm; constriction here, of course, is counterproductive. A tight psoas muscle is the common cause. To check the arm length is easy. With the person lying face up, hold both hands with Your thumbs on their pisiform bones – at the base of both hands below the little finger, really they are one of the wrist bones. With both hands directly overhead and parallel to the body, give a few jiggles to loosen the shoulder muscles. Then make a sweep bringing both hands out to the sides, and then bring palms together at the Heart – fingers touching, pointing straight. Compare the two pisiforms. A short arm indicates the side of psoas tightness and diaphragmatic fixation.

Have the person bend the leg on the short-arm side, so the foot is flat on the table. Position Yourself on the opposite side. With one hand secure the knee; the other hand lies flat on the abdomen with the fingers pointing toward the inguinal area. Push the knee away from You, as far as comfortable, and as You bring it toward You, with the other hand press into the abdomen and massage toward the inguinal area; bring the knee as far as You comfortably can toward You, while massaging the abdomen. Then push the knee away again; repeat five more times. Recheck the arm length making sure they are equal; repeat if necessary.

Conclude by Directing the Vagal Energy with Your right hand directly under the sternum, gently moving head to feet, while both visualize clear crystal, with 3X3 Sacred Breaths.

D3 relates to respiratory function. Tenderness at D3 with breathing challenges or allergies is an indicator to consider diet. Avoid dairy, flour, sugar, and refined processed foods. Lymphatic drainage relieves the mucus congestion – see also: **D7**.

With the person face up on the table, stand on one side and hold the top of the head – fingers on one side and thumb on the other, so You can rotate the head. Turn the face toward You, and with the other hand, reach up to the top of the neck and the base of the skull. As You stroke downward toward the center/base of the neck, turn the head toward the side being stroked. Repeat five more times. On the other side of the table, same procedure. Then standing at the head of the table, with the index and middle fingers of both hands, massage the spaces between the first five ribs, on both sides of the sternum. Repeat five more times.

Then ask the person to place their thumbs on the edge of the shoulders, bringing their fingertips to the chest. This is roughly the beginning of the lung meridian. Have the person find the tender areas and lightly massage them while You complete the procedure.

Conclude by Directing the Vagal Energy with Your right hand flat on the abdomen pointing up to, and fingertips

just touching the outside corner of the ribcage, moving up and down, head to feet, for 3 minutes; then do the same on the other side for 3 minutes, while both of You visualize medium rose, with 3X3 Sacred Breaths.

D4 relates to gall bladder function. Tenderness at D4, or a sore right shoulder, elbow or wrist, yellowing of the whites of the eyes, palms of the hands or soles of the feet, are all indicators.

With the person lying face up, stand on the right side. With Your left thumb and forefinger, work the sore spot at the web of the person's right hand; with the index and middle finger of Your right hand, contact a point two inches below and two inches to the right of the navel. Gently massage for 3 minutes.

Then move to the left side of the table and have the person cross the right ankle over the left knee. With Your left thumb, find the tender spot at the center of the right foot; with Your right index and middle fingers contact the point two inches below and two inches to the right of the navel. Massage the foot vigorously, and the abdomen gently… for 3 minutes.

Conclude by Directing the Vagal Energy with the index and middle fingers of Your right hand at the point where the eighth rib joins the sternum on the right side, about an inch or two down from and to the right of the tip of the sternum. Hold this contact for 3 minutes, while both of You visualize dark burgundy, with 3X3 Sacred Breaths.

D5 relates to stomach function. Tenderness at D5, or left shoulder pain possibly extending down to the fifth anterior rib, tenderness at the left thumb web, or the area above the navel may feel like a rock. {Pain after eating is caused by gastritis, or malignancy. Pain relieved by eating is usually an ulcer.}

Stand on the left. With Your left index finger and thumb, grasp the person's left thumb web at the tender point. With the fingertips of Your right hand, find the hard or tender spot between the tip of the sternum and the navel. Massage the web on the hand until the other spot relaxes.

Conclude by Directing the Vagal Energy with Your right hand on the area under the left ribcage. Move up and down, head to feet, for 3 minutes, while both of You visualize violet light, with 3X3 Sacred Breaths.

D6 relates to pancreatic function. Tenderness at D6, any sugar discrepancy... whether hypoglycemia – low blood sugar: dizziness when standing up... or hyperglycemia – diabetes... irritability, frequent urination, abnormal thirst or weakness, are all indicators to look for with tenderness at the *right* thenar pad. There are 3 areas: #1 is closer to the wrist and relates to the enzyme producing function of the pancreas; #2 is the middle of the thenar pad and relates to pancreas / brain communication, regulating pH of the body; #3 is closer to the thumb relating to insulin producing functions of the pancreas.

Massage the tender point with Your left thumb, while Your right hand makes 3 separate contacts: 1st Your right hand lies flat, centered just below the sternum, moving gently up and down, head to feet, for one minute; 2nd Your right hand rests on the right lower rib cage, with Your right thumb under the ribcage holding with 3 lbs of pressure, for one minute; 3rd make contact with Your index and middle fingers two inches below and two inches to the right of the navel; hold this contact for one minute, while You continue massaging the right thenar pad.

Then to further strengthen the pancreas, have the person bring both feet up on the table, bending their knees to give some slack to the abdomen. Grasp the abdominal tissue using thumb and fingers at the midline, with both hands – one above the navel and one below the navel – and as the person exhales, lift towards the ceiling and direct the tissues headward. Repeat five more times.

Conclude by Directing the Vagal Energy with Your right hand below the sternum, gently moving up and down, head to feet, for 3 minutes while both of You visualize deep blue, with 3X3 Sacred Breaths.

D7 relates to spleen and immune function. Tenderness at D7, fatigue, irritability, memory challenges, pain in the axillary or groin, pain one inch below the navel with pressure in a headward direction, are all indicators to encourage lymphatic drainage.

With the person face up on the table, stand on one side and hold the top of the head – fingers on one side and thumb on the other so You can rotate the head. Turn the face toward You, and with the other hand, reach up to the top of the neck and the base of the skull. Stroking downward toward the center/base of the neck, turn the head toward the side being stroked. Repeat five more times. On the other side of the table do the same procedure. Then standing at the head of the table, with the index and middle fingers of both hands, massage the spaces between the first five ribs, on both sides of the sternum. Repeat five more times.

Then press with Your thumbs bilaterally on the superior border of the clavicle moving from medial to lateral. Repeat five more times, deeper with each stroke.

Then have the person wrap a towel around the hand a couple of times and stick this wad in the opposite axilla, while You take that arm by the wrist and make a pumping action moving from the outside and across the chest as far as comfortable. Do this at least five more times. Switch hands and do the opposite side.

Then gently press with Your left hand on the lower sternum in a pumping motion, while Your right thumb contacts the spot one inch below the navel, until the tissues soften.

Conclude by Directing the Vagal Energy with Your right hand over the spleen – the bottom, left side of the ribcage. Move gently up and down for 3 minutes while both visualize lavender, with 3X3 Sacred Breaths.

D8 relates to liver function. Deeply reflecting our feeling body, congested emotions reflect congestion in the liver – the Harmonizer of All the Elements. Fortunately, we can reboot the liver bringing emotional support. Indicators: tenderness at the 8th dorsal vertebra; persistent or recurrent headaches; shifting pains affecting various parts of the body; stiff muscles when resting, requiring a warm-up period to get going. Check for tenderness at the web between the thumb and index finger of the right hand, as well as the right foot at the liver point, below the ball of the foot under the two little toes.

The following procedure is also suitable for a healthy person, to energize the liver. Vary the pressure used when squeezing the liver. If the person is debilitated, the procedure may still be performed using gentle pressure. Contraindications: abdominal *pain* associated with a gastric ulcer, or associated with fever; sharp pain at the lower right rib cage; or a tender pea-sized nodule in the right thumb web, which can indicate gallstones. Except for these instances, this procedure is safe and beneficial, even when pregnant.

Begin by Directing the Vagal Energy... of the 12 Cranial Nerves, #10 the Vagus, the Wanderer leaves the skull down both sides of the neck with many branches, innervating every organ and gland. The Vagus is the primary parasympathetic nerve – digest, rest and repair! The therapist can direct the flow of energy by placing the receptive left hand on the shoulder inviting the energies to circle the heart, then going out the right hand to any organ or gland.

Reboot the liver: with the left hand on their right shoulder – fingers around the back, thumb along the clavicle – and right hand over the liver, fingers pointing toward center. Gently move Your right hand head to foot nurturing the liver. You are actually waking a slumbering organ. Hold this contact while both of You visualize rose-purple, taking 3X3 Sacred Breaths – roughly, 90 seconds.

With Your left hand, reach around the back – between their scapula and vertebrae, looking for a tender spot to the right of the 3rd 4th or 5th dorsal vertebra. Hold this contact with the index and middle fingertips of Your left hand. With none being tender, contact the 4th space.

Then with the index and middle fingertips of the right hand, locate the spaces between the 1st four ribs, just to the right of their sternum. Determine the tender point. If all are tender or if none, make contact at the middle space – between 2nd and 3rd ribs.

Massage these points until the pain is released or – in the absence of pain – for 3 Sacred Breaths. This re-establishes connection between kidneys and the liver.

Then bring Your left hand from behind the back, and place the index and middle fingertips of Your left hand at the point Your right hand was massaging in the front. Move Your right hand to the lower right rib cage, hand flat – fingers pointing to center – moving head to foot for 3 Sacred Breaths.

Now the energetic stage has been set to wring out the liver – treating it like a sponge, so to speak – driving out *stale* blood. Bring Your left hand from the point of contact at the ribs, and place the palm at the *side* of the right lower rib cage, with fingers pointing toward center. Move Your right hand to the lower right abdominal cavity, over the cecal area of the large intestine; the palm of Your right hand is now medial to the right crest of the hip, the bony protuberance... with fingers pointing toward the liver.

Have the person take a deep breath and as the person exhales, press against the rib cage with the palm of Your left hand, and down on the rib cage with the fingers of the same hand, effectively compressing the liver. At the same time, create a wavelike pressure extending from the palm of Your right hand moving to the fingertips; the motion is into the gut, and toward the liver. **Hold** both contacts, and ask the person to take another deep breath. Exhaling the 2nd time, compress the liver from above and below, even more. Hold this pressure asking the person to take a 3rd deep breath. As the person exhales the 3rd time, press down on the ribcage even more – see if the fingertips of the right hand can move under the ribs. Ask the person to take a *deep* breath... as *deep* as possible. At this point it may be a bit uncomfortable so encourage the person by saying **deeper** a couple of times, until the person is full. Then with this exhalation release both hands suddenly – as though powerful springs were pushing You away. Fresh, oxygenated blood now fills the liver!

Conclude by Directing the Vagal Energy with Your hands as they were at the beginning: left hand on right shoulder, right hand over the liver. Gently nurture the liver. Hold this contact while both of You visualize rose-purple, taking 3X3 Sacred Breaths.

Recheck the liver reflex point. The pain is probably gone. If still somewhat present, resume the Vagal contact for another 3 Sacred Breaths and check the reflex point again. If it still persists, do this procedure in another 3 days; it may be done 2-3X a week as part of a protocol to help rebuild the liver. After this procedure, the person may be somewhat dizzy when sitting up; before standing, recommend a mOMent to relax and regain composure.

A 5-minute brisk walk, hopefully barefoot, with arms freely swinging will collate and integrate the total experience, thus concluding the session. The next day, it is common to have an unusually dark or foul stool – as the body celebrates the release of old, stale blood from the liver, showering Blessings on Your Journey!

D9 relates to adrenal function. Whatever side of D9 is tender indicates the adrenal gland under stress. Nodes in the joints of the hands, high or low blood pressure – indicating over active or under active adrenals; fatigue, arthritis, poor calcium metabolism, are all indicators.

Place both thumbs together in the midline two inches below the sternum, with fingertips resting on the lower ribs of each side. The motion alternates in a wavelike fashion: press (2 lbs) the thumbs, then release as You press the fingertips... then release as You press the thumbs... continuing for 3 minutes. Caution: With high blood pressure, the movement is slow; with low blood pressure, the movement is with less force, yet rapid.

Then with the index and middle fingers of Your left hand, contact the center of the sternum; with the index and middle fingers of the right hand find the points one inch above the navel and two inches on either side. Hold the abdominal contact lightly for low blood pressure, firmly for high blood pressure for 3 minutes.

Conclude by Directing the Vagal Energy with Your right hand pointing sideways covering the area one inch above the navel, and holding for 3 minutes, while both visualize dark burgundy, with 3X3 Sacred Breaths.

D10 relates to the small intestine. Tenderness at D10, parasites, elimination challenges, tenderness within a four-inch circle around the navel, are all indicators.

Stand on the side of abdominal tenderness. Hold the shoulder on that side with one hand, while the index and middle fingers of the other hand are on the tender spot. Massage with 3 pounds of pressure until tenderness dissipates.

Then contact the right thumb web with Your thumb and index finger of Your left hand, while the index and middle fingertips of Your right hand contact the point 2 inches below and 2 inches to the right of the navel.

Follow with the procedure at **D8** above, to rejuvenate the liver. Then to further strengthen the intestines, have the person bring both feet on the table, bending their knees to give slack to the abdomen. Then grasp the abdominal tissue with thumb and fingers at the midline with both hands – one above the navel and one below the navel – and as the person exhales, lift towards the ceiling and direct the tissues headward. Repeat five more times.

Conclude by Directing the Vagal Energy with Your right hand resting on the navel for two minutes, while both of You visualize mist blue, with 3X3 Sacred Breaths.

D11-12 relates to kidney function. Tenderness on either side of D11-12, swelling around the eyes or cheeks, pitting edema of the ankles, clubby hands with short brittle nails, are all indicators.

Find a tender spot on the right or the left, one inch above the navel and four inches to the side. Depending on which side is tender, stand so the index and middle fingers of one hand are on the lateral collarbone, with the index and middle fingers of the other hand on the tender spot. Hold that contact for 3 minutes until the tenderness dissipates. When that happens, move Your superior hand to contact with the index and middle fingers at the central sternum. Hold that contact with two pounds of pressure for two minutes. Check the arm length, as noted in **D2** above.

Conclude by Directing the Vagal Energy with Your right hand one inch above the navel, pointing sideways. Hold this contact for 3 minutes while both of You visualize all the colors of fire with 3X3 Sacred Breaths.
L1 relates to the ileocecal valve. Tenderness at L1, or when asked to raise the right arm the person tilts the head to the right, or thin ribbon-like stools, are all indicators.

The index and middle fingers of Your right hand contact the area two inches below and two inches to the right of the navel. Your left hand grasps the right shoulder, with the thumb massaging the painful point at the top of the humerus in the front, until the pain goes away. Then push Your fingers downward and test for strength. Weak? Push Your fingers upward. Strong? Hold Your fingers in that position, with Your left hand over the shoulder for 3 deep breaths.

Conclude by Directing the Vagal Energy with Your right hand gently resting at the abdominal area that You were just contacting, and hold for 2 minutes while both of You visualize ultraviolet, with 3X3 Sacred Breaths.

L2 relates to the cecum. Tenderness at L2, or arthritis – gout, torticollis, lumbago, enlarged finger joints, are all indicators; with acute pain in the right lower abdominal area, always suspect appendicitis.

With the left fingertips around the right shoulder, contact the trapezius insertions in the back, at the top of the shoulder; the right index and middle fingers contact the area 3 inches below and 2 inches to the right of the navel – massage both points until tenderness dissolves. Then move the index and middle fingers of the left hand to the center of the sternum; keep the right-hand contact in place, applying 5 lbs of pressure headward until the tissues soften.

Conclude by Directing the Vagal Energy resting Your right hand gently over the point You were working for two minutes, while both of You visualize lavender, with 3X3 Sacred Breaths.

L3 relates to the ovaries / testes. Tenderness at L3, or joint pains, muscle weakness, indecisiveness, heart challenges, nervousness and being emotionally distraught, are all indicators.

With Your left hand over the right shoulder, make a contact with Your right hand: the thumb on one side of the pubic bone and the index and middle fingers on the other. Squeeze gently for one minute, then relax... 3X.

Conclude by Directing the Vagal Energy with Your right hand placed over the pubic bone for 3 minutes, while both of You visualize medium rose.

Glandular aberrations may be normalized by reconnecting energies: have the person hold their left hand over their right shoulder, with the right hand cupping the genitals; this may be done several times a day to balance and normalize glandular secretions. Visualize medium rose, with 3X3 Sacred Breaths.

L4 relates to the colon. Tenderness at L4, or irregular bowel habits are indicators. Tenderness on the underside of the most lateral part of the clavicle is present with constipation; with diarrhea, the medial part is tender.

Stand on the left with Your right hand contacting the middle of the left descending colon, and Your left hand contacting the middle of the right ascending colon. Work both hands in unison for accurate results. Start at the middle and move towards the feet; then return to the middle and move towards the head, and then across the transverse. Select the most painful area with the index and middle fingers of Your right hand, while the left hand goes over the shoulder, with the

thumb contacting the painful spot on the clavicle. Massage until both points relax.

Conclude by Directing the Vagal Energy with Your right hand resting gently over the abdominal area You were working for 3 minutes, both of You visualize lavender, with 3X3 Sacred Breaths.

L5 relates to the uterus / prostate. Tenderness at L5, or pain at the top of the head or the pubic area, burning pain across the small of the back or hips, and breast pain, are all indicators.

Check the inguinal ligament on both sides for the most painful area. Contact that area while Your other hand contacts the tender spot on the trapezius on the same side, around the top of the shoulder. Use gentle pressure until both pains dissolve. Then keeping the inguinal contact, move Your hand from shoulder to mid-sternum and hold for 3 minutes.

Check the arm length as in **D2**; do the procedure at **L1**, and then **D8**.

Conclude by Directing the Vagal Energy with Your right hand gently resting at the pubic bone for two minutes, while both visualize frost, with 3X3 Sacred Breaths.

These procedures are from the chiropractic philosophy of Sacral-Occipital Technique {SOT}. For further explorations: *Energy Medicine: Balancing Your Body's Energies for Optimal Health, Joy, and Vitality* by Donna Eden with David Feinstein, PhD. If symptoms persist, see a holistic physician or health practitioner.

Relationships
Your physical form is the expression of Great Spirit – You Are the Word Made Flesh! Each One of us explores human consciousness, experiencing *feelings* from their own individual point of view. The individual *experience* with one's physical vehicle through nurturance and sensuality, makes *us* our first and most precious partner in the world. Self-care cultivates acceptance, trust, respect and love – all qualities which translate immediately into Your actions with Others – who are *also* expressions of Great Spirit exploring human consciousness. Experiencing their own feelings. Being kind to Yourself brings kindness into the world. Your feeling body, Your thinking body and Your acting body are Gardens... in which You grow

Gifts... to first offer Self... and then offer to Others... ultimately, to offer Your Significant Other.

Until we learn how to discover our true Self... and relate to Self with Love... we will be co-dependent with Others: lover, children, business partner, healer, and everyOne. To enter into and nurture relationship with Self... we will benefit from Meditation, Fasting and Mirror Therapy. The latter is simple: stand close to the mirror looking deeply in Your own eyes offering words of appreciation and love... for You... for the wonderful blessings Life gives You... and the blessings You give Life. Look closely in Your own eyes... stripped to Your core... recognizing Beauty within... trusting the process of Life... at Peace... *feeling*... I Am that I Am... I Am whole and complete!

I Am, speaks to Your thinking body. **You Are**, speaks to Your feeling body. John Diamond, MD says speak in the **3rd person** making a "news" announcement to the Universe! Use either Your given name, or the nick-name You use when speaking to Yourself. {While my nick-name is Bobby Tony, I say Bobby for simplicity.} Dr Diamond claims this is the most effective use of affirmations. Speak to ALL with a slight **smile**... with feelings of **excitement!** Whether doing affirmations in the mirror, or when using the Wand of Light - Intention is paramount. {See above: **Grounding:** design Your own **Med-Bed**.}

My Glands and My Organs... My Muscles and Bones... and All My Systems* Are Happy and Healthy... Doing an Excellent Job Keeping My HeartMindBodySpirit in Balance. My Life of Service Continues to Be One Blessing After anOther! **YES!!! THANK YOU!!!**

Your Glands and Your Organs Your Muscles and Bones and All Your Systems* Are Happy and Healthy... Doing an Excellent Job Keeping Your HeartMindBodySpirit in Balance. Your Life of Service Continues to Be One Blessing After anOther! **YES!!! THANK YOU!!!**

Bobby's Glands and his Organs... his Muscles and Bones and All his Systems* Are Happy and Healthy... Doing an Excellent Job Keeping Bobby's HeartMindBodySpirit in Balance. Bobby's Life of Service Continues to Be One Blessing After anOther! **YES!!! THANK YOU!!!**

* Body Systems:
Cardiovascular
Cerebral-Spinal-Nerves
Digestive-Excretory
Endocrine-Hormonal
Immune-Lymphatic
Integumentary
Musculo-Skeletal
Reproductive
Respiratory
Urinary

These messages and the experience – looking in Your own eyes, are integrated and collated by Your corpus collosum... and Your HeartMindBodySpirit resonates!

Until we arrive at this point – Pure Love of Self – we are looking for someone to fulfill our dreams, to make us complete. When we truly love our Self there is possibility for a true relationship by Gifting our complete and contented Self to the Other.

When the Other also recognizes completeness and wholeness at all levels of Self, and thus exchanges the Gifting of Self... we can experience an inter-dependent relationship – one that recognizes, honors, and accepts the "I Am that I Am" in the Self, in the Other, in all Others.

To facilitate conscious relationships...
Be clear about what You choose to create.
Be clear about what gets to change in Your life.
Stand in Your Wish Fulfilled... *feel* Yourself *there.*
Expect... Listen... and allow the Universe to deliver.
The Universe conspires for Your Success!

Clarity is required. Specificity **+** Feelings **=** Manifestation! Clarity is Vital. The mind wanders... and meditation gives a certain focus to Monkey-mind. While it is proper and responsible to be concerned with the details of Life... if we choose to harvest vegetables, we get to plant specific seeds and care for them... it is the same with meditation. We attend to details by releasing worry... and keeping our focus. While it is natural to be concerned about our little ones – with clothes and school supplies in order, etc... as well as with personal projects – with details set in motion, presume things are going brilliantly... surround these situations with Love and Light... keeping Your focus on Your Wish Fulfilled. Needless worry and anxiety only serve to energize and attract what we worry about.

The way we think is the way we feel.
The way we feel is the way we vibrate.
The way we vibrate is the way we attract.

When old habits of worry or anxiety visit Monkey-mind... nip things in the bud saying: I Am so blessed! ... Focus on and recount all Your blessings. Make a list of 31 things You appreciate about Yourself, assigning one to each day of the month. Should negative thoughts or feelings appear, simply substitute the appreciation for the day; put a smile on Your face, and stand in Your Wish Fulfilled.

After that month of appreciation, begin a week of *feeling* Gratitude... then a week of *feeling* Amusement... then a week of *feeling* Enthusiasm... then a week of *feeling* Reverence for All Life Everywhere. After two months, old habits are history. You are closer to Your Wish Fulfilled.

Affirm what You choose to create and keep Your Awareness focused throughout the day:

I Am in a relationship based on Trust and Integrity. Our lives are filled with fun and laughter. We have easy communication about everything... from the mundane to the intellectual.

We are a team – enthusiastic about Life. We share a deep esteem for Mother Earth and Her Natural Processes.

We assist each other in conscious living, keeping Our focus on the Energies around Us... and within Us.
We appreciate the Divine within Our Self and each Other as expressions of the One Creative Power... expressions of Infinite Mind... Be-ing in Action.

We assist each other as We stand in... and create... Our Wish Fulfilled. We have a lavish, steady, dependable income, consistent with integrity and mutual benefit for All.

We are a Source of Inspiration for Each Other... Our Children, and All Children Everywhere. We *are* so Blessed. Our Life of Service continues to be One Blessing after anOther!

Rice and Arsenic: Catch 22
It is usually recommended to use whole grain rice for its antioxidants, B-complex, fiber, heart health, etc, whether long-grain, short-grain, brown, red or whole grain white basmati rice. Unfortunately, it has more inorganic arsenic than refined, white rice! Use **caution**. When preparing rice, first wash it several times and then soak it overnight – or through the day – giving the soak water to Your plants. Add **6** times the amount of water and boil for 30 minutes; throw that water away with the residual arsenic, which has cooked out from the bran. Rinse and then steam until tender.

There are other "healthy" foods that have surprisingly high amounts of inorganic arsenic. Cruciferous vegetables, especially Brussel sprouts – as well as broccoli, cauliflower and kale – are rich in sulfur compounds that attract the inorganic arsenic from the soil! Having Brussel sprouts once a month at times of festive celebrations is generally regarded as safe.

The body efficiently excretes inorganic arsenic through keratin – in our hair and especially in our toenails. Tissue analysis can determine toxicity levels. Otherwise, if Your Inner Voice Intuition prompts You, do the Sway Test... You can facilitate elimination; the homeopathic protocol may safely be followed as found above: **Alzheimer's, Aluminum, Mercury & Other Heavy Metals** using quantum physics to bring balance.

Ritalin: Natural Alternatives
The United States and other countries classify Ritalin in the 2nd highest category of addictive and controlled substances. Yet, Ritalin is sold illegally on the streets. A street drug, crank – like speed, chemically known as methamphetamine – is prescribed for children as Desoxyn®! Taking prescriptions teaches children drugs are the way to cope with Life. As with other amphetamine-like drugs, Ritalin has dangerous side effects. Withdrawal or reducing dosage can cause life-threatening situations. According to the *Diagnostic and Statistical Manual (DSM-IIIR)*, psychiatrists state suicide is the major complication of withdrawal from Ritalin and similar drugs. Interestingly enough, the Armed Forces consider recent use of Ritalin in the same category as cocaine and heroin... excluding people as "medically rejected"! Put into perspective, let's assess the causes, and resolve the crises!

What makes people hyper? The first focus was dangers found in sugar... then the artificial colors, flavors and other "chemical junk" added to foods. While the FDA conducted some tests, and has a list of additives that are on the GRAS list – <u>G</u>enerally <u>R</u>ecognized <u>A</u>s <u>S</u>afe – these tests have been done *only* on an individual basis. No tests have been done on multiple additives, or even the *common mixtures* found in today's foods. When a food at the grocery lists the ingredients using more than 3 lines, put it back on the shelf. As much as possible eat whole grains and vegetables at one meal, and fruits at another meal. Nuts and seeds combine with fruit *or* vegetables… they digest easier when germinated.

A Florida university study following co-eds through four years found those who drank diet sodas averaged a 20-point drop in their IQ! (See: **Sweet Poison** below) Besides avoiding caffeine and processed foods – irritating the central nervous system – eat foods low on the food chain that support neurotransmitters in the brain, the most abundant source being edible fresh-water and marine algae. Looking for energy… replace caffeine with algae or, double-bag peppermint tea.

ADD means: Algae Deficient Diet. The Japanese, known to be voracious algae eaters, have the highest average IQ of any country in the world at 106. The US is in the low 90s. Algae… the very bottom of the food chain… have been around for 3 billion years! The macroalgae in seaweed, as well as microalgae from Klamath Lake, are wild-grown and superior.
ADD, rather than a Ritalin deficiency, is truly a neuropeptide / neurotransmitter deficiency – gram for gram, the most nutrient-rich, wild-grown plant source of amino acids to create neuropeptides – precursors to neurotransmitters – is found in seaweed and microalgae from Klamath Lake. Also offering great benefit: spirulina and chlorella. (See: **AFA** above.)

There are many varieties of ocean vegetables also known as seaweeds. Explore the different tastes and textures, adding to salads and soups. If it leaves something to be desired, give small baggies to friends so they can choose what they consider tasty.

Rules of Life
Great minds talk about ideas.
Average minds talk about things.
Small minds talk about other people.

Tell the truth – there's less to remember.

The best things in life aren't things.

Speak softly and wear a loud shirt –
You're bound to brighten someone's day.

The one who dies with the most toys – still dies.

Age is relative – when You're over the hill,
You pick up speed.

There are 2 ways to be rich: make more, or desire less.

Beauty is internal and eternal.

Why judge a day by the weather?
No rain… no rainbows! ~.~*

Sacred Breath See above: **Breath: Physical – Sacred (3X3 Breaths)**

Sacred Geometry
"By the Greeks geometry was held in the very highest honor, and none were more illustrious than mathematicians. But we Romans have limited the practice of this art to its usefulness in measurement and calculation." Cicero, 106-43 BCE

Pythagoras based his teachings on Mathematics, Music and Astronomy – calling these the Triangular Foundation of all the arts and sciences. Affirming that Mathematics could exist without the other two – yet, nothing could exist without Number – Pythagoras placed Mathematics at the top of the Triangular Foundation. Consider:

"In ancient Greece, advanced students of the philosopher Pythagoras, who engaged in deep studies of natural science and self-understanding, were called *mathematikoi* – 'those who studied all.' The word *mathema* signified 'learning in general'. If only we could see **numbers** and **shapes** as the ancients did: **symbols of principles** – available to teach us about the natural structure and processes of the universe, and thus to give us perspective on human nature! Instead, 'math education' for children demands rote memorization of procedures to get one 'right answer' and pass 'skill tests' to prove superficial mastery… before moving on to the next isolated topic. Fortunately, when I was 16 one of my teachers mentioned mathematics can be found in nature: a 6-sided snowflake is shaped like a bee's cell… and quartz crystal as well. I was stunned to make the connection. Nature wasn't what it was made out to be... an antagonist to fear, conquer, and exploit... but a garden of wonder and a patient teacher... worthy of great respect. This book is a fanning of little sparks of philosophy from deep antiquity to introduce the general reader to another view of mathematics, nature, and ourselves; this is our heritage, our natural birthright. Plato says all knowledge is already deep within us, so no one can really teach us anything new. But we can remind each other of the archetypal principles of number and nature we already know but may have forgotten. This book is intended as that reminder to guide You through this world of wisdom, beauty, uplift and delight... and to remind You of the gentle, wise principles by which the universe is designed. What is taught in schools is secular mathematics. 'Symbolic' or 'philosophical mathematics' recognizes simple *numbers* and *shapes* relate to each other in harmonious recurring patterns. According to ancient mathematical philosophers, the simple counting numbers from one to ten and the shapes that represent them – circle, line, triangle, and square – express a consistent, comprehensible **language**. The ten numbers are a complete, archetypal sourcebook. They are the original ten patents for designs found all through the universe, from small subatomic particles to the largest galactic clusters, crystals, plants, fruits, vegetables, weather patterns, animal and humans.

"In 1611 Galileo wrote: 'Philosophy is written in this grand book – I mean the universe – that stands continually open to our gaze... but it cannot be understood unless one first learns to comprehend the language... and interpret the characters in which it is written. It is written in the language of mathematics, and its characters are triangles, circles, and geometrical figures, without which it is humanly impossible to understand a single word of it... without these, one is wandering about in a dark labyrinth!' So, why didn't school teach us when we see the same spiral shape in shells, galaxies, and watery whirlpools we are witnessing the principle of balance through motion? Or that the hexagonal cells of beehives package the maximum space using the least materials, energy and time? Nature labels everything with a cosmic calligraphy, but generally we hardly suspect even the existence of the language. To see more deeply into this design alphabet... we must be conversant in Nature's native tongue, the language of symbolic mathematics." –*A Beginner's Guide to Constructing the Universe: The Mathematical Archetypes of Nature, Art and Science*, by Michael S. Schneider. Ch 7: The Language of Number.

Secret of the Spheres

Our Sun – merely One of the stars in the vast Milky Way – radiates Life through Mother Earth, and along with her moon and the planets, they are all spheres; and so are You! **O** the sphere is the source of creation. Two spheres come together to form the vesica pisces – the basic building block of Sacred Geometry, from which comes the Seed of Life. As this bud opens and matures, the Flower of Life unfolds, based on the Golden Mean Rectangle and the phi ratio – found everywhere in nature, such as the pattern of seeds in a sunflower. The phi ratio is also found in the Fibonacci sequence, which begins with the sphere: **O** 1 1 2 3 5 8 13 21 34 55 89 144 &etc. Divide 34 by 55 and there's the phi ratio – 0.618 and the same with 55 divided by 89, and 89 by 144 – to infinity**!**

Everything begins with the sphere. Everything is from sOurce: the zerO – which e e cummings calls "the no of all nothing" which contains everything. Under proper circumstances, the Ovum meets the spherOid-with-a-tail... and bOOm – it's You! Imagine... 23 chromosomes from that single sperm broke through the protective, female shield... and began to jitterbug with the 23 chromosomes from the wom(b)an. What a Rush being a *fertilized egg*... a zygote... You develop into the mOrula – again, all spheres - now actually considering, where shall we implant, and call hOMe? As the embryO develOps, the Only remaining spheres are Your eyes, allowing You to lOOk at the KingdOm *within* as One with All... and All as One. OM is hOMe! Welcome aboard. The Kingdom of Heaven truly is within You. All–ways available here & nOw... which is anytime... anyplace... You happen to becOMe aware of Your Sacred Breath. Home Sweet hOMe!

Secret Santa

Santa is usually associated with Saint Nick, who believed "Christmas is more than a day. Christmas is a Way of Life!" While many Secret Santas come forth during the Thanksgiving and Christmas holidays, there are many who saw the movie *Pay It Forward* and take the message to heart.

Numerous people follow the philosophy of St Nicholas and keep a crisp $20 and $100 in their pocket, perhaps folded twice for convenience; when they see a deserving situation, such as a Mother and child who look like they could use a boost, they simply walk over, hand them one or the other bill saying, "Here's a gift for You to get something special for You and the little one... Blessings on Your Sacred Journey!" Feelings of Joy course through and nurture their Hearts... and Ours... truly realizing we are One. ~.~*

Sleeping Pills
While on rare occasion, a sleeping pill may be tolerable, taken >2 weeks can cause chronic insomnia. When they lose effectiveness, people increase the dosage... leading to addiction. Stopping can lead to nightmares, severe for two nights, then diminished over the next few days; these drugs suppress rapid eye movements (REM) of normal dreaming... and nightmares are the rebound effect.

Alcohol taken as a sedative can cause restless sleep, especially the second half. Instead have a cup of chamomile tea, double-strength if required, at 9:30 and go to bed at 10. Healing-rest happens before midnight. Set this rhythm, and Your internal clock will sort things out. Meanwhile: SomaRest™ may be helpful.

As a homeopathic remedy: Mother Tincture of *Passiflora incarnata*, 10 drops in an ounce of water, 3X/day, to regulate the pineal gland. Melatonin from food: almonds: rich in magnesium, walnuts, also rich in calcium; dark leafy greens – rich in calcium and micronutrients. Oranges contain B-Vitamins and calcium; the white, fibrous tissue found between the segments and on the insides of the skin are rich in bio-flavonoids; banana, pineapple, orange bell pepper, tomato - also support melatonin production.

Smell as a Diagnostic Tool
Once upon a time, doctors used smell for a precise diagnosis. During the 19th century, if a person had the smell of a butcher's shop, yellow fever was suspected. With a rash and a fever – exuding the aroma of freshly baked bread – nurses would confidently diagnose typhoid fever. Characteristically sweetish odors come with diphtheria. The smell of rotten apples indicates gas gangrene. If a wound gave off the smell of grapes, there was infection with *pseudomonas* bacteria. A whiff of ammonia from an old man suggests an enlarged prostate; acetone at any age suggests diabetes.

The medical interest in smells focuses on the unpleasant and pathological; there is also a physiological function. The characteristic smell exuded by newborns make baby more kissable, encouraging bonding with the mother; sebum is produced by the sweat glands, secreted in prodigious quantities in the first few weeks, then tapers off after about 6 months.

Intake = Output. Rather than anxiety hormones produced by violence, stress and fear... with a natural diet, living a natural lifestyle, and more focused on meditation and love, our pheromones exude a sweet fragrance. Each flower has its fragrance, as do humans – which can become rancid, sour or even putrid – with dietary indiscretions... as well as a charged, stressful, emotional atmosphere of judgment and coercion. For a natural sweetness: Be Here Now with 3X3 Sacred Breaths.

Smoking
The brain knows from habit... when we inhale... we bring in smoke – along with an extra dose of oxygen. Ironically, when the brain requires oxygen, the smoker reaches for the nearest pack. Instead, take a few deep breaths and breathe out **forcefully**, through *pursed* lips. This creates backpressure driving oxygen from the lungs into the bloodstream. After 3 deep breaths of this nature, the craving for a cigarette greatly diminishes. Homeopathic remedies are also effective:

Nux vomica: for a wide variety of addictions, especially those with a sedentary lifestyle, and mental exertion.
Tabacum: for those with anemia, asthma, cholera, seasickness, tetanus and esophageal stricture.
Staphysagria: for hypersensitivity to touch, noise and smell; for sleeplessness, or compressive, stupefying headaches.
Ignatia amara: for mood changes and irritability.
Lobelia inflata: for spasmodic coughs, stomach ache and nausea.
Chionanthus virginicus: for pressure headaches and nausea.
Choose one or two; use 30C 3X/day, 15 minutes apart from food or drink; taking more than one remedy – take them 15 minutes apart.

Sneezing
Sneezing is the body's way of eliminating dust or other foreign matter in a sudden and forceful way. We have been taught to cover our mouths when sneezing as a common courtesy, and sometimes we have been taught to suppress the sneeze when possible – dangerous advice, because it builds up tremendous

pressure in the blood vessels and can lead to stroke. Let the sneeze come out, as gracefully as possible.

If You are in a situation where You would like to interfere with Your sneezing mechanism, simply place the tip of Your index finger under Your nose – which we do almost by instinct – and press against Your upper gum. This pressure point greatly relieves one's urge to sneeze.

Coughing may be delayed as well. Take a deep breath and, with lips closed... clear Your throat... appropriate at the theatre and elsewhere. Muffle the sound of a sneeze or a cough into the crook of Your elbow.

Soy

Digesting soy products such as infant formula, ice cream, milk, oil, even TVP, brings challenges. The reason may be found in history. The early Chinese pictograph for soybean emphasizes the root, because soy was first introduced to *fix nitrogen* in the soil. Emperor Sheng-nong (2967-2579 BCE) spoke of the benefits of soy in *The Yellow Emperor's Classic of Internal Medicine*. The discovery of fermentation techniques in the Chou Dynasty (1134-246 BCE) led to the creation of tempeh, miso and tamari. Tofu, or bean curd, was introduced much later around 700 CE.

Tempeh when first introduced, was enzyme-rich and beneficial to intestinal flora. Commercially made tempeh lacks life-enhancing enzymes and friendly bacteria, as most companies are interested in speed and profits rather than natural health benefits.

Miso can have its enzymes intact. You can tell because it says non-pasteurized and *requires* refrigeration. Anything that sits on a shelf has been pasteurized.

Soy sauce is chemically fermented with added refined salt. Tamari is naturally fermented with added sea salt. Purists prefer Nama Shoyu™ organic, unpasteurized soy sauce. For soy or salt sensitivities, use kelp powder – a whole food rich in minerals.

Tofu, tolerated by most on occasion, is of questionable benefit. The reason: phytates in the form of phytic acid interfere with calcium, magnesium, iron and zinc absorption. In addition, non-fermented soy products can contain enzyme inhibitors, rancid fatty acids and denatured protein. Mash soft or silken tofu, sprinkling in 1 capsule probiotic to induce The Lazarus Effect –

resurrecting enzyme activity – then create Your favorite soy dish for later.

Cooked soy oil can be carcinogenic, especially in a weakened system... including soy meats and ice cream. Have these products rarely... if at all.

Soy protein isolates in protein powders and Texturized Vegetable Protein (TVP) are created with high pressure and high temperatures. TVP contains artificial flavorings, and since it is the by-product of soy oil production may contain remnants of hexane used in extraction. Hydrolyzed vegetable protein (HVP) also extracted from soy, has monosodium glutamate (MSG). It is wise to avoid TVP, HVP and MSG, and the *high estrogen in soy* altogether; for special occasions, have either fermented or sprouted soy.

Stevia

Stevia rebaudiana is 30-40 times sweeter than sucrose... well-paid lobbyists have made it illegal to advertise Stevia as a sweetener! Natural physicians recommend it as a healthy substitute for sugar, honey, maple syrup, cane syrup, even Sucanat™ – which is dehydrated sugar cane from the natural juice. **Caution: refined stevia** – clear liquid or white powder – while offering sweetness with 1 drop / 8 oz, has *lost* its healing energetics! Natural physicians said unrefined **Stevia concentrate** supports healing for both pancreas and liver... and so, it has been taken off the market! Grow Your Own... in Your kitchen and Garden of Eatin'! A little leaf goes a long way. Completely safe, it leaves blood sugar levels unaffected. Mother Nature's healing sweetener is unrefined Stevia powder made from the whole-leaf.

Sun Therapy

Whole body air and sun bathing, especially while stretching, is invigorating. At sunrise and sunset, we can nourish our eyes by staring at the sun. Called sun-gazing, it is safe up to 45 min after sunrise, and again beginning 45 min before sunset. At other times, hold Your hand over one eye and look a couple of inches above the sun with the sun as the center of a clock, and You are looking at 12 on the dial. Look for a second, blink; then look at 1 o'clock, blink; then 2 o'clock, blink; and work Your way around the clock. Then switch hands and repeat nurturing the other eye.

To avoid jet lag and re-set the internal clock when crossing time zones – sun-gazing toward evening with bare feet on the ground works wonders!

Supernatural Breathing with the Human Halo: Variations on a Theme by Dr Joe Dispenza

Classical composers of music have often found their creative juices flowing while listening to works of other composers. Dr Joe Dispenza explains Supernatural Breathing: how to stimulate movement of the sacrum, the Sacred Bone, to accentuate the flow of cerebrospinal fluid {CSF} and to experience the Light of Love within.

Inspirations came from my own background as a chiropractor specializing in Harmonics, a branch of Sacral-Occipital-Technique {S.O.T.} specializing in CSF flow, including the recommended humming exercises to increase cranial neurovascular energetics – stimulating blood flow throughout the brain, including the Circle of Willis where 70% of strokes occur. Stimulating the cranial nerves awakens the hypothalamus – the Motherboard of the brain – allowing access to Your subconscious, enabling You to Reprogram Your Inner Child and Rehabilitate Your Life… Creating Your Wish Fulfilled!

Dr Joe's approach is to dig Your index finger into the crown of Your head to bring attention to this sacred energy point. Then remove Your finger while keeping Your *focus* there; as You breathe in, contract the genital-anal muscles of the pelvic floor, reminiscent of Kegel exercises; when the inhale is complete, hold Your breath for a few seconds while contracting the lower abdominal muscles, then contract the upper abdominal muscles; exhale. After several repetitions of this breathing technique, You enhance the flow of CSF… and enhance Your experience of the Kingdom of Heaven within.

Relaxing as I exhaled – and continuing to caress the roof of my mouth, which completes the microcosmic circuit between the Central and Governing Vessels – I let out a soft humming sound, similar to the ending of an OM chant. It was exhilarating… experiencing Universal Consciousness… losing track of time.

Further inspiration came recalling the teachings of Drunvalo Melchizedek. While the top of the head is, indeed, a primary energy point leading to the crown energy center and the pituitary gland, producing vital hormones… it is the entrance point for a tube of light energy that travels through to the perineum – another sacred energy point associated with the gonads, also producing vital hormones. Furthermore, there are four other tubes of light energy that comprise what may be called a halo. One tube of light travels horizontally through the area at the temples; another tube of light travels horizontally through the Third Eye area, an inch above and between the eyebrows, out the back of the skull; another tube of light travels from the hairline diagonally through the skull exiting at the area of the brain-stem; the fourth also travels diagonally through the skull exiting through the chin. These tubes of light energy vary in size. You can visualize Yours by joining Your thumb to the tip of Your middle finger.

These tubes of light energy extend a hand's length from the skull – measuring from the base of the palm to the tip of the middle finger – as well as from the perineum. This measurement is known as Your primary aura, and extends from Your entire body – torso, arms and legs. Your secondary aura measures from 4-12' depending on spiritual development. Your tertiary aura, verified by Drunvalo at NASA, extends 55' from Your heart energy center. We *all* have a Human Halo… indeed, we are *all* the Word made flesh. Jesus said "You shall do greater things than I." The Essene master also said: "I and the Father are One, and You are One with Me as I am One with You!"

One of the most gifted and inspired Renaissance artists was Fra Angelico: The Adoration of the Magi, Detail of the Christ Child and The Transfiguration, among many others, clearly show details of the Human Halo – at least from a two-dimensional view – the one going from the top down, the other going horizontally. Many artists, even other cultures, have depicted the halo in their works. Truly we *are* photon energy in the flesh! And so… doing Supernatural Breathing, I brought the fingertips and thumb of each hand together, as when doing EFT tapping, and placed them at the horizontal tube of light, at the temples… and finally, bringing both hands together at the crown of the head. Feeling the flow of inner energies may lead to visions or insights. Explore where the quest may lead.

Exploring… You may like to follow advice of renowned yogi, BKS Iyengar, author of *Light on Yoga*. Claiming most westerners simply were missing something from their DNA to allow them to do strenuous asanas, including the full or half lotus for long meditations, he suggested *savasana* – traditionally called the *Corpse* Pose. With the body ready to receive the next insight into Reality, *savasana* truly is the *Receptive* Pose of Yoga – entangling, energizing, and uniting HeartMindBodySpirit as One.

On a somewhat firm mat – arms and legs slightly apart – tighten every muscle: raising head, arms and legs as long as possible, then relax; become aware of Sacred Breath. Deeper breathing – technically called diaphragmatic breathing – involves the diaphragm, the muscle sheet separating thorax from abdomen. Allowing lungs to totally fill and empty offers a rhythmic massage for the small and large intestines – creating an experience of the Buddha-belly by slowly filling completely, and then slowly emptying completely. Breathe... Be Aware. See where this may lead enhancing Your meditation experience.

Serious Students Seeking Inner ExplOrations
Meditation for some advanced practitioners is a blissful exercise in Nirvana; sometimes twice a day... in a heartbeat, they are able to focus within and experience Pure Bliss. Others are beginners who may be helped by the advice found on the previous pages. The following is offered for those exploring Ancient Wisdom. While breath is paramount, the meditation experience may be enhanced by the position of one's hands... among other things, such as visualizations. These suggestions are offered for the serious student to explore inner energetics. While inner explorations may take place in *savasana*... traditionally be seated, whether in the lotus or half-lotus, on a cushion, or on the edge of a chair with feet flat on the floor, or even with Your back somewhat supported by the chair; whichever way, *always* have the *spine erect* allowing free flow of Energy. First, settle down; take 3, 6, or 9 slow, deep breaths alerting Monkey-mind and Monkey-heart the Intention is to explore within.

Ancient yogic traditions suggest touching tip of the tongue to the palate, completing the *microcosmic circuit* and enhancing the free flow of *energy*, in acupuncture referred to as chi. The microcosmic circuit aka the Master Meridians are in charge of the other five *paired* meridians: liver / gall bladder, heart / small intestine, spleen / stomach, lungs / large intestine, kidneys / bladder. The Master Meridians are called the Central or Conception Vessel {CV} which begins at the perineum and flows up through the soft tissues at the front of the body, ending at the tip of the tongue... and

the Governing Vessel {GV} which begins at the perineum and flows up the hard, bony tissues at the back of the body through the vertebrae, up the back, over the top of the skull, ending at the maxilla under the nose: maxilla bones fuse, forming the hard palate.

Caressing the hard palate stimulates branches of the palatine nerve which connect to the Pineal center. Furthermore, the tissue at the root of the tongue is embryologically connected to the mesoderm tissue that forms the pericardial sac, which holds the heart. Connecting the *microcosmic circuit* unites Heart / Pineal energy centers, with the HeartMindBodySpirit as One. The *microcosmic circuit* complete, we direct the flow of energy through this *microcosmic orbit*:

Exploring inner energetics {chi} – a microcosm of the macrocosm – take 36 disciplined breaths: 9 breaths at each of the **4** hand positions – 18 minutes.

The **1st** of Your four hand positions is at the lower hara or power center, located just below the navel. Place Your left hand on top of the right, palms up, with thumbs touching; bring the insides of Your hands – from baby fingers to the wrists – to make skin contact at Your hara. Ancient Wisdom says the left hand on top allows You to *empty* anything less than Your highest choice... making room energetically after the first 9 breaths, for the **2nd** hand position – when You place Your right hand on top, thumbs together, for 9 breaths. As You *receive* and *restore* pristine energies. Rather than count breaths from 1-9, many find it easier to keep track by counting from 1-3 and repeat 1-3 again, and again. You will begin to feel Your breath... Your Heart... Your energy... as One.

As You slowly breathe in, slightly *pressing* the tip of the tongue against the bump at the middle of the hard palate, *contract* the muscles of the pelvic floor with eyes closed yet directed toward the 3rd Eye; visualize energy rising from the perineum, going up the spine through the Governing Vessel to the crown of Your head; take 9 seconds or so for the slow inhale, and when lungs are comfortably full, hold for about 6 seconds – gently pressing and contracting. Enjoy the feeling of fullness.

As You slowly breathe out, rather than press with the tongue, gently *caress* the bump with the tip of the tongue, *relax* the muscles of the pelvic floor with eyes closed yet directed downward toward Your nose;

visualize energy descending from the crown, down the front through the Central Vessel returning to Your perineum; take 9 seconds to slowly exhale, and with lungs comfortably empty, hold for about 6 seconds – totally relaxed. Enjoy the feeling of emptiness.

The **3rd** hand position is with Your fingertips and tips of Your thumbs touching – fingers and thumbs spread apart from each other. With wrists touching the skin at Your hara, follow directions for the 9 breaths.

The **4th** hand position allows Your fingers to relax and interlace with thumbs crossing, wrists touching the skin at Your hara. This traditional pose has fingers of both hands crossing the midline, allowing access to the subconscious. With wrists touching the skin at Your hara, follow directions for the final 9 breaths.

According to ancient Taoist wisdom – teaching alchemy and immortality – these techniques subdue Monkey-mind, soothe Monkey-heart, and tie up the running horse of intellect, all of which serves to curtail past and future desires and anxieties. As the heart gets used to this condition, it will be free from all illusions culminating in the resurrection of the Spirit. In this state of serenity, Spirit vibrates within as You gather the microcosmic alchemical substance and swallow the nectar of immortality.

Having completed the flow of energy throughout the *microcosmic orbit*… Be Still… And Know… I Am God! After these 36 breaths, roll Your closed eyes left to right clockwise 9X. Between Your eyebrows, You may witness white light – the Seed of Vitality perhaps with golden or reddish-yellow light in the middle – the Seed of Immortality similar to the male and female organs of a flower, the union of which bears fruit. Prepare for Harvest as You begin exploring… breathing… or being still… as directed by Your Inner Voice Intuition… comfortable with All That Is on Your Sacred Journey.

Whatever form of meditation You enjoy, to exercise and refresh Your lungs, always begin with 9 deep breaths exhaling completely. There is a subtle connection between the rhythm of our breath and the rhythm of the flow of cerebrospinal fluid {CSF} which Taoist Wisdom calls the **microcosmic inner alchemical agent** transmuting Vitality into Spirit. Taoist Alchemy retains the generative force in the body for purification and transmutation into positive vitality

restoring primordial Spirit, and the primal Immortal State. https://www.summum.us/

Super Sprouts… Quantum Sprouts!
If humankind only knew the power of 3s… 6s… and 9s it would be a completely different Universe.
-Nikola Tesla

Having read this quote 3, 6, or 9X… perhaps 9_{99}X… Inner Guidance… Inspiration… Inner Voice Intuition… began prompting Awareness – when stirring a pot – among other mundane chores… clockwise… 3, 6, or 9X… or making motions of a figure eight on its side ∞ the Infinity symbol… consciously tapping into Infinite Source: *being aware* of Being Aware… knOwing All–Ways: OM… as *vibration* truly is Home Sweet hOMe!

Exploring the Quantum arena to understand *how* to grow quantum sprouts requires clarity. Our daily **MEDS** support our Journey. **M** = Meditation, the Foundation; focus on Sacred Breath; experience the Force Field… and the quanta supporting that Vibration.

Sacred Breath is abundant with Blessings… even as we prepare sprouts. Tasty, easy, long-lasting sprouts are found with Roland Foods – Green Lentils. {Roland historically supports conscious agriculture practices.} Being Aware of *being aware*: finally… after decades of growing sprouts… Inner Voice Intuition gave a nudge: when soaking seeds, add Himalayan pink salt to the soak water mimicking minerals found in Nature.
Triple-wash the seeds *focusing* on Sacred Breath… in a large bowl filled with water, lovingly lift them with both hands 3X. **1st** wash has non-viable floaters dumped with the somewhat cloudy bathwater; **2nd** wash, loving and lifting 3X – less floaters, less cloudy; **3rd** wash few floaters and clear water. Then fill with water adding 1Tbs unbleached sea salt; let them sit for **6** hrs.

Pour through a large colander slightly tilted for drainage; cover with a plate to maintain moisture and warmth in the ecosystem. In the morning, babies go for a rinse; then back in the covered colander, tilted. Repeat this morning ritual until vibrant tails appear; then after the final rinse, refrigerate in the colander allowing air to flow in the sides, cover with a saturated cotton washcloth to maintain moisture; depending on humidity: 2-3 days. Grown with Love-felt Sacred Breath… every step of the way… they last for a week.

Awareness of Sacred Breath brings Peace to every activity: preparing food, dining, cleaning up…

preparing for a commute... going for a brisk walk in the park or along the beach... settling down with a book... getting to the nitty-gritty out in Your Garden of Eatin'... begin with 3 Sacred Breaths 3X... to set the tone. Bringing 5D Awareness to the 3D world blesses Your Sacred Journey and those with You on the Path – transforming Your Life and Theirs!

Consciousness... **IS**... All That Is.
Pure Consciousness... Pure Vibration...
feminine **V**ision and **I**magination...
masculine **B**e-ing and **A**ction
expl**O**ring as **Y**ou... and as **M**e!
Kn**O**wing we a**R**e **O**ne Vibration...
creates Inner Peace and Harmony
within and around You...
nourished by Sacred Breath: **3X3**.

Sweet Poison

Sugar paralyzes the immune response system, the artificial colors and flavors *with* the sugars contribute to hyperactivity and sickness, as well as behavioral and learning challenges. Sodas are notoriously loaded, and most contain caffeine. If something is sugar free, *how* is it sweetened? Aspartame or NutraSweet aka Equal has 3 molecules: phenylalanine... aspartic acid (both amino acids) and methyl alcohol (methanol), a *human specific, highly toxic poison.* Methyl alcohol is converted into formaldehyde and formic acid; both are highly carcinogenic having a toxic effect on the immune response system – specifically affecting the thymus gland – as well as affecting the brain and central nervous system, the heart and lungs. Children and pregnant women are vulnerable to the cumulative effects. Methyl alcohol, toxic to the fetus, can cause malformation, even death.

After entering the body, the components of Aspartame are rapidly released into the bloodstream. Methanol, a deadly metabolic poison, is apparently the first to be separated. Rarely found in its free form, methyl alcohol is usually derived or produced from other substances. It can cause serious tissue damage, blindness, even death. *Since the body lacks the necessary enzymes to detoxify it, methanol is toxic. Its rate of elimination is five times slower than a similar amount of ethyl alcohol – in beer, wine and distilled spirits.* For Aspartame to be eliminated, the body converts it to **formaldehyde**, then to formic acid, and ultimately to carbon dioxide.

Dr Richard Wurtman, professor of neuroendocrinology at MIT, says that phenylalanine is known to be toxic to the brain in large doses. This amino acid can cause mental retardation and seizures with phenylketonuria (PKU) a genetic disorder. Their numbers are relatively small (1 in 15,000); they must avoid phenylalanine.

An estimated 2% of the US population has one of the two genes required for PKU. While free from the disease, they may have *sensitivities*. They have yet to discover a test for this one-gene condition. Someone who drinks 4-5 Aspartame-sweetened drinks a day might introduce enough phenylalanine into the brain to affect the synthesis of neurotransmitters, possibly leading to moodiness, irritability, anxiety, depression, insomnia, headaches, high blood pressure, increased appetite, even seizures. The concentration of phenylalanine and aspartic acid – the two amino acids in aspartame – is ten times higher than found in foods. Searching aspartame dangers, or aspartame alert; You will find: "Aspartame (L-Aspartyl / L-phenylalanine Methyl Ester) is an artificial sweetener, 200X sweeter than sugar "accidentally" discovered by the **Searle Drug Company** in 1965.

The story of duplicity by which Searle Co. managed to gain approval to market Aspartame is reprehensible... and also a matter of Public Record. The FDA, defending itself, states that no food additive went through a longer period of examination; indeed, that is true. Fact is: Boards of Inquiry, investigative panels and renowned scientists, over a lengthy 6-year period, *unanimously* recommended *against* approval. A newly appointed Director of the FDA overruled them! He later resigned under charges of bribery.

In examining the tests submitted by Searle, the investigators found systematic attempts to deceive the FDA. Negative results were deliberately withheld, many tests were so badly botched that no conclusions could be ascertained, untagged test animals in unmarked cages were mixed up with control groups, tumors were cut out and not examined for malignancy, and lab rats were substituted from unrelated tests. At one point, there was an official demand that Searle be indicted by a Federal Grand Jury for fraud; in the end, however, Searle did not even have to submit new tests to prove the safety of Aspartame as required by law. As the law now stands, only the company requesting approval for a food additive need supply test results to the FDA, **who do no testing to verify**, unlike the more stringent regulations for a drug. Under that same law, Searle (now the NutraSweet Co.) is not required to monitor or report any adverse symptoms that result from the use of its product.

Aspartame, known commercially as NutraSweet or Equal, sweetens several thousand different products and is used by >100 million people in the US. It is consumed most commonly in so-called diet sodas. The FDA and NutraSweet Co. quickly reassure us: we ingest methanol in fruit juices and some vegetables; neglecting to point out in these natural products, methanol is bound by pectin that our body enzymes cannot break down – in addition to being accompanied by ethanol in far greater amounts, which effectively buffers methanol's ability to cause damage.

Big Buck$ are being made from Aspartame sweetened drinks; simply put... sugar and sweets are addictive and Aspartame creates an increased thirst. The NutraSweet hangover consists of malaise, nausea, headache, dizziness; sometimes visual disturbances, even convulsions, and possible severe mood swings. These also can occur because of the methyl alcohol in cigarette smoke and alcohol. Methyl alcohol intoxication is suspected in mental aberrations, seizures, suicidal tendencies, behavioral disorders, urinary tract infections, skin lesions and de-myelinating diseases such as MS and ALS.

Experiment: cleanse Your system from all these hangover symptoms, drink plenty of re-mineralized and re-energized distilled or r/o water, avoid this sweet poison for 30 days and see how You feel. As the body cleanses, the first few days may show an increase in symptoms; this is normal, and tapers off... You will feel great relief. After 30 days, if there is any doubt about the effects... ingest some and see the results. Be glad You know the difference... and know... that You are in control of what You take in... and how You feel! Be Consciously Aware.

Tanning/sun beds
Experience is showing the use of ultra-violet sun beds may activate and accelerate the growth of HIV as well as other infections. UV-A radiation can cause increased skin wrinkling, irregular pigmentation, altered skin texture aka photo-aging, skin fragility and deeply pigmented freckles. This artificial tan gives little protection from natural burning. Some say sun beds are like a microwave, cooking You from the inside out.

Thymus Thump
Did Tarzan's innate wisdom lead him to pound his chest? As part of our endocrine energy system, interestingly enough, the thymus gland lies behind the sternum, and pounding or even tapping the sternum actually activates production of T-cells! Many people have heard of and gratefully utilize the thymus thump. There are more benefits to consider when You make the optimal energetic connection with Your tongue.

Tip of the Tongue at the Roof of the Mouth
This practice is taught in all the Martial Arts, many forms of meditation and yoga, and by many natural healers. First hearing about the practice while learning Raja yoga meditation in the early '70s, the effect was obvious. Then in the late '70s when the first AIDS / HIV headlines appeared – while studying the Immune response system at Palmer College! – the professor mentioned this simple technique called the **Thymus Thump**: tapping the sternum stimulates the thymus gland to produce T-cells and enhances the immune response system. The practice of keeping the tip of the tongue at the roof of the mouth is also widely known to maintain focus, keeping One calm and centered. It is easy to explain with corroborating evidence.

Acupuncture dates back millennia. 6 paired meridians energize our organ systems. One pair – known as the Master Meridians – are in charge of all the rest. They are the Conception or Central Vessel {CV} and the Governing Vessel {GV}. The fact they are called vessels gives a clue. While a meridian is a line of energy; a vessel is a container. The Master Meridians "contain" the secret of energy and vitality, known as chi. Both meridians begin at the perineum, between the anus and the genitals. The Central Vessel travels up the front – through the soft tissues of the body – ending at the tip of the tongue. The Governing Vessel travels up the back – through the hard, bony tissues of the vertebrae, over the bones of the cranium – ending at the maxilla forming the roof of the mouth.

With the tip of the tongue at the roof of the mouth, completing the "microcosmic circuit" between CV and GV Chi or Energy flows. Doing so while tapping the sternum *directs* this flowing energy to the thymus gland, stimulating its function – producing T-cells – enhancing the immune response. Tapping under the jaw sends vibrations to the tonsils and they produce T-cells as well. Completing this circuit allowing free flow of energy, tap over the right lower rib cage to stimulates the liver... tap the cranium to stimulate the brain... and so forth. Keeping the tip of the tongue at the roof of the mouth is a Blessing, with the potential of keeping One focused on the Sacred Breath... in the Here & Now. When asked about *dentures*, my response in the past has been: Intention is of primary importance, so hold Your intention, and let go of worry. Now I **know**... and answer differently. Technology can be useful in ways You least expect.

In the Oasis Spa at Hippocrates Health Institute in West Palm Beach, there is a machine called the H-wave. Contracting muscles and reducing pain, relieving lymphatic and circulatory congestion, the H-wave continues to save many amputations. I gave a talk at the Institute about Vibrational Energy Medicine mentioning the tip of the tongue at the roof of the mouth. A few days later one of the guests said, "It really works!" Thinking she observed calming effects as many do... I inquired.

She was on the H-wave and her mind was wandering. She remembered... and thought: "This would be a perfect time to have my tongue there; I'll be attached to this machine for ½ hour." As soon as she put the tip of her tongue to the roof of her mouth, the contractions were noticeably more vigorous. Skeptical that such a simple thing could have such a profound effect – thinking her muscles were now warmed up, and able to move easier – she took her tongue away. She was shocked when the contractions reduced intensity. So, she kept her tongue where it belongs for the rest of the therapy, and now keeps that habit throughout the day.

She was at the Institute with her daughter and her mother. Mentioning this experience to her daughter, she performed her own experiment and confirmed the results. When Mother's turn came, she noticed no difference. Then, realizing Mother was wearing dentures, the daughter asked her to remove them. Sure enough, she could clearly see the difference. If anyone asks about dentures, the answer is simple: always remove synthetic dentures when doing therapeutic work or meditation, allowing the free flow of energy through the "microcosmic circuit" or, with a permanent bridge, touch any part of the palate. Unless eating, drinking or talking – when it's impossible – keep the tip of the tongue at the roof of the mouth for focused attention... Be Here Now... with this Sacred Breath!

The tip of the tongue at the hard palate establishes the connection between the Central & Governing Vessels, allowing free flow of energy through the meridians and... profoundly establishes a connection with the heart itself. Tissues at the base of the tongue and the tissues of the pericardial sac have an embryological connection. Meditating in this manner, You can enter the Sacred Space of Your Heart... and the Tiny Space of Your Heart. {See below: **Tongue Awareness**}

Tithing
Regularly Gifting 10%, 5% or 1% of earnings for spiritual purposes is an ancient practice. *Pay It Forward* is a modern option for Gifting to others. Remember to tithe a part of the day... 10% of 24 hours is 2½ hours; discounting the time we sleep, 10% is 1½ hours. Make time every day and Gift Your Self! R&R restores and replenishes Your spiritual energies.

Rather than being caught up in the busy-ness of the day, take care of Your Self – especially if it means putting it in Your schedule: Get Outdoors! Meditate... Be One with the sounds of Nature... whether the ocean surf, waves at the lake, splashing waters of a river or creek, a breeze blowing through the cottonwoods, or simply songbirds in the park... Breathe. Be One with Self. Know Thyself! Remember: tithe... take time for... Oneself. Your business acumen and Your efficiency will heighten, easing all the other factors of Your Life.

A tithe, meaning a tenth, is a Gift of Your income for spiritual purposes, typically to a religious or charitable institution. Certain Jewish and Christian groups practice tithing, as does Sikhism; other spiritual groups such as Buddhism or Confucianism promote charitable caring for others as one of their basic tenets. Tithing is called by many names, such as Dasvandh among Sikhs; the principle is that if You give to the Infinite... Infinity, in turn, gives back to You. It is a spiritual practice through which You build Trust in the ability of the Infinite to respond to the flow of love and energy that You give. This energy then expands tenfold and flows back to You in abundance. Sikhs began bringing offerings during the time of the first Sikh Guru, Guru Nanak (1469-1539) founder of the Sikh Path, who promoted the concept and virtue of Dasvandh.

The Buddhist suttas are full of stories of businesspeople, courtesans, even paupers... who made a practice of giving 10% of what they receive from their efforts and received a hundredfold in return;

in this manner, they attained stages of Awakening in their lifetimes – while also... even some beggars... became very wealthy in the process!

Many will tithe directly to a needy family... or small group outside the IRS, yet with larger contributions many wish it could be tax-deductible, rather than pay taxes... which contribute to our present-day War Economy. Some find in convenient to tithe to a *reputable* tax-deductible organization, if You can find one – they are rare! Previously thinking the reputation of the Salvation Army was sacrosanct: "every penny will help addicts recover" – current research sadly proves what others have long suspected. The Reality is W.T. Stead, co-founder of the Salvation Army, supported British Imperialism promoted by the Pilgrims Society, is involved in human trafficking! W.T. Stead is the "Father of Tabloid Journalism" where fact and opinion are intertwined into a confusing muddle.

Research! Rather than using Google which is part of the Mockingbird Matrix Media... use another search engine, such as https://duckduckgo.com/ or... simply muscle test or Sway Test to discern Truth. Explore: https://aim4truth.org/ Here is an option for tithing.

As a physician and minister of the Essene tradition, Holistic Lifestyle Medicine and Mother Nature's Ways are taught by the Church of Compassionate Service and the Order of Compassionate Service; we offer tax-deductible donations through Compassionate Service Charities, Inc – a 501(c)3 which can be dedicated to: Holistic Essene Ministries. See: **Appendix B**.

Tolerance
"While I may disagree with what You have to say... I shall defend to the death, Your right to say it." (Voltaire 1763, *Essay on Tolerance*, one of the basic principles of Freedom and Independence. To refresh our memory it would be a Blessing for Americans and every person of every Culture, to read the Constitution of the United States and the Bill of Rights to understand why the Founding Families *had to revolt* against British Imperialist Control. As for current events in the 2020s... Plato's *Republic*, written as a collection of conversations between friends with Plato's teacher, Socrates, gives insights into human behavior amazingly similar to our times... hence, controversial. https://counter-currents.com/2017/03/plato-hitler-totalitarianism/

With a closed mind – whether a totalitarian political situation or an authoritarian, dogmatic religious one – there is constant judgment, which is quite comforting to those with low self-esteem who continually reassure themselves they are "right" and anyone who disagrees is foolish or crazy. Unfortunately, this mind-set stifles Spirit, nurturing decay and leading to death.

When we allow free expression of thought, belief, opinion and speculation... when we weigh and consider the words of others, even those with whom we think we disagree, we may end up with a real appreciation of who we are, and what we are about: enriching self-esteem and Self Knowledge. We may end up refining and polishing our concepts, growing and developing, evolving our Own conscious awareness and Empowerment experiences! The Master said: "If You love those who love You, what right have You to claim any credit? But I say this to You: love Your enemies, love those who hate You, bless those who persecute You. In this way You become perfect."

Seeking to follow the Master... seeking to "become perfect" Emperor Frederick II of the Holy Roman Empire had a revelation – how tolerance and appreciation benefits everyOne. His experience has profound implications for the Middle East today. This bit of his-story was discovered researching Bio-Dynamic Gardening! "There is nothing new about the original work of an innovative and non-reductionist scientist being overlooked, whether German, English, American, Hebrew, or Arab. In fact, most innovative Arab researchers of the past have been overlooked and completely discarded by the West.

"The only thing the **Crusaders** ever accomplished – other than killing a lot of innocent people – was to **bring Arab science to the West**. In the 12th century, the crusader Frederick II invented bird banding to investigate bird migration. He was also the first to use nicotine sulfate on the wings of his hunting falcons to kill bird lice. I have never seen credit given to him for either of these modern scientific endeavors. The Arab people understood bird migration and poisons of all sorts long before western Europeans ever thought about such fields of study. Frederick II learned much from his contacts with Middle Eastern Arabs. He went east to fight – and discovering killing in the name of God is a dastardly occupation – he stayed to study. He became a friend of the sultan he was supposed to kill...

sometimes things really do turn out right in Life! The white flowing robes and gray beards of Arab and Hebrew philosophers from Jerusalem, Baghdad and Syria were a common sight at Frederick's court at Apulia in southern Italy.

"His love of farming is attested to by the fact that he grew oats, millet, hemp, cotton, corn, wheat, grapes and olives. His advisors were the Cistercian monks – the scientific farmers of those days. {Cistercians were reformed Benedictines, who founded an abbey in Cistercium [Citeaux] France in 1098.} These monks developed new breeds of animals and plants using crossing methods later perfected by the monk Mendel – now called the science of genetics. Cistercians experimented with soil types as did the father of the study of soil erosion, Ewald Wollny." *Paramagnetism: Rediscovering Nature's Secret Force of Growth*, Philip S. Callahan, PhD.

Additional advancements in science, mathematics and language were brought to the West from the Arab world, exemplified by Sacred Geometry. *Thinking* and *art* of the East is based on the 6-*petal*ed Flower of Life... rounded lines and female, right brain energy. *Thinking* and *art* of the West is based on the 6-*point*ed Star Tetrahedron... straight lines and male, left brain energy. Interestingly enough, both of these art forms center on the Golden Mean Rectangle, based on the phi ratio 0.618 which is the Heart of Sacred Geometry. Perhaps peace in the Middle East is as simple as finding diplomats who have developed their talents exercising their brain, their corpus callosum – integrating Thinking... Feeling... and... Acting.

It is Truly Astonishing to realize Jews... Christians... and Arabs... all look to Abraham as their spiritual father. The story is told in *Genesis*. Yahweh promised Abraham he would actually be what his name meant (Father of a multitude); yet, in their advanced old age, he and his wife Sara (Princess Mother of Kings) never had a child. Sara suggested Abraham take her Egyptian maidservant, Hagar (Forsaken), as his wife and through her have progeny. {According to Mesopotamian Law a barren wife could present one of her female slaves to her husband and consider the child as her own.} Abraham was 86 when Hagar bore Ishmael (Yahweh has heard). Then 13 years later when Abraham was 99 and Sara was 90, Sara gave birth to Isaac (Laughter – which was Sara's reaction when told she would bear a child at her advanced age).

Ishmael had 12 sons becoming chiefs of 12 Arab tribes, among many other tribes. Isaac gave birth to Jacob (May Yahweh protect) who had 12 sons who became chiefs of the 12 tribes of Israel (He who struggles with God – Jacob wrestled with an angel, and had his name changed to Israel). They seem to be struggling to this day**!**

Our current problem has roots in Sara's pride. After she gave birth to Isaac, she banished Hagar and Ishmael trying to pretend they never existed. She was in denial; she wished Hagar and Ishmael were back in Egypt – maybe on a boat, floating down d'Nile! Despite her denial, it is a clear fact that **Arabs are the first children of Abraham.** Perhaps Jews... still feeling Sara's pride... resent that**?!?** The answer is... recognizing that we are all "kissin' kin"! When we learn to lay aside our petty differences, we honor our father Abraham, and Peace on Earth prevails. Actually, Abraham was neither Jew nor Arab, rather a resident of Ur in Sumeria, son of the High Priest Terah. We are all on a Journey... searching for Truth... and 95% of the things we thought were Truth, turn out False. Meanwhile we are killing for our beliefs... for what we *think* is the truth. We kill "infidels" ignoring the basic commandment: Thou shalt not kill.

Non-resistance is the Key. *Ahimsa* literally means Free from Force. When we resist, we give recognition, strength and determination to the "enemy." Loving our "enemies" we overpower any negative aspect; surrender allows inner truth to prevail... and Love conquers all. Love recognizes everyOne as Pure Awareness exploring human consciousness. Each of us with Our Sunny-side as well as Our Shadow-side have Free Will to choose explorations: with both ends of the continuum from Brilliant Light to Dazzling Darkness... and everyone and everything in between.

Few of us kill people for violating our beliefs. Yet, how many of us support the Matrix with tax dollars and votes? How many support politicians who, in the name of business and financial remuneration, incarcerate people – thereby killing their spirit and the spirits of their Loved Ones for consensual "crimes" causing no harm to anyone's person or property**?** Our Founding Families would be horrified to say the least. Our distorted reaction to these so-called crimes – such as cannabis, now world-wide recognized for its healing powers – overtaxes our police, courts, jails, and communal psyche fostering the growth of organized crime. Explore the Bible, the Constitution and the Bill of Rights. See what they really say: all captured eloquently in *Ain't Nobody's Business If You Do: The Absurdity of Consensual Crimes in a Free Society*, by Peter McWilliams. The World would Benefit from a **born-again NAACP: The National Association for the Advancement of Conscious People.**

Tongue Awareness

We've all had the experience... eating, slowly chewing and swallowing until it's gone... then, with our napkin, we discreetly remove a small piece of onion skin that accidentally was in the salad. We can thank the massive nerve and vascular network of the tongue to sort things properly. Add the ability to make sounds and the tongue gets A for intelligence and performance. Metaphysically, the tongue gets A+!

Through Martial Arts, Meditation, and Yoga, most people have heard about touching the tip of the tongue to the roof of the mouth – completing the microcosmic circuit between the Central and Governing Vessels. In a 70s meditation group, someone accidentally made a discovery. What we call the roof of the mouth is really the ceiling! Stretching, the tongue can actually reach behind the uvula, enter the nasal cavity, and rest *on* the real roof of the mouth. You can feel the cartilage at the nasal septum. Rising... the tongue is free... in the Akasha!

This is called the Khechari mudra... meaning, the posture for creative energy. It can be maintained after leaving the meditation *place* to maintain the meditation *space*: while preparing food, walking down the street, driving, &etc. Developing this practice – or simply caressing the bump at the roof of Your mouth – is a reminder to Be Here Now... with the Sacred Breath... *in* the meditation *space*.

Ancient Wisdom teaches there is a bump {a tiny % have a small hole} at the hard palate which can be found with the tip of the tongue; first reach back to the soft palate; then bring it forward and just after contact with the hard palate... the bump is in the middle. Slowly caressing with the tongue over and around the bump, it expands and becomes firm much like the nipple of Your Beloved; with the nerves stimulated, blood flows. This hyper-sensitive area has been studied. Drunvalo Melchizedek amazed NASA hooked up to their EEG. By massaging each quadrant of that area with the tip of his tongue, he could light up different areas of the brain. They initially thought it was a fluke... experimenting further, they could only conclude there is a definite connection.

There is more. The tip of the tongue at the hard palate establishes the connection between the Central and Governing Vessels – encouraging free flow of chi energy along the meridians – and establishes a connection with the Heart itself. There is an embryological connection between the tissue at the root of the tongue and the tissue forming the pericardial sac that holds the Heart. Meditating, simply caressing and being aware of Your Sacred Breath, allows entry into Your Heart of Hearts. You can gently move Your tongue, caressing the bump – swallowing nectar as required – and experience the Kingdom of Heaven within... making Love to YourSelf... connecting with High Self... Experiencing Oneness.

Skeptics reading this may say hyperbole... metaphor. Experience is the only test of this Truth. Simply visit Your favorite Sacred Spot in Nature – spend some time barefoot, breathing slowly and caressing: Love Yourself. 3X3 Sacred Breaths. You will experience Peace defying description. Be Patient. You can enter the Sacred Space of Your Heart, as well as the Tiny Space of Your Heart. After a while, many experience a buildup and release of Energy... compared to the pleasurable waves that follow orgasm. Breathe. Enjoy.

TV: From Global Village to Global Brainwash

TV screen-time for the average child 2-5 years of age: 3½ hours/day; the average adult watches 5 hours. This adds up to >21,000 commercials a year. Other than work and sleep, the screen – especially with computers and phones – is the main attraction in life; for most in our society, it is part of our Standard American Diet (SAD)! Activities, conversations, dress, mannerisms, even meals revolve around what is seen on the screen or other devices and gadgets. The global brainwash is complete with >50% of TV outside the US being American re-runs – spreading worldwide monoculture.

100 corporations (out of 450,000 corporations in the US) sponsor 75% of commercial network TV. This means they have effective censorship of what people watch, hear, think and do. These corporations manufacture drugs, chemicals, cosmetics, packaged and processed foods, cars and oil. Take a simple example with aspirin; there seems to be freedom of choice with Advil, Anacin, Bayer, Bufferin, Excedrin, St.

Joseph's... baby aspirin. Yet, whether You buy this or that... satisfaction seems to come from consuming the commodities these corporations have to offer.

In a truly free society, we would be warned: chronic aspirin use depletes folic acid as well as iron, potassium, sodium and Vitamin C... and told the sources of headaches are usually found in diet or dehydration, or stress... and given suggestions about changes in diet or Lifestyle to prevent headaches... or told about white willow bark or meadowsweet tea, from which aspirin was isolated. Alas, we live in a controlled society... far from Free!

TV = Tell-lies-with-Vision... programs are exactly that – *programming* – from basic values to food choices... most of which are far less than optimal for us, as well as for Mother Earth. Commercials and promos simply add insult to injury. Screen-time is hypnotic and addictive. Scientists who study brain-wave activity report with an increase in time, the brain slips into alpha, the brain's receptive mode. Who needs subliminal advertising? Australian National University calls it "sleep teaching" - mnemonic learning - free from conscious participation. One of the contributing factors is lack of eye movement; people blankly stare at the screen; eye movement equals mental and/or thought stimulation. Complicating matters, light on the screen flickers on and off many times per second!

Screen-time accelerates the nervous system. The ANU researchers also tell us it leads to hyperactivity among children. Many children are told, "Settle down; go watch some TV." All the violence, especially in cartoons where we are encouraged to laugh at violence (sic!) increases our fight or flight hormones, and the stored-up energy eventually bursts forth. TV acts as a mood-altering drug and actually prepares for harder drugs. TV trains us for drug dependency... as well as commodity co-dependency: "I can be happy, if only I can get..." The rapidly changing visual imagery shortens our attention span, overwhelms our brain circuitry and results in stupor, nurturing stupidity. The rapid world of TV imagery makes life seem dull by comparison; anxiety sets in. The natural world seems slow, unreal and boring. With our nervous system at high speed, we experience the antithesis of being in Nature, feeling calm. The remedy: spend time reading a physical book; build a library; be with humankind – especially out with Mother Nature.

During any war, how much coverage is given to the peacemakers, or the skills of negotiation, or alternative politics promoting peace? Instead, TV serves as psychic numbing to the psychotic nonsense of Doublespeak and War Profiteering. Presidents referred to MX missiles as "peacekeepers" saying "the goal of the war is peace." Military leaders have said, "We had to destroy the village to save it." When our presidents "lead the way" and speak "in forked tongue" we must Beware – we must beAware. Suggested reading: *In the Absence of the Sacred: The Failure of Technology & the Survival of the Indian Nations* (1991) and *Four Arguments for the Elimination of Television* (1978) by Jerry Mander... thoughtful reading.

In his classic work *Health and Light*, John Ott demonstrated lab mice exposed to agitating radiation from a TV set would at first become overexcited; later the same mice would become inert and lethargic, eventually developing degenerative diseases. The author gives examples where aggressive behavior among breeding animals, such as mink and aquarium fish, was eliminated by removing commercial fluorescent lights. Similar effects with school children; some teachers simply eliminate disruptive behavior by turning off fluorescent lights! Similar reactions are observed among children who inordinately watch: they busy themselves with other things, while the TV drones on. Families exhibit this behavior; few really care what is actually on – only that something is on – interfering with inter-acting and real communication. Being a couch potato is a comfortable escape from an unhappy social or family life.

Tests by Herbert Krugman show: while viewers were watching TV, right-brain activity outnumbered left-brain activity by a ratio of 2:1. In other words, viewers were in an altered state more often than not. They were entranced, getting a beta-endorphin fix. To measure attention spans, a psychophysiologist at the VA Hospital in Bedford, MA, Thomas Mulholland, attached young viewers to an EEG machine wired to shut off the TV whenever the children's brains produced alpha waves. Although the children were instructed to concentrate, only a few could keep the set on more than 30 seconds! Most viewers are already hypnotized. Deepening the trance is easy. Simply place a blank, black frame every 32 frames of the film, creating a 45-beats-per-minute pulsation perceived only by the subconscious mind; this is an ideal pace to generate deep hypnosis. Commercials or suggestions presented following this alpha-producing broadcast are more likely to be accepted by the viewer. A high % of the viewing audience accepted suggestions, if they refrained from asking to do something contrary to morals, religion or self-preservation.

The medium for takeover is here. By 16, most children spend more hours of screen-time than school-work. We are engaged in an alpha-level world, where the placid, glassy-eyed masses respond obediently to instruction. Researcher Jacob Jacoby, a psychologist at Purdue University, found that of 2,700 tested... 90% misunderstood simple viewing fare: Barnaby Jones. Minutes after watching, the typical viewer missed 23-36% of questions about what was seen. They were going in and out of trance. If You go into a deep trance, You must be instructed to remember – otherwise You automatically forget. How many are living, yet "watching unaware" as life slips by?

TV programs are simply that: programming! Insidious? Here's how deep it can get... suitable for Ripley's **Believe It or Not!** There is a "teething toy" the shape of a TV remote {sic! – in the full sense of the term: truly, sick!}. Push a button and it sings a jingle:
> "I've got a remote... and I'm ready to roll...
> making things happen... 'cause *I'm in control*!"

This *programs* infants and older siblings as well, and anyone else within earshot... even adults who hear the repetitive meme... thus influencing the subconscious of society, our collective consciousness. Messages are clear: as long as You have the remote, You are in control of Your life. You are in charge of Your Reality!

Push another button... and yet another jingle ends with: "changing channels is such fun!" Channel-surfing is thus promoted as one of Life's fun-filled experiences. Since this "toy" nurtures short attention spans... and zombies, I threw it in the plastic recycling container; hopefully it gets turned into something useful – such as an asphalt substitute.

This graphic example – perhaps poignantly, a pornographic portrayal – shows how The Mockingbird Matrix Media... in a velvety, smooth way... conspires to establish Aldous Huxley's *Brave New World*! Although there is a mute switch on the side of the "toy" the babysitter and siblings kept switching it back on, perhaps thinking it amuses the fussing baby, rather than cuddling or walking. Discovering this fact, the only reasonable solution was to recycle the plastic... as well

as recycle the old consciousness with conscious Awareness. Beware... Be Aware!

Twelve Steps and Beyond
Many Roads, One Journey: Moving Beyond the 12 Steps by Charlotte Kasl offers 16 Steps for Discovery and Empowerment:

1) We affirm we have the power to take charge of our lives and stop being dependent on substances, or others, for our self-esteem and security.

2) We come to believe Great Spirit – a High Power – Universe – awakens healing wisdom within, when we open ourselves to that Power.

3) We choose to become our authentic selves and trust in the healing power of the truth.

4) We examine our beliefs, addictions, and dependent behavior in the context of living in a hierarchical, patriarchal culture.

5) We share with another person and the Universe all those things inside of us for which we feel shame and guilt.

6) We affirm and enjoy our strengths, talents and creativity... rather than hiding these qualities to protect other egos.
7) We become willing to let go of shame, guilt and any behavior that keeps us from loving self, and others.

8) We make a list of those we have harmed, and those who have harmed us, and take steps to clear out negative energy by making amends and sharing our grievances respectfully.

9) We express love and gratitude to others, and increasingly appreciate the wonders of life and the blessings we have.

10) We continue to trust our reality and daily affirm that we see what we see, we know what we know, and we feel what we feel.

11) We promptly acknowledge our mistakes and make amends when appropriate, and avoid apologizing for things done by others, as well as covering up, analyzing, or taking responsibility for the shortcomings of others.

12) We seek out situations, jobs, and those who affirm our intelligence, perceptions, and self-worth, and avoid situations or those who are hurtful, harmful or demeaning to us.

13) We take steps to heal our physical bodies, organize our lives, reduce stress and have fun.

14) We find our inward calling, and develop the will and the wisdom to follow it.

15) We accept the ups and downs of life as natural events to be used as lessons for growth.

16) We grow in awareness that we are interrelated with all living things… and we contribute to restoring peace, balance and harmony on the planet… beginning with home and family.

Vaccinations

While people firmly believe vaccinations are responsible for eradication of disease, the British Association for the Advancement of Science (1971) and *Scientific American* (1973) presented records documenting facts: 90% of all contagious disease was eliminated by vastly improved *sanitation, water systems, refrigeration, nutrition,* as well as humane living and working conditions.

Vaccinations and antibiotics were introduced a century *after* that enormous period of decline (1850-1940) and yet is given *full* credit! US Congress' Office of Technology Assessment's report entitled: *Assessing the Efficacy and Safety of Medical Technologies* states, "It has been estimated **only** 10-20% of all procedures currently used in medical practice have been shown to be efficacious by *controlled* trial." Meaning 80-90% of all drugs, devices and surgeries in daily use are *unproven*. The report adds **almost every surgery subjected to controlled medical study has been abandoned!**

Vaccination (technically minor surgery) remains unproven because authorities say it's unethical to not vaccinate. Vaccinating the entire population would destroy evidence to prove or disprove the theory.

Dr Leon Chaitow has reported in testimony under oath, British army medical personnel were instructed by their authorities to *re-diagnose* any disease that occurred (and was not supposed to) as a result of the mandatory vaccinations. Statistics are used to manipulate public trust. World health records from England, Germany, Italy, Mexico, Philippines and British India document devastating epidemics after mass vaccination.

Clearly: Health results from proper management of multiple stress factors: personal hygiene, nutrition, environment, and nurturing social relationships.

Normal metabolism is two-sided: *anabolism* builds up and *catabolism* breaks down; we eliminate waste material through our bowels, our tonsils – part of the lymphatic system which empties into the large intestine – our lungs and our skin. Bacteria fluctuate to deal with available waste materials; they decompose and recycle wastes to sanitize the area. The wastes create conditions for bacteria to multiply. Bacteria are present in greater numbers in the second and third stages of disease. Do bacteria cause disease… or does disease create an environment favorable to the proliferation of bacteria… *demanding* they multiply**?** Rather than a deficiency of some synthetic drug – many being coal-tar derivatives – disease is really the body curing itself. To facilitate the process of cure: drink extra water to rinse out; take extra enzymes with meals and in between meals on an empty stomach; take enemas and salt baths to facilitate the elimination process… and get more rest – get horizontal during the day, meditating or listening to Nature sounds.

One thing is clear; bacteria do not cause disease. Throat cultures from healthy people show multiple bacteria, such as diphtheria, staph, strep, etc. A healthy immune response system holds them in check; they are unable to flourish and cause disease, or any dis-ease, dis-comfort. Unfortunately, it is "normal" for vaccinated children to be plagued with rashes or fever, earaches and sore throats. Even with lowered vitality, their bodies seek the quickest route – skin, ears, and tonsils – to expel toxic vaccine material and waste created by the vaccine's damage. Antibiotics only suppress symptoms driving toxins deeper and complicate elimination. Vaccines lower immune response and vitality… a proven Fact of Life!

It is interesting to note the greatest rise in polio (1952) was five years *after* the introduction of the pertussis vaccine. This rate declined greatly over the next 3 years *before* the introduction of the Salk vaccine (1956). The Sabin vaccine was introduced in 1962. William F. Koch, scientist and physician, stated in his experience, individuals who had been vaccinated with other vaccines ran as much as 400% greater risk of contracting polio. Facts are clear; see above: **Polio**.

When choosing an informed decision about vaccines, consider the fact that pharmaceutical / drug / chemical companies are the most pervasive and powerful businesses on earth. These companies fund medical schools and determine the curriculum, the texts, and sometimes even the professors! Can we expect unbiased information from their students and promoters? Would You go to a butcher to find out about vegetarianism? The Matrix Medical Mainstream Mafia influences with Fear, tending to overshadow logic, intelligence, and protective instincts. Most parents are intimidated, sweet-talked and bullied into giving uninformed consent, to get it done in a hurry. Fortunately, thanks to COVID19(84), parents are beginning to realize vaccination is not emergency care; they are making an informed choice, even with tremendous pressure from authorities, friends and family. Responsible informed choice requires time to uncover facts, acknowledge our feelings, and find moral support meeting with some unvaccinated children, adults and their families – offering parents a clear picture of our natural abilities, seeing illness as strengthening for our immune response system and, ultimately, bringing long-term optimal health. When will we return to the previous "scientific standard" 3-5year double-blind studies to know what is safe?

Many people avoid taking their children for any shots by saying, "It is against my religious and spiritual beliefs." What beliefs? "Ancient Wisdom follows Mother Nature's Ways!" Indeed, why should other parents be upset because some choose to exercise their Freedom and keep their children free from vaccinations? If my children get sick, I deal with it. Rather than drugs for childhood illnesses, some parents give plenty of pure water to drink on a daily basis… enemas when a child has a fever to facilitate the body's efforts eliminating toxins… and monthly salt baths to allow the skin, our largest eliminative organ, opportunity to discard excess acids. This strengthens the immune response system, and prepares children for the onslaught to come in later years.

Others are free to use vaccines, drugs or surgery when they are sick. If they believe in the efficacy of drugs and vaccines, then they are protected from whatever causes the disease or sickness… as well as from others keeping their children free from these coal-tar derived, synthetic pollutants. The reason for their discomfort is clearly evident; they intuitively understand. They are uneasy.

As for developments in the 2020s, inquire about ingredients. WI-38 is code for cell lines from a female aborted fetus used to cultivate vaccine viral components. Injecting DNA from a female (carrying two X chromosomes) into a male (who *already* carries one X chromosome and a weaker Y chromosome) there is an overload of the X chromosome. Now we have an onslaught of boys who think they should be girls. Do we have male DNA in vaccines? Yes! MRC-5 is code for cell lines from a male aborted fetus also used to cultivate vaccine viral components. Do we have girls thinking they are boys? Yes! Is it as prominent as boys wanting to be girls? No! Why? Because girls have two dominant X chromosomes. When they are injected with a vaccine containing MRC-5, they are getting a Y chromosome, and also *another* dominant X chromosome, on top of the two they already have. That's why we have less girls wanting to be boys, as the other way around. The Baphomet, half-male – half-female, blurs the lines, yet is in charge of those mandating vaccines that either kill, maim, or confuse our society. We had 3 shots given children 50 years ago and 72 given today. When did society become gender confused? About the *same time* farmers were giving hormone shots to their cows so they would give gallons instead of quarts. Hormonal residues get sloughed off in the secretions and concentrated: it takes 1 gallon of milk to make 1 lb of cheese! Think… Gender confusion is far from accidental, designed by the Matrix to further disintegrate Family Life and Values.

In addition to male and female aborted fetal DNA, the COVID19(84) injections called "vaccines" – although they fail to create anti-bodies or offer immunity which previous vaccines did – they are in Reality 'mRNA-vaccines' and actually *experimental* synthetic drugs affecting our DNA. BEWARE the Trojan Horse – which is a Bioweapon! COVID19(84) vaccines contains untested, synthetic mRNA, among other dangerous substances. Staggering numbers of doctors and scientists are speaking out, alarmed; as children are over-vaccinated, their immune response systems create allergies, and autoimmunity**!**

Explore the controversy. https://www.drtenpenny.com/ where "Penny for Your Thoughts" is taken to the next Order of Magnitude by Sherri Tenpenny, DO. Those who promote vaccines unabashedly proclaim they will help **reduce** the population by 10-15%! Truly, the Grand Plan is to reduce population approximately 93%, as per: Georgia Guidestones: Who Paid for It and Why? | Historic Mysteries. Why was it fire-bombed and then demolished, much like the Twin Towers? Explore: https://911truth.org, https://stateofthenation.co/ at which Search: FUNVAX. Explore: No Jab For Me! Are these crazy theories? Documentation regarding the Matrix and their Grand Plan is abundant: https://aim4truth.org/

Why the "Global Emergency" to vaccinate, especially considering 2020 has been, for all intents and purposes, an "average" flu season… with a 99% Survival Rate?

Why were there zer**O** reported deaths from "the flu" in 2020/2021? Is COVID19(84) the antidote for the flu?

Please test all of this information for **T**ruth or **F**alsehood! See above: **Muscle Testing… Pendulums… Sway Test... and Switched Energies** See the results Yourself. Explore Your Inner Voice Intuition. Meditate. Be Wise. Realize Who You Are and Why You Are Here… Now at this time in history!

2020, our collective **Year of 20/20 Vision**, invites us to Learn about Nature! Grow Your Own Garden of Eatin'! Take Charge of Your Life with: Appreciation. Gratitude. Care. Compassion. Minimalism. Permaculture. Return to Mother Nature's Ways! The Essene Tradition nurturing HeartMindBodySpirit as One, is holistic. Harmonious Healing and Ancient Wisdom in Modern Times helps One find the Way back hOMe!

Rather than go down the Primrose Path… be informed. Make an informed choice. Indeed, My Body. My Choice! Beware the Trojan Horse of the British Pilgrims Society which promotes British Imperialism. Since Google is the **M**ockingbird **M**edia **M**ainstream **M**atrix **P**rimrose **P**ath, search through another source such as: DuckDuckGo — Privacy, simplified. Compare results with what comes up on Google using the same topic, and see the difference. Be a-**maze**-d: taken out of the "**maze**" and off the devious **MMMMPP!**

Vegan Life and Religions

While religions purport to make their followers responsible citizens, most religions have little to say about Compassion – toward other species. Religions around the world preach: "Thou shalt not kill" as one of the most important Laws. Yet, every day the faithful sit with plates of dead bodies, blessing their murdered food in the name of the Deity that commanded them to refrain from killing! Christ, Buddha, Mohammed, Bible scholars, ancient authors of the Vedas and Dead Sea Scrolls, urge their followers to live with compassion and love, putting up their swords… living in Peace.

Unfortunately, the scriptures that record the lives and teachings of the enlightened masters are vague. To complicate things, many scriptures are modified. Before the internet, computers and printers… there were mimeograph machines or duplicating machines. Before that, there were printing presses. Johann Gutenberg tinkered with movable type in 1444… finally, suitable for mass production, creating the Gutenberg Bible in 1455. Before that, everything was hand-written by scribes – the most famous being monks dedicated to the monastic life. We now know over the course of centuries, some monks wrote border notations to facilitate an understanding of the text, based on *their* interpretations. The next monk years later thought the original scribe was distracted, and inserted the notation as part of the text.

An even more blatant compromise of the message of the scriptures is in the Christian religion, adopted as the state religion of the Roman Empire in the 4th century. Flavius Valerius Aurelius Constantinus crowned himself Emperor in 306 after the death of his father, Emperor Constantius. As Emperor of the Holy Roman Empire, Constantine issued his Edict of Milan in 313 along with Emperor Licinius, of the eastern parts, giving freedom of worship and equal rights to all religious groups. Constantine, in 325, convened the 1st Ecumenical Council, known as the Council of Nicaea. With his blessing, early Christians came out of hiding from their underground gatherings. Conceding to His Graciousness, the priests and politicians re-wrote the scriptures to make them acceptable to Roman liking, particularly in regard to eating meat and drinking. These changes are clearly seen when we read the Dead Sea Scrolls, the pre-Roman documents discovered in 1947, and the Nag Hammadi Library discovered a year earlier in Egypt. Even more will be revealed as the Church gathers the courage to release all ancient scrolls... and open the Archives of the Vatican. Meanwhile we learn from translations made by Edmond Bordeaux Szekely among others, that are now freely available to all: download on a thumb drive. https://www.thenazareneway.com/from_enoch_to_the _dead_sea_scrolls.htm

As an Essene Master... Jesus exhorts his followers: "Be considerate, be kind, be tender, be merciful; not to Your kind alone, but every creature in Your care; for You are to them as gods, to whom they look to fulfill their needs." Texts from the Old Testament used in defense of meat eating are used out of context, or are compromises permitted in crisis situations – such as after the flood. Rigid delineated guidelines for kosher killing are followed with instructions on how to deal with leprosy, as if saying: "If You are going to eat this way, then prepare Yourself for the consequences." And after years of emphasis on animal foods, we do suffer the consequences of wide-spread, chronic, degenerative diseases. Vegetarian, vegan communities in the Holy Land, and holy lands everywhere attest to the Truth. Vegan living is becoming popular among discerning people around the globe as sustainable for us and for Gaia. Physicians Committee for Responsible Medicine has done the research: https://www.pcrm.org/

The Vedas were written in Sanskrit, the ancient language upon which all Indo-European languages are based, including Greek, Latin, German, English. Buddhists, Christians, Hindus and Muslims alike, espouse vegetarianism as the spiritual ideal. There are 1000s of injunctions against meat eating in the Vedas: "By refraining from killing any living being, one becomes fit for salvation." The Vedas are ancient hymns, considered the ancestors of all world religious scripture. Jesus surely studied them as a boy in Egypt, and again on his travels to the East in search of the lost tribes of Israel, who were taken as slaves by the Assyrians centuries before. This is confirmed by the Government of India which is similar to BBC, who produced a 1 hr intriguing documentary: The Rauzabal Shrine of Srinagar – The Tomb of Jesus in Kashmir: https://www.youtube.com/watch?v=hup6fe_JFJE

Further supporting this idea, Steven Hairfield, PhD, a U.S. author and Zen priest, has done research in various monasteries concerning the Wise Man from the West known as Issa or Yuza Asaf. He studied Buddhist Principles which are repeatedly found in the Gospels. Consider Jesus' Secret Life in India – 2 parts:

https://www.youtube.com/watch?v=8SugTSaVk7Q
https://www.youtube.com/watch?v=hZJ5hW9x7zE

Vegetarian Power
The word vegetarian has confusing connotations. "Yes, I'm a vegetarian; I eat lots of vegetables, and once in a while a little chicken." "I'm a pisco-vegetarian, so I also eat fish." "I'm a lacto-ovo-vegetarian. I also eat dairy and eggs." "I'm a sanguino-vegetarian. I have duck-blood soup during the holidays." Free from qualifiers, vegetarians include preferably raw, dairy and perhaps some eggs. While vegans who thrive on a plant-based diet and lifestyle, eschew even honey!

The British Vegetarian Society coined the term (1840s) and the word vegetarian has little to do with vegetables. The Society's Founders based their name on the Latin word *vegetus*, meaning active, lively, or vigorous. At the time, the word veget was used in England to describe a robust, healthy person. According to the BVS, the diet conducive to a healthy, vigorous life is free from animal foods. As a reason-able person is able to reason... a veget-able diet is able to impart veget – vigor. Today, many people feel a plant-based diet supports an active, vigorous lifestyle – and science supports their theory, which is evidenced by The China Health Project and the Physicians Committee for Responsible Medicine https://www.pcrm.org/.

Most people can get along well on a vegetarian diet, yet... doesn't it stand to reason athletes need meat to keep up strength and stamina? ...that growing athletes need extra protein to build muscles? It might seem reasonable, but in fact that kind of reasoning makes as much sense as our primitive ancestors thinking that eating hearts and ground up teeth of lions, ingesting their tough or 'hearty' organs, they would also take in the animal's courage and strength.

Athletes throughout history have believed meat, being muscle itself, was a logical source of muscle power. By the 1860s, when the Oxford rowing crew in England stoked up on bread, beer, undercooked beef and mutton, it was known that muscles – meat – were made up of protein. The practice seemed to have scientific support. "Then in 1865, two German scientists went mountain climbing. By measuring nitrogen in their urine throughout the expedition, they found the extra exertion did not use up extra protein. Other experimenters confirmed these findings: muscle exertion used carbohydrate, not protein, regarded as a landmark in nutrition history.

"In 1907, another now famous study at Yale University put 49 men through a series of exercises and found the vegetarians among them had more than *twice* the endurance. Countless studies confirmed these early findings. Scientists and sports doctors agree strenuous muscle work is fueled by *complex carbohydrates*. Strong muscles are built up by exercise, rather than extra protein. A high protein diet does not improve athletic performance. What's more, it doesn't matter whether the protein is from animals or plants... in fact, the fat in steak is especially hard to digest and can cause cramps if it is eaten a few hours before any heavy exercise. And instead of increasing strength or endurance, extra protein can increase the urge to urinate – in the middle of a competition. Worse, doctors warn: high-protein diets can be hard on the kidneys." (*The Case Against Meat*, p.174.)

Gabriel Cousens, MD, holistic physician, Essene bishop, rabbi and author of *Conscious Eating*, mentions studies relating to vegetarian power. He reports Dr Irving Fisher concluded in the Yale Medical Journal in 1917, a vegetarian diet helps the body function at an endurance rate approximately *twice* that of a flesh-centered diet. Even sedentary vegetarians had more endurance than meat eating athletes! In a study confirming that... Dr Joteyko of the Academy of Medicine in Paris compared vegetarians and non-vegetarians from all walks of life: vegetarians had 2-3X the endurance, and took one-fifth the time to recover! In a Danish study in 1968, the performance of the *same* people on 3 different diets showed on a strictly vegetarian diet they averaged 167 minutes on a bicycle endurance test compared to 57 minutes on high meat and dairy diet. In Belgium, research comparing handgrip strength showed vegetarians averaged 69 squeezes as compared to 38 squeezes for non-vegetarians. Vegetarians also had a faster recovery time. Researchers said one of the reasons meat-eaters had less strength and endurance as well as slower recovery is because the protein breakdown products – uric acid, urea and purines – poison and interfere with muscle and nerve function.

If eating muscle made muscles, why don't the cattle ranchers feed their herds meat? Why don't dairy farmers feed their cows milkweed? Why don't students eat head cheese – made from sheep brain – to

enhance cognitive potential? 80% of muscle is water; protein is made from amino acids. To build muscle: drink plenty of re-mineralized and re-energized distilled or r/o water, have complex carbohydrates such as the high-protein alkaline grains – quinoa and amaranth, preferably germinated. Easily assimilated foods such as salt-water and fresh-water algae – amino acid ratios comparable to human milk – provide optimal nutrition. Athletes tell their story: Vimeo | The Game Changers (gamechangersmovie.com)

Violence and its Causes
Arun Gandhi, grandson / student of Mohandas K. Gandhi and *ahimsa*, attributes eight causes for all violence:

Wealth without work...
Pleasure without conscience...
Knowledge without character...
Commerce without morality...
Science without humanity...
Worship without sacrifice...
Politics without principles...
Rights without responsibilities.

All violence can be resolved through respect, understanding, acceptance and appreciation. Violence can happen under our own roof! Peace on Earth begins at home, *especially* in the kitchen. As long as we have blood on our cutting boards, we will have blood in our streets. Once we look in the eyes of an animal and recognize consciousness, we become deeply aware of the consciousness that takes its own perceptions through *our* eyes.

With great Honor and Respect for other animals, especially other mammals, we Gratefully look to the plant kingdom for sustenance. Every nutritive substance we require is found in the plant kingdom, if we know where to look – macroalgae and microalgae, germinated nuts and seeds, enzymes and probiotics in various fermented foods. Simply put – Living Foods have Everything everyOne Requires! AnyOne doubtful, can simply take the Conscious-Vegan Challenge! While there can be junk food vegans... Twinkies & soda... conscious vegans eat 80% raw and living foods: fruits, veggies, and sprouts, germinated nuts and seeds – that would grow if planted, and 20% cooked, preferably steamed to retain nutrients. Follow these guidelines 30-Days. See how You feel. How You look in the mirror.

Vitaflex Foot Reflexology

Stanley Burroughs, 20th century naturist and renegade, popularized Vitaflex particularly – foot reflexology based on the piezoelectric properties of the human skin. Vitaflex is a specialized form of manual stimulation at specific reflex points, using the pads and nails of the fingers in a rolling motion to produce therapeutic electrical voltages and currents. Vitaflex massage, an ancient modality originating in India and Tibet, is used with many protocols. *Healing for the Age of Enlightenment: Balanced Nutrition, Vitaflex and Color Therapy* offers effective detox with his Master Cleanse, a guide to reflex points on the body: >5,000, and color used in healing.

Weight

First... give Yourself permission to love Yourself as You are, releasing guilt patterns associated with food. Love Yourself. See the beauty of who You are, what You do. Accept Yourself. See room for improvement.

Next... imagine what can be, visualizing Your beautiful physical body full of vitality, strength and health. Imagine the constant flow of Joy and Love going through Your body. Imagine. Practice.

Changing nutritional habits comes about easily when guided by Inner Vision, so relax and breathe deeply. Bring the tip of Your thumb to the tip of Your middle finger. Visualize a column of light that size coming through the top of Your head and the base of Your spine as a toroidal field... joining and flowing out from Your heart center – circling and re-uniting once again with the columns of light, above and below.

Mother Nature is in a state of constant Joy and Love for Life, enjoying every second! You feel it when You walk in Nature, listen to the chanting of a river, the songs of the birds, and witnessing squirrels playing in the trees. Nature receives everything directly from the sun, air, water and the earth. Animals naturally eat whole, raw foods; and move toward the fire of the sun, feeling radiating warmth; they understand instinctively the fires *we* create are life destroying; they run from those fires which decimate worms and beetles. Likewise, cooking destroys the life force of food and denatures the structure of proteins and major minerals. We are wise to observe Mother Nature and eat whole, living foods.

To experience change in Your Life requires serious adjustment in the Way You do things. **Fact of Life**:

> If You always do... what You've always done –
> You'll always get... what You've always gotten!

Old, learned habits repeat old aches, pains and problems – such is the nature of patterns based on competition, isolation, and death. You are invited by Mother Nature to remember life-giving patterns. There is always **Choice**. For example, some people overeat out of Fear... there may not be enough later or tomorrow. Perhaps not really hungry in the morning, they eat anyway because they fear to be hungry at 11 o'clock. Rather than eat by instinct, they eat by ideas. Eating like this habitually creates imbalance in the acting body... affecting the feeling body and thinking body, creating anguish!

Create a new perspective in nutrition... accept Yourself as You are, and accept everything You do. You are a work in progress: a conscious Creation of Infinite Being... a Being of Radiant Light exploring Divine Love on the human plane. Visualize a bright future with a healthy body. Experience choice... change habits... discover new ways of eating, with living foods and natural love as foundation stones. When experiencing new ways of eating... remember to give Yourself permission to step back when necessary. Enjoy! Celebrate Life! If You feel some regression – rather than beat Yourself up – Congratulate Yourself for all You have accomplished, and give Yourself credit. Commit again to Your outcome. Know Thyself ~ Love Yourself. Breathe. Enjoy Life!

Rather than saying: "I will never do that again" say: "I Am free to do whatever I choose at every moment." Before doing something, take a moment to feel why You do it. Is it a real requirement for Your body, a way to escape physical fatigue... or emotional discomfort? Stimulating, artificial substances, fried or animal foods, sugary stress foods, caffeine or alcohol are pleasant for a moment – they *stimulate* Your body to fight, to eliminate. Later, body forces depleted, You feel tired. So, become aware of What You do and Why.

Some people fear change in this area – fearing to lose the freedom their pleasures seem to bring: the cigarette or the drink, the restaurant, the cafe, the meat, the pastries, the casual acquaintances. Consider Your explorations of something new an open-door experience. You can go back to Your old jail anytime.

Truly, the ways of eating enjoyed by most is like a jail built by fear patterns and ignorance, breeding disease – this servitude empowers and enriches the unhealthy Disease Management System at Your expen$e!

Opt-out. Empower Yourself. Create Your own health maintenance system. Explore the power of natural food. Discover the Joy of living foods and the Love they support You in feeling. These are pleasurable, indeed, and sometimes can be addictive! The purpose of Nature is to make human beings Happy, filled with Love and Joy. Suffering and disease are creations of twisted minds. Change Your mind. Change Your habits. Enjoy Life. You can experience ever-expanding discovery of Self... as a being of light feeling free. increasing Your consciousness beyond the limits of social patterning. You are built for health, joy and love; You are here to enjoy... so have fun! Some, caught between the old and the new patterns, find temporary solace in chewing the foods they choose to eliminate and, rather than swallowing, discarding it. If You find Yourself doing this, rather than chide Yourself – enjoy it, and smile... Laugh! Let the animals find it, or let it compost into the soil. Focus on the new patterns You choose to create... Consciousness of the New You!

Optimal body weight is obscured by weight charts that give a variance of 20-30 lbs according to one's height, compounded by the nebulous issue of small-boned and big-boned people. Weight charts offer such broad latitude because they are based on the normal weight of the average person, rather than the optimal weight of healthy people. Use the Body Mass Index. To determine BMI, divide weight in kilograms by height in meters, squared. The supposed ideal for women is 18.1 – 23.6; for men, 20.1 – 25. If the figure comes to >25 = overweight; if it is 30-34.9 = obese; 35-39.9 = very obese; >40 extreme obesity. For example, a man weighs 145 lbs; divide by 2.2 to convert to kg – he weighs 65.9 kg. He is 6' tall; to convert to meters divide inches 72 by 39.37 and we find the person is 1.83 m in height, squared = 3.34. Divide 65.9 by 3.34 and the person has a BMI of 19.7 – decent, optimal weight.

Rather than optimal weight... You can figure optimal measurements based on Ancient Greek proportions of Beauty: twice around the wrist equals once around the lower neck; twice around the lower neck equals once around the waist. Simple formula!

What is the primary cause of excess weight – particularly among those whose challenge is getting in shape and staying that way? Some factors include under active pituitary or thyroid, and excessive high calorie foods. The leading cause is toxicity. With a congested liver, its role as a blood detoxifier is compromised. Why? The body surrounds toxins with a layer of fat to avoid harming organs and tissues. When someone diets by reducing calories or fasts, the fat is metabolized and weight is shed. The toxins remain unless the body is given long-standing support through enemas or colonics, salt baths, drinking plenty of re-mineralized and re-energized distilled or r/o water and chlorophyll-rich foods and juices. If toxins remain suspended in the circulatory and the lymphatic system because of a congested liver – when normal eating is resumed, even small amounts – fats surround those toxins for protection and weight returns. Hence, the rationale for systemic enzymes am/pm on an empty stomach, and ½ hr before meals.

To attain Your ideal weight, drink plenty of re-mineralized and re-energized distilled or r/o water. For the underweight, drink a minimum of two quarts, building muscle tissue. For the overweight, a minimum of 3 quarts brings multiple benefits. Rather than think more water means more weight, actually, water naturally suppresses the appetite and metabolizes stored fats. Studies clearly indicate a decrease in water consumption causes fat deposits to increase, while an increase in water consumption reduces fat deposits. To understand the mechanism behind this fact, we turn to the liver. When we lack sufficient water, the kidneys filter poorly and some of their load is dumped on the liver. One of the liver's major functions is to metabolize stored fat into usable energy. Having to carry the excess load of the kidneys, the liver functions poorly as well... meaning it metabolizes less fat, which results in more fat being stored. With fluid retention... drinking water is the remedy. With less water, the brain sees a threat to survival and conserves every drop. Diuretics force out water as well as nutrients. The brain sees this as a threat, replacing water at the first opportunity.

The #1 cause of chronic fluid retention is over-acid diet. The body retains water to dilute the acids, so it can maintain proper pH in the blood, to remain between 7.35 – 7.45, slightly alkaline. Avoiding animal foods, cooked foods, alcohol and sodas... while including more living, enzyme-rich foods, eliminates this cause of water retention, and gradually the body returns to normal metabolism. Another cause of chronic fluid retention is excess table salt – sodium chloride with a dose of aluminum to keep it free-flowing, perhaps a dash of dextrose to counter the bitter taste of the aluminum. Drinking re-mineralized and re-energized distilled or r/o water flushes out this chemical sodium.

The question is how much water? The average person can use two quarts a day. The overweight can use one extra eight-ounce glass per twenty-five pounds of excess weight – more if You exercise briskly, or if the weather is hot and/or dry. Some people divide their weight in half and drink that many ounces of water per day. Drinking cold water on an empty stomach before exercise can burn some extra calories… however, the stomach likes to be around 101° to secrete digestive juices, to function smoothly. So, yes if You drink cold water, it will increase Your metabolism… and, simply remember to wait an hour to eat, so Your stomach can adjust the thermostat and resume its normal temperature to secrete HCL, pepsin and other digestive factors, adequately digesting the meal.

Start Your day with water. Delay eating as long as possible. Having water before and during exercise forces Your body to burn fat as a source of energy. Experiment. You will be surprised with Your capabilities, and pleased with Your results.

Many people report improved digestion, as well as mood and weight regulation by taking large amounts of plant-based enzymes. The enzyme *serrapeptase* was derived originally from silkworm, now from yeast fermentation; it helps dissolve fibrin and scars. Take 3 plant-based enzymes before and between meals. Ask Your body. Muscle test. Be patient; watch and feel the improvement.

Facilitate Your journey with lymphatic exercises – such as the rebounder, jumping rope or at least, a chi machine for passive stimulation of the one-way valves that regulate lymphatic flow – You can stretch and exercise, loosening joints – while You are on the machine for 15 minutes. Make it a meditation. Enjoy!

Massage with organic hemp seed oil; it has the proper balance of Omega 3s, 6s & 9s and the full-spectrum Family of Omegas. Enjoy happy thoughts. Visualize. Be in Your outcome. Breathe deeply… exhale completely! Develop the habit of 3X3 Sacred Breaths whenever feasible and feel the Joy! To facilitate Your

process, see above: **Rejuvenation of Organs** D-8; support Your liver.

White Chocolate

White chocolate is rich in sugar, milk solids, artificial colors and flavors. Since they all compromise the immune response system, avoid these polluting and congesting factors. For the occasional celebration… Enjoy organic, dark chocolate with 70% cacao.

Who is Robert Anthony Kreucher?
Exploring Numerology

As an octogenarian reflecting on the vagaries of Life… I am so Blessed beginning with parents in a loving, happy relationship caring for me as I transitioned from the Spirit World in this physical vehicle. I have been ultimately blessed to have cared for them during their transitions back to the Spirit World. Rose Mae passed at 101 lucid and happy… I then left the Great Lakes for the great tropics – one of the Blue Zones, Nicoya Peninsula – living at Viktoras' Essene Sanctuary - Montezuma, Costa Rica. We met 40 years ago. Back in the day, our spouses practiced the sacred art of Belly Dance – White Dove as adept teacher with White Rose as star student. Victor and I were colleagues in holistic healing – promoting Health and Happiness for HeartMindBodySpirit at Hippocrates Health Institute in West Palm Beach, where I was their first chiropractor.

Viktoras co-founded HHI in Boston in the mid-60s with Dr Ann Wigmore, where he met David A Phillips, PhD who told him so much about himself in 90 minutes, he knew he had to explore **Numerology** {see above}. Viktoras was R&D with Dr Ann for several years until his parents called him to care for Grandmother – who was bedridden for a few months with Alzheimer's and told she would never walk again. After 5 weeks, she was "up & about" cooking breakfast at 2am as normal for her daughter, who was off to work at the bakery! Viktoras (23 Feb 1939) stayed for a while with Grandma; she pulled him through the war-torn streets of Lithuania at 5 years of age… *seeing* people shot, stepping over bodies and around blood puddles. Invaded by Russia, the Germans brought them to freedom and they lived in a refugee camp for five years, before emigrating to the USA. Viktoras landed in Connecticut, knowing little English at age 10. Victor and I were born 2 years apart… and 2 worlds apart.

Robert Anthony Kreucher landed (4Nov1941) next to the Detroit River, across from Windsor, Ontario –

birthplace of his maternal Grandfather. Named after his father, Robert and paternal Grandfather Anthony, Robert has a name adding to 111. Normally, Pythagorean numerology reduces to a single digit, except for the Master Numbers 10, 11, 22 and 33 – 111 would reduce to 3, yet as Master Number of the Mystery Schools **1** is the beginning after Unity, the sphere – **O** – referred to by e e cummings as the "nO of all nOthing". **111** - Wake-Up! Pay Attention to Energy Flow… a new beginning, cycle… or perhaps Initiation in the Mystery Schools.

According to *The Complete Book of Numerology: Discovering the Inner Self*, by David A Phillips, PhD: **Robert** = **33** a Master number of Creation because 3 begins the mental plane of 3 6 9… thought is the beginning of all creation; 3 also governs memory.

One's Soul Urge – someone's spiritual sensitivity, fortitude and drive – is determined by the vowels: **o+e** = 6+5 = **11** offering valuable intuitive strength, especially beneficial for individuals without 2 5 8 on their birth chart, *or* as part of their Ruling number. 11 serves to increase compassion.

One's Outer Expression is determined by the consonants: **R+b+r+t** = 9+2+9+2 = **22** with an exceptionally strong power for organizing, especially working in compassionate fields… such as benefitting under-privileged children.

The Ruling number – the foundational driving vibration – is from the birth date: 4+1+1+1+9+4+1 = 21 = **3** – the first number of the mental plane sparking Creativity. Four 1s and two 4s show an attraction to the physical world, yearning to explore Mother Nature. With one extra 4 and three extra 1s which add to 7… Robert has an honorary Line of Practicality. 3s are fairly witty.
When someone has 3 5 *and* 7 = the Line of Spirituality. Robert, without any of those numbers = the Line of the Skeptic, or the Line of the Inquirer – often assuming the role of Devil's Advocate. When someone has 2 5 *and* 8 = the Line of Emotional Balance. Robert, without any of those numbers = the Line of Hypersensitivity – easily hurt in younger years, may become shy – their natural sensitivity indicates a loving and tender nature.

Robert Anthony was born to: Robert John (3Dec1915) = Master# 22 with the Line of the Planner and the Line of Determination. Rose Mae (2July1915) = Ruling# 7 – student and teacher – with the Line of Determination.

Teen-agers in the 1929 Crash, Robert put in a couple of short school years – only during the cold winter months – to help Anthony in his construction business after losing, with the Depression, 11 houses – "ready for market."

Both were proud to be part of The Arsenal of Democracy, as Detroit was known. They went to Tuesday novenas to Our Mother of Perpetual Help at Holy Redeemer in Detroit, a basilica church with a huge downstairs chapel that were both packed! {Baskets were passed only on Sundays; these were entirely devotional events.} Keeping their spirits up with revelry and song, Rose Mae and Robert listened to Big Band sounds on the radio… blessed with these experiences in my 1st 10 years of Life.

At about the same time on my Sacred Journey – age 10, 1951 – I learned Independence. Despite the jokes, many Catholics believed, although far from official dogma, only *they* would be allowed in Heaven; *others* went to Limbo. I was privileged to go to private school at St. Cecilia's as did most playmates. Even though some went to public school, everyone was at church except one lad who went to another church, and the fact was obvious – *he* was the real Peacemaker - breaking up fights, soothing tensions. How could he go anywhere *but* Heaven? I chose to believe differently. Had I lost my Faith or had I found it?

Also, at the tender age of 10, I was brought to the doctor. "He eats like a horse and hasn't put on a pound. What's wrong?" Rose Mae weighed 104, and Robert, with his love of white potatoes, continuously struggled to stay under 200 to look reasonably professional as a detective with DPD. Several tests indicated a high basal metabolism, yet completely normal. I began wondering about the Charles Atlas ads on the inside covers of comic books. I joined the 5th & 6th grade basketball team. Christmas morning, I found a bicycle and the next Spring I found Freedom… riding with a couple of friends 5 miles north to the Zoo, or 5 miles south to the Detroit River.

My 3rd discovery at age 10 was tobacco. Having seen cowboy movies and Indian Chiefs with the ever-present peace pipe, Rosemary (2 yrs older) and I were watching 2 toddlers who were sleeping; she knew Bobby Tony's mischievous, exploring ways and presented a cigarette butt from the ashtray. She choked and coughed. I thought it tasted great! We each had 2 puffs. Those were the days: "9 out of 10 doctors recommend Camels!" – a pack of 20 was 23¢! Europeans gave the Indians alcohol, which became an addiction. Indians gave the Europeans tobacco, which became an addiction. Little did we realize. We knew Camels were a blend of Domestic and Turkish tobaccos and had a rich flavor. Kools were rumored to have a dash of codeine along with menthol, for those who enjoy that "outdoors" flavor.

Every plant has many uses. CoQ10 is derived from mold, actually cultivated on tobacco leaf. There are also homeopathic preparations of tobacco. Tobacco brought me from the world of competition to the world of relaxation in Nature, shifting from Type A to Type B personality. Kicked off the 6th grade basketball team for smoking, and really enjoying an occasional cigarette, I'd ride my bike to the river, soon packing basic fishing gear. As a paperboy making $12/wk, by 16 I had a 5.5 horse Johnson motor, took the family car out to the lake, rented a boat for $2 sometimes enjoying a sunrise cigarette.

Another formative influence... by 16 I was a day-student at Sacred Heart Seminary {1/2 hr bus ride} and quite aware of the church's complicity of silence with Rosa Parks and the civil rights movement, spearheaded by Dr Martin Luther King, Jr. That's when I began to understand the 3 City-States – City of London, Vatican City and Washington, DC: control through usurious finances, control through guilt and fear, control through military might! Sharing what I knew, I had lovely experiences at 3 parishes. Then after 5 years: Change! Experimenting with a plant-based diet for 30 days changed my Life as did exploring fasting from the New to the Full Moon in Appalachia, in a pre-Civil War log cabin... learning Mother Nature's Ways in the ashrams of Europe and India. I returned to school, graduating as Doctor of Chiropractic – licensed as a Primary Care Practitioner in Florida in 1981.

In my clinical years, I was attracted to the gentle ways of Sacral Occipital Technique {SOT} developed by Dr M B DeJarnette, close friend of William Garner Sutherland, DO of craniosacral fame. The Major 23Dec1899 has amazing numerology, including the Line of Greatness.

Dr George Joseph Goodheart, a Major in the Army at age 26, was awarded the Bronze Star for inventing a bombing release mechanism. He worked with his father as a DC; he was the first official US Olympic team chiropractor. Even at the end of his life, will be remembered as a gentleman with unflappable optimism. He had a lifelong passion for tennis, and would remind opponents of his Detroit City Parks & Rec. championships. He was still skiing in the Alps at the age of 83. His trademark Corvette and khaki suits made him recognizable throughout Grosse Pointe.

Thank You Great Spirit... all of these formative forces forged my future. Further details are found in: *ABRACADABRA Your Wish IS Fulfilled! How to Create Magic and Miracles in Your Life: Reprogram Your Subconscious, Rehabilitate Your Inner Child, Recreate Your Life!* **Appendix 3: Self-Knowledge: Know Thyself!** ॐ **My Journey in Consciousness** ☮

Confessions of a Radical Priest

Women's Issues
Women on Hormone Replacement Therapy ingest pregnant mare's urine (Pre-mar-in) or other synthetic hormones, with side-effects of blood clots, fluid retention, salt build-up, breast and uterine cancer. Alternatively use *Dioscorea* or Wild Yam, recommended as a homeopathic remedy, or as a high-quality cream. Side effects come from synthetics because the molecular structure is foreign to the body. The progesterone taken from the wild yam is nearly identical to what the body produces, and the body easily converts it into the identical molecule, strengthening the bones and balancing mood. Another homeopathic remedy to assist female *stress* at Life's change, and other times: Mother Tincture of *Caulophyllum* or Blue Cohosh – 10 drops in 1oz water 3x/day. As a *toning* remedy for the uterus, especially after multiple births or miscarriages, Mother Tincture of *Aletris Farinosa* or Stargrass – 10 drops in 1oz water 3x/day.

To supplement the energies of *Dioscorea*, soybeans are appropriate when sprouted and/or made into tempeh. Some people consume soy and have gas, indicating lack of tolerance. Asians who use sprouted or fermented soy products are less likely than Westerners to develop breast or ovarian cancers, and problems of menopause – such as hot flashes – because of a plant hormone called genistein, which reduces blood cholesterol. Soy sauce, soy oil and soy-based ice cream, however, lack genistein; besides, cooked soy oil may be carcinogenic. Get Your Vitamin E from sprouted seeds, nuts, grains, avocado, or 800 IU of mixed-tocopherols; 1-3 Dong Quai tablets per day, more with age. Do the Sway Test. Black cohosh is a helpful addition. Other plant sources of isoflavones (phytoestrogen) are found in greens: baby sunflower and buckwheat greens, sugar snap peas, green beans, and green peas.

The pineal makes melatonin in darkness, and serotonin in the light. There is a relationship between increased electrical exposure in the home, office and stores, and a decrease in melatonin levels. Women with jobs in the electrical industry increase risk of estrogen-related illnesses... and possible death from breast cancer.

If PMS remains after dietary changes and using *Dioscorea* cream, use *Agnus castus* aka chasteberry (Vitex). A wonderful balancing energy for most female conditions, it is to be avoided during pregnancy; small amounts during lactation help increase production.

If fibroids are an issue, make dietary and lifestyle changes, use *Dioscorea* cream, eat seaweed, increase walking, and visualization. Alternate every other day between ginger compresses on the lower abdomen, and castor oil packs on the liver. Take ½ C fresh grated ginger root or 2 Tsp dried; soak in ½ C hot water for 3 minutes. Soak a cloth in this liquid, and place on the abdomen; cover with plastic, hot water bottle, a towel and a blanket. Visualize, meditate or read uplifting material for 1 hour; same protocol with cloth saturated in hexane-free castor oil placed over the right lower ribcage energizes the liver.

TSS – Toxic Shock Syndrome could be a temperature >102° with diarrhea, sore throat, headache, muscle pains, skin rash, dizziness or fainting. Tampons create the perfect environment for bacteria to produce toxins known as TSS. Of those affected, 2/3 are under 25. To avoid TSS, avoid tampons. A safe alternative is found in a sea sponge, available in health food stores; this cosmetic sponge may be used after washing thoroughly and rinsing several times, cleaning out any sand or grit; boil to sterilize. Safe... it can be rinsed in a sink and re-used again and again.

A wonderful book for every woman: *Dressed to Kill*, by Sydney Ross Singer and Soma Grismaijer. The title makes one think about several things: high heels –

invented by men – to tilt the pelvis forward, extending and accentuating the derriere... or makeup and hairspray loaded with chemicals that absorb through the skin. While these issues are serious enough, the real danger is brassieres. Evolution, in this regard, gives us cause for thanks... and a precaution. Bras are only about 100 years old taking their origin from corsets – much more dangerous. Corsets were designed to rearrange things, to create the "desired" hourglass figure. They caused much undesired digestive distress and back problems, as well as the real danger for which bras still reign supreme. Enough women rebelled; the corset gave way to the bra.

As discussed in the sections on aerobic exercise and the lymph system, the areas under the arms – from the elbow to mid-chest – are loaded with lymphatic vessels providing drainage for toxins. Wearing a bra constricts the lymph flow in this vital, secondary waste removal system. This book documents how constriction causes stagnation of the lymphatic system, building up waste... leading to problems.

Some think wearing a bra keep breasts from sagging, which is really a function of the pectoral muscles – kept in shape with regular exercise. Nevertheless, some women faithfully wear a bra... some day and night... and still report sagging breasts. Fact: cultures without bras are basically also without breast cancer, especially those cultures that thrive of plant-based foods. Taking off the bra, *any* marks on the skin means it is too tight. Anyone having a lymph massage is amazed at the lightness of touch, because lymphatic vessels are close to the skin surface. Whenever possible be bra-free. Wear a bralette, or loose-fitting camisole. Be aware of what You wear. Dare to be free. Let the girls come out and play! Enjoy Your sensuality, a Gift from sOurce. Feel what You feel. Enjoy Life! Respect and Honor Your Divine Feminine; that's Who You Are!

Yin // Yang...
Jane // Tarzan...
Right Brain // Left Brain
Yin, Jane, Right Brain // Yang, Tarzan, Left Brain
Dark, cold, winter // Light, heat, summer
Descending sap // Rising sap
Down, horizontal, rotund // Up, vertical, slender
Expanding downward, drooping // Expanding, upward, swelling
Moon:reflective/absorptive // Sun: radiative/expansive

White, blue (indirect light) // Black, red (indirect light)

Black, red (direct light) // White blue (direct light)

Dull, underside // Shiny, topside

Inside // Outside

Center, backward, past // Periphery, forward, future

Mass, form // Energy, function

Slow // Fast

Bent, decelerating, round // Straight, accelerating, square

Space, Here // Time, Now

Intact, concave (spoon) // Separated, convex (fork)

Body, root // Head, leaf

Centripetal growth // Centrifugal growth

Salt // Sugar

Shorter // Taller

Slower // Faster

Quieter // Louder

Softer (more fat) // Harder (more muscle)

Less hairy // Hairier

Lower expanded (hips) // Upper expanded (shoulders)

Stronger anabolically // Stronger catabolically

Controlling protecting center // Aggressive expand territory

Internal sexual organs // External sexual organs

Orgasm: Contraction, absorption // Expansion, ejaculation

Ovum: solitary, spherical, slow // Sperm: many, elongated, swift

Position: under or inside // Position: topside, external

Right Brain // Left Brain

Non-verbal, analogue, geometric // Verbal, digital, linear

Subjective, emotional // Objective, rational

Associative, meaning, pattern // Concrete, information,

Synthesizing, overview // Analytic, component

Symbolic, whole, color // Logical, part, form

Body language: being, intuitive // doing, tangible

Arts, synchronicity // Sciences, separate events

Background, interconnected, space // Foreground, separate, time.

Zen

I gained nothing at all
from supreme Enlightenment…
that's why it's called supreme Enlightenment.
-Buddha

A young Zen student in The Big Apple for a seminar; knowing You can get anything Your Heart desires in NYC, he walked outside… and the first thing to catch his eye was a hot dog vendor. He immediately walked over and said: "Make me One with everything!"

His fellow Zen student shrugged: "I'd like to offer You something to help… but in the Zen school, we don't have a single thing!"

According to the Zen master: Everyone can benefit from a 20-minute meditation. Unless You're too busy… then make it an hour!

People into Zen crave awarefulness rather than busyness. The self-discovered person is respected and honored. Zen may be described as a teaching without scriptures, beyond words and letters. Pointing to the Divine Mind as the essence of humankind… seeing directly into One's Nature, Enlightenment is Experienced by Be-ing the Observer.

With distinct disregard of formalism… Zen is self-searching, realizing one's true nature through meditation – all the while tending to self-discipline, simplicity of living, understanding and peace… free from guilt, fear, unnecessary cravings or extreme emotions… enJoying Life – tranquil Bliss. The most illustrious Zen Masters are Buddha and Jesus. Their teaching is: We Are All One: Expressions of the Divine Presence: One, here and now at this point of Infinity – this time of no-time and space of no-space – in which Infinite Being continues to explore on a finite level, with mindful breathing… inhaling & exhaling completely; experiencing Sacred Breath. 3X3.

Zinc

Promoting healthy eyesight and sexual vitality, zinc is abundant in sunflower and pumpkin seeds. A word of Caution: copper and zinc are antagonistic, while small amounts of copper are also important in a balanced diet, taking a man-made copper / zinc supplement is throwing money away – they negate each other. Always look for nutrients from natural whole foods. Nuts and seeds are rich in zinc, magnesium, iron, phosphorus, calcium, copper, Vitamin A, and B complex. As whole, germinated foods, they are almost 100% easily assimilated – a wise choice, along with seaweed and microalgae for minerals and trace elements.

Zip Lock Bags

These little bags can be a lifesaver, especially traveling… great for soaking and sprouting mung beans or lentils; wheat, rye, spelt or kamut; almonds, sunflower or pumpkin. Place 1/3 capacity with nuts or seeds of Your choice, then fill the bag with water and zip it shut, letting them soak for 8-24hrs, depending on size. For safety, keep these bags in a waterproof container, such as a small plastic tub. After soaking, pour the water off, rinse, and snip a tiny opening at the corners of the bag to allow for complete drainage to avoid rot. Rinse once a day and... while You're traveling, Your lunch is growing... traveling along with You; that's about as fresh as it gets, optimal fast-food with optimal results. You can also bring a container of slightly fermented nut or seed dressing with herbs and spices; a Royal treat ready when You are!

Another use for plastic bags / containers is storing greens. Sometimes people put a head of lettuce or a bunch of parsley in a plastic bag at the store, and before it's all used – it starts to get slimy, and much of it gets thrown away. Why? Like synthetic clothing... plastic does not breathe. The solution appears to be simple. Put the greens in a paper bag. Soon, however, the greens lose their luster and are wilted. What happened? The paper bag absorbs the moisture from the greens! The trick: use them both. Saturate the paper bag with water; place the greens inside and place the entire thing in a plastic bag or container. The paper bag is far from being thirsty, so the greens retain their moisture, and may even refresh themselves! The plastic bag surrounding them protects the paper bag from the drying effect of the refrigerator. The same theory may be used to refresh vegetables, such as asparagus... cut off the bottom inch, place in a glass jar with a couple of inches of water and a pinch of whole salt for nourishment; cover with a wet paper bag, then protect it with a plastic bag covering the entire thing – leaving a bit of breathing room at the bottom.

Zwieback
Pronounced ZWYbok, it means twice baked. You can enjoy Your favorite bread on occasion... such as French black-olive sour-dough rye... and facilitate digestion by baking it twice, breaking down starches, converting them to simple sugars. Slice the bread about ½" thick and set it in the sun, turning until perfectly dry – it snaps when You break it; or place in the dehydrator or the oven on low heat.

Bread of this nature is sometimes given to teething babies – minus the black olives, or anything else the baby could choke on. While babies only produce the starch-digesting enzyme amylase after all 20 teeth are in, this form of pre-digested starch as a treat, rather than a daily diet, is usually tolerated: Celebrate Life! Everyday fare for a teething baby: a stick onion, or Spring onion; spiciness soothes those aching gums!

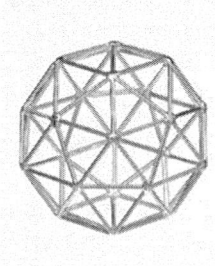

APPENDIX A
Essene Communions with the Angels

Cosmos is Our Home...
Universe is Our Way...
Love is Our Law...
Peace is Our Shelter...
Experience is Our School...
Obstacle is Our Lesson...
Difficulty is Our Stimulant...
Pain is Our Warning...
Work is Our Blessing...
Balance is Our Attitude...
Harmony is Our Nature...
Perfection is Our Destiny...
OM is Our Home Sweet hOMe.

Essenes know in their HeartMindBodySpirit that We are the Word made flesh in a multitude of forms. Throughout the ages, Knowledge of the ancients was kept and guarded by select organizations of the chosen few. The order called the White Brotherhood formed in ancient Egypt to preserve the record of Truth – so-called because male and female members wore pure white garments symbolizing purity of their teachings, and they met at the time of the Full Moon which is also white.

Master Moses was an initiate of the White Brotherhood and when it was time for him to leave his physical body, he called together a few chosen Ones to entrust the guardianship of the Truth. It was their duty to preserve the purity of Truth through centuries of turmoil – through the darkness and savagery of the Arian Age... and to prepare for the Master of the Piscean Age. Jesus led people into the Light of Truth openly proclaiming Unity Consciousness: I and the Father are One. You are One with Me... as I Am One with You! Thus, Jesus explicitly stated what was implied in the Book of Enoch: Be still and know I Am God! The Master taught the Kingdom of Heaven is *within* introducing the World Consciousness to quantum physics!

Prepared from the age of 3 to be the mother of Jesus, Mary, like Joseph and her nephew John the Baptist, as well as many of Jesus' disciples, were Essenes who congregated around Mt Carmel and the Sea of Galilee. Essenes, as part of their daily discipline, communed with guardian angels. When Herod learned of the birth of a great king and sought to destroy him, an angel appeared in a dream with a dire warning. Essenes were aware; they provided safe passage along the way, and made sure the child was safely hidden in Egypt until Herod's death.

Jesus – Jeshua Ben Joseph – was sheltered and educated by the Therapeutae of Egypt, part of the Essene Order. Schooled in the ancient traditions, at the age of 12 Jesus was initiated into the Essene Order and given the name of Issa, which in the Far East literally means Divine Salvation, the Anointed Savior {Messiah} or Master of Masters.

At 17, Jesus and his cousin John the Baptist went for further training and initiation studying at Heliopolis, near the Great Pyramid, for the highest of Brotherhood degrees; here their life mission was revealed along with Knowledge – Self-Realization. Salvation is found by *experiencing* the Knowledge, the Power, that is within. The only real Peace that You can ever experience is within You. Practicing meditation, the student learns how to still the mind and find quiet space; with practice student becomes Master – keeping the meditation "space", when moving *from* the meditation "place".

Following this, Jesus – as Issa, Master of Masters – traveled countries of the known world studying the ways of humankind various philosophies and religions. The purpose of his travels was to evaluate consciousness among the masses... and learn how to reach them. The name Issa – sometimes Saint Issa – is recorded in some ancient monasteries as a Wise Man from the West; he traveled to Persia, India, Tibet, China and Japan. Throughout his travels people were concentrating on him as a person, obscuring his message as the Christed One. Being *christened* means being *anointed*, or dedicated with chrism –

usually olive oil as used for sacred ceremonies. Christening with oil was common – dedicating an article used in sacred rites, or dedicating a person whose life is to be one of sacred service, such as a temple priest or a monarch.

Jesus was to redeem humankind from their narrowminded perceptions meant to keep them living in guilt and fear; he was to redeem humankind from the sin of ignorance. The powerful message of Jesus redeems us from past ignorance and fills us with Knowledge that can only truly be mastered within each individual Heart – Knowledge that is far from factual. Knowledge attained by a total paradigm shift – Knowledge of Conscious Awareness. The ancient message to the world was clear: every single person is the Word {Vibration} made flesh, each One having an individual personality, with potential to be Anointed or Christened by Consciousness, as Jesus was anointed by Self-Realization – Know Thyself! He spoke *clearly*: I and the Father are One, and You are One with Me, as I Am One with You! In terms of quantum physics, he taught: Singularity Consciousness!

Jesus retreated to Egypt, training a few chosen Masters in the Truth. These Masters would preserve the purity of the Knowledge taking charge, teaching all of humankind. Mark the Elder – different from the apostle Mark – and the apostle Thomas went with Jesus to Egypt. To preserve the pure philosophy preparing the way for the Aquarian Age Messiah. Jesus founded the Coptic Order in Egypt. Under his guidance and direction, Mark the Elder and Thomas established the Coptic Templar Order in Cairo in 40 CE. To make the teachings available to the outer world, to those who were ready for it, Mark and Thomas established an outer temple in Alexandria, Egypt in 70 CE, which developed into what is known as the Coptic Orthodox Church, established in Cairo in 117 CE.

Essene writings found in the Archives of the Vatican contain Communions with the Angels, offering the opportunity to focus on Love, Truth and Beauty, Trust, Harmony and Peace. With the first conscious breath of morning, we call upon the Earthly Mother and Her Angelic Forces. Our first thought is empowering... especially as we recall that thought throughout the morning. At mid-day, we call upon the Heavenly Father and His Angelic Forces. With the last conscious breath of evening, we call upon the Angels who protect us through the night, and guide us on our Sacred Journey. Those last thoughts before sleep seed our subconscious – sprouting abundant blessings that show up as the creative energies of our lives.

As Children of Infinite Being communing with the Forces of the Earthly Mother, the Heavenly Father and our Guardian Angels, we begin to recognize ourselves as Infinite Being, being infinitely *inquisitive* as we explOre our options in this finite wOrld of pOlarity.

Empowered by these Communions, those on the spiritual path can approach all interactions with others in harmonious, peaceful, creative ways. Free from any judgment or coercion, we recognize All as Be-ing somewhere on the Divine Spectrum between Brilliant Light and Dazzling Darkness. We are Pure Awareness exploring various aspects of human consciousness… each in our own way.

Learning our Lessons… and with the Gift of Free Will… we are able to *choose* how we feel, think and act at any given moment – thus *creating* our Reality.

Blessings on Your Sacred Journey!
One Day at a time.
Breath by Sacred Breath.

The Essenes And Their Teaching
(thenazareneway.com)

From Enoch to the Dead Sea Scrolls
(thenazareneway.com)

Who Really Was Jesus Christ? The Reality
Revolution podcast (player.fm)

Butterflies are Free to Fly – A New and Radical
Approach to Spiritual Evolution (butterfliesfree.com)

Essene Daily Communions
Prologue before each morning, afternoon and evening communion:

I enter the Eternal and Infinite Garden with reverence to the Divine Presence, Great Spirit – the Heavenly Father, the Earthly Mother – and the Great Masters… with reverence to the wholly pure and saving Teaching… with reverence to the Children of Light!

Friday evening: THE HEAVENLY FATHER AND I ARE ONE.

This communion unites us with the eternal cosmic ocean of superior radiations from all planets. Feeling the cosmic consciousness awakened, the Individual is One with Supreme Power.

Saturday morning: THE EARTHLY MOTHER AND I ARE ONE. SHE GIVES THE FOOD OF LIFE TO MY WHOLE BODY.
This communion unites us with all edible plants, trees, grasses, grains and fruits. Feeling the currents of Life flowing… the Individual enhances the metabolism of the acting body.

Saturday noon: HEAVENLY FATHER, SEND TO ALL YOUR ANGEL OF PEACE. TO YOUR KINGDOM, HEAVENLY FATHER, SEND YOUR ANGEL OF ETERNAL LIFE.
In this communion we experience Peace with the Kingdom of our Heavenly Father.

Saturday evening: ANGEL OF ETERNAL LIFE DESCEND UPON ME, GIVING ETERNAL LIFE TO MY SPIRIT.
This communion unites us with the currents of thought of the superior planets. Overcoming the sphere of gravitation of earthly currents of thought, the Individual is One with Divine Thought.

Sunday morning: ANGEL OF EARTH ENTER MY GENERATIVE ORGANS AND REGENERATE MY WHOLE BODY.
This communion unites us with the life-generating soil and growing grass. Feeling currents of the Angel of Earth transforms sexual energy-> regenerative forces.

Sunday noon: HEAVENLY FATHER, SEND TO ALL YOUR ANGEL OF PEACE. TO THE KINGDOM OF OUR EARTHLY MOTHER, SEND THE ANGEL OF JOY.
In this communion we experience Peace with the Kingdom of our Earthly Mother.

Sunday evening: ANGEL OF CREATIVE WORK DESCEND UPON HUMANITY AND GIVE ABUNDANCE TO ALL.
Like bees at work, we feel the creative work of humanity in all spheres of existence.

Monday morning: ANGEL OF LIFE ENTER MY LIMBS AND GIVE STRENGTH TO MY WHOLE BODY.

This communion unites us with the trees. We feel ourselves absorbing vital forces of trees and forests.

Monday noon: HEAVENLY FATHER SEND TO ALL YOUR ANGEL OF PEACE. TO OUR KNOWLEDGE, SEND YOUR ANGEL OF WISDOM.
In this communion we experience Peace with our Culture.

Monday evening: PEACE... PEACE... PEACE... ANGEL OF PEACE BE ALWAYS EVERYWHERE.
In this communion we are united with the moon and moonlight, experiencing a feeling of universal peace in all spheres of existence.

Tuesday morning: ANGEL OF JOY DESCEND UPON EARTH AND GIVE BEAUTY TO ALL BEINGS.
This communion unites us with vibrations of joy in the beauties of Nature. We feel the colors of sunrise and sunset, the song of a bird, the fragrance of a flower, the strength and tenacity of a blade of grass.

Tuesday noon: HEAVENLY FATHER SEND TO ALL YOUR ANGEL OF PEACE. TO HUMANKIND, SEND YOUR ANGEL OF WORK.
In this communion we experience Peace with our Community and within our Society.

Tuesday evening: ANGEL OF POWER DESCEND UPON MY ACTING BODY AND DIRECT ALL MY ACTS.
This communion unites us with the radiations of the stars and the Cosmic Ocean of Life. We feel the cosmic vital forces from the stars being absorbed by the nervous system of the acting body.

Wednesday morning: ANGEL OF SUN ENTER MY SOLAR CENTER AND GIVE THE FIRE OF LIFE TO MY WHOLE BODY.

This communion unites us with the rising sun feeling accumulated solar forces radiating through the solar plexus, reaching all parts of the body.

Wednesday noon: HEAVENLY FATHER SEND TO ALL YOUR ANGEL OF PEACE. TO OUR FAMILY AND FRIENDS, SEND YOUR ANGEL OF LOVE.
In this communion we experience Peace with our Family.

Wednesday evening: ANGEL OF LOVE DESCEND UPON MY FEELING BODY AND PURIFY ALL MY FEELINGS.
This communion unites us with the feeling body sending and receiving currents of feeling to and from all beings on Earth... all beings everywhere in the Cosmic Ocean of Love.

Thursday morning: ANGEL OF WATER ENTER MY BLOOD... AND GIVE THE WATER OF LIFE TO MY WHOLE BODY.
This communion unites us with the waters of the Earthly Mother found in clouds, rain, rivers, lakes and oceans. We feel the Angel of Water directing the currents and tides in our body fluids.

Thursday noon: HEAVENLY FATHER SEND TO ALL YOUR ANGEL OF PEACE. TO OUR MIND, SEND YOUR ANGEL OF POWER.
In this communion we experience Peace with the Mind.

Thursday evening: ANGEL OF WISDOM DESCEND UPON MY THINKING BODY AND ENLIGHTEN ALL MY THOUGHTS.
This communion unites us with the thinking body sending and receiving currents of thought to and from all beings on Earth... all beings everywhere in the Cosmic Ocean of Thought.

Friday morning: ANGEL OF AIR ENTER MY LUNGS AND GIVE THE AIR OF LIFE TO MY WHOLE BODY.
This communion unites us with the atmosphere, feeling Energy with the inbreathings and outbreathings of the Spirit of Life.

Friday noon: HEAVENLY FATHER SEND TO ALL YOUR ANGEL OF PEACE. TO OUR BODY, SEND YOUR ANGEL OF LIFE.
In this communion we experience Peace with the Body.

Crossing the Threshold of Faith
The Essene Tradition promotes Peace in HeartMindBodySpirit. As holistic healers – making whOle, experiencing Oneness with each Other and Mother Earth – we expand our Conscious Awareness, and we cross the threshold of faith. When all the Children of Abraham... Jews, Christians and Muslims... realize we are "kissin' kin" and greet each other as such: "Namaste!" "The Divine within Me

recognizes and honors the Divine within You!" – then a powerful message is sent to the rest of humankind, and we can all begin to live as the Family of Love.

The Spiritual Visions of Our Planet actually confirm and illumine Each Other. As they developed throughout history... each One has profound contributions:

The Sevenfold Peace of the Essenes
The Cosmic Greatness of Hinduism
The Moral Issues of Zoroaster
The Poetry of Shinto
The One God of Israel
The Simple Love of Tao
The Joy in Truth of Buddha
The Spiritual Victory of Jainism
The Wisdom of Confucius
The Redeeming Radiance of Christianity
The Glory of God of Islam
The Harmony of the Sikhs
The Singularity of the New World Awakening

Great Poems in different languages have different values, yet all are poetry.

These Spiritual Visions all come from One Light and in Them... We have Lamps of Fire that Glorify Infinite Being – the Essence of Love, Truth and Beauty, Trust, Harmony and Peace.

There Will Be Peace on Earth when there is Peace among the World's religions! ~.~*

APPENDIX B
Sprouting Essene Healing CommUnities
The origin of the name Essene remains somewhat of a mystery. Aramaic is the closest to any language: 'yssyn means healer. It may be understood as those who practice a wholesome, holy – holistic – Way of Life, integrating the physical, emotional, mental and spiritual aspects of HeartMindBodySpirit...thus healing our whole Be-ing... as One. As such, Essenes were the primal holistic healers, facilitating understanding of the relationships between our feeling body, our thinking body and our acting body.

Essenes of Mt Carmel and Qumran were healers and teachers who shared daily work in the fields, with Gardens that were known as places where humankind could retreat and re-connect with true Self. They freely shared Knowledge of the Sacred Journey within, and how to Experience the I Am Presence: the Source of All. Gardens were places to connect with Earthly Mother... with Heavenly Father... as well as with Each Other... as Sisters and Brothers. Essene communities traditionally are places where everyOne supports the highest potential for each Individual, and the highest potential for All to express their loving talents and their resources. Essenes continue to grow bountiful Gardens sharing Abundance, giving freely to others.

Custodians of Ancient Wisdom, Essenes knew they had to write things down; we discovered, and now call them Dead Sea Scrolls, which were wrapped in cloths, stored in clay containers with lids, and hidden in the caves at Qumran. The scrolls were planted as seeds to be found for posterity; as it happened, they were discovered by a Bedouin boy throwing rocks in caves searching for a lost lamb in 1947. This is similar to the scrolls discovered in Egypt in 1946 by a farmer in search of rich, composted soil for his fields. Called the Nag Hammadi Library, they are an extraordinary collection of ancient manuscripts hidden centuries before, probably by monks from the nearby Monastery of St Pachomius to preserve them from destruction ordered by the rigid Roman church as part of its violent expunging of heterodoxy and heresy – interestingly, *heresy* literally means, choices; *heterodoxy* literally means, other teachings or traditions.

The inspired translations of ancient Aramaic manuscripts held in the Vatican Archives, and other writings by Professor Edmond Bordeaux Szekely capture the essence of the Essene message. Fluent in ten languages, he researched original documents of Roman historians and others who wrote about the Essenes and their timeless message, something unique to offer every generation.

In 325 CE Emperor Constantine compromised the original message of the Essenes and their Masters – including John the Baptist and Jesus. (See Ch 10: **Vegan Life and Religions**) References to vegetarianism, reincarnation and the Feminine Aspect of the Mother-Father God have all but been deleted; notably only a few references to Jesus mentioning re-incarnation remain – Mt 11: 13-15, and Mt 17: 1-13. We find reference in the Nag Hammadi Library to Jesus in the Garden of Gethsemane the night before his death, crying: Abba, Amma – Father God, Mother Goddess.

We are rediscovering much of this ancient knowledge encouraging us to live a natural, harmonious life with our sisters and brothers – and with the whole of creation. Realizing we are all Infinite Beings having a wide variety of physical experiences, as we explore finite reality – Essenes recognize we are all in this together – realizing *I Am That*, long before the book!

From earlier writings discovered in Nag Hammadi, we learn the ancients communed with God, the Creator of All as a genderless GOD: **G**enerator, **O**perator, **D**estroyer called Great Spirit or Infinite Mind. God is simply The Divine Presence, the vibrational frequency Sustaining All. Quantum Physics would define The Divine Presence as The Divine Wavicle – both wave and particle – and when the idea for Creation surfaced in Infinite Mind... a Divine Particle slipped out as Mother-Goddess and a Divine Particle slipped out as Father-God – All of Creation flows from both forces.

We are made in that image and likeness as exemplified by our right brain {feminine energies: Vision and Imagination} and our left brain {masculine energies: Be-ing and Action}. While a woman's ovaries produce estrogen... her adrenals produce testosterone – likewise, a man's testes produce testosterone, and his adrenals produce estrogen! Scriptures say: God made them all male and female – engaging the next Order of Magnitude, intertwining HeartMindBodySpirit as One!

Ancient writings honor Great Spirit, the Creator of All Life Everywhere, beginning creation with Divine Feminine and Divine Masculine energies – in all Their Magnificent Glory. Also recounted in these scrolls, the original commandments: Honor Heavenly Father and Earthly Mother by respecting the Life in every living being. Ancients were attuned to the pulsations and vibrations around them. Nicholas of Cusa said: "Divinity is the enfolding and unfolding of everything that is. Divinity is in all things in such a way that all things are in divinity."

We can facilitate that Experience by communing with the Angels of the Heavenly Father and Earthly Mother, bathing in the Fountain of Light, and merging with the Sea of Eternity as the Infinite finite Be-ing – That I Am.

Tat tvam asi –
You ARE That!

Since You truly Are – You will enjoy explOring All That Is: History of Non-dual Meditation Methods.pdf (uned.es)

The Discovery of the Essene Gospel of Peace

In addition to Sanskrit, Aramaic, Greek and Latin, Professor Edmond Bordeaux Szekely fluently spoke 10 modern languages. Studying in Rome, he found his way into the Archives of the Vatican in 1927 through the Prefect Msgr Mercati. He also gained entrance to the Archives of the Benedictine Monastery of Monte Cassino, where Szekely claimed he had discovered *The Essene Gospel of Peace* – two decades before the discovery of the Dead Sea Scrolls. In the Essene Gospel, Jesus speaks of the power of benedictions and fasting, and he describes the Communions with the Angels as bridges to be built with patience, every day. Angels are the branches and roots of a tree and we are the trunk. These Communions or Invocations link to natural and cosmic forces. From the Source of All, through the Angelic realms, we draw energy for healing, rejuvenation, and spiritual growth.

In the story of his discovery, the Professor claimed copies of *The Essene Gospel of Peace* can also be found in the Library of the Hapsburgs and the British Museum. People who go, have been told the document does not exist. We can only conclude the document has been suppressed in both places or, perhaps more likely, *The Essene Gospel of Peace* is the Professor's own literary creation – a bit of revisionist history. Either way, it is well-written prose capturing the Quintessence of the Essene Way of Life – well-worth reading, at least from that perspective. See the Professor's writings: https://www.thenazareneway.com/from_enoch_to_the_dead_sea_scrolls.htm

Carrying on the Traditions

Essenes, authors of the Dead Sea Scrolls and Coptics, the compilers of the Nag Hammadi Library, traditionally offer places for people to rejuvenate getting their hands in the soil... connecting with The Divine Presence – the Source of All – with Father Sun and Mother Earth – and with Each Other as Sisters and Brothers: All as One! In 1972, I had barely heard of the Dead Sea Scrolls written by the Essenes. After five years as a Catholic priest in Detroit, I heard of Arnold Ehret, Austrian naturist, who promoted a plant-based diet and water fasting. Impressed and intrigued by the difference I felt only half-way through the 30-day Vegan Challenge, I was amazed – compelled to do a two-week water fast in the mountains from New Moon to Full Moon. After these revelations, traveling overland around the globe 5 years, witnessing Realities of natural healing... I returned to school to prepare for my new Service as a natural primary care physician, as a Doctor of Chiropractic, practicing S.O.T. Sacral-Occipital-Technique: specializing in Harmonics – Vibrational Energy Medicine practiced from ancient times at a Home-Office in Coconut Grove in 1980.

On Valentine's Day '92... 25 years after being ordained a priest in Detroit... I was ordained a second time as Essene minister; Bishop Viktoras Kulvinskas, DD, PhD invited me to expand my scope of service. Currently affiliated with the Church of Compassionate Service {CoCS} a Free-Church – neither a 501c3 nor a 508c1a, as other churches are – we are outside the IRS Tax Code altogether. CoCS as a Free-Church, rather than having a tax *exemption* as other churches, has a *mandatory* tax **exception**. CoCS also facilitates Compassionate Service Charities, Inc: a 501c3 suitable for tax-deductible donations to carry on the Essene tradition through Holistic Ministries.

Do We Have as Much Sense as a Goose?
Geese fly in **V** formation for a reason. As each bird flaps its wings, it creates uplift for the bird immediately following. Flying in V formation, the flock adds 71% greater flying range... than if each bird flew on its own.

Basic Truth #1: People who share common direction and a sense of community get where they are going quicker and easier... because they travel on the thrust of one another.

Whenever a goose falls out of formation, it suddenly feels the drag and resistance of trying to go it alone... and quickly gets back into formation to take advantage of the lifting power of the bird immediately in front.

Basic Truth #2: If we have as much sense as a goose, we stay in formation... with those headed in the same direction.

When the lead goose gets tired, s/he rotates back in the wing and another goose takes point position.

Basic Truth #3: It pays to take turns doing hard jobs – with geese flying – or people proceeding toward their goals.

The geese honk from behind to encourage those up front to keep up their speed.

Basic Truth #4: Be careful what is said when honking from behind... being mindful of Verbal Diet, make everyday a Non-Judgment Day.

Finally, when a goose is sick or is wounded from gunshot and falls out, two geese fall out of formation and follow to help or to protect. They stay until she is able to fly or until dead... then they catch up with the group, or join another formation.

Final Truth: Sharing the sense of the goose... we stand by each other... We truly are One!

Having the sense of a goose... perhaps also with a sense of history, as well as a sense of urgency... Holistic Ministries and the Church of Compassionate Service are dedicated to creating healing retreats and wholistic Sanctuaries, establishing Essene Healing Communities. If You are attracted to this venture and can support this effort, we look forward to partnering with You. Together we can co-create Harmonious Healing: Ancient Wisdom in Modern Times and carry on the Essene tradition: providing a Doorway to experience HeartMindBodySpirit as One.

The mOMent of Creation
At the mOMent of Creation "God *said*, 'Let there be light.' And there was light!" The spoken word is sound, which is vibration... from which all creation flows. When we speak, our vocal cords vibrate. Our ears take in those vibrations. The bones in the ears vibrate. And communication happens. Sound is the essence of creation. Today we "capture" sound on paper with a musical staff and notes. From time immemorial, the ancients captured sound through Sacred Geometry based on the *phi ratio* and the *golden mean rectangle* – which architects continue to use. Plato in *Timaeus* equated the *tetrahedron* with fire, the *cube* with earth, the *octahedron* with air, the *icosahedron* with water, and the *dodecahedron* with the ether – of which the constellations and heavens were made. Seeking explanations, here we have the seeds of Plasma Cosmology. Science has determined the Universe is 99.999% plasma! Yet, the "problem" of Consciousness continues to puzzle inquisitive minds. Professor Robert Temple talking about a New Science of Heaven - YouTube with Pam Gregory, astrologer, mention that while Pythagoras and Plato said mathematics and

number are the Fundamentals of nature, Plasma Cosmology points to angles and ratios – the building blocks of Fractality – even more basic Fundamentals. *A New Science of Heaven* by Professor Temple opens an avenue into the Cosmos worth exploring. Infinite Mind expresses in mysterious ways.

From time immemorial, Lovers of Wisdom have been intrigued by mystical experiences... mysteries of the stars... and their Source... leading them to consider and explore... discussing the Nature of Source with great *enthusiasm* – a word that literally derives from the Greek: *en theos* – referring to "Source or Great Spirit" hence, we have the study of theology: *theologos* "one discoursing on the gods"! As long as the focus is on "externals" such as the Milky Way, much discussion is in the area of speculation – theory. Then again on the practical side, referred to as Practical Theology, the focus is on "internals" – the focus is within... and so, the great Masters of all Ages say: the Kingdom of Heaven is within You!

At the Heart of the Essene tradition are Peace and Blessings – far more practical than theories of number and fractals. Our life on Earth is a search for the Peace that, ultimately, only is found within, and for all the Blessings required to support our Sacred Journey. There have been prophets and masters to guide us in every culture, pointing the way. Perhaps the most widely known Essene Master is Jesus who retreated to the peace of the desert to fast, and went to the mountains to teach. His famous sermon, The Beatitudes aka the Sermon on the Mount, teaches the essence of Christ Consciousness – remarkably similar to the essence of the Buddhist Suttas – bearing zerO resemblance to the Church of Rome and any other corporate State Religions; crassly vying for the $alvation of the masse$ through Guilt & Fear, they seek world control as witnessed by UN Agenda 2030.

Sacred to the Essene community is Mt Carmel... far from the congestion and corruption found in cities, where people tend to live out of balance with Mother Nature – subsequently experiencing many dis-eases. Peace and Blessings are rare in cities, and quite abundant in the country-side. From time immemorial, Essenes offered sanctuaries from the separation and competition ruling society, offering *choices* for those who would Know the Self and explOre their Heart of Hearts. This focused, Sacred Space naturally calls You in Gratitude to put Your hands in the fertile soil of Mother Earth – and Your arms around each Other as sisters and brothers – loving All as One.

Essenes knOw and deeply feel each One of us is an expression of Pure Awareness explOring human consciousness in our own particular style, our own way. Indeed, Jesus quotes Psalm 82:6, "I once said: You, too, are gods... all of You." A little later Jesus, addressing a paternalistic culture, says, "I Am in the Father and the Father is in me. Understand, I Am in my Father, and You in me and I in You!" Speaking more to the point he said, "Whatsoever You do to the least of these, that You do unto me!" When we understand and apply Singularity... Peace on Earth prevails.

The Essene mission is to expand Conscious Awareness of who we are and why we are here. As One Infinite Being exploring infinite possibilities in the complete spectrum of human consciousness – the good, the bad, the ugly and the beautiful – we are here with Free Will to express Infinite Mind as our particular soul dictates... to learn our own Lessons as each soul progresses to perfection, following the advice of the prophet Jesus: "Be perfect!" How do we begin the process of perfection?

Since we are spiritual beings having a physical experience, we begin at the physical level. We have 7 hormone-producing endocrine glands, each surrounded by blood vessels and a ganglion or bundle of nerves, which creates a vortex of energy – all under the direction of the hypothalamus – taking cues from the Heart. These glands keep us in balance until being exposed to traumas, toxins, negativity or stress.

Traditionally, these seven endocrine energy centers have been re-calibrated and harmonized... which re-establishes homeostasis or balance... by using the seven colors of the rainbow, the seven notes of the musical scale, and vibrational frequencies emitted by stones, fragrances, and the frequencies of our *words* – affirming our chosen reality: We Voice our Choice. This is the essence of Vibrational Energy Medicine. Now we take energetics to the next Order of Magnitude with the quantum Energy, Scalar Wave, Wand of Light. I Am available to assist Your Quest to Create Your Own **Med-Bed** and to explOre Your internal energetics: Your connection to Source... experiencing yourSelf as expressing Source – in the Here and Now!

3Ds for Success in our 3D world:
Dedication to Your **P**rinciples engages the thinking body. **D**evotion to Your Heart's **P**urpose engages the feeling body. **D**iscipline with Your **P**rotocol engages the acting body.

Know Thyself!
Be Aware of Yourself as Pure Consciousness
explOring Pure Awareness
Creating the New You!
We Are the Ones We've Been Waiting For!

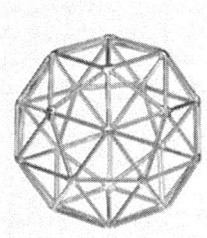

Peace and Blessings on Your Sacred Journey!

http://realdoctor.blogspot.com/

drbobkreucher@gmail.com